T0201939

OXFORD MEDICAL PUBLICATIONS

Oxford Handbook of
Nutrition and
Dietetics

Published and forthcoming Oxford Handbooks

Oxford Handbook for the Foundation Programme 5e

Oxford Handbook of Acute Medicine 4e

Oxford Handbook of Anaesthesia 4e

Oxford Handbook of Cardiology 2e

Oxford Handbook of Clinical and Healthcare Research

Oxford Handbook of Clinical and Laboratory Investigation 4e

Oxford Handbook of Clinical Dentistry 6e

Oxford Handbook of Clinical Diagnosis 3e

Oxford Handbook of Clinical Examination and Practical Skills 2e

Oxford Handbook of Clinical Haematology 4e

Oxford Handbook of Clinical Immunology and Allergy 4e

Oxford Handbook of Clinical Medicine—Mini Edition 10e

Oxford Handbook of Clinical Medicine 10e

Oxford Handbook of Clinical Pathology

Oxford Handbook of Clinical Pharmacy 3e

Oxford Handbook of Clinical Specialties 10e

Oxford Handbook of Clinical Surgery 4e

Oxford Handbook of Complementary Medicine

Oxford Handbook of Critical Care 3e

Oxford Handbook of Dental Patient Care

Oxford Handbook of Dialysis 4e

Oxford Handbook of Emergency Medicine 4e

Oxford Handbook of Endocrinology and Diabetes 3e

Oxford Handbook of ENT and Head and Neck Surgery 3e

Oxford Handbook of Epidemiology for Clinicians

Oxford Handbook of Expedition and Wilderness Medicine 2e

Oxford Handbook of Forensic Medicine

Oxford Handbook of Gastroenterology & Hepatology 2e

Oxford Handbook of General Practice 4e

Oxford Handbook of Genetics

Oxford Handbook of Genitourinary Medicine, HIV, and Sexual Health 3e

Oxford Handbook of Geriatric Medicine 3e

Oxford Handbook of Infectious Diseases and Microbiology 2e

Oxford Handbook of Integrated Dental Biosciences 2e

Oxford Handbook of Humanitarian Medicine

Oxford Handbook of Key Clinical Evidence 2e

Oxford Handbook of Medical Dermatology 2e

Oxford Handbook of Medical Imaging

Oxford Handbook of Medical Sciences 2e

Oxford Handbook for Medical School

Oxford Handbook of Medical Statistics

Oxford Handbook of Neonatology 2e

Oxford Handbook of Nephrology and Hypertension 2e

Oxford Handbook of Neurology 2e

Oxford Handbook of Nutrition and Dietetics 2e

Oxford Handbook of Obstetrics and Gynaecology 3c

Oxford Handbook of Occupational Health 2e

Oxford Handbook of Oncology 3e

Oxford Handbook of Operative Surgery 3e

Oxford Handbook of Ophthalmology 4e

Oxford Handbook of Oral and Maxillofacial Surgery 2e

Oxford Handbook of Orthopaedics and Trauma

Oxford Handbook of Paediatrics 2e

Oxford Handbook of Pain Management

Oxford Handbook of Palliative Care 3e

Oxford Handbook of Practical Drug Therapy 2e

Oxford Handbook of Pre-Hospital Care

Oxford Handbook of Psychiatry 4e

Oxford Handbook of Public Health Practice 3e

Oxford Handbook of Rehabilitation Medicine 3e

Oxford Handbook of Reproductive Medicine & Family Planning 2e

Oxford Handbook of Respiratory Medicine 3e

Oxford Handbook of Rheumatology 4e

Oxford Handbook of Sport and Exercise Medicine 2e

Handbook of Surgical Consent

Oxford Handbook of Tropical Medicine 4e

Oxford Handbook of Urology 4e

Oxford Handbook of
Nutrition and Dietetics

THIRD EDITION

Edited by

Joan Webster-Gandy
Freelance Dietitian, London, UK

Angela Madden
Principal Lecturer in Nutrition and Dietetics
University of Hertfordshire
Herts, UK

Michelle Holdsworth
Professor in Public Health (Honorary)
School of Health & Related Research
University of Sheffield, UK
and
Chargée de Recherche, French National
Research Institute for Sustainable
Development (IRD),
Montpellier, France

OXFORD
UNIVERSITY PRESS

Great Clarendon Street, Oxford, OX2 6DP,
United Kingdom

Oxford University Press is a department of the University of Oxford.
It furthers the University's objective of excellence in research, scholarship,
and education by publishing worldwide. Oxford is a registered trade mark of
Oxford University Press in the UK and in certain other countries

First Edition published in 2006
Second Edition published in 2012
Third Edition published in 2020

Impression: 3

Published in the United States of America by Oxford University Press
198 Madison Avenue, New York, NY 10016, United States of America

British Library Cataloguing in Publication Data
Data available

Library of Congress Control Number: 2019957199

ISBN 978–0–19–880013–2

Printed and bound in Italy by L.E.G.O. S.p.A. Lavis (TN)

To Beth, Didier, Catherine, Jane, Ottilie, Matthew, Milo, Paula, Vivienne, and Will, with much love.

Foreword

Both health professionals and the general public now realize that good nutrition is essential for good health. Indeed, nutrition is the health topic on which the lay public receives the most advice from popular books and magazines, but often this advice is unsound. It is therefore essential that healthcare workers have readily available reliable information about all aspects of nutrition. This includes nutritional science, public health nutrition, and therapeutic nutrition.

This handbook provides, in concise format, the information about nutrition needed by those training to be dietitians (RD), nutritionists (RNutr), or doctors or nurses in all settings. It will continue to be a valuable resource after graduation, because the scope of modern nutrition is so large that a specialist in one field (say, public health nutrition) cannot hope to have instantly accessible all the necessary information about therapeutic diets, or nutritional sciences, and vice versa.

The three authors of this handbook are all registered dietitians, each of whom has a solid research record, as well as extensive experience of the nutritional problems that dietitians, hospital doctors, general practitioners, and specialist nurses will encounter. I am confident that readers will be thankful to have this book in their pocket to guide them to the correct immediate response to a nutritional problem, even if later they have to consult a senior dietitian or textbook for more detailed advice.

John Garrow, MD, PhD, FRCP
Emeritus Professor of Human Nutrition
University of London
(1929–2016)

Preface

When we were approached to write this handbook the original idea was to write a book for general practice. However, we all remember being student dietitians and all created our own handbook of useful information that we carried around with us and were totally lost without. On reflection of what textbooks are now available in nutrition or dietetics, it became clear that, although there are now concise pocketbooks written for dietitians working predominantly in a clinical setting, there was a need for a user friendly handbook of nutrition and dietetics for a wider audience that included doctors, nurses, nutritionists, and other healthcare professionals. The available textbooks are, by necessity, large tomes or series that are unlikely to adorn the shelves of many doctors or nurses whether in primary or secondary care.

As a result, we have tried to present nutritional science, therapeutics, and community public health nutrition in a concise and integrated manner. While writing the text we have tried to identify what information would be useful to different professionals in a variety of settings. For example a doctor or nurse may want information on obesity and will find a ready reckoner for the calculation of body mass index (BMI), information on associated problems and treatment options. Dietitians working in the community or public health will have this information, but will find the sections on the measurements of obesity or nutrition interventions more informative. How well we have achieved this is for the reader to decide.

Nutrition is fascinating for many reasons, one of which is the fact that it is a very dynamic discipline. We have tried very hard to be contemporary, but there will inevitably be changes in basic science, practice, and policy as the discipline continues to evolve. Major developments and changes will be posted on the relevant page of the OUP web site. For us it has been a very enjoyable, if at times rather demanding, process and we hope that this book is useful to all healthcare professionals.

J.W-G.
A.M.M.
M.H.

Acknowledgements

Special thanks go to everyone who has helped and supported us during the production of this book. We are particularly grateful to: Alison Culkin, Clare Soulsby, and Liz Weekes.

Finally, thanks to the medical division at OUP for all the encouragement and support.

Contents

Contributors *xv*
Symbols and abbreviations *xix*

1	Introduction to nutrition	1
2	Dietary reference values and food-based dietary guidelines	21
3	Current dietary patterns in the UK	33
4	Nutrition assessment	37
5	Macronutrients and energy balance	61
6	Micronutrients	99
7	Electrolytes and fluid balance	175
8	Food labelling, functional foods, nutrigenetics, and nutrigenomics and food supplements	187
9	Non-nutrient components of food	205
10	Nutrition and catering in institutions	219
11	Popular diets	231
12	Diet before and during pregnancy	237
13	Infants and preschool children	257
14	School-aged children and adolescents	303
15	Older people	321
16	Nutrition in vulnerable population groups	337
17	Nutrition interventions with patients and individuals	365
18	Nutrition policy	391
19	Healthy and sustainable diets	423
20	Global nutrition	435
21	Obesity	469

22 Diabetes   493

23 Cardiovascular disease   519

24 Cancer   541

25 Nutrition support   555

26 Nutrition in gastrointestinal diseases   621

27 Pancreatic disease   679

28 Liver disease   689

29 Kidney disease   703

30 Respiratory disease and cystic fibrosis   735

31 Human immunodeficiency virus (HIV) infection   745

32 Nutrition in mental health   753

33 Nutrition in neurological conditions   781

34 Rheumatology, dermatology, and bone health   799

35 Palliative care   811

36 Inherited metabolic disorders   815

37 Food hypersensitivity   825

38 Drug–nutrient interactions and prescription
    of nutritional products   833

    Appendix 1 843
    Appendix 2 847
    Appendix 3 867
    Appendix 4 871
    Appendix 5 873
    Appendix 6 875
    Appendix 7 883
    Appendix 8 891
    Index 893

Contributors

Alison Culkin
Lead Intestinal Failure
Dietitian
St Mark's Hospital,
Harrow, UK

Alastair Duncan
Senior Lecturer
School of Medicine,
Diabetes and Nutritional
Sciences Division,
King's College London,
London, UK

Pam Dyson
Research Dietitian
Oxford Centre for Diabetes,
Endocrinology and
Metabolism,
Churchill Hospital,
University of Oxford,
Oxford, UK

Fiona Graham
Research Associate,
Institute of Health & Society,
Newcastle University, UK

Vanessa Halliday
Senior Lecturer in Public
Health
School of Health and Related
Research,
University of Sheffield,
Sheffield, UK

Anne Holdoway
Freelance Dietitian
Bath, UK

Michelle Holdsworth
Professor of Public Health
School of Health and Related
Research,
University of Sheffield,
Sheffield, UK
and
Chargée de Recherche, French
National Research Institute for
Sustainable Development (IRD),
Montpellier, France

Emma Jordan
Senior Paediatric Dietitian
Leicestershire Nutrition &
Dietetic Service,
Leicestershire Partnership
NHS Trust,
Leicestershire, UK

Natasha Kershaw
Burns Dietitian
St Andrew's Centre for Plastic
Surgery and Burns,
Mid Essex Hospital Services
NHS Trust,
Chelmsford, Essex, UK

Edwige Landais
Research Associate, UMR
NUTRIPASS
Institut de Recherche pour le
Développement- IRD,
Montpellier, France

Miranda Lomer
Senior Consultant Dietitian in
Gastroenterology
Guy's and St Thomas' NHS
Foundation Trust,
London, UK

Angela M. Madden
Principal Lecturer in Nutrition
and Dietetics
University of Hertfordshire,
Hertfordshire, UK

Bruno Mafrici
Lead Renal Dietitian/Team
Leader
Department of Dietetics and
Nutrition,
Nottingham University Hospitals
NHS Trust,
Nottingham, UK

Yvonne McKenzie
Specialist Dietitian in
Gastrointestinal Nutrition and IBS
Oxford, UK

Kate Moffat
Head of Nutrition & Dietetic
Services,
South London and Maudsley
NHS Foundation Trust,
London, UK

Hilda Mulrooney
Associate Professor of Nutrition
Kingston University,
Kingston upon
Thames, UK

Elizabeth Neal
Specialist Ketogenic Dietitian and
Honorary Research Associate
Institute of Child Health,
London, UK

Fionna Page
Freelance Dietitian
First Page Nutrition Ltd,
Great Somerford, Wiltshire, UK

Mary Phillips
Advanced Specialist Dietitian
(Hepato-pancreato-biliary
Surgery)
Royal Surrey County Hospital,
Guildford, Surrey, UK

Rebecca Pradeilles
Senior Research Associate in
Public Health Nutrition,
School of Sport, Exercise and
Health Sciences,
Loughborough University
Loughborough, UK

Kath Roberts
Honorary Lecturer,
School of Health and Related
Research,
University of Sheffield,
Sheffield, UK

Louise Robertson
Specialist Dietitian in Inherited
Metabolic Disorders
Department of Nutrition and
Dietetics,
University Hospitals Birmingham
NHS Foundation Trust,
Birmingham, UK

Clare Shaw
Consultant Dietitian
Department of Nutrition and
Dietetics,
The Royal Marsden NHS
Foundation Trust,
London and Sutton, UK

Lisa Sinfield
Senior Dietitian
Leicestershire Nutrition &
Dietetic Service,
Leicestershire Partnership
NHS Trust,
Leicestershire, UK

Isabel Skypala
Consultant Allergy Dietitian and
Director of Rehabilitation and
Therapies,
Royal Brompton & Harefield
NHS Trust,
London, UK

Clare Soulsby
Senior Dietitian
Liverpool University Hospitals
NHS Foundation Trust,
Liverpool, UK

Nikki Stewart
Clinical and Operational Lead
Dietitian,
Hertfordshire Community
NHS Trust,
UK

Lisa Waddell
Community Paediatric Allergy
Dietitian
Director of Food Allergy
Nottingham Service Ltd,
Nottingham, UK

Joan Webster-Gandy
Freelance Dietitian
London, UK

C Elizabeth Weekes
Senior Consultant Dietitian
Department of Nutrition and
Dietetics,
Guy's and St Thomas' NHS
Foundation Trust,
London, UK

Kevin Whelan
Professor Nutritional Sciences
School of Medicine, Diabetes
and Nutritional Sciences
Division, King's College London,
London, UK

Rhys White
Principal Oncology Dietitian
Department of Nutrition and
Dietetics,
Guy's and St Thomas' NHS
Foundation Trust,
London, UK

Kirsten Whitehead
Freelance Dietitian, UK

Symbols and abbreviations

↑	increased
↓	decreased
→	leading to
❶	caution
∴	therefore
ℛ	website
♀	female
♂	male
☛	controversial topic
1°	primary
2°	secondary
5FU	5-fluorouracil
AA	amino acid
AAA	abdominal aortic aneurysm
AAD	antibiotic-associated diarrhoea
abv	alcohol by volume
ACE	angiotensin-converting enzyme
AcP	acute pancreatitis
AD	Alzheimer's disease
ADₕH	alcohol dehydrogenase
ADH	antidiuretic hormone
ADHD	attention deficit hyperactivity disorder
ADP	air-displacement plethysmography
AED	anti-epilepsy drug
AfN	Association for Nutrition
AI	adequate intake
AIDS	acquired immune deficiency syndrome
AKI	acute kidney injury
ALA	alpha-linolenic acid
ALDH	aldehyde dehydrogenase
AN	anorexia nervosa
AP	assistant practitioners
Arg	arginine
ART	antiretroviral therapy

ARV	antiretroviral
ASA24	automated self-administered 24-hour recall
ASD	autism spectrum disorders
Assoc Nutr	associate nutritionist
ATP	adenosine triphosphate
BAPEN	British Association for Parenteral and Enteral Nutrition
BCS	behaviour change strategies
BDA	British Dietetic Association
BED	binge eating disorder
BFI	baby friendly initiative
BHA	butylated hydroxyanisole
BHF	Better Hospital Food
BHT	butylated hydroxytoluene
BIA	bioelectrical impedance analysis
BMA	British Medical Association
BMI	body mass index
BMR	basal metabolic rate
BMT	bone marrow transplantation
BN	bulimia nervosa
BNF	British National Formulary
BPD	bilio-pancreatic diversion
BPD-DS	bilio-pancreatic diversion with duodenal switch
BSA	body surface area burn
BV	body volume
BWt	body weight
CBT	cognitive behavioural therapy
CBT-ED	cognitive behavioural therapy
CC	critical care
CD	Crohn's disease
CF	cystic fibrosis
CHART	continuous hyperfractionated accelerated radiotherapy
CHD	coronary heart disease

CHO	carbohydrates
CI	Consumer International
CKD	chronic kidney disease
CI	chlorine
CLA	conjugated linoleic acid
CMAM	community-based management of acute malnutrition
CNS	central nervous system
CoD	coeliac disease
COMA	Committee on Medical Aspects of Food Policy
CP	chronic pancreatitis
CQC	Care and Quality Commission
CRD	component-resolved diagnosis
CRP	C-reactive protein
CRRT	continuous renal replacement therapy
CSSI	continuous sub-cutaneous insulin infusion
CT	computed tomography
CVA	cerebrovascular accident
CVD	cardiovascular disease
DASH	dietary approaches to stop hypertension
DBP	diastolic blood pressure
DEFRA	Department for Environment, Food and Rural Affairs
DES	dietary energy supply
DESM	diabetes education and self-management
DfE	Department for Education
DH	Department of Health
DHA	docosahexaenoic acid
DHp	dermatitis herpetiformis
DIT	dietary induced thermogenesis
DM	diabetes mellitus
DNA	deoxyribonucleic acid
DOM	Dietitians in Obesity Management
DRV	dietary reference value
DS	duodenal switch
DSW	dietetic support worker

DXA	dual-energy X-ray absorptiometry
EAR	estimated average requirements
EB	epidermolysis bullosa
ECF	extracellular fluid
EE	energy expenditure
EFA	essential fatty acids
EFAD	European Federation of the Associations of dietitians
EFS	Expenditure and Food Survey
EFSA	European Food Safety Authority
EGRA	erythrocyte glutathione reductase activity
EMA	endomysial antibodies
EPA	eicosapentaenoic acid
EPAFF	Export Panel on Armed Forces Feeding
ER	emergency regimen
ERF	established renal failure
EU	European Union
EUFIC	European Food Information Council
FAD	flavin adenine dinucleotide
FAO	Food & Agriculture Organization (UN)
FBDG	food-based dietary guidelines
FBS	food balance sheets
FDEIA	food-dependent, exercise-induced anaphylaxis
FFM	fat free mass
FFQ	food frequency questionnaire
FFST	fat-free soft tissue
FFW	food for work
FH	familial hypercholesterolaemia
FHS	food hypersensitivity
FIRSSt	Food Intake Recording Software System
FIVE	familial isolated vitamin E
FIVR	food intake visual and voice recognizer
FM	fat mass
FMN	flavin mononucleotide

FOS	fructo-oligosaccharides		IDL	intermediate density lipoproteins
FPIES	food-induced proctitis and enterocolitis		IDPN	intradialytic parenteral nutrition
FSA	Food Standards Agency		IF	intestinal failure
FSP	Food in Schools Programme		IFE	infant feeding in emergencies
GAM	global acute malnutrition		IGD	Institute of Grocery Distribution
GDA	guideline daily amounts		IgE	immunoglobulin E
GDM	gestational diabetes		IMD	inherited metabolic diseases
GF	gluten free		IMF	International Monetary Fund
GFD	general food distribution		INR	international normalized ratio
GFR	glomerular filtration rate		INS	International Numbering System
GI	gastrointestinal, also glycaemic index		IOM	Institute of Medicine
GL	glycaemic load		ISAK	International Society for the Advancement of Kinanthropometry
Gln	glutamine			
GM	genetically modified		IVNAA	in vivo neutron activation analysis
GMO	genetically modified organisms			
GOR	gastro-oesophageal reflux		J	Joule
GORD	gastro-oesophageal reflux disease		kcal	kilocalories
			KD	ketogenic diet
GOS	galacto-oligosaccharides		kJ	kilojoules
GTF	glucose tolerance factor		LBW	low birth weight
GTN	glyceryl trinitrate		LCP	long chain fatty acids
GVHD	graft vs. host disease		LCT	long chain triglycerides
HbA1c	glycated haemoglobin		LDL	low-density lipoprotein
HCPC	Health & Care Professions Council		LFT	liver function test
			LIDNS	Low Income Diet and Nutrition Survey
HD	haemodialysis			
HDL	high density lipoproteins		LGIT	low glycaemic index treatment
HFE	high fat or energy		LP(a)	lipoprotein (a)
HFSS	high fat, sugar or salt		LRNI	lower reference nutrient intake
HIV	human immune virus			
HR	heart rate		LTP	lipid transfer proteins
HT	hypertension		MAC	midarm circumference
Ht	height		MAD	modified Atkins diet
IA	insulin analogues		MAM	moderate acute malnutrition
IBD	irritable bowel disease		MAMC	midarm muscle circumference
ICCID	International Council for Control of Iodine Deficiency		MANTRA	Maudsley Anorexia Nervosa Treatment for Adults
ICF	intracellular fluid			
IDA	iron deficiency anaemia		MAOI	monoamine oxidase inhibitors
IDD	iodine deficiency disorder			

MAS	milk alkali syndrome	NCHS	National Center for Health Statistics
MBD	mineral bone disease	NDNS	National Diet and Nutrition Survey
MCH	mean cell haemoglobin		
MCT	medium chain triglycerides	NE	niacin equivalent
MCV	mean corpuscular volume	NFS	National Food Survey
MDG	millennium development goals	NG	nasogastric
MDI	multiple daily injections	NGA	non-governmental agency
MDT	multi-disciplinary team	NHANES	National Health and Nutrition Examination Surveys
MEOS	microsomal ethanol-oxidizing system	NHS	National Health service
MHRA	Medicines and Healthcare products Regulatory Agency	NICE	National Institute for Health and Clinical Excellence
MI	motivational interviewing	NIE	nutrition in emergencies
MIMS	Monthly Index of Medical Specialties	NIRI	near infrared interactance
MIYCN	maternal, infant, and young child nutrition	NJ	nasojejunal
		NMES	non-milk extrinsic sugars
MJ	megajoules	NMN	N^1-methylnicotinamide
MND	motor neurone disease	NS	nephrotic syndrome
MoD	Ministry of Defence	NS-SEC	National Statistics Socio-economic Classification
MPFR	mobile phone food record		
MRC	Medical Research Council	NSP	non-starch polysaccharides
MRI	magnetic resonance imaging	NTD	neural tube defects
MS	multiple sclerosis	OA	osteoarthritis
MTCT	mother-to-child transmission	OCD	obsessive compulsive disorder
MUAC	mid-upper arm circumference	OFC	occipito-frontal head circumference
MUFA	monounsaturated fatty acids	Ofsted	Office for Standards in Education, Children's Services and Skills
MUST	malnutrition universal screening tool		
Na	sodium	ONS	Office for National Statistics
NAD	nicotinamide adenine dinucleotide	ORP	operational ration packs
NADP	nicotinamide adenine dinucleotide phosphate	OSFED	other specified feeding or eating disorder
NAFLD	non-alcoholic fatty liver	PA	physical activity
NASH	non-alcoholic steatohepatitis	PABA	para-aminobenzoic acid
NatCen	National Centre for Social Research	PAD	peripheral arterial disease
		PAL	physical activity level
NATO	North Atlantic Treaty Organization	PAR	physical activity ratios
		PAYD	Pay as You Dine
NCCTSL	non-carious cervical tooth surface loss	PCB	polychlorinated biphenyl
		PCHR	Personal Child Health Record
NCD	non-communicable diseases	PCOS	polycystic ovary syndrome

PCR	protein catabolic rate		RNI	reference nutrient intake
PCSG	Primary Care Society for Gastroenterology		RQ	respiratory quotient
PD	peritoneal dialysis		RQIA	Regulation and Quality Improvement Authority
PDA	personal digital assistant		RS	resistant starch
PDis	Parkinson's disease		RUTF	ready to use therapeutic food
PEG	percutaneous endoscopic gastrostomy		SACN	Scientific Advisory Committee on Nutrition
PEJ	percutaneous endoscopic jejunostomy		SAM	severe acute malnutrition
			SAP	severe acute pancreatitis
PERT	pancreatic enzyme replacement therapy		SBGM	self-blood glucose monitoring
PFS	Pollen Food Syndrome		SBP	systolic blood pressure
PHCT	primary health care teams		SBS	short bowel syndrome
Phe	phenylalanine		SCF	Scientific Committee for Food
PHE	Public Health England		SCI	spinal cord injury
PI	pancreatic insufficiency		SD	standard deviation
PICC	peripherally inserted central catheter		SDC	Sustainable Development Commission
PKU	phenylketonuria		SDS	slowly digestible starch
PMTCT	prevention of mother to child transmission		SEMS	self-expanding metal stent
PN	parenteral nutrition		SENr	Sport and Exercise Nutrition Register
PNI	protective nutrient intake		SFA	saturated fatty acids
PRG	percutaneous radiological gastrostomy		SFT	School Food Trust
			SGA	subjective global assessment
PSE	portal systemic encephalopathy		SGLT-2	sodium-glucose co-transporter-2
PUFA	polyunsaturated fatty acids		SLE	systemic lupus erythematosus
PWS	Prader–Willi syndrome		SMI	serious mental illness
QUID	quantitative ingredient declaration		SPT	skin prick test
			SSB	sugar sweetened beverages
R. Nutr.	registered nutritionist		TBK	total body potassium
RD	registered dietitian		TBSA	total body surface area
RDA	recommended dietary amount		TBW	total body water
RDis	Refsum's disease		TEE	total energy expenditure
RDS	rapidly digestible starch		TG	triglyceride/triacylglyceride
REE	resting energy expenditure		TPN	total parenteral nutrition
RfS	refeeding syndrome		TPP	thiamine pyrophosphate
RIG	radiologically inserted gastrostomy		TSF	triceps skin-fold
RMR	resting metabolic rate		TSH	thyroid-stimulating hormone
RNA	ribonucleic acid		tTGA	IgA tissue transglutaminase

TVP	textured vegetable protein
UC	ulcerative colitis
UF	ultrafiltration
UL	upper limit
UNU	United Nations University
US	ultrasound

VAD	vitamin A deficiency
VLCD	very low calorie diets
VLDL	very low-density lipoproteins
WHO	World Health Organization
Wt	weight

Chapter 1

Introduction to nutrition

Definitions 2
Components of the diet 4
Food composition tables 8
Titles 12
Digestion 16

Definitions

Nutrition

'*Nutrition is the branch of science that studies the process by which living organisms take in and use food for the maintenance of life, growth, reproduction, the functioning of organs and tissues, and the production of energy.*'[1]

Public health nutrition

Usually described as '*the promotion of good health through nutrition and the primary prevention of nutrition-related illness in the population*'. Emphasis is on maintaining the wellness of the population through applying public health principles to influence food and nutrition systems. There is no internationally agreed definition.

1 Bender, A.E., Bender, D.A. (1995). *Oxford dictionary of food and nutrition*. Oxford University Press, Oxford.

Components of the diet

Diet

Diet is what a person habitually eats and drinks, so everyone is always on a diet. One of the most important and difficult tasks in nutritional medicine is to estimate accurately the habitual nutritional intake and diet of the patient. These difficulties arise because a person's diet may vary widely from day to day, food processing may greatly affect the nutrient content of foods s/he eats, and hardly anyone with a nutritional problem can accurately recall what s/he has eaten.

Dietary value

Dietary value is assessed by the measured energy and nutrient content of a particular diet and often in reference to dietary reference values (see ➔ Chapter 2 'Dietary reference values', p. 21) or recommendations. Foods and diets also have many other kinds of value including political, economic, social, and cultural values (see ➔ Chapter 14 'Influences on children's food choices', p. 318). In most societies where people live above starvation level, effort is put into diversifying meals and the overall diet, e.g.:

- use of food in rituals, e.g. birthday and wedding cakes, also fasting (Ramadan and Lent);
- use of food to express values and social relationships, e.g. sharing food, preparing special foods as expression of love, etc.;
- prestige foods, e.g. champagne and caviar as symbols of wealth and privilege.

Components of the diet

Diets are composed of food and drinks that contain nutrients: macronutrients (protein, fats, carbohydrates, and alcohol), micronutrients (vitamins, minerals, and trace elements), and water. They also contain many non-nutritional, but biologically active substances. These include toxins and contaminants, such as alkaloids and aflatoxins, which are detrimental to health, as well as constituents, such as phytochemicals, that may be health-promoting. As consumers we do not eat nutrients, but meals and foods. These are the components of diet that are most meaningful to the public and usually the basis of food choice.

Food groups

Foods vary in their energy and nutrient content. Food groups are a classification of foods on the basis of the nutrient profile (see ➔ Chapter 2 'The Eatwell Guide', p. 27 and Table 1.1). Commonly used food groups are:

- high protein foods, e.g. meat, fish, eggs, dairy products, pulses/legumes;
- carbohydrate-rich foods, e.g. cereals, roots, and tubers;
- dairy foods;
- fruit and vegetables;
- foods rich in fat or oil.

Food groups are widely used in the formulation of dietary guidelines and for nutrition education messages of various kinds, such as eat five portions of fruit and vegetables a day (a UK health message). Although useful, such classifications are also somewhat arbitrary; some foods can be placed in more than one food group.

Table 1.1 Nutrient profiles of the main food groups

Food group	Fat	Carbo-hydrate	Protein	Fat-soluble vitamins	Water-soluble vitamins	Minerals
Cereals		+++	++		++ (Bs) but variable	+
Roots and tubers		+++	+ but variable		++ (C) but variable	
Legumes / pulses	Variable	+++	++		++ (Bs)	+
Meat, fish, eggs	+		+++	++	+ (Bs)	+
Dairy products	+		++	++	+ (C)	++
Fruits		+			+++ (C)	
Vegetables			++		+++ (C, folate)	++
Sugar		+++				
Fats and oils	+++			+++ but variable		

+, This food group is a source of the nutrient(s) in most human diets; ++, this food group is an important source of the nutrient(s) in most human diets; +++, this food group is a major source of the nutrient(s) in most human diets.

Staple foods

Traditionally, a staple food is one that forms the basis of the diet in terms of both quantity and frequency of consumption, and that provides the highest proportion of energy. In developed countries it is not always easy to specify one particular food as the staple. Staple foods vary with geographic region, but in global terms the most important staple foods are the following.

- *Cereals:* globally, cereals supply approximately 51% of the world's dietary energy supply (DES) with rice, maize, and wheat being the most important, although other cereals, such as millet and sorghum, are also important in some regions. Cereals are a good source of carbohydrate, but also contain reasonable amounts of protein, and, depending on variety and processing, some micronutrients, e.g. Fe and some B vitamins.
- *Roots and tubers, and particularly cassava or manioc:* in sub-Saharan Africa these supply 22% of the DES, with this figure rising to over 70% in individual countries, such as the Democratic Republic of Congo. Other important roots are potatoes, yams, sweet potatoes, and taro. They are high in carbohydrate, but low in fat, protein, and, with some important exceptions e.g. sweet potatoes, micronutrients.

Other less common staple foods are sago eaten in parts of Malaysia and Indonesia, and plantain and bananas in many tropical countries (sub-Saharan Africa, Asia, Caribbean, and South America). The importance of staple foods has declined in industrialized countries (e.g. in industrialized countries cereals only supply 26% of the DES), but they remain important in many low-income countries. In Nepal, 77% of the DES is derived from cereals (predominantly rice), while in the USA only 23% of the DES is derived from cereals (as a mixture of rice, wheat, and maize).

Meals

Most foods are eaten as part of meals. Meals may differ in the following ways.

- The combination of foods eaten, e.g. the traditional British meal of 'meat and two veg'.
- How they are processed, prepared, and cooked. This can have an impact on the nutritional value of food, e.g. steaming, rather than boiling vegetables reduces the loss of water-soluble vitamins.
- The order in which particular items or dishes are consumed. In most European countries a formal meal is a three-course sequence pattern of starter, main course, and pudding or dessert, whereas in Chinese banquets many dishes may be served at once.
- How food is eaten. With hands or implements, from separate dishes or a common bowl. This is largely a matter of social etiquette, but can be important in child feeding, e.g. if small children are fed from a common pot, rather than given an individual serving.
- Who eats with whom and the allocation of food within the household. In some societies men and women eat separately, and there is also an unequal division of food between the sexes, including children.

These meal patterns may impact on the dietary intake of individuals within a household.

Snacks

Snacks are foods that are not eaten as part of meals. The place of snacks in individual diets and their contribution to overall dietary intake are variable.

Food composition tables

The food composition tables used in the UK are those of McCance and Widdowson. The 7th edition was published in 2014 by the Food Standards Agency (℘ www.food.gov.uk) and Public Health England (PHE) (℘ www. gov.uk/government/organisations/public-health-england).[2] The UK Composition of Foods Integrated Dataset (CoFID) is regularly updated and available on the PHE website. Food tables may be country-specific to account for country-specific food laws, e.g. fortification. An EU-funded project (EuroFIR, ℘ www.eurofir.org) has made some progress towards the development of a comprehensive, validated databank providing a single, authoritative source of food composition data for Europe.

Food composition tables list the energy, macronutrient, and selected micronutrient content of selected foods. Mean values are derived from representative samples of each type of food and expressed in standard units of 100 g per food type. Values are usually expressed in terms of the edible portion of the food, although 'as purchased' values may be given. The contents are arranged by food groups: cereals and cereal products, dairy products, eggs, meat and meat products, etc. Foods are given an individual code. Supplements are available for specific foods, e.g. fish, fats, and oils.

Food composition tables are used to analyse the foods and diets of individuals and groups; the values obtained are often then compared with dietary reference values (DRVs) and reference nutrient intakes (RNI). Other uses of food composition tables include:

- the planning and assessment of food supplies, e.g. during famines or war;
- designing institutional and therapeutic diets, e.g. in schools or hospitals;
- prescription of diets in clinical practice;
- modifying diets to ↑ or ↓ particular nutrients;
- health promotion and teaching;
- nutrition labelling;
- food regulations and consumer protection;
- research on relationships between diet and disease.

Food composition tables are compiled by laboratory analyses of selected samples of foods and cooked recipe dishes. They may also be compiled from published results in the literature.

❶ Tables usually include an introduction explaining how they are compiled; it is important to read this section. ❶ The printed version of McCance and Widdowson does not include a complete list of foods; more comprehensive data are included in the supplements and in the online dataset.

Calculation of energy values

The gross energies of foods are measured using a ballistic bomb calorimeter, but the values used in the tables are the energy available for the body to metabolize—metabolizable energy. Metabolizable energy accounts for faecal and urinary losses. The difference between gross energy and

---

2 Food Standards Agency & Public Health England (2014). *McCance and Widdowson's the The Composition of Food*, 7th Seventh summary edn. Royal Society of Chemistry, Cambridge.

metabolizable energy is about 5%. The direct measurement of metaboliz-able energy required human trials. Energy conversion factors, e.g. Atwater factors are used (see Table 1.2). These factors are derived from elaborate human studies.

Calculation of protein content

Most tables give protein and amino acid analyses. Protein content is usually derived from nitrogen content. It is assumed that, on average, protein is 16% nitrogen. Therefore, the nitrogen content is multiplied by 6.25 (100/16) to derive protein content, but there are limitations:

- the nitrogen content of food proteins varies;
- the nitrogen content varies with amino acid composition;
- other food constituents contain nitrogen, e.g. purines, urea, pyrimidines, and dipeptides.

Calculation of fat content

Most tables give total fat and fatty acid analyses. Before determining the fat content of foods it is necessary to extract the fat with alcohol, which can be done by a variety of methods, e.g. Soxhlet extraction. Each method of extraction will vary in the extent to which different fats are extracted, so introducing a possible error.

Calculation of carbohydrate content

Some tables report carbohydrate content by difference, i.e. carbohy-drate = 100 − amounts of protein, water, fat, and ash. This assumes that all carbohydrates have equal digestibility, which is not correct. Other tables summarize measured values of total available carbohydrate (the sum of sugars and starches); this is usually reliable, but the ↑ use of glucose and high fructose syrups may → overestimation of sucrose. Dietary fibre is de-termined by one of two methods (Englyst and Southgate) and values from the methods should not be mixed.

Table 1.2 Energy conversion factors

Nutrient	kcal/g	kJ/g	Comments
Protein	4	17	
Fat	9	37	Original Atwater factor was 8.9 kcal, ∴ the lower kJ figure is preferable
Carbohydrate	3.75	16	Value is for available carbohydrate expressed as monosaccharides. If carbohydrate is expressed directly or by difference 4 kcal/g is used
Sugar alcohols	2.4	10	Mean value used in food labelling
Ethyl alcohol	7	29	
Glycerol	4.31	18	Assumes complete metabolism

Calculation of micronutrient content

There are many methods for measuring micronutrients and these have variable accuracy. Some micronutrients have a variety of forms that are biologically active, e.g. folate. No single assay gives total free folate activity in foods.

Limitations of food tables

Real variation in energy and nutrient content All foods vary in energy and nutrient content because of many factors—variety or strain, sex and age of animals, agricultural processes, environmental factors, e.g. soil and climate, conditions and duration of storage, processing, and preparation. There is less variation in macronutrients than micronutrients, with the exception of fat. The cut of meat will influence fat content as will personal preference of the consumer.

Variation in water content Water content is one of the most significant sources of variation in nutrients. Dry cereal grains have relatively little water, but their content is variable and the amount of water absorbed in preparation is variable, e.g. cooked rice has water content of between 65% and 80%.

Sampling errors The sample analysed must be representative of the average composition of particular foods. This needs to take into account seasonal or regional variations. This is particularly true of processed foods, where the recipe and process is variable. Different recipes will add another layer of inaccuracy. Recipes are often given in food composition tables or the recipe used should be calculated from raw ingredients.

Inappropriate methods The choice of analytical method is important and should be reported. Some methods used for the determination of a nutrient may not be interchangeable, e.g. fibre.

Laboratory errors Laboratories and/or processes are standardized, but errors may still occur.

Use of conversion factors Conversion factors may introduce errors as described before.

Bioavailability This is not an error, but it is important to consider the bioavailability of specific nutrients.

Errors in coding and calculation Calculation of the nutrient content of foods requires precise information on the amounts of food eaten. Often, average portion sizes are used, which will introduce errors as average portion sizes vary with age and between countries, cultures, etc. Average portion sizes have been published for some countries. Errors may also occur in the coding of foods and calculation of nutrient content.

Studies have compared values obtained directly and by using food tables, and found that energy and protein values varied by 10–15% and that values for micronutrients varied by up to 50%. Provided the limitations of the use of food tables are understood, they are invaluable tools for nutritionists and dietitians.

Food composition analysis programmes are now available that make the calculations less arduous, e.g. CompEat, Dietplan 6.

Titles

Dietitian (dietician)

The titles dietitian and dietician are protected by law in the UK; anyone using these titles must be registered with the Health & Care Professions Council (HCPC). Anyone using these titles without registration is liable to prosecution. Registered dietitians are also able to use the post-nominal letters RD. The European Federation of the Associations of Dietitians (EFAD) has defined the role of the dietitian as follows.

- A dietitian is a person with a qualification in nutrition and dietetics recognized by national authorities. The dietitian applies the science of nutrition to the feeding and education of groups of people and individuals in health and disease.
- The scope of dietetic practice is such that dietitians may work in a variety of settings and have a variety of work functions.

European academic and practitioner standards for dietetics can be found on the EFAD website (℧ www.efad.org).

Many dietitians work in the National Health Service (NHS) and may specialize in specific areas, e.g. oncology, renal disease. They are employed in all sectors of healthcare and are a key part of the healthcare team. Dietitians also work outside the NHS in areas such as industry, sport, education, journalism, and research.

Health Professions Council

More information about the Health Professions Council (HPC) is available at ℧ www.hpc-uk.org.

British Dietetic Association

The British Dietetic Association (BDA) is the professional body representing dietitians and was established in 1936 to:

- advance the science and practice of dietetics and associated subjects;
- promote training and education in the science and practice of dietetics and associated subjects;
- regulate the relations between dietitians and their employer through the BDA trade union.

Specialist groups within the BDA cover areas of specialist interest, e.g. Paediatric Group, Dietitians in Obesity Management (DOM) UK. Full membership is available to RDs; other membership categories are available for dietetic assistants, students, and affiliates. The BDA is responsible for the curriculum framework for the education and training of dietitians. More information about the BDA is available at ℧ www.bda.uk.com. The BDA is one of the 24 full member associations, and 3 affiliate members, of EFAD ℧ www.efad.org. It is also one of over 40 national dietetic associations that are members of the International Confederation of Dietetic Associations (ICDA) (℧ www.internationaldietetics.org).

Dietetic support workers and assistant practitioners

Dietetic support workers (DSW) and assistant practitioners (AP)[3] work under the direct supervision of a RD. Their roles may include administration and dietetic tasks as delegated by the RD. In a hospital setting these may include assisting patients requiring special diets to choose from the hospital menu, and collecting and recording information regarding the patient's food consumption and weight. In primary care they may include providing dietary consultation, under the direction of the dietitian, and liaising with the RD regarding the patient's progress. Within a community setting they may include assisting the dietitian to assess the food and health needs of local residents, and enabling people to eat a healthier diet to prevent disease, offering guidance in relation to food selection and preparation, planning menus, standardizing recipes, and testing new products. Individual tasks undertaken by DSWs, and even more so by APs, may be exactly the same as the band 5 dietitian, with the difference being in the detail of the task/activity and the level of autonomy. Unlike the dietitian, a DSW or AP would have established and predetermined protocols for which referrals they are able to accept, and for which conditions, and at what point they would need to hand over to a dietitian. There would be pre-agreed treatment options and a DSW or AP would not have the autonomy to move away from these options without first checking this with a dietitian. Again in project work, e.g. healthy eating session or diet sheet/resource development, it would be expected that the dietitian would oversee the project once delegated, and then sign off the information/project plan at the end. The level of both experience and formal education achieved are what differentiate between a DSW and an AP, and the complexity of the work expected of them. National Vocational Qualification level 3 courses are available in allied health professional support (dietetics).

Nutritionist

The title 'nutritionist' has no legal standing and no educational requirements are necessary for a person to be called a 'nutritionist'. The Association for Nutrition is endeavouring to regulate the field of nutrition and protect the title 'nutritionist'.

The Nutrition Society

The Nutrition Society (🔊 www.nutritionsociety.org) was established in 1941 'to advance the scientific study of nutrition and its application to the maintenance of human and animal health'. Until 2010 the Nutrition Society was responsible for the UK Voluntary Register of Nutritionists; this was transferred to the Association for Nutrition.

The Association for Nutrition

The Association for Nutrition (AfN) is a professional body for the regulation and registration of nutritionists (including public health nutritionists and animal nutritionists). The AfN 'governs the UK Voluntary Register of

---

3 The British Dietetic Association (2010). *Dietetic Support Worker and Assistant Practitioner Roles*. Available at: 🔊https://www.bda.uk.com/publications/apdswcareer.

Nutritionists (UKVRN) to distinguish nutrition practitioners who meet rigorously applied training, competence and professional practice criteria. Its purpose is to protect the public and assure the credibility of nutrition as a responsible profession.' Registrants must demonstrate high ethical and quality standards, founded on evidence-based science. The AfN sets proficiency and competency criteria, promotes continuing professional development and safe conduct, and will accredit university undergraduate and postgraduate nutrition courses. The association awards the titles Associate Nutritionist (ANutr), Registered Nutritionist (RNutr) and Fellow of AfN (FAfN). Only practitioners registered with AfN may use these titles. Further details can be obtained at ℘ http://www.associationfornutrition.org

Registered Public Health Nutritionist

The title Registered Public Health Nutritionist (RPHNutr) is now defunct. AfN registrants who were registered as RPHNutr now use the title RNutr.

Registered Sport and Exercise Nutritionist

The Sport and Exercise Nutrition Register (SENr) (℘ http://www.senr. org.uk) is a voluntary register designed to accredit suitably qualified and experienced individuals who have the competency to work autonomously as a Sport and Exercise Nutritionist with performance-orientated athletes, as well as those participating in physical activity, sport, and exercise for health. The register is administered by BDA on behalf of the SENr Board; all registrants are required to be a member of the BDA.

Digestion

Food is broken down by mechanical and chemical mechanisms in the gastro-intestinal (GI) tract before nutrients can be absorbed into the body. The GI tract is a continuous tube from the mouth to the anus and is approximately 7 m in length (Fig. 1.1). Food is transported through the lumen of the tract as it is digested.

The mouth and oesophagus

Food is chewed by teeth and mixed with saliva, which is produced by salivary glands (parotid, submaxillary, and sublingual glands). Saliva contains the enzyme amylase, which starts the digestion of starch. The food is mixed with saliva, fluid, and mucus to form a bolus that is pushed into the pharynx by the tongue. The pharyngeal muscle contracts to swallow the bolus of food. The bolus is moved down the oesophagus into the stomach by peristalsis.

The stomach

The cardiac sphincter is found at the junction of the oesophagus and stomach and contracts to prevent food leaving the stomach and re-entering the oesophagus. The stomach is a muscular organ that further breaks down the bolus by mechanical, chemical, and enzymatic actions. Parietal cells in the stomach wall secrete hydrochloric acid, which helps break down the food, denatures protein, and converts the inactive pepsinogen into active

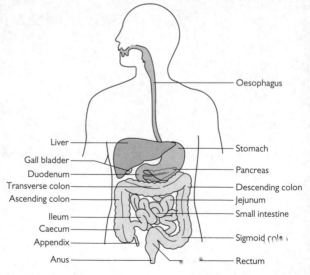

Fig. 1.1 The gastrointestinal tract.

pepsin. Chief cells in the stomach secrete pepsinogen. Pepsin begins the breakdown of proteins. Enzymes, protease and lipase, break down protein and fat, respectively. Goblet cells secrete mucin, which protects the stomach from hydrochloric acid. The food is converted into chyme in the stomach, which then passes into the small intestine.

The small intestine

The pyloric sphincter is a circular muscle at the junction of the stomach and small intestine that controls the release of chyme into the small intestine. The small intestine consists of the duodenum, jejunum, and the ileum. Chyme is transported along the small intestine by slow muscular contractions known as peristalsis. It can take up to 5 hours to complete the movement through the small intestine; this slow transition aids absorption. The surface area of the small intestine is large to facilitate digestion and absorption. Villi and microvilli are finger-like projections lining the lumen. Enzymes lactase, maltase, and sucrase complete carbohydrate digestion into monosaccharides. The villi have thin walls through which nutrients are absorbed into capillaries (carbohydrates and proteins) and lacteals (fat absorption, Fig. 1.2). The lacteals connect with the lymphatic system. Proteins are further broken down in the small intestine into amino acids, which can be absorbed through the villi wall.

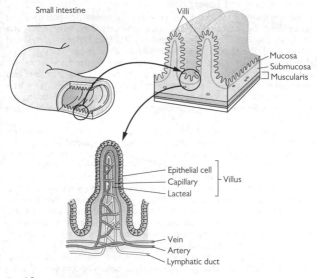

Fig. 1.2 Villi of the small intestine.

The pancreas secretes a mixture of enzymes that continue digestion; trypsin, chymotrypsin, and carboxypeptidase break down proteins and polypeptides into amino acids, and lipase breaks down fats into fatty acids and glycerol. Bile is secreted by the liver and stored and concentrated by the gall bladder. Bile dilutes and buffers the chyme, and emulsifies fat so enabling lipase to break down the fat. Water-soluble nutrients (amino acids, mono-saccharides, and water-soluble micronutrients), and short and medium chain fatty acids are taken to the liver via the portal vein. Fat-soluble nutrients are transported in the lymphatic system and enter the blood system at the left subclavian vein.

The large intestine

The remaining chyme passes into the large intestine through the ileocaecal sphincter, a circular muscle that separates the small and large intestines. The large intestine consists of the caecum (and appendix), colon (ascending, transverse, descending, and sigmoid), rectum, and anus. Less than 10% of digestion occurs in the large intestine. Water is reabsorbed to conserve water and to form faeces. Some vitamins including vitamin K and biotin are absorbed in the large intestine. The microbiota of the colon ferment dietary resistant starches and fibre to produce short chain fatty acids. These are increasingly being recognized as important in reducing the risk of conditions including gastrointestinal disorders. Faeces consist of undigested food, particularly insoluble fibre, and are expelled from the rectum through the anus by powerful contractions. The anal sphincter controls defaecation.

Fat digestion and absorption

Most dietary fat is in the form of triacylglycerides (triglycerides) and is digested by pancreatic lipase into non-esterified fatty acids and monacylglycerides. Phospholipid digestion yields lysophosphoglyceride and a fatty acid. Cholesterol is hydrolysed before absorption. Triacylglyceride digestion is very efficient, with 95% of fat being digested and absorbed; only 40% cholesterol is absorbed. The products of fat digestion pass into 'mixed micelles': molecular aggregates of monoacylglycerides, large fatty acids, bile salts, and phospholipids. Cholesterol, carotenoids, tocopherols, and some undigested triacylglycerides are taken into the hydrophobic core of the micelles (Fig. 1.3).

Lipid absorption occurs mainly in the jejunum. The digestion products of fats pass from the micelles into the enterocyte's membrane by passive diffusion. A fatty acid binding protein binds to fatty acids and they are rapidly re-esterified to monoacylglycerides. Cholesterol is re-esterified by acyl-CoA:cholesterol acyltransferase or by reversal of cholesterol esterase. Cholesterol esterase is induced by high levels of dietary cholesterol. Fats are packaged into chylomicrons and taken into lacteals, and then they circulate via the lymphatic system and are mainly removed in adipose tissue by lipoprotein lipase. The chylomicrons are not completely consumed by the enzyme, but are degraded to smaller particles, that are removed by the liver. Short and medium chain fatty acids are directly absorbed into the portal vein. Lipids are synthesized in the liver and those delivered by chylomicron remnants are packaged into very low density lipoproteins (VLDL) and secreted into the blood.

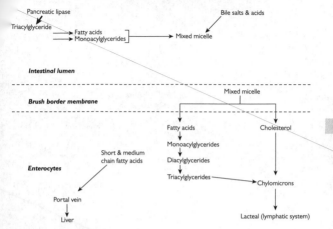

Fig. 1.3 Fat digestion and absorption.

Chapter 2

Dietary reference values and food-based dietary guidelines

Dietary reference values 22
Food-based dietary guidelines 26

Dietary reference values

Dietary reference values (DRVs) are established within a population as a measure of nutritional adequacy. The first DRVs were established in the late nineteenth century and international values were established by the League of Nations in 1936–8 to prevent deficiencies in population groups. Many countries have their own values and international values have been published by Food & Agriculture Organization (UN) (FAO)/World Health Organization (WHO)/United Nations University (UNU). DRVs for food and nutrients for the UK (report of the Panel on DRVs of the Committee on Medical Aspects of Food Policy [COMA]) were last completely revised in 1991.[1] DRVs for energy were revised in 2011 (Scientific Advisory Committee on Nutrition [SACN] ℘www.gov.uk/government/groups/scientific-advisory-committee-on-nutrition).[2] SACN have more recently produced revised recommendations for energy, carbohydrate, and vitamin D. UK DRVs are given for energy and nutrients in ⮞ Chapter 5, 'Macronutrients and energy balance: introduction p. 61' and ⮞ Chapter 6, 'Micronutrients, p. 99', and are summarized in Appendix 6.

DRVs are based on the assumption that the individual requirements for a nutrient within a population or group are normally distributed and that 95% of the population will have requirements within 2 standard deviations (SD) of the mean, as shown in Fig. 2.1. They assume that individuals are healthy, and also consider gender, age, growth, and physiological status, i.e. pregnancy and lactation.

Limitations of DRVs

Although DRVs can be useful, they can be misused and the inherent problems associated with making recommendations for the whole population should be appreciated.

- A standard distribution of nutrient requirements is assumed; the distribution may not be normal or insufficient data may be available to establish normality.
- Good data are required for the panel to evaluate requirements; these data may be derived from balance studies, tissue levels, pool size, etc., amount required to prevent symptoms of deficiency, or a measure of function of the nutrient (see Fig. 2.2). Such data are not always available and at times the panel has decided that the data are insufficient to set requirements and has ∴ recommended a 'safe level' of intake.

Factors affecting dietary requirements

- Metabolic requirement including:
  - age, gender, body size;
  - lifestyle (smoking, obesity, physical activity, etc.);
  - disease, e.g. fever, catabolism;
  - trauma;
  - growth.

1 Department of Health (1991). *Dietary reference values for food and nutrients for the United Kingdom.* HMSO, London.

2 Scientific Advisory Committee on Nutrition (2011). *Dietary reference values for energy.* TSO, London.

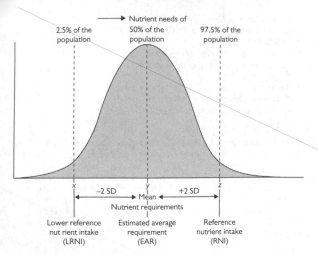

Nutrient needs of 50% of the population

2.5% of the population

97.5% of the population

x   −2 SD   y   +2 SD   z
Mean
Nutrient requirements

Lower reference
nutrient intake
(LRNI)

Estimated average
requirement
(EAR)

Reference
nutrient intake
(RNI)

Fig. 2.1 Derivation and definition of dietary reference values in the UK. (Adapted from Department of Health. Dietary reference values for food and nutrients for the United Kingdom. London, UK: Her Majesty's Stationery Office. © Crown Copyright 1991. Available at ⅁ https://assets.publishing.service.gov.uk/government/uploads/system/uploads/attachment_data/file/743790/Dietary_Reference_Values_-_A_Guide__1991_.pdf. Contains public sector information licensed under the Open Government Licence v3.0.)

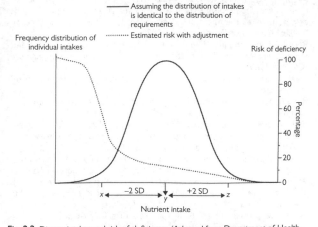

Assuming the distribution of intakes is identical to the distribution of requirements
······· Estimated risk with adjustment

Frequency distribution of individual intakes

Risk of deficiency

Percentage

100
80
60
40
20
0

x   −2 SD   y   +2 SD   z
Nutrient intake

Fig. 2.2 Dietary intakes and risk of deficiency. (Adapted from Department of Health. Dietary reference values for food and nutrients for the United Kingdom. London, UK: Her Majesty's Stationery Office. © Crown Copyright 1991. Available at ⅁ https://assets.publishing.service.gov.uk/government/uploads/system/uploads/attachment_data/file/743790/Dietary_Reference_Values_-_A_Guide__1991_.pdf. Contains public sector information licensed under the Open Government Licence v3.0.)

- Bioavailability including:
  - altered absorption, e.g. milk Ca is better absorbed than non-milk Ca;
  - reduced utilization;
  - ↑ losses, e.g. diarrhoea, burns, renal disease;
  - environment, e.g. heating of nutrients;
  - drugs, e.g. diuretics;
  - dietary concentration;
  - dietary interactions;
  - drug–nutrient interactions.

Uses of DRVs

- Dietary assessment of individuals, although it must be noted that DRVs are based on populations and groups not individuals. Other factors may need to be considered.
- Dietary assessment of groups or populations; it is important that the population is comparable with that for which the recommendations are derived.
- Prescription of diets and provision of supplies, e.g. school meals.
- Food labelling.
- Food formulation.

Definitions

⚠ The definitions will vary according to the country or organization responsible for the recommendation.

UK

- See the recommendations given by the Department of Health.[3]

Recommended Daily Amount (RDA) 'The average amount of the nutrient which should be provided per head in a group of people if needs of practically all members of the group are to be met' (Committee on Medical Aspects of Food [COMA], 1979).[4]

Recommended intakes 'The amounts sufficient, or more than sufficient, for the nutritional needs of practically all healthy persons in a population' (COMA, 1969).[5]

'Intake' emphasizes that the recommendations relate to food actually eaten.

Requirement The amount of a nutrient that needs to be consumed to maintain normal nutritional status.

Estimated average requirement (EAR) (point *y* in Fig. 2.1) The mean requirement of a nutrient for a population or group of people. On average, 50% will consume more than the EAR and 50% less.

Lower reference nutrient intake (LRNI) (point *x* in Fig. 2.1) The level at which only approximately 2.5% of the population or group will have an adequate intake; it will not be enough for most people. An individual with this intake may be meeting their requirement, but it is highly probable that they are not.

Reference nutrient intake (RNI) (point *z* in Fig. 2.1) At this level intake will be adequate for 97.5% of the group or population. It is possible that an individual's intake will not meet their requirement at this level, but is highly improbable. RNIs for micronutrients are given in Appendix 6 and as appropriate throughout the handbook.

Safe level Given when insufficient information is available to derive requirements. It is an average requirement plus 20%, and is believed to be adequate for most people's needs. The COMA judged that there was no risk of deficiency at this level and that there is no risk of undesirable effects above this level.

FAO/WHO

Estimated average requirement (EAR) As for 'UK'.[6]

Recommended nutrient intake (RNI) As for 'FAO/WHO'.

Protective nutrient intake (PNI) An amount > RNI for some micronutrients that may be protective against a specified health or nutritional risk of public health relevance. PNI are expressed as daily value or an amount to be consumed with a meal.

Upper tolerable nutrient intake level (upper limit [UL]) The maximum intake of some micronutrients that is unlikely to pose risk of adverse health effects in almost all (97.5%) apparently healthy individuals in a gender- and age-specific population.

USA

Recommended dietary amount (RDA) Average daily dietary intake that meets the requirements of nearly all (97–98%) healthy persons.[7]

Adequate intake (AI) Established for a nutrient when available data are insufficient to estimate an intake that would maintain adequacy. The AI is based on observed intakes by a group of healthy persons.

Tolerable upper intake limit (UL) As for 'FAO/WHO'.

Estimated average requirement (EAR) As for 'UK'.

3 Department of Health (1991). *Dietary reference values for food and nutrients for the United Kingdom.* HMSO, London.

4 Department of Health & Social Security (1979). *Recommended daily amounts of food energy and nutrients for groups of people in the United Kingdom.* Reports on Health and Social Subjects, 15. HMSO, London.

5 Department of Health & Social Security (1969). *Recommended intakes of nutrients for the United Kingdom.* Reports on Public Health and Medical Subjects, 120. HMSO, London.

6 FAO/WHO (1988). *Expert consultation on human vitamin and mineral requirements.* WHO, Geneva.

7 National Academy of Sciences, Institute of Medicine, Food and Nutrition Board (2006). *Dietary reference intakes: the essential guide to nutrient requirements.* National Academies Press, Washington.

Food-based dietary guidelines

Historically, dietary guidelines were nutrient-based; food-based dietary guidelines (FBDG) were developed to facilitate the teaching of 'healthy eating' and nutrition to population groups. FBDG focus on foods, rather than nutrients, and are intended for use by the general public. They are designed to be understandable to most consumers. FBDG give practical information on 'healthy eating' and intakes of nutrients to meet DRVs of macro- and micronutrients (see ⊃ Appendix 6, p. 875). FBDG are designed to be appropriate to each population group; they may be country, age, or culturally specific.

Development of FBDG

The FAO/European Food Information Council (EUFIC) report on the development of FBDG is available on the websites ℛ http://www.fao.org and ℛ http://www.eufic.org.

Key concepts

The following points should be considered in development of FBDG.

Dietary patterns

- Total diet, rather than nutrients.
- Reflect food patterns, rather than numeric nutrient goals.
- Various dietary patterns can be compatible with health.

Practical considerations

- Food should be affordable, widely available, and accessible.
- FBDG should recognize social, environmental, and agricultural conditions affecting foods and eating patterns.
- They should be flexible such that they can be used by people with different lifestyles, ages, and physiological conditions, e.g. pregnancy.

Comprehensibility

- Should be easily understood.
- Food groups should make sense.
- Should include visual representations.
- Testing is essential before dissemination.

Cultural acceptability

- Foods and colours should be culturally appropriate.
- Should be sensitive to cultural and religious considerations.
- Avoid racial changes in current practice.
- Use appropriate dialect or language.
- Should be positive and encourage enjoyment.

Underlying assumptions

- Foods are more than nutrients—food has cultural, social, ethnic, and family messages.
- Biological functions may not be fully elucidated. Foods may be more beneficial than nutrients alone.
- Combinations of nutrients in foods can have different metabolic effects.
- Food processing and preparation influence nutritional values.
- Specific dietary patterns can be associated with reduced risk of specific diseases.

- FBDG are based on scientific knowledge and principles from science-based disciplines including:
  - nutrition;
  - food science;
  - behaviour;
  - communication;
  - agriculture.

Nutrition concepts

These concepts are generic and recommended by FAO. Country-specific concepts are developed.

ⓘThese concepts may be different to UK's dietary recommendations **➜** later in this chapter Table 2.1 p. 28.

- Energy:
  - aims to prevent excess or deficiency;
  - promotes appropriate energy intakes by encouraging appropriate food choices;
  - physical activity is also encouraged.
- Protein:
  - *high quality protein*: 8–10% total energy;
  - *vegetable-based mixed diet*: 10–12% of total energy;
  - *elderly where energy intake low*: 12–14% total energy.
- Fat:
  - at least 15% energy from fats and oils;
  - childbearing age women at least 20% to ensure adequate essential fatty acids;
  - active non-obese <35% total energy (saturated fatty acids [SFA] <10%);
  - sedentary <30% total energy;
  - SFA <10% total fat.
- Carbohydrate:
  - main energy source >50%;
  - fibre 15 g for 2–5 y, 20 g 5–11 y, 25 g 11–15 y, 30 g adults in the UK;
  - sugar usually ↑ acceptability and energy density. Inversely related to fat intake. Moderate intakes compatible with a varied nutritious diet. WHO recommend <5–10% total energy. UK recommend free sugars <5% of total energy.
- Micronutrients:
  - compounds with different metabolic activities;
  - essential for normal growth, development, and health;
  - important in preventing infectious and chronic diseases.

A summary of the recommendations for the UK is shown in Table 2.1.

The Eatwell Guide

'The Eatwell Guide' (an interactive version is available at ℘ http://www.nhs.uk/Livewell/Goodfood/Pages/the-eatwell-guide.aspx) is the pictorial representation of FBDG in the UK (Fig. 2.3). It is applicable to most people including minority ethnic groups, vegetarians, and people of all ages except children <2 years. It is based on five food groups:

- potatoes, bread, rice, pasta, and other starchy carbohydrates;
- fruit and vegetables;
- beans, pulses, fish, eggs, meat, and other proteins;
- dairy and alternatives;
- oil and spreads.

Table 2.1 A summary of the dietary recommendations for the UK*

Recommendation		Population group	Reason for recommendation
Fruit and veg	>5 × 80 g/day (400 g)	Adults	↓ Risk of some cancers, CVD, and other chronic conditions
Oily fish	>1 portion/ week (140 g)	Adults	↓ Risk of CVD
Red and processed meat	<70 g/day	All red meat consumers	↓ Cancer risk
Free sugars	<5% food energy†	All	Free sugars ↑ risk dental caries, high energy intake, ↑ sugar sweetened beverages ↑ risk type 2 diabetes
Fat	<35% food energy	All	↓ Risk CVD, ↓ energy density of diet
Sat. fat	<11% food energy	All	↓ Risk CVD, ↓ energy density of diet
Fibre	>18 g/day	Adults	↓ Risk CVD, bowel cancer, hypertension type 2 diabetes
Alcohol	<3–4 units/ day men <2–3 units/ day women	Adults (>18 years)	↓ Risk liver disease, CVD, cancer, injury from violence or accidents
Salt	<6 g/day	Adults	↓ risk hypertension and CVD
Vitamins and minerals	DRVs	All	To prevent deficiencies and promote growth
Dietary vitamin D	RNI for children >4 years, adults >65 years, pregnant and breastfeeding women. Others with limited sun exposure also require dietary vitamin D‡	All	To prevent deficiency

Table 2.1 (*Contd.*)

Recommendation		Population group	Reason for recommendation
Supplements	Vitamin D	May be needed in autumn and winter. People from African, Afro-Caribbean, and S. Asian backgrounds may need supplements all year. Older adults, housebound or living in institutions, or who eat no meat or oily fish	To achieve adequate vitamin D status and ↓ risk of poor bone health

*Source: data from the Nutritional Wellbeing of the British Population (2008) Scientific Advisory Committee on Nutrition.

†Energy consumed as food and drink excluding alcohol.

‡Vitamin D supplements are also recommended for pregnant and lactating women.

Other information on the guide includes:
- Choose wholegrain or higher fibre versions with less added fat, salt, and sugar.
- Eat at least five portions of a variety of fruit and vegetables every day.
- Eat more beans and pulses, two portions of sustainably sourced fish/week, one of which is oily. Eat less red and processed meat.
- Choose lower fat and lower sugar dairy and alternative options.
- Eat less foods high in fat, sugar, and salt, i.e. cakes, sweets, chocolate, crisps, etc.
- Check the label on packaged foods; choose foods lower in fat, salt, and sugars.
- Drink plenty of fluids: six to eight glasses of fluids/day, including water, lower fat milk, sugar-free drinks including tea and coffee. Limit fruit juice and/or smoothies to <150 mL/day.

MyPlate

MyPlate (Fig. 2.4) is the pictorial representation of the USA FBDG (℞ http://www.choosemyplate.gov). It was released in June 2011 by the United States Department of Agriculture's Center for Nutrition Policy & Promotion. MyPlate is intended as 'a reminder to find your healthy eating style and build it throughout your lifetime. Everything you eat and drink matters. The right mix can help you be healthier now and in the future'. This is achieved by:
- Focusing on variety, amount, and nutrition.
- Choosing foods and beverages with less saturated fat, sodium, and added sugars.
- Starting with small changes to build healthier eating styles.
- Supporting family eating for everyone.

The website has resources and tools to help consumers of all ages, including students, make healthier food choices and increase their physical activity.

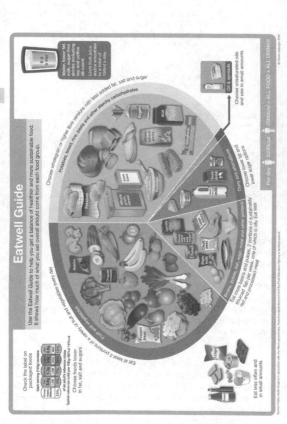

Fig. 2.3 The 'Eatwell Guide'. (Reproduced from Public Health England in association with the Welsh Government, Food Standards Scotland, and the Food Standards Agency in Northern Ireland. Eatwell Guide. London, UK: Public Health England. © Crown Copyright 2016. Available at https://assets. publishing.service.gov.uk/government/uploads/system/uploads/attachment_data/file/528193/Eatwell_guide_colour.pdf. Contains public sector information licensed under the Open Government Licence v3.0.)

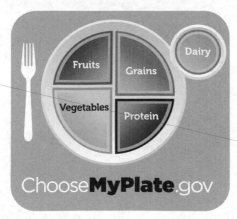

Fig. 2.4 MyPlate food-based dietary guidance for USA (U.S. Department of Agriculture).

Current dietary patterns in the UK

Current dietary patterns *34*

Current dietary patterns

Information on current dietary patterns in the UK is taken from the National Diet and Nutrition Survey (NDNS).[1] NDNS is a rolling programme commissioned by the Food Standards Agency (FSA) and Public Health England (PHE) and surveys people aged 1.5 years and older living in private households. Combined intakes from 2014–15 and 2015–16 with additional information from the previous surveys are reported as appropriate. Updates are available at ℘ https://www.gov.uk/government/collections/national-diet-and-nutrition-survey.

❶ Previous adult NDNS surveys have slightly different methodologies ∴ be cautious when making comparisons.

Fruit and vegetable consumption

The mean fruit and vegetable consumption was 4.2 portions/day for adults and 2.7 portions/day for children aged 11–18 years.

Fewer than 31% of adults eat the recommended intake of 5 portions/day; only 8% of 11–18 year olds meet the recommendation.

In 2000/01 households receiving state benefit consumed on average
- 1 less portion of fruit and vegetables/day.
- Oily fish
  - All age groups consumed <1 portion (140g)/week.
- Red and processed meat
  - On average adults exceeded the recommendation to eat <70g/day.
- Sugar sweetened soft drinks
  - Men consumed an average of 159 g/day and women consumed 100 g/day. Children consumed on average 37 g/day in the 1.5–3 years category; 83 g/day and 191 g/day in the 4–10 and 11–18 years categories, respectively.

Energy and nutrient intakes for adults

- See Table 3.1.
- Average protein intakes were above the reference nutrient intake (RNI).
- The mean percentage energy derived from free sugars was more than twice the recommended value
- The mean daily intake of fibre was below the recommended average intake of 18 g/day for men and women.
- The daily food energy intake from fat was near the recommended intake of <35%.
- The mean food energy derived from saturated fat was above the recommended level of 11%.
- The intake of trans fatty acids was below the recommended intake for men and women.

Alcohol consumption

- Men are more likely to consume alcohol than women.
- Men drank an average of 16.7 g/day when non-consumers were included in the analysis; this increased to 29.2 g/day when the

1 Public Health England & Food Standards Agency (2018). *The National Diet and Nutrition Survey*: results from Years 7 & 8 of the Rolling Programme (2014/2015–2015/2016). Public Health England, London.

Table 3.1 Average intake of macronutrients and energy (2014–15 and 2015–16) (NDNS)* compared with DRVs

Energy/nutrient	Men	Women
Total energy intake (MJ) (kcal)	8.79 (2101)	6.87 (1641)
% EAR	81%	79%
Protein (g)	87.4	66.6
% RNI	164%	143%
Total carbohydrate (g)	249	199
% Food energy	47.6	47.7
Free sugars (g)	64.3	50.0
% Food energy	11.9	11.6
DRV (% food energy)	<5%	<5%
Fibre† (g)	15.1	12.9
DRV (g)	30	30
Total fat (g)	76.6	62.4
% Food energy	34.4	35.0
DRV (% food energy)	<35.0	<35.0
Saturated fatty acids (g)	27.5	22.8
% Food energy	12.3	12.7
DRV (% food energy)	<11%	<11%
Trans fatty acids (g)	1.1	0.9
% Food energy	<0.5	<0.5
DRV (% food energy)	<2%	<2%

*Source: data from Public Health England & Food Standards Agency (2016). *The National Diet and Nutrition Survey: Results from Years 5 and 6 (combined) of the Rolling Programme (2012/2013–2013/2014)*. Public Health England, London.

†Association of Official Analytical Chemists (AOAC) fibre.

non-consumers were excluded. The means for women were 8.6 g/day and 17.8 g/day, respectively.
- When non-consumers were excluded, mean intakes for men and women exceed the recommendation to drink <14 units (56 g/week). The mean daily energy intake from alcohol in adults was 8.4% of total energy.

Vitamin and mineral intakes
- Mean intakes for most vitamins were close to or exceeded the RNI for men and women.
- Of adults aged 19–64 years, 17% had intakes less than the RNI for vitamin D from food sources.
- Substantial proportions of the population had red cell folate levels indicating deficiency; this was particularly apparent in older girls and women of childbearing age.

Vegetarianism/veganism
- Data from 2011–12 NDNS.
- Of those surveyed, 2% reported being vegetarian and <1% reported being vegan; the Vegan Society now estimate this to be slightly >1%.
- Vegetarianism/veganism was particularly popular in women aged 19–34 years.
- All avoided red meat, 92% avoided white meat, 29% avoided all animal products.

Nutrition assessment

Nutrition assessment: introduction 38
Dietary assessment 40
Individual assessment 44
Body composition 50
Anthropometry 54

Nutrition assessment: introduction

This chapter considers dietary assessment of populations and groups, and nutrition assessment of the individual. Assessment of physical activity and energy expenditure can be found in Chapter 5, 'Macronutrients and energy balance', p. 61. Individual nutritional assessment should be structured, focused, and standardized; it usually follows the ABCDEF format:

• Anthropometry, body composition.
• Biochemical, haematological tests.
• Clinical, physical.
• Dietary.
• Environmental, behavioural, and social.
• Functional.

Dietary assessment

Dietary assessment is an imprecise procedure; the imprecision can be minimized using the appropriate technique and by understanding the errors implicit in the methodology. Dietary assessment is further hampered by the fact that diet can and does change. Precision varies from very precise techniques, such as metabolic balance studies to the broad estimates of population studies. The methodology chosen must be appropriate for the nutrient/s and the individual or population being assessed. The timing of the assessment is also important and must consider cultural variations, such as differences in the week (weekday vs. weekend day), seasons (wet vs. dry season), and special occasions, e.g. Ramadan, Christmas.

This section gives a brief description of the methods used to assess diet; fuller descriptions and methods of assessing validity are described by Margetts and Nelson (1997)[1] and Gibson (2005).[2]

Country level assessment

Information is available on a national level on food production and agriculture; but this does not consider imports and exports. Food balance sheets (FBS, see Box 4.1), per country, are published annually by FAO ($\mathcal{N}$ http://www.fao.org/faostat/en/#data/FBS) and estimate a country's food supply (Table 4.1). Data are collated on domestic food production, food imports, and food taken from storage. Food *per capita* data can be derived as shown below and these can also be converted into nutrient values.

Per capita supply = total production + imports

- + adjustment for storage levels
- – exports – animal use – seeds
- – losses (storage, transport, and processing)

> ## Box 4.1 Food balance sheets (FAO methodology)
> *Strengths*
> - Information available in over 160 countries, since 1961.
> - Data routinely collected in the countries.
> - Does not entail implementation of special surveys.
> - Assesses long-term trends.
> - Provides global information on undernourishment.
> - Provides information comparable across countries and across time.
> - Is timely: estimates produced rapidly.
> - Provides global information on dietary patterns.
>
> *Weaknesses*
> - Does not measure actual energy intake or utilization.
> - Inaccuracy of country food balance data.
> - In some countries estimates not consistent with socio-economic indicators.
> - Underestimates actual energy needs in poor countries.
> - Data on equality of food distribution not available.
> - No disaggregation at subnational level.
> - Does not take into account all food available for consumption, such as game or subsistence agriculture.

1 Margetts B, Nelson M, eds. Design concepts in nutritional epidemiology. Oxford, Oxon: Oxford University Press; 1996.
2 Gibson RS Principles of Nutritional Assessment. Oxford, Oxon: Oxford University Press; 2005.

Table 4.1 Strengths and limitations of household survey data*

Method	Strengths	Limitations
Food account	1. Cheap: data collected by government and readily available for analysis	i. Home foods only unless family members collect data
	2. Representative: national sample	ii. Incomplete; may not include sweets, alcohol, soft drinks
	3. Possible subgroup analysis—by region, income, etc.	iii. No individual data
	4. Provides information on food consumption patterns	iv. Based on food composition tables see 'Food composition tables', ➲ Chapter 1 (p. 8)
		v. No knowledge of change in food stocks
		vi. Bias of over purchasing especially in elderly or low-income households
Inventory	1–3 plus:	i–iv plus:
	5. Considers changes in larder stocks	v. Larder inventory may distort usual purchasing patterns
	6. Measures actual home food consumption	
Household record	3, 5, and 6 plus:	i, iii, and iv plus:
	7. Used in societies with low levels of literacy	vi. Observer presence may distort normal patterns
	8. Can be modified to measure individual consumption	vii. Seasonal variation in food availability may limit comparisons between groups
List-recall	1–3, and 6 plus:	i–iv plus:
	9. Based on single interview	viii. Memory errors
	10. Measures food use	ix. Observer presence may bias responses
	11. Retrospective; reflects actual patterns	

*Adapted from Garrow, J.S., James, W.P.T., and Ralph, A. (2000) *Human Nutrition and Dietetics* 10th edition, Table 17.1, p. 315, Churchill Livingstone: London with permission from Elsevier.

This information can be used to study the links between diet and disease and can aid the development of food-based dietary guidelines (FBDG) (see ➲ Chapter 2, 'Dietary reference values and food-based dietary guidelines', p. 22), but the FBS only give information on availability not consumption. FBS give an estimate for the country as a whole and show no patterns of variation within the country.

Household-based surveys

Examples of this type of survey, conducted on a regular basis, include the UK National Diet and Nutrition Survey (NDNS) (℘www.gov.uk) and dietary surveys that are part of the National Health and Nutrition Examination Surveys (NHANES). NHANES is conducted by the Center for Disease Control and Prevention (CDC), USA (℘ http://www.cdc.gov). The limitations and strengths of each method are shown in Table 4.1.

Food account

Food accounts are also known as budget household surveys. The main respondent notes all food that is purchased, grown, or received as gifts, assuming no change in stocks. Foods taken out of the household may be recorded. Waste is assumed to be 5-10%. The amounts of different food groups at the household level are deducted from the price paid for each food group. The amount can be divided by the number of people living in the household according to their gender, age, or body size. Records are usually kept for 1–2 weeks, which may not reflect the full dietary cycle of the household. The degree of disaggregation of food codes affects the precision of the study, e.g. 50 groups, will be less precise than a survey, which uses 500 food groups.

Inventory

This is similar to a food account, with the addition of a larder inventory at the start and finish of the survey period. Over short periods the survey may be distorted as attention is drawn to larder items that would not normally be consumed.

Household record

Foods are weighed or estimated using household measures with an allowance for waste. An interviewer visits after breakfast and foods consumed at breakfast are recalled. Food for further meals is weighed or estimated. An afternoon or evening visit may be made to establish waste. This method is most useful in developing countries where most food is home produced and levels of literacy are low.

List recall

This survey is based on the recall of foods consumed in a household over a set period, usually 1 week. It does not estimate individual consumption.

Individual assessment

The assessment of an individual's diet is susceptible to many possible errors including under- or over-reporting by subjects, recall difficulties, measurement errors, coding and calculation errors. Estimation of portion sizes may also introduce inaccuracies. Assessment may be prospective or retrospective; the strengths and limitations of each method are summarized in Tables 4.2 and 4.3, and the steps in choosing a method are given in Fig. 4.1.

Prospective methods

Duplicate diet

Subjects weigh and record food at the time of consumption and a duplicate of the diet is weighed and stored for direct chemical analysis; it does not require the use of food composition tables. This method usually uses metabolic units so the onus of weighing, etc., is not on the subject. Aliquot

Table 4.2 Strengths and limitations of prospective measurements of individual food consumption*

Measurement	Strengths	Limitations
General features	Current diet	Labour-intensive
	Direct observation of what is eaten	Requires numeracy and literacy skills
		Subjects need to be well motivated
	Duration may be varied to meet requirements of estimates of food consumption or nutrient intake	Usual consumption may change because of:
		• inconvenience of recording;
		• choice of foods that are easy to record;
		• beliefs regarding which foods are healthy or unhealthy.
		Overweight subjects tend to under-report
		Coding and data entry errors are common
Duplicate diet	Direct analysis of nutrients (not dependent on food composition tables)	Very expensive
		Intense supervision required
	Required for metabolic balance studies	May not be usual diet
Weighed inventory	Widely used ∴ able to compare studies	Food composition tables are used
	Precision of portion sizes	
Household measures	No scales needed	Loss of precision compared with weighed inventory

* Reproduced from Garrow, J.S., James, W.P.T., and Ralph, A. (2000) *Human Nutrition and Dietetics*, 10th Edition, Table 17.2, p. 317, Churchill Livingstone: London, with permission from Elsevier.

Table 4.3 Strengths and limitations of retrospective measurements of individual food consumption*

Measurement	Strengths	Limitations
General features	Inexpensive	Biases caused by: • errors in memory, conceptualization of food portion sizes, perception; • presence of observer
	Quick	Daily variation not usually assessed
	Lower respondent burden	Dependent on regular eating habits
	Can assess typical or past diet	Food composition tables used to estimate nutrients
Diet history	Assesses usual diet	Over-reporting of foods believed to be healthy
24-hour recall	Very quick	Prone to underestimate consumption because of omissions
	Can be repeated to gain measure of daily variation and improve precision	Single observation provides poor measure of individual intake
Food frequency questionnaires	Suitable for large-scale surveys	Requires validation in relation to reference measure
	Can be posted	Literacy and numeracy skills required if self-completed
	Short versions (or screeners) can focus on specific foods, e.g. fruit and vegetables	

*Adapted from Garrow, J.S., James, W.P.T., and Ralph, A. (2000). *Human Nutrition and Dietetics*, 10th edition, Table 17.2, p. 317, Churchill Livingstone, Edinburgh.

sampling and equivalent composite are both duplicate diet methods. In aliquot sampling a sample, usually 10%, is taken, rather than an exact duplicate. This is less wasteful, but introduces possible sampling errors. In equivalent composite assessment an investigator prepares a duplicate diet from the list of ingredients used by the subjects which is analysed chemically.

Weighed inventory

This method is widely used: subjects weigh and record all food prepared and waste. The major advantage of this method is that it does not rely on assumptions of portion size. Food composition tables are used to estimate nutrient intake from the records.

Household measures

This method is similar to the weighed inventory except that food portions are estimated. Photographs or household measures, e.g. spoons and cups, may be used to aid portion size estimation. This method requires less effort by the subject than the weighed inventory, but is more prone to error.

Steps and tips on choosing a dietary assessment method

STEP 1 Defining the objective
The method is determined by the reason for the assessment—is it part of a research study or to clarify an individual's deficiency?
⇓

STEP 2 Foods and/or nutrients?
Are data needed at the nutrient level or will a description of food patterns suffice?
⇓

STEP 3 Decide the conceptual timeframe of dietary intake
Past, present, usual?
Will a retrospective or prospective method be most applicable?
⇓

STEP 4 Decide the actual timeframe of dietary survey
Day, week, or year?
Number of interviews (e.g. multiple 24 hr recalls),
Consecutive days? Weekdays and/or weekends?
Account for seasonality?
⇓

STEP 5 Who will be interviewed and by whom?
e.g. children (interview parent or the child directly?)
Who will conduct the dietary assessment? Do they need training?
Who will record the information? (Interviewer or interviewee?)
⇓

STEP 6 What type of foods and drink need to be assessed?
If all, then a prescribed method like a FFQ may be inappropriate.
Is information needed on whether foods are raw or cooked and the cooking methods used?
⇓

STEP 7 Estimating how much is eaten and/or how often
Is frequency of intake enough to meet the objectives?
If the aim is to estimate nutrient intake then quantities will be needed. What method is best adapted to the context?
- Direct quantification: weigh, measure volume
- Indirect quantification: household measures, estimated with utensils and food containers
- Standard food portions
- Actual dimensions of the food
- Food models (2 or 3 dimensional)
- Photos of foods with a range of portion sizes
- A count of handfuls, e.g. with a shared dish
- Proportion of the prepared meal that was consumed, e.g. household intake
⇓

STEP 8 Comparing intake with recommendations
If data includes nutrient analysis: are all foods available in food composition tables? Which dietary analysis programme should be used? Dietary patterns could be explored or diet scores created to compare with FBDGs.

Fig. 4.1 Steps and tips on choosing a dietary assessment method.

Retrospective methods

24-hour recall

A trained interviewer guides the subject through their food intake over the previous 24 hours. It is a quick method, but cannot be used to classify a subject's usual intake as it is not necessarily representative of the subject's normal eating pattern. Two 24-hour recalls may be used in population surveys.

Diet history

A diet history is an extension of a 24-hour recall and gives more detailed information about the usual diet; it can typically take 2 hours. The reliability of the results is dependent on the skills of the interviewer.

Food frequency questionnaire

Printed questionnaires are used and subjects (or interviewer) tick the category that approximates to their usual consumption of a list of foods, i.e. never eaten, eaten once a month, eaten once a fortnight, number of times eaten per week. This is quantified and intake is estimated; the questionnaires can be sent and returned in the post. The number of foods can vary; sometimes only a few are used when assessing a food group or nutrient, e.g. fruit. These are sometimes called screeners. Food frequency questionnaires (FFQs) are often used in large surveys. It is necessary to validate FFQs against a more precise method such as weighed food intake. There are three main types of FFQ:
• qualitative—no portion size;
• semi-quantitative—standard portion size is used;
• quantitative—subjects are asked to record data on portion size.

Computer-based dietary assessment methods

Many computer-based or Internet-based methods to assess dietary intake have been developed; usually based on FFQs and 24-hour recalls e.g.
• Food Intake Recording Software System (FIRSSt).
• EPIC-SOFT (widely used in Europe) (⌖http://epic.iarc.fr/).
• Automated self-administered 24-hour recall (ASA24; ⌖http://appliedresearch.cancer.gov/asa24/).

They aim to reduce the burden of data collection, data coding, and data management, and to standardize data collection.

New approaches using technologies to assess dietary intakes

New methods are currently being developed and tested to improve the accuracy of estimation of dietary intake using technologies such as mobile phones with a camera, personal digital assistants (PDA), and microphones, e.g.
• food intake visual and voice recognizer (FIVR).
• mobile phone food record (MPFR) project.

Physical assessment

Observation of an individual may offer a gross assessment of nutritional status (see ⮊ Chapter 25, 'Nutrition screening', p. 558).

- Physical appearance: e.g. pallor, emaciation, and hair changes may be indicative of long-term energy deficit; loose dentures and loose clothing may indicate recent weight loss; xanthoma or corneal arcus in some types of hyperlipidaemia; nail and teeth changes may occur in bulimia nervosa.
- Oedema: may be present following protein depletion.
- Pressure sores or poor wound healing: may be the result of immune response abnormalities or undernutrition.
- Breathlessness: may be the result of anaemia.
- Mobility: may be reduced following ↓ in muscle mass caused by immobilization, which may present difficulties in food purchasing and preparation.
- Mood: e.g. apathy and depression, may be present in patients with eating disorders and other causes of undernutrition.

Biochemical and haematological assessment

Various parameters of nutritional status can be measured by analysis of serum, plasma, whole blood, urine, and faeces. Some measures are dynamic and reflect very recent changes, not long-term nutritional status. See sections on specific nutrients in ➔ Chapter 5, 'Macronutrients and energy balance' (p. 61), ➔ Chapter 6, 'Micronutrients' (p. 99), and ➔ Chapter 25, 'Nutrition screening' (p. 558).

- Vitamin and mineral status: may be assessed by circulating levels, although deficiency of some micronutrients must be prolonged before blood levels are affected. For other micronutrients the body is very finely balanced and a dietary deficiency is balanced by mobilization from tissues, e.g. phosphate, or excretion.
- Protein status: may be reflected by serum proteins such as albumin, although levels do not truly reflect changes in protein status; levels are affected by other factors, e.g. infection, C-reactive protein levels. Serum transferrin and rapid turnover proteins, e.g. thyroxine, are reasonable markers of protein status, but are also affected by metabolic stress and may not be very specific.

Body composition

Body composition can be used to establish nutritional status, especially when measuring adiposity. Most methods are based on a limited number of cadaver analyses. Only a few cadavers have been analysed, and these varied in ethnicity, age, gender, and cause of death. While unsystematic cadaver selection may confound the validity of data obtained, the enormity and difficulty of the task involved, and significant ethical considerations, make these remarkable analyses unlikely to be repeated. Therefore, existing assumptions are used as references for most modern techniques in body composition, ensuring a degree of consistency, at least, even if absolute accuracy cannot be wholly guaranteed. Modern body composition analysis may be perceived at five interactive levels: atomic, molecular, cellular, tissue/organ, and whole body.

Theoretical models

Theoretical models are used to derive reference data for the development of indirect methods, e.g. anthropometry. The body is divided into compartments; the classic two-compartment model divides the body into fat mass (FM) and fat-free mass (FFM). FM consists of all extractable lipids and the remainder is FFM. Cadaver analysis was used to derive properties of FM and FFM.

- Density of FM = 0.901 g/mL.
- Density of FFM = 1.10 g/mL.
- Densities of FM and FFM are constant within and between individuals.
- FFM is assumed to be 73.8% water, 19.4% protein, and approximately 7% mineral.

Other models require a combination of techniques to isolate the specified component of FFM.

- The three-compartment model estimates FM + total body water (TBW) + 'dry' FFM (protein and mineral).
- The four-compartment model is FM + TBW + protein + mineral.

Methods used to derive each compartment vary, with more sophisticated methods being needed to differentiate between compartments. Table 4.4 summarizes the methods available. Multi-component models are expensive, time-consuming, and difficult to use in field conditions; so alternative techniques may be more appropriate.

Independent methods

Each individual method can be used in multi-component models or used individually, provided it is applied appropriately and that the limitations are recognized.

Hydro-densitometry or under-water weighing

Body weight (BWt) is measured in air and during a procedure involving water displacement with the subject submerged, and with a correction for lung volume, to provide under-water weight (UWW). Body volume (BV) is calculated as BWt − UWW, and density (d) = BWt/BV, from which body fat and FFM may be obtained, as above.

Table 4.4 Summary of methods for the determination of body composition*

Method	Accuracy	Cost	Radiation	Time	Convenience for subject
Cadaver analysis	+++	–		–	
IVNAA	+++	–	–	++	++
Densitometry	++	+		++	+/–
Dilution	++	+/–	(–)	+	++
TBK	++	–		++	++
DEXA	+++	+/–	–	++	++
CT scanning	++	–	–	++	++
MRI scanning	++	–		++	+
Anthropometry	+	+++		++	+
Infrared interactance	+	++		++	++
BIA	+	+		+++	+++
TOBEC	+	–		++	++
Urinary metabolites	+	+		–	–

* Republished with permission of John Wiley and Sons Inc from *Introduction to Human Nutrition* 2nd edition. MJ Gibney *et al.* Copyright © 2009 John Wiley and Sons Inc; permission conveyed through Copyright Clearance Center, Inc.

+++, Excellent; ++, very good; +, good; +/– reasonable; – bad.

IVNAA, *In vivo* neutron activation analysis; TBK, total body potassium; DEXA, dual energy X–ray absorptiometry; CT, computer-assisted tomography; MRI, magnetic resonance imaging; BIA, bioelectrical impedance analysis; TOBEC, total body electrical conductivity.

Air-displacement plethysmography

BV can also be determined using air-displacement plethysmography (ADP), consisting of a chamber in which the subject sits comfortably and breathes normally. ADP measures chamber volume with and without the subject present by generating and measuring small pressure changes. BV is assessed by the difference in pressure changes with corrections for air in the lungs and adjacent to skin. To derive percentage body fat, body density is substituted into appropriate equations, e.g. Siri.

Siri formula: % Body fat = (495/body density) − 450.

As above, BV and weight obtained during both these techniques are also integral to the three- and four-component models if required.

Isotope dilution techniques

Total body water (TBW) may be measured using isotope dilution techniques in which labelled water is administered. Deuterium (^{2}H) dilution is the technique of choice as it is a safe stable isotope, which occurs naturally in the water. Oxygen-18 (^{18}O) is also a stable isotope and potentially more accurate for TBW estimation; however, ^{18}O-labelled water is more expensive and less readily available than ^{2}H-labelled water. In health, hydration of FFM is relatively constant, usually between about 72% and 74%, depending on factors, such as age.

❶ Caution is necessary in patients with abnormal hydration, e.g. liver and kidney diseases.

Dual-energy X-ray absorptiometry

X-rays at two distinct energies are used to differentiate bone, fat, and fat-free soft tissue (FFST), and so may be considered a specific three-component model. Therefore, dual-energy X-ray absorptiometry (DEXA) can provide estimates of FM and FFM, which are quite accurate and precise, at least in health. DEXA may be less accurate or precise in extremes of body dimensions (e.g. obesity and anorexia) and disproportionate changes in body chemistry (e.g. oedema), and may not assess changes accurately (e.g. in weight loss).

Although DEXA directs ionizing radiation, the exposure is considered to be relatively low, depending on the particular manufacturer and model, making it relatively safe. However, DEXA should not be used in pregnant women and there may be ethical issues in children.

Other methods

There are a number of methods that can be used to gather important body composition information in health and disease. However, caution is advised to ensure that estimates provided are appropriate to requirements, otherwise substantial errors are possible. Many indirect techniques depend on assumptions that may be uncertain, leading to such errors.

Bioelectrical impedance analysis

An electrical current flows predominantly through tissues containing water and ions, but not through fat, which is an insulator, therefore body resistance or impedance (Z) was originally used as an index of TBW. However, because of complex differential electrical properties of tissues, and lack of uniformity of body shape and dimensions, an essentially empirical approach was adopted. Whole body impedance was regressed against reference measures of TBW, which were then extended to FFM and fat, producing equations claimed to estimate or 'predict' body composition.

In practice, bioelectrical impedance analysis (BIA), which is now in widespread use, applies measures of impedance between hand and foot, usually, but foot to foot or hand to hand equipment are also widely available.

Impedance is commonly adjusted for an index of height (often Ht^2/Z) and then a derived equation to predict body composition. Often with other anthropometric measures incorporated, $\therefore$ a very large number of different BIA prediction equations is available.

❶ Caution is needed when using or interpreting BIA, as prediction equations are often originated, and applied, inappropriately, and without sufficient understanding.

Although useful for large-scale epidemiology and field studies, because of portability and low cost, BIA may be relatively ineffective in different population groups and certain disease states because it may be insensitive to underlying variability between individuals (e.g. males vs. females, adults vs. children) or fundamental changes caused by disease. See Smith & Madden (2016) for a comprehensive review of BIA.[1]

---

1 Smith, S., Madden, A.M. (2016). Body composition and functional assessment of nutritional status in adults: a narrative review of imaging, impedance, strength and functional techniques. *J. Hum. Nutr. Diet.* **29**, 714–32.

Total body potassium counting
Total body potassium (TBK) can be used to provide estimates of body composition, as TBK is present only in FFM with 98% in cells and its concentration is assumed to be relatively constant, but slightly different in males and females. A known proportion (0.012%) of natural potassium occurs as a radioactive isotope, ^{40}K, the radioactive decay of which produces γ-emissions detectable using whole body counters. Therefore, it is possible to estimate TBK and then to derive FFM from it in a non-invasive process that may take only 20–30 minutes, depending on the type of counter. Whole body counters are rarely available, are expensive, and can be affected by variations in body shape and dimensions, and environmental contamination.

Imaging techniques: computed tomography, magnetic resonance imaging, and ultrasound
Assessments of segmental and whole body tissues by computed tomography (CT) and magnetic resonance imaging (MRI) are very accurate, and extremely valuable measures in their own right, and may complement body composition estimates from other techniques. Estimates of gross body composition (e.g. body fat) are also possible, but these generally require the use of assumptions. MRI and CT are expensive and CT exposes the subject to relatively high doses of radiation, which has major ethical considerations.

Ultrasound (US) is a safe technique for complementing body composition methodology by providing relative dimensions of body tissues, e.g. adipose tissue and muscle, particularly tissue depths. Recent developments enable three-dimensional (3-D) assessments of tissues and organs.

Urinary metabolites
Excreted metabolic end products can be used to provide estimates of FFM. Twenty-four hour collections of urinary nitrogen (for protein turnover), creatinine (the constant spontaneous degradation product of creatine, found only in muscle), and N-methyl-histidine (N-MH; specific end product of muscle protein degradation) have all been used as indices of FFM. As urinary excretion is variable and physical losses of urine are known to occur, resulting in a major source of error, completeness of 24-hour urine collection may be confirmed by use of orally administered para-aminobenzoic acid (PABA). Creatine and N-MH measurement require the subject to be essentially on a meat-free diet. Nitrogen balance is representative of FFM, but also requires determination of faecal nitrogen. This technique is rarely used outside metabolic units.

Anthropometry and derived prediction equations
Body mass index (BMI) can be calculated from weight (Wt) and height (Ht); $BMI = Wt/Ht^2$. BMI is in itself precise and informative, particularly at the group level, but Wt and Ht, or BMI are not considered accurate or precise enough to be used independently to predict or estimate body composition, especially for individuals.

Skin-fold thicknesses obtained at various sites are used as indices of subcutaneous adipose tissue and can also be integrated to give predictions of body fat, but these estimates are not considered accurate or precise enough for estimating body composition. (See ➔ this Chapter, 'Anthropometry', p. 54.)

Anthropometry

Anthropometry simply means the measurement of man and involves measurement of height, weight, skin-fold thicknesses, circumferences, and various lengths and breadths of the body. These techniques require relatively cheap equipment and are ∴ widely used in clinical practice. The techniques for some anthropometric measurements are shown in Tables 4.5 and 4.6.

Children

See ➓ Chapter 13, 'Growth reference charts' (p. 258), ➓ Appendix 2 (p. 861).

WHO growth charts

The WHO produced new growth charts in 2006 for children aged 0–5 years, representing growth standards of healthy breastfed children in optimal conditions using data collected in the WHO Multicentre Growth Reference Study. These were extended in 2007 for children and adolescents aged 5–19 years (𝒮www.who.int/childgrowth/en/). The WHO Reference 2007 is a reconstruction of the 1977 National Center for Health Statistics (NCHS)/WHO reference. It uses the original NCHS data set supplemented with data from the WHO child growth standards sample for children aged <5 years.

UK 0–4 years charts

UK-WHO Growth Charts for children from birth to 4 years of age were introduced in 2009 (England) and in 2010 (Scotland). The charts combine UK90 and WHO data, and replace previous UK90 charts for age ≤4 years. Features include an adult height predictor, a BMI conversion chart, and guidance on gestational age correction. The UK90 charts should still be used for all children aged >4 years. They are included in the UK Personal Child Health Record (PCHR) or 'red book' issued to each newborn (see Appendix 2, p. 861). (See 𝒮 http://www.rcpch.ac.uk/Research/UK-WHO-Growth-Charts.) BMI percentiles should be used to identify overweight and obesity, and the new chart is recommended for routine clinical diagnosis of growth faltering. Overweight is classified as ≥91st centile and obesity ≥98th centile of the UK-WHO charts. Epidemiological studies use an internationally acceptable definition to classify prevalence of child overweight and obesity[2] or the WHO estimates of overweight from WHO growth charts for BMI-for-age.

Z-score

Anthropometric measurements can be expressed as Z-scores. A Z-score is the standard deviation (SD) score; the deviation of the value for an individual from the median value of the reference population divided by the SD for the reference population:

$$Z\text{-score} = (\text{observed value} - \text{median reference value}) /$$
$$\text{SD reference population}$$

2 Cole, T.J., et al. (2000). Establishing a standard definition for child overweight and obesity worldwide: international survey. BMJ **320**, 1240–3.

Table 4.5 Standardized anthropometric measurements: circumferences*

Site	Anatomical reference	Measurement
Waist	Narrowest part of torso**	Apply tape snugly around waist. Take measure at end of natural expiration
Hip (buttocks)	Maximum posterior extension of buttocks	Apply tape snugly around buttocks
MAC (biceps)	Midpoint between acromion process of scapula and olecranon process of ulna	Arms hanging freely with palms facing thighs

*Adapted from Heyward, V.H. and Stolarczyk, L.M. (1996). *Applied Body Composition Assessment*, Table 2.1 (pp. 28–9) and S.1 (pp. 71–4). (Copyright 1996, Human Kinetics).

**With increasing obesity this may be difficult to find, ∴ the midpoint between the top of the hip bone and bottom of the ribs may be used.

Table 4.6 Standardized anthropometric measurements: skin-fold measurements*

Site	Direction of fold	Anatomical reference	Measurement
Subscapular	Diagonal	Inferior angle of subscapular	Fold is natural cleavage line just inferior to interior angle of scapula with calliper applied 1 cm below
Supra-iliac	Oblique	Iliac crest	Fold is grasped behind to mid-axillary line and above iliac crest
Triceps	Vertical	As circumference above	Midpoint is measured and fold is 1 cm above line on posterior aspect of arm
Biceps	Vertical	Biceps brachii	Fold is lifted over the belly of biceps at line marked for triceps; calliper is applied 1 cm below fingers

*Adapted from Heyward, V.H., and Stolarczyk, L.M. (1996). *Applied Body Composition Assessment*, Tables 2.1 (pp. 28–9) and S.1 (pp. 71–4). (Copyright 1996, Human Kinetics). Permission requested from Dr Timothy Lohman.

Adults

Weight

Body weight is not a measure of body composition; scales require regular calibration and servicing, and weight may vary between scales. Monitoring of weight over a period can be a useful indicator of nutritional status.

Height

- A stadiometer is used or the subject is measured against a wall. The floor should be uncarpeted.

- The subject should be barefoot, with weight evenly distributed between both feet.
- Arms should hang loosely.
- Heels should be together, touching the vertical board or stadiometer. Head, scapula, and buttocks should be touching the vertical board or wall.
- Head should be held head erect with eyes focused straight ahead (Frankfurt Plane).
- The subject should inhale.
- The rod is lowered to the most superior point, compressing hair.

Surrogate measures of height

- Recall height may be used in bed-bound patients. This tends to overestimate height by 7 mm, but this does not affect BMI categorization except in the elderly.
- Ulna length can be measured by bending the left arm across the chest with the palm facing inwards and the fingers pointing to the shoulder. The measurement is taken between the central and post prominent parts of the styloid process and the tip of the olecranon. Details on how to convert ulna length to height are given in Elia (2003).[3]
- Knee height is measured in sitting subjects. The knee and ankle are bent to 90° and the observer's hand is placed flat on the thigh. The tape measure is held between the fingers and the height measured to the floor, on the lateral plane of the leg, in the same plane as the lateral malleolus (prediction equations are given in Table 4.7).
- Demispan can be measured in patients sitting in a chair or supine. The right arm is raised until it is horizontal with the wrist in natural flexion and rotation. The tape is placed between the middle and ring finger and runs smoothly along the arm. The measurement is taken from the tip of the finger to the centre of the sternal notch (prediction equations are shown in Table 4.7).

Body mass index

BMI reflects body fat stores and is calculated as: $BMI = Wt\ (kg)/Ht\ (m)^2$.

BMI is correlated to the risk of obesity and underweight-associated morbidity. Overweight subjects have an ↑ risk of associated health problems, this risk ↑ with ↑ BMI. The WHO cut-offs for the definition of overweight and obesity are given in Table 4.8 (see ➔ Chapter 21, p. 469).

BMI is a useful clinical and epidemiological tool. It should be used with caution in the elderly and in muscular subjects. Cut-off values will vary depending on ethnicity.

Circumferences

Waist circumference and waist–hip ratio have been proposed as measures of risk of obesity-associated morbidity. The WHO cut-offs for waist circumference are shown in Table 4.9.

❶ The precise sites used will vary depending on which manual is followed. The examples in this chapter may differ from those used by the International Society for the Advancement of Kinanthropometry (ISAK) or WHO.

3 Elia, M. (2003). *Development and use of the Malnutrition Universal Screening Tool ('MUST') for adults.* BAPEN, Basingstoke.

Table 4.7 Equations for the estimation of height*

Knee height			
Gender	Age, years	Ethnicity	Equation
Men	18–60	Black USA	Height = [knee height × 1.79] + 73.42
		White USA	Height = [knee height × 1.88] + 71.85
Women	18–60	Black USA	Height = [knee height × 1.86] − [age × 0.06] + 68.10
		White USA	Height = [knee height × 1.87] − [age × 0.06] + 70.25
Men	≥60	Black USA	Height = [knee height × 1.85] − [age × 0.14] + 79.69
		White USA	Height = [knee height × 1.94] − [age × 0.14] + 78.31
Women	≥60	Black USA	Height = [knee height × 1.61] − [age × 0.17] + 89.58
		White USA	Height = [knee height × 1.85] − [age × 0.21] + 82.21

Demi-span			
Gender	Age, years	Population	Equation
Men	20-45+	European	Height = 57.8 + [1.40 × demi-span]
Women		Nottingham, UK (n=125)	Height = 60.1 + [1.35 × demi-span]
Men	≥65	Living at home (Health Survey for England); 98% white; England, UK (n=2469)	Height = 73.0 + [1.30 × demi-span] − [0.10 × age]
Women			Height = 85.7 + [1.12 × demi-span] − [0.15 × age]

*Reproduced with permission. Madden & Hoffman (2019) Nutrition assessment. In *Manual of Dietetic Practice* sixth edition. Ed J Gandy. Wiley Blackwell

Table 4.8 International BMI classification*

BMI		Weight status
<18.5		Underweight
18.5–24.9		Normal
25.0–29.9		Pre-obesity
≥30.0		Obese
	30.0–34.9	Obese class I
	35.0–39.9	Obese class II
≥40		Obese class III

*World Health Organization (2018). Body mass index - BMI. Available at ℬ http://www.euro.who.int/en/health-topics/disease-prevention/nutrition/a-healthy-lifestyle/body-mass-index-bmi.

Table 4.9 Waist circumference cut-offs associated with disease risk*

Country or ethnic group	Gender	Waist circumference, cm
Europid	Men	>94
	Women	>80
South Asian	Men	>90
	Women	>80
Chinese	Men	>90
	Women	>80
Japanese	Men	>90
	Women	>80

*WHO (2008) *Waist circumference and waist hip ratio*. WHO, Switzerland.

Skin-fold thickness measurements

Most of the body's fat is stored subcutaneously. The thicknesses of skin-folds at specific sites are measured (at least 3 measurements are needed at each site) by callipers (Figs 4.2 and 4.3) and can be used to estimate total subcutaneous fat. The most commonly used sites are subscapular, supra-iliac, biceps, and triceps. Total skin-folds from these sites can be substituted into prediction equations to give an estimate of % FM. The most commonly used equations are those derived by Durnin and Womersley (1974).[4] Equations that are appropriate for specific ages and ethnic groups are available. Skin-fold measurements are cheap and quick, but the technique requires training and skill. Ideally practitioners should attend an accredited course, e.g. ISAK (🖰 http://www.isakonline.com).

Arm muscle measurement

Midarm circumference (MAC) can be measured as shown in Table 4.5. It is assumed that the arm is a cylinder of muscle covered by adipose tissue and that the double thickness of the fat layer is measured by triceps skin-fold (TSF) thickness. Midarm muscle circumference (MAMC) can be calculated:

$$MAMC(cm) = MAC - (3.14) \times TSF(cm).$$

This estimate of FM and FFM is used clinically to monitor nutritional status. Appendix 2 (p. 847) gives reference values.

4 Durnin, J.V.G.A., Womersley, J. (1974). Body fat assessed from total body density and its estimation from skinfold thickness: measurements on 481 men and women aged from 16 to 72 years. *Br. J. Nutr.* **32**, 77–97.

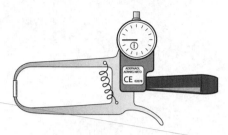

Fig. 4.2 Diagram of callipers.

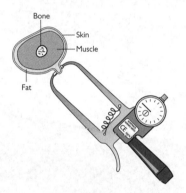

Fig. 4.3 Diagram of skin-fold measurement.

Resource: Madden A.M. & Hoffman Assessment of nutritional status. Manual of Dietetic Practice 6th edition. Ed Joan Gandy. Wiley Blackwell, Oxford, Oxon.

Madden, A.M. & Smith, S. (2016) Body composition and morphological assessment of nutritional status in adults: a review of anthropometric variables. Journal of Human Nutrition and Dietetics 29, 7–25.

Macronutrients and energy balance

Macronutrients: introduction 62
Protein 64
Fats 70
Carbohydrate 78
Energy balance 86

Macronutrients: introduction

The macronutrients are protein, fat, and carbohydrate, and they are required in gram amounts. They are major sources of energy as well as providing essential nutrients such as some fatty and amino acids.

Protein

Protein provides approximately 10–15% of the energy in the diet. Protein is essential for numerous structural and functional purposes and is essential for growth and repair of the body. In adults, approximately 16% of body weight is protein. 43% of this is muscle, 15% skin, and 16% blood. Protein is in a constant state of flux in the body with protein being synthesized and degraded continuously.

Protein flux (Q) can be described by the following equation:

$$Q = I + D + S + O$$

where I = intake, D = degradation, S = synthesis, and O = oxidation to CO_2 and urinary nitrogen.

Function

Protein has numerous functions in the body. Recent research has increasingly been focused on the role of amino acids in metabolism, e.g. the role of branch chain amino acids in glucose homeostasis, particularly insulin resistance. Examples of the different functions of protein are as follows.

- *Structural:* Protein is important for the structure of the body and about half of the body's protein is found in structural tissues such as skin and muscle. These structural proteins are collagen (25% of the body's protein), actin, and myosin.
- *Transport:* Proteins act as transport carriers in the blood and body fluids for many molecules and nutrients, e.g. haemoglobin, lipoproteins.
- *Hormonal:* Hormones and peptides are proteins or amino acid chains, e.g. insulin, pancreatic polypeptide.
- *Enzymes:* All enzymes are proteins. Extracellular enzymic proteins include the digestive enzymes, e.g. amylase. Intracellular enzymes are involved in metabolic pathways, e.g. glycogen synthase.
- *Immune function:* Antibodies are protein molecules. Proteins are also involved in the acute phase response to inflammation.
- *Buffering function:* The protein albumin acts as a buffer in the maintenance of blood pH.

Structure

Proteins are macromolecules consisting of amino acid chains. Amino acids are joined to each other by peptide bonds (Fig. 5.1). Amino acids form peptide chains of various lengths from two amino acids (dipeptide), four to ten peptides (oligopeptides) and more than ten amino acids (polypeptides). Reactive side groups of the amino acids combine to form links between amino acids in the chain and other peptide chains. The polypeptides form β pleated sheets or α helices. Polypeptides fold and cross-links form between amino acids to stabilize the folds. Proteins are formed by the combination of polypeptides. These cross-links give the peptide a distinctive function and shape (Fig. 5.2). There are approximately 20 amino acids and each has a different side group, size, and different properties, e.g. pH, hydrophilic or hydrophobic. These properties are used in the analysis of amino acids.

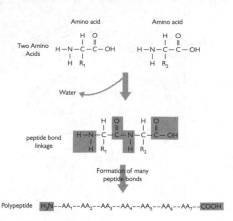

Fig. 5.1 Formation of a polypeptide.

Indispensable (essential) amino acids

Some amino acids can be synthesized by the body but others must be supplied by the diet. These are known as indispensable or essential amino acids;
there are eight essential amino acids (Table 5.1). Some amino acids are only
essential in specific circumstances and are classified as conditionally indispensable. In childhood, other amino acids are essential that are not essential
in adults (arginine, histidine, cysteine, glycine, tyrosine, glutamine, proline).
These amino acids are essential in children because they are required in
amounts larger than can be synthesized because of high demand, immature
biological pathways, or a combination of these. Conditionally indispensable
or essential amino acids only become essential in circumstances when the
requirement is ↑, e.g. glutamine in certain clinical conditions.

Requirements

The amino acid content of a protein determines its biological value. Proteins
that contain all the indispensable amino acids in sufficient quantities have
high biological value. High biological value proteins are from animal sources,
e.g. meat, eggs, milk, dairy products, and fish. If one, or more, indispensable amino acid(s) is absent from a protein, it will have low biological value.
Generally, plant proteins are of low biological value. The indispensable
amino acid that is in shortest supply is known as the limiting amino acid.
By combining foods with low biological value, it is possible to provide all
indispensable amino acids in the diet; this is important in vegan diets. For
example, the limiting amino acid in wheat is lysine and in pulses it is methionine. A diet combining wheat products such as bread with pulses will
provide all the indispensable amino acids, e.g. pitta bread and dhal.

As already stated, protein is constantly being turned over; 3–4 g of protein are turned over per kg of body weight per day. Each day 10–15 g of
nitrogen are excreted in urine (6.25 g protein is equivalent to 1 g nitrogen).

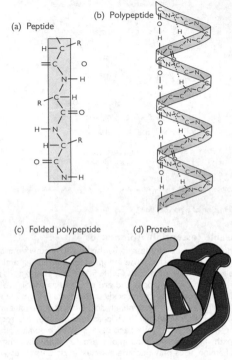

(a) Peptide

(b) Polypeptide

(c) Folded polypeptide

(d) Protein

Fig. 5.2 Formation of a protein.

Table 5.1 Classification of amino acids

Indispensable/essential amino acids	Indispensable (conditionally essential) amino acids	Dispensable (non-essential) amino acids
Leucine (Leu)	Tyrosine (Tyr)	Glutamic acid (Glu)
Isoleucine (Ile)	Glycine (Gly)	Alanine (Ala)
Valine (Val)	Cysteine (Cys)	Aspartic acid (Asp)
Phenylalanine (Phe)	Arginine (Arg)	
Threonine (Thr)	Proline (Pro)	
Methionine (Met)	Histidine (His)	
Tryptophan (Trp)	Glutamine	
Lysine (Lys)	Serine (Ser)	
	Asparagine (Asn)	

Small amounts are lost in faeces and skin. When nitrogen (protein) intake equals nitrogen excretion, the body is said to be in nitrogen balance. Healthy adults will be in positive nitrogen balance. Nitrogen balance studies have been used to derive the recommended requirements listed in Table 5.2.

Deficiency

If energy intake is insufficient, protein will be degraded to produce energy; ∴ protein deficiency can occur when the diet does not provide

Table 5.2 Recommended nutrient intake of protein for all age groups and average daily intakes of protein of adult men and women in the UK*

Age	Weight, kg	RNI, g/day
Children (both sexes)		
0–3 months	5.9	12.5
4–6 months	7.7	12.7
7–9 months	8.8	13.7
10–12 months	9.7	14.9
1–3 years	12.5	14.5
4–6 years	17.8	19.7
7–10 years	28.3	28.3
Males		
11–14 years	43.0	42.1
15–18 years	64.5	55.2
19–50 years	74.0	55.5
50+ years	71.0	53.3
Females		
11–14 years	43.8	41.2
15–18 years	55.5	45.4
19–50 years	60.0	45.0
50+ years	62.0	46.5
Additional RNI required for females		
During pregnancy		+6.0
Lactation: 0–6 months		+11.0
Lactation: 6+ months		+8.0
Adults (19-64 years)	Average daily intake UK, g/d	
Men	87.4	
Women	66.6	

*Source: data for RNIs, Department of Health (1991). *Dietary reference values for food and nutrients for the United Kingdom.* HMSO, London. Source: data for average daily intakes for adults, Public Health England & Food Standards Agency (2018). *The National Diet and Nutrition Survey: Results from Years 7 and 8 (combined) of the Rolling Programme (2014/2015–2015/2016).* Public Health England, London.

enough protein or energy or a combination of both. Protein energy malnutrition (PEM) is a major cause for concern in developing countries (see ⊃ Chapter 20, 'Global nutrition', p. 435), but does occur in the UK amongst at risk groups. These include immunocompromised individuals (e.g. AIDS), people with anorexia nervosa, and cancer patients with cachexia. Mild PEM is fairly common amongst surgical or elderly hospital patients. Protein deficiency can also occur as the result of ↑ losses in renal disease, ↑ catabolism in trauma, burns, or sepsis, or malabsorption. Protein deficiency results in muscle wasting, stunted growth, poor wound healing, and susceptibility to infection, oedema, and fatty liver.

Sources of dietary protein

In the typical UK diet, 60% of protein intake has high biological value. High biological protein is supplied by meat and meat products, fish, eggs, and milk and dairy products (Table 5.3). Plants such as cereals and pulses supply proteins of low biological value.

Table 5.3 Contribution of food sources to protein intake in UK adults*

Food group	% Daily intake
Cereals and cereal products (including bread)	22
Red meat (all meat excluding chicken and turkey)	20
Chicken, turkey and dishes	17
Milk and milk products	13
Bread	11
Fish and fish dishes	7

*Source: data from Public Health England & Food Standards Agency (2018). *The National Diet and Nutrition Survey*: Results from Years 7 and 8 (combined) of the Rolling Programme (2014/2015–2015/2016). Public Health England, London.

Fats

Fats are often referred to as lipids. Lipids are described by chemists as substances that are poorly soluble or insoluble in water but are soluble in organic solvents. Fat is the term most often used when discussing foods and lipid metabolism. Over 95% of dietary fats are triglycerides (triacylglycerols); other types of fat include cholesterol, phospholipids, and sterols.

Function

The functions of fat in the diet are:
- Energy source—fat provides 37 kJ (8.8 kcal) per gram.
- Fat provides essential fatty acids.
- Fat is a carrier for fat soluble vitamins A, D, E, and K.
- ↑ Palatability by improving taste perception and appearance of food.
- Some fats are important constituents of cell membranes and can be converted to biologically active compounds, such as steroid hormones, interleukins, thromboxanes, and prostaglandins.
- Cholesterol is converted to bile acids, which are important in digestion.

Fatty acids

Fats consist of fatty acids that have carbon chains containing up to 22 carbon molecules in the chain. The type of fatty acid attached to the glycerol molecule determines its physical properties, nutritional function, and physiological function. Hydrogen is added to unsaturated fatty acids to make them more solid when manufacturing some food products such as vegetable spreads; this process is known as hydrogenation.

Fatty acids are carbon molecules with a methyl group at one end and a carboxyl acid at the other (Fig. 5.3). They can have chains of 4–22 carbon molecules, although most have 16–18. Hydrogen atoms are attached to the carbon chain; the number of hydrogen atoms determines the degree of saturation (with hydrogen atoms) of the fatty acid. A fatty acid with hydrogen atoms on every arm is 'saturated'. Unsaturated fatty acids contain double carbon bonds where there is no hydrogen (Fig. 5.3). If there is only one double bond, the fatty acid is monounsaturated. When more than one double bond is present, the fatty acid will be polyunsaturated.

Fatty acids have a common name, e.g. linoleic acid, a systematic name, and a notational name. The systematic name reflects the number of carbon atoms, and the number of double bonds, so that linoleic acid becomes octadecadienoic acid. This represents 18 carbons (octadeca-) and two double bonds (di-). The notational name for linoleic acid is 18:2 n6 or 18:2 ω 6; again this represents 18 carbon atoms and two double is also represented as :2 after 18. The position is relative to the methyl (or omega) end of the carbon chain. Linoleic acid has its first double bond between the sixth and seventh carbons. Common names, systematic names, and notational names are shown in Table 5.4. Table 5.5 shows the average intakes of fat and DRVs. Table 5.6 shows the main sources of fat in the UK adult diet.

Saturated fatty acids

Saturated fatty acids (SFA) contain carbon atoms linked by single bonds and hydrogen on all available arms; they have a relatively high melting point and tend to be solid at room temperature. SFA are obtained from animal storage fats and their products, e.g. meat fat, lard, milk, butter, cheese, and cream. Fats from plant origin tend to be unsaturated with the exception of coconut oil and palm oil. Some manufactured margarines and spreads contain significant amounts of SFA. Plasma low-density lipoprotein (LDL) cholesterol, and ∴ plasma cholesterol, tends to be raised by dietary SFA. High intakes of SFA are associated with atherogenesis and cardiovascular disease.

Monounsaturated fatty acids

Monounsaturated fatty acids (MUFA) contain only one double bond and are usually liquid (oil) at room temperature. Olive oil and rapeseed oil are

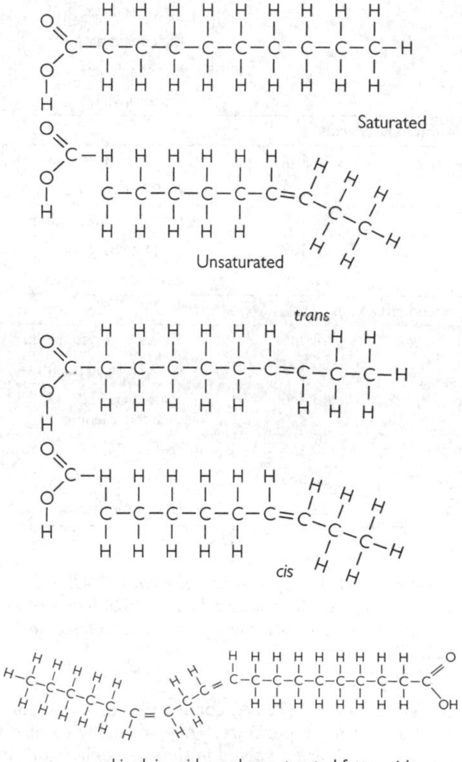

Linoleic acid, a polyunsaturated fatty acid.
Both double bonds are *cis*

Fig. 5.3 Structure of fatty acids.

Table 5.4 Nomenclature of fatty acids

Common name	Notational name	Systematic name
Saturated fatty acids		
Butyric	4:0	Tetranoic
Caproic	6:0	Hexanoic
Caprylic	8:0	Octanoic
Capric	10:0	Decanoic
Lauric	12:0	Dodecanoic
Myristic	14:0	Tetradecanoic
Palmitic	16:0	Hexadecanoic
Stearic	18:0	Octadecanoic
Arachidic	20:0	Eicosanoic
Behenic	22:0	Docosanic
Monounsaturated fatty acids		
Palmitoleic	16:1n7	cis-9 hexadecenoic
Oleic	18:1n9	cis-9 octadecenoic
Elaidic	18:1n9	trans-9 octadecenoic
Eicosenoic	20:1n9	cis-11 eicosaenoic
Erucic	22:1n9	cis-13 docosaenoic
Polyunsaturated fatty acids		
Linoleic	18:2n6	cis, cis-9,12 octadecadienoic
α-linolenic	18:3n3	cis-9,12,15 all octadecatrienoic
γ-linolenic	18.3n6	trans-5, cis-9, cis-12 octadecatrienoic
Arachidonic	20:4n6	cis-5, 8, 11, 14 eicosatetraenoic
EPA	20:5n3	Eicosapentaenoic
DHA	22:6n3	Docosahexaenoic

the most concentrated dietary sources of MUFA. MUFA are present in many foods, including meat fat and lard. Dietary MUFA do not raise plasma cholesterol, and lower LDL without a detrimental effect on high-density lipoproteins (HDL).

Polyunsaturated fatty acids

Polyunsaturated fatty acids (PUFA) contain two or more double bonds and are liquid at room temperature. They are easily oxidized in foods and in the body. PUFA are involved in the metabolism of cholesterol, are components of phospholipids in cell membranes, and are precursors of biologically active compounds such as prostaglandins, interleukins, and thromboxanes. Therefore, they have a vital role in the immune response, blood clotting, and inflammation. PUFA are derived from the

Table 5.5 Average intake for adults compared with DRVs for fat for adults (as a percentage of daily food energy intake) in the UK*

	Average intake (% daily food energy)		DRV (% food energy intake)
	Men	Women	
Total fat	34.4	35.0	35
Saturated fat	12.3	12.7	11
Trans fatty acids	1.1	0.9	<1.2

*Source for average daily intakes for adults, Public Health England & Food Standards Agency (2018). The National Diet and Nutrition Survey: Results from Years 7 and 8 (combined) of the Rolling Programme (2014/2015–2015/2016). Public Health England, London.

Table 5.6 Sources of total fat, saturated and trans fatty acids in the diet of adults in the UK (NDNS)*

Food	Total fat, %	Saturated fatty acids, %	Trans fatty acids, %
Meat, meat products, and meat dishes	22	23	28
Cereal and cereal products	21	21	18
Milk and milk products	12	21	30
Vegetables, potatoes	12	5	7
Fat spreads	8	8	9

*Source for average daily intakes for adults, Public Health England & Food Standards Agency (2018). The National Diet and Nutrition Survey: Results from Years 7 and 8 (combined) of the Rolling Programme (2014/2015–2015/2016). Public Health England, London.

essential fatty acids linoleic acid (n6 or ω6) and α-linoleic acid (n3 or ω3), and are ∴ divided into omega 3 (ω3) or omega 6 (ω6) groups of PUFA. Essential fatty acids (EFA), eicosapentaenoic acid (EPA), and docosahexaenoic acid (DHA) are important in neural development of the fetus and infant. PUFA occur as cis or trans forms depending on the way the hydrogen atoms are arranged. In cis formation the hydrogen atoms are bonded to either end of the double bond on the same side; whereas, in the trans form the hydrogen atoms are on opposite sides (Fig. 5.3). Most naturally occurring fats are in the cis form.

Omega (ω) 3 PUFA

ω3 PUFA (and parent essential fatty acid α-linoleic acid) are found in fish and fish oils and their health benefits are being more fully explored. The health benefits of ↑ consumption of oily fish include improved cardiovascular risk factors. The Western diet contains a high ratio of ω6:ω3 PUFA; a lower ratio is recommended. Research studies have shown benefits in cognitive function but epidemiological studies are required.

Trans fatty acids

Trans fatty acids are rare in naturally occurring fats. Some are made in the rumen of cows and sheep, and ∴ are found in lamb, beef, milk, and cheese. However, the most significant source of *trans* fatty acids in the diet is through hydrogenation of PUFA to produce more solid forms of vegetable oils for spreads, margarines, and some food products. *Trans* fatty acids have been associated with adverse effects on lipoprotein status by elevating LDL and depressing HDL, although further research is required. It is recommended that intake should not exceed 1.2% of total energy intake.

Essential fatty acids

Linoleic and α-linoleic acids are essential fatty acids. Other longer chain fatty acids such as arachidonic, EPA, and DHA are physiologically important but can be synthesized to a limited extent from linoleic and α-linoleic acids. These longer chain fatty acids are not essential fatty acids but their intake may become critical in fatty acid deficiency. EFA are most commonly found in plant and fish oils. Deficiency of linoleic acid has been demonstrated in children, although a deficiency of α-linoleic acid has not been seen in healthy people. This has → debate about the essentiality of α-linoleic acid. Deficiency is characterized by a scaly dermatitis. The recommended intake of linoleic acid is at least 11% of total energy and 0.2% for α-linoleic acid.

Sterols

Sterols are relatively simple molecules; the most common sterol is the wax-like cholesterol. Cholesterol and cholesterol ester (cholesterol to which a fatty acid is attached) are only found in animal foods. Phytosterols are found in plant foods. Cholesterol has structural roles in lipoproteins and membranes and is a precursor for bile acids, steroid hormones, and vitamin D. Dietary cholesterol has little influence on plasma levels as most circulating cholesterol is endogenous. Reduction of intake of saturated fat results in lower plasma cholesterol levels.

Lipid transport

Fat digestion and absorption are covered in ➋ Chapter 1, 'Digestion' p. 16. Lipids are not soluble in water, and ∴ complex with apolipoproteins to form water-miscible compounds. Approximately 2% of total plasma lipids are free fatty acids and are transported as compounds of albumin. The remainder of the lipids are carried in the blood as lipoproteins. Lipoproteins are identified by the apoliprotein that is present (apo A, apo B, apo C, apo D, apo E, apo F, apo H, and apo L). There are five classes of lipoproteins, which vary in density:

- Chylomicrons.
- Very low-density lipoproteins (VLDL).
- Low-density lipoproteins (LDL).
- Intermediate density lipoprotein (IDL).
- High-density lipoproteins (HDL).

In addition, lipoprotein (a) complex of LDL with apolipoproteins (A), may be formed; this particle is highly atherogenic.

Table 5.7 Dietary sources of cholesterol

Cholesterol content	Food
High	Liver, offal
	Eggs, mayonnaise
	Shellfish
	Fish roe
Medium	Meat fat
	Full fat milk and dairy produce, e.g. cream, cheese, butter
	Meat and fish products
	Manufactured meat products, e.g. pies
Low	Skinless poultry
	Skimmed milk and dairy products, e.g. cottage cheese, low fat yoghurt
Cholesterol free	Fruit (including avocados and olives) and vegetables
	Vegetable oils
	Cereals, pasta
	Rice
	Egg white
	Sugar

High and low levels of the lipoproteins have adverse effects on health. High levels of LDL are associated with ↑ health problems and LDL is colloquially known as 'bad cholesterol'. HDL is colloquially known as 'good cholesterol' (see Table 5.7 for dietary sources).

Chylomicrons

Chylomicrons mainly consist of triglycerides as they transport dietary lipids. Plasma levels rise after eating and are negligible in the fasting state. Chylomicrons leave the enterocytes of the small intestine and enter the lymphatic system before transferring to blood vessels. The triglycerides are hydrolysed by lipoprotein lipase, so releasing fatty acids that are used for energy or stored in adipose tissue. The life cycle of a chylomicron is 15–20 minutes and the liver clears the remnant from the blood. Fat-soluble vitamins reach the liver as part of the remnant.

Very low-density lipoproteins

VLDL are synthesized in the liver and are large particles that are rich in triglycerides. They deliver fatty acids to adipose tissue, muscles, and heart where lipoprotein lipase facilitates their release from triglycerides. The enzyme in the heart has a high affinity for triglyceride and, when triglyceride concentrations are low, they are preferentially released into heart tissue. Following release of triglycerides the remaining remnants

Table 5.8 Functions of plasma lipoproteins

Lipoprotein	Function
Chylomicrons	Transport dietary lipids to peripheral tissues and liver
VLDL	Transports lipids from liver to peripheral tissues
LDL	Transports cholesterol to peripheral tissues and liver
HDL	Removes cholesterol from peripheral tissues to the liver

are intermediate-density lipoproteins (IDL), which are the precursors of LDL (see Table 5.8).

IDL

IDL are formed from the degradation of VLDL; they are either degraded further to LDL or are rapidly cleared by the liver.

LDL

LDL contain mainly cholesterol and cholesterol ester as they are the end product of VLDL metabolism. They carry approximately 70% of plasma cholesterol and are taken up by the liver and other tissues.

HDL

The liver and intestine synthesize and secrete HDL. HDL is involved in the reverse transport of cholesterol from tissues, especially arteries and arterioles, to the liver or transfers it to other lipoproteins.

Carbohydrate

Carbohydrates are the most significant source of energy in the diet (see ➔ this Chapter 'Energy balance', p. 86). In developing countries up to 85% of energy in the diet is provided by carbohydrate; this figure is as low as 40% in some developed countries. The relationship between dietary carbohydrates and fat is usually reciprocal. Diets rich in fat will have low levels of carbohydrates and vice versa.

Structure and classification

The empirical formula for carbohydrates is $C_x(H_2O)_y$; glucose is the simplest carbohydrate ($C_6H_{12}O_6$ or $C_6(H_2O)_6$) (Fig. 5.4). Simple carbohydrates (monosaccharides) can combine to form disaccharides, e.g. sucrose ($C_{12}H_{22}O_{11}$) from two disaccharides, oligosaccharides, e.g. raffinose which is formed from three to nine monosaccharides, or polysaccharides, which form from ten or more saccharides, e.g. starches.

❶ It is important to recognize that the physical effects (food matrix) of a carbohydrate may influence its nutritional properties.

Carbohydrates that can be digested and absorbed in the small intestine and → ↑ in blood glucose levels are referred to as glycaemic carbohydrates (Table 5.9). Plant polysaccharides that cannot be digested (non-glycaemic) are referred to as fibre or non-starch polysaccharides (NSP). Sugar alcohols,

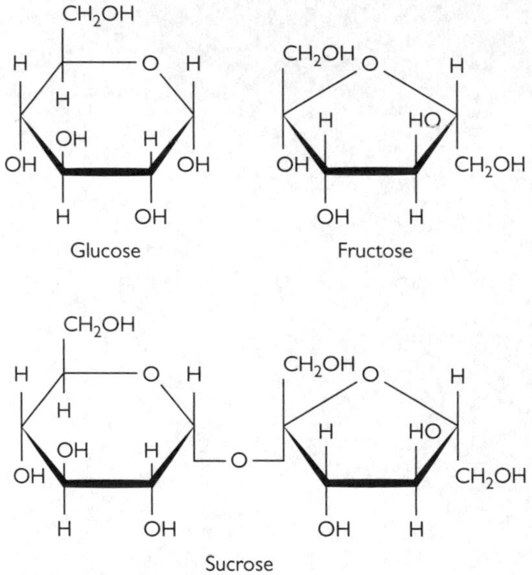

Fig. 5.4 Carbohydrate molecules.

Table 5.9 Classification of carbohydrates in the diet (FAO/WHO 1998)*

Glycaemic	Non-glycaemic
Monosaccharides	**Oligosaccharides**
Glucose	Raffinose, stachyose, verbascose
Fructose	Human milk oligosaccharides
Galactose	Fructo-oligosaccharides
	Inulin
Disaccharides	
Sucrose	
Lactose	
Maltose	
Trehalose	
Polysaccharides	**Non-starch polysaccharides**
Starch—amylopectin, amylose, modified food starches	Cellulose (insoluble)
	Hemicellulose (soluble and insoluble forms)
	β-glucans (mainly soluble)
	Fructans, e.g. inulin (not assayed by current methods)
	Gums (soluble)
	Mucilages (soluble)
	Algal polysaccharides (soluble)
Sugar alcohols†	
Sorbitol	
Xylitol	
Mannitol	

*Source: data from WHO/FAO (1998). *Carbohydrates in human nutrition*, FAO food and nutrition paper no.66. FAO, Rome.

†Sugar alcohols are only partially absorbed.

e.g. sorbitol, are also classified as carbohydrates, although their empirical formula is slightly different.

Sugars (mono- and disaccharides)

Monosaccharides include glucose, fructose, and galactose. The monosaccharide glucose is found in small amounts in fruit and vegetables, but is not abundant in natural foods. It is made from starch and used commercially. Fructose is found in honey, fruit, and vegetables and is manufactured from fructose-rich corn syrup for the food industry. Sucrose is the commonest disaccharide and is extracted from sugar beet or sugar cane. Table sugar is 99% sucrose and the major dietary source of disaccharides. Sucrose is hydrolysed into glucose and fructose. Lactose is found in milk and milk products. It is hydrolysed to glucose and galactose. Maltose is present in malted wheat and barley. Malt extract is used in brewing and in malted products.

Oligosaccharides

Raffinose, stachyose, and verbascose are oligosaccharides that are made of galactose, glucose, and fructose. They are found in legumes and seeds. Humans do not have the enzyme needed to digest them but they may be fermented in the colon. Fructo-oligosaccharides and inulin have been shown to stimulate growth of the potentially beneficial bifidobacteria in the colon.

Polyols

Sorbitol, inositol, and mannitol are polyols (sugar alcohols) that are only partially absorbed and ∴ provide less energy than the corresponding sugars. They have been used as sugar substitutes. Small amounts occur naturally, but significant amounts in the diet come only from manufactured foods. Large amounts can cause osmotic diarrhoea.

Starch

Starch is the main storage polysaccharide in plant cells and is found in large quantities in cereal grains, potatoes, and plantains. Starch is the largest source of carbohydrate in the diet. Starch consists of two glucose polysaccharides: amylose and amylopectin. The linkages between the glucose molecules are hydrolysed by the action of saliva and pancreatic amylases. Many factors affect the rate at which hydrolysation occurs so that some starches are readily digested while others pass undigested into the colon. This has resulted in the classification of starches (Table 5.10) into rapidly digestible starch (RDS), slowly digestible starch (SDS), and resistant starch (RS). Both RDS and SDS are digested in the small intestine while RS passes undigested into the colon where it is available for fermentation.

Fibre

Dietary fibre as defined by the Scientific Advisory Committee on Nutrition (SACN)[1] '...encompasses all carbohydrates that are naturally integrated components of foods and that are neither digested nor absorbed in the small intestine and have a degree of polymerisation of three or more monomeric units, plus lignin'. SACN also recommended that the term fibre be used rather than non-starch polysaccharide. Fibre can be classified as soluble (in water at pH 7.0) or insoluble, and it is this classification that categorizes the function of these polysaccharides. Insoluble fibre consists mainly of cellulose and some hemicelluloses. Insoluble fibre binds to water in the colon and swells. This stimulates peristalsis so ↑ transit time in the colon thereby reducing the risk of constipation and possibly reducing the risk of colon cancer. Soluble fibre blunts the response of blood glucose to ingestion. The reabsorption of bile acids is slowed by soluble fibre so ↑ cholesterol losses in faeces and reducing blood cholesterol levels. Diets high in fibre are associated with ↑ risk of bowel cancer, type 2 diabetes, and cardiovascular disease (CVD). Table 5.11 lists sources of soluble and insoluble fibre in the diet.

Intrinsic sugars

These are sugars that are present in intact cells, e.g. fructose in whole fruit and sugars in milk, i.e. lactose and galactose.

Free sugars

Sugars that are in a free or readily absorbable state, e.g. added sugars (usually sucrose), or released from disrupted cells, e.g. fructose in fruit puree or juice. Previously known as non-milk extrinsic sugars (NMES). Diets high in

1 SACN (2015) Carbohydrates and Health report and supporting documents are available at ℜ www.gov.uk/government/publications/sacn-carbohydrates-and-health-report

Table 5.10 Classification of starch

Class	Glycaemic response	Food source
Rapidly digestible starch	Large	Cooked starchy cereals, warm potatoes
Slowly digestible starch	Small	Muesli, oats, pasta, legumes
Resistant starch	None	Unripe bananas, whole grains, starchy foods e.g. potatoes that have been cooked and cooled

Table 5.11 Dietary sources of soluble and insoluble fibre in the diet

Soluble fibre	Insoluble fibre
Apples	Beans
Barley	Brown rice
Citrus fruits	Fruits with edible seeds
Guar gum	Lentils
Legumes	Maize
Oats	Oats
Pears	Pulses
Strawberries	Wheat bran
	Wholemeal breads
	Wholemeal cereals
	Wholemeal pasta
	Whole wheat flour
	Peas

free sugars are associated with ↑ risk of dental caries, obesity, and type 2 diabetes, and contribute to the development of dental caries.

Recommended intakes

Sugar and starch
SACN recommended that the average intake of free sugars should be <5% of the daily food energy. Starches, intrinsic sugars, and milk sugars should provide the balance of dietary energy not provided by alcohol, protein fat, and free sugar, which is on average 36.2% in the UK (Tables 5.12–5.14).

Fibre
It is recommended that the adult diet contain 30 g/day (see Table 5.15).

Glycaemic index

The glycaemic index (GI) is a method of ranking foods and carbohydrates based on their immediate effect on blood glucose levels. The FAO/WHO (1998)[2] define the GI as 'the incremental area under the blood glucose

2 WHO/FAO (1998). *Carbohydrates in human nutrition*, FAO food and nutrition paper no.66. FAO, Rome.

Table 5.12 Daily carbohydrate and NMES intake of adults (NDNS)*

	Men	Women
Total carbohydrate, g/day	249	199
% food energy	47.6	47.7
DRV, % food energy	50.0	50.0
Free sugars, g/day	64.3	50.0
% food energy	11.9	11.6
DRV, % food energy	<5	<5
AOAC Fibre, g/day	20.7	17.4
DRV, g/day	30	30

*Source for average daily intakes for adults, Public Health England & Food Standards Agency (2018). *The National Diet and Nutrition Survey*: Results from Years 7 and 8 (combined) of the Rolling Programme (2014/2015–2015/2016). Public Health England, London.

Table 5.13 Sources of carbohydrate in the diet (NDNS)*

Food group	% Daily intake
Cereals and cereal products including bread	46
Bread	18
Potatoes and savoury snacks	10
Non-alcoholic beverages	7
Alcoholic beverages	3

*Source for average daily intakes for adults, Public Health England & Food Standards Agency (2018). *The National Diet and Nutrition Survey*: Results from Years 7 and 8 (combined) of the Rolling Programme (2014/2015–2015/2016). Public Health England, London.

Table 5.14 Sources of free sugars in the diet (NDNS)*

Food group	Specific foods	% Intake
Sugar, preserves, and confectionery		25
	Table sugar, preserves, and sweet spreads	16
Cereals and cereal products		24
Non-alcoholic beverages		21
Alcoholic beverages		9

*Source for average daily intakes for adults, Public Health England & Food Standards Agency (2018). *The National Diet and Nutrition Survey*: Results from Years 7 and 8 (combined) of the Rolling Programme (2014/2015–2015/2016). Public Health England, London.

Table 5.15 Sources of fibre in the diet (NDNS)*

Food group	Selected food	% intake
Cereals and cereal products		38
	Breakfast cereals	6
Vegetables (excluding potatoes)		20
	Potatoes and savoury snacks	12
Fruits, seeds, and nuts		10

*Source for average daily intakes for adults, Public Health England & Food Standards Agency (2018). *The National Diet and Nutrition Survey*: Results from Years 7 and 8 (combined) of the Rolling Programme (2014/2015–2015/2016). Public Health England, London.

response curve of one 50 g carbohydrate portion of a test food expressed as a percentage of response to the same amount of carbohydrate from a standard food taken by the same subject'. The standard carbohydrate is glucose, which has a GI of 100. Foods with a high glycaemic index are readily absorbed and raised blood glucose quickly. Low glycaemic index foods are digested and absorbed slowly and raise blood glucose levels slowly. The GI can only be determined by *in vivo* measurement. Foods are categorized as:
- Low GI: ≤55.
- Medium GI: 56–69.
- High GI: ≥70.

Table 5.16 lists examples of GI of these categories. A list of foods that have been tested was published by Foster-Powell et al. (2002)[3]; more information is available at the Glycemic Index Foundation ℘http://www.gisymbol. com/. A list of commercially available products in the UK was published by Henry et al. (2005).[4] The way a food is processed, prepared, and cooked will affect the GI of the food. The overall GI of the diet is important rather than aiming to introduce a few low GI foods. The health benefits of a low GI diet include:
- improved diabetic glucose control (see ➜ Chapter 22, p. 493);
- improved risk factors for heart disease (see ➜ Chapter 23, p. 519);
- weight reduction (see ➜ Chapter 21, 'Obesity', p. 469);
- there is some evidence to suggest ↓ risk of some cancers.

3 Foster-Powell, K., et al.. (2002). International table of glycaemic index and glycaemic load. *Am. J. Clin. Nutr.* **76**, 5–56.

4 Henry, C.J.K., et al. (2005). Glycaemic index and glycaemic load values of commercially available products in the UK. *Br. J. Nutr.* **94**, 922–930.

Table 5.16 Examples of low, medium, and high GI foods

Low GI	Medium GI	High GI
Apples, oranges, pears, peaches	Honey	Glucose
Beans and lentils	Jam	White and wholemeal bread
Pasta (all types made from durum wheat)	Shredded Wheat	Brown rice, cooked
	Weetabix	White rice, cooked
Sweet potato, peeled and boiled	Ice cream	Cornflakes
	New potatoes, peeled and boiled	Baked potato
Sweet corn		Mashed potato
Porridge	White basmati rice, cooked	
Custard	Pitta bread	
Noodles	Couscous	
All Bran, Special K, Sultana Bran		

Glycaemic load (GL)

GL extends the concept of GI by considering the effect that GI and the amount of a carbohydrate have on postprandial blood glucose levels.

$$(GL = \text{Carbohydrate in food portion (g)} \times GI)/100$$

Blood glucose levels rise more rapidly after a high GL meal than a low GL meal. It is recommended that a healthy diet should have a low GI and a low GL.

Energy balance

To maintain body weight, energy intake must equal energy expenditure (EE). If EE exceeds energy intake, body weight will be lost. Weight loss is achieved by ↑ EE or ↓ energy intake. To gain weight the equation is reversed.

The SI unit of energy is the joule (J); the joule is a small amount of energy. Energy in food is usually expressed as kilojoules (kJ) and EE is expressed as kJ or megajoules (MJ). In practice many people continue to express energy in kilocalories (kcal). A calorie can be defined in several ways, although the most frequently used definition is:

- the energy required to raise the temperature of 1 g of water from 14.5°C to 15.5°C.

EE can be expressed per unit of time, e.g. kJ per minute or MJ/day or in Watts (W) (see Box 5.1 for a summary of units).

EE

Total energy expenditure (TEE) has the following components:
basal metabolic rate (BMR), 50–75%;
physical activity (PA), 20–40%;
dietary induced thermogenesis (DIT), 10%.

Growth, pregnancy, lactation, injury, and fever are energy-requiring processes that will ↑ EE and → ↑ energy intake.

BMR

BMR is the amount of energy expended by the body to maintain normal physiological functions. It remains constant throughout the day, under normal conditions, and constitutes 50–75% of TEE; it is the largest component of TEE.

BMR is affected by many factors:

- Body weight: BMR ↑ or ↓ with ↑ or ↓ body weight.
- Body composition: Fat mass is relatively metabolically inactive and expends less energy gram for gram than fat free mass (FFM). Men have a higher FFM to fat ratio than women and ∴ have a higher BMR than women of the same age and weight.
- Age: children have a higher BMR per kg than adults as a result of the energy requirement of growth. As adults age, metabolism slows and FFM ↓ ∴ ↓ BMR.

Box 5.1 Units used in energy balance

- 1000 joules = 1kJ
- 1000 kJ = 1MJ
- 1 kcal = 4.184 kJ*
- 1 kJ = 0.239 kcal
- 1 W = 1 joule per second
- 0.06 W = 1 kJ per min
- 86.4 W = kJ per 24 h

*The Royal Society (London) recommended conversion factor.

- Gender: men generally have a higher BMR because of differences in body weight and body composition. The BMR of a 65 kg man will be approximately 1 MJ/day higher than a weight- and age-matched woman.
- Genetic factors: BMR can vary by up to 10% between subjects of the same age, sex, and body weight. Recent research has shown that there are ethnic differences in BMR.
- Physiological changes: BMR ↑ during pregnancy and lactation.
- Disease and trauma: fever, sepsis, infection, and surgical and physical trauma ↑ BMR.
- Nutritional status: the body adapts to changes in energy intake by altering body weight and/or body composition. An individual who is consuming more energy than is required will ↑ weight and ↑ BMR so making further weight gain impossible unless there is further intake ↑ or ↓ PA.
- Environment: the energy cost of maintaining body temperature is influenced by ambient temperature, wind speed, radiant temperature of the surrounding, and clothing.
- Hormonal status: several hormonal factors influence BMR, especially thyroid function. BMR is ↑ in hyperthyroidism and ↓ in hypothyroidism. There are small cyclical changes during the menstrual cycle of some women, with a rise after ovulation.
- Pharmacological effects: therapeutic drugs and substances such as caffeine and capsaicin can modulate BMR.
- Psychological effects: anxiety will ↑ EE in the short term. Longer term effects of stress and anxiety have not been established.

Measurement of BMR
- BMR must be measured under standard conditions.
- Post-absorptive state: at least 12 hours after last food or drink. This should also include other stimulants such as caffeine or smoking.
- Thermoneutral environment: 20–25°C; comfortably warm.
- Supine: sitting up will ↑ EE slightly.
- Awake but in a state of complete physical and mental relaxation.
- Heavy PA on the day before the measurement may influence the BMR and should be avoided.

In practice BMR is usually measured first thing in the morning before eating and drinking or undertaking PA. If any of the conditions are not met, the measurement is termed resting metabolic rate (RMR). RMR is slightly higher than BMR while sleeping metabolic rate is 5–10% lower than BMR.

Measurements of EE
EE can be measured directly (the measurement of heat production), in-directly (the measurement of O_2 consumption), or by non-calorimetric methods, e.g. heart rate (HR) monitoring. Methods have also been developed that are indirect measures of gaseous exchange (O_2 consumption), i.e. doubly labelled water technique.

Direct calorimetry
Direct calorimetry is the measurement of heat produced by the body. Subjects are placed in an insulated chamber and heat loss is measured over

a period of at least 24 hours. Direct calorimetry is difficult in practice as the chamber must be capable of detecting all heat generated within the chamber and other sources of heat must be eliminated or accounted for. Direct calorimeters are very precise instruments but are expensive and difficult to build and maintain and few are available; $\therefore$ this method is not frequently used.

Indirect calorimetry

Indirect calorimetry is based on the principle that food is oxidized in the body to produce energy and that by measuring oxygen consumption it is possible to calculate EE. The following equation demonstrates the amount of energy produced by the oxidation of 1 mole of glucose:

$$C_6H_{12}O_6 \quad + \quad 6O_2 \quad \rightarrow \quad 6CO_2 \quad + \quad 6H_2O \quad + \quad heat$$

$$(180\ g) \quad (6 \times 22.41L) \quad (6 \times 22.31L) \quad (6 \times 18g) \quad (2.78MJ)$$

The energy produced by the oxidation of 1 g glucose is $\therefore$ 15.4 kJ (2780/180) and 1L of oxygen is equivalent to the production of 20.7 kJ (2780/(6×22.4)). Therefore, if the amount of oxygen used is known, it is possible to calculate the amount of energy or heat produced. Similar calculations can be made for protein, fat, and alcohol.

Respiratory quotient (RQ) is the ratio of CO_2 produced to O_2 used. From the RQ it is possible to estimate the macronutrient composition of the diet (see Table 5.17). The energy content of a mixed diet is approximately 35% fat, 50% carbohydrate, and $\therefore$ has an RQ of 0.87. To improve the accuracy of the calculations, an estimate of nitrogen excretion is used. Substitution into a formula yields EE. The formulae most frequently used are those of Weir (1949),[5] or Elia and Livesey (1992)[6] despite limitations (see Box 5.2).

Indirect calorimetry equipment

A variety of apparatuses are available to measure oxygen consumption. The simplest method is the Douglas bag where expired air is collected in a strong non-permeable bag. The volume of expired air over a set period is measured using a dry gas meter and the expired gases are analysed and compared to the ambient air. From this, it is possible to calculate O_2 consumption and CO_2 production rates and $\therefore$ calculate EE. In clinical situations, a ventilated hood, canopy, or tent, e.g. Deltatrac, Gem, Sensormedics, is used which measures gaseous exchange continuously and has a processor to calculate EE. Other systems are available that can be used during exercise. Respiration chambers are used by some research units; these are small chambers in which a subject stays for several hours or days and gaseous exchange is measured continuously. These chambers are expensive to build and use, but give precise measurements.

5 Weir, J.B. (1949). New methods for calculating metabolic rate with special reference to protein metabolism. *J. Physiol. (Lond.)* **109**, 1–9.

6 Elia, M., Livesey, G. (1992). Energy expenditure and fuel selections in biological systems: the theory and practice of calculations based on indirect calorimetry and tracer methods. In *Metabolic Control of Eating, Energy Expenditure and the Bioenergetics of Obesity* (ed. A.P. Simonopoulos), pp. 68–131. Karger, Basel.

Table 5.17 Energy values for oxidation of nutrients*

Nutrient	O_2 consumption, L/g	CO_2 production, L/g[†]	RQ	Energy released, kJ/g	Energy released, kJ/L O_2
Starch	0.829	0.832	0.994	17.49	21.10
Glucose	0.746	0.742	0.995	15.44	20.70
Fat	1.975	1.402	0.710	39.12	19.81
Protein	0.962	0.775	0.806	18.52	19.25
Alcohol	1.429	0.966	0.663	29.75	20.40

*Reproduced from Garrow, J.S., James, W.P.T., Ralph, A. (1999). *Human Nutrition and Dietetics*, Table 3.4, p. 28. With permission from Elsevier.

[†]CO_2 is not an ideal gas, 1 mole at STP occupies 22.26 L not 22.4 L.

Box 5.2 Weir, and Elia and Livesey formulae

Weir formula

$$EE\ (kJ) = 16.489\ VO_2\ (L) + 4.628\ VCO_2\ (L) - 9.079\ N\ (g)$$

If nitrogen cannot be measured, protein is assumed to be 15% of the energy of the diet and the formula becomes:

$$EE\ (kJ) = 16.318\ VO_2\ (L) + 4.602\ VCO_2\ (L)$$

Elia and Livesey formula

$$EE\ (kcal/24\ h) = \left((15.913\ VO_2\ (L) + 5.207\ VCO_2\ (L))\right.$$
$$\left. \times\ 1.44 - 4.464\ N\ (g)\right) \times 0.239$$

where VO_2 = O_2 consumed, VCO_2 = CO_2 produced, and N = urinary nitrogen excretion

Non-calorimetric methods
- HR is related to EE and this relationship has been used to estimate EE, although the results are not very reliable, particularly at low activity levels.
- Accelerometers are often used to measure PA; they are small computer motion analysers that measure duration, frequency, and intensity of PA. They are used in conjunction with log books that enable the full analysis of activities.

Doubly labelled water
Data are collected on free-living subjects over a period of 10–20 days. This does not require extensive equipment for the collection of gases and ∴ does not restrict the subject. Subjects are given an oral dose of water that has known amounts of the stable isotopes deuterium (^2H) and ^{18}O. These

isotopes mix with the body's water and, as energy is used, CO_2 and H_2O are produced. As ^{18}O is in both H_2O and CO_2 it is lost more rapidly than ^2H, which is only lost in H_2O. The difference between the rate of loss of ^2H and ^{18}O reflects the rate at which CO_2 is produced. From this, it is possible to calculate EE. This method requires collection of body fluid, either blood, urine, or saliva, before the test period and samples at specified times during the study. It is possible to use this method in babies, hospital patients, field work, and other groups in whom it is difficult to measure EE by other methods. Specialist equipment is required for the analysis of blood and urine samples and, because of a world shortage of ^{18}O, this method is expensive.

Estimation of energy requirements

Energy requirements are estimated by using prediction equations such as the Henry equations (2005), see Appendix 4, p. 871. Table 5.18 shows the Henry equations with additional data on men aged 60–70 years (DH 1991).[7] Regression analysis of measured BMR against gender, age, and weight was used to generate the equations. Numerous equations are available; ideally they should be population-specific. They are developed for use in healthy groups; in individuals the accuracy may be ±10–20%. If equations are extended for use in illness, the accuracy may be reduced by 50%.

Traditionally, TEE is calculated using a physical activity level (PAL) that has been derived from experimental studies, often using doubly labelled water; this is known as the factorial method.

For example, a sedentary male worker, aged 40 years, weight 90 kg, with an inactive lifestyle would have PAL of 1.4 (Table 5.19); ∴ his TEE would be

BMR from prediction equations (7.808 MJ) x 1.4 = 10.93 MJ.

Table 5.18 Formulae for the estimation of BMR*

	Age, years	BMR prediction equation, MJ/d†
Males	<3	0.255 (w) −0.141
	3–10	0.0937 (w) +2.15
	10–18	0.0769 (w) +2.43
	18–30	0.0669 (w) +2.28
	30–60	0.0592 (w) +2.48
	**>60	0.0563 (w) +2.15
Females	<3	0.246 (w) −0.0965
	3–10	0.0842 (w) +2.12
	10–18	0.0465 (w) +3.18
	18–30	0.0546 (w) +2.33
	30–60	0.0407 (w) +2.90
	**>60	0.0424 (w) +2.38

*Henry, C.J. (2005) Basal metabolic rate studies in humans: measurement and development of new equations. *Public Health Nutr.* **8**, 1133–1152.

** Department of Health (1991). Dietary reference values for food and nutrients for the United Kingdom. HMSO, London.

†w Weight in kg.

7 Department of Health (1991). Dietary reference values for food and nutrients for the United Kingdom. HMSO, London.

Table 5.19 Calculated PAL values for light, moderate, and heavy activity (occupational and non-occupational)*

Non-occupational activity level	Occupational activity level					
	Light		Moderate		Heavy	
	M	F	M	F	M	F
Sedentary	1.4	1.4	1.6	1.5	1.7	1.5
Moderately active	1.5	1.5	1.7	1.6	1.8	1.6
Very active	1.6	1.6	1.8	1.7	1.9	1.7

*Source: data from Department of Health (1991). *Dietary reference values for food and nutrients for the United Kingdom*. HMSO, London.

If an activity diary has been kept, it is possible to calculate TEE more accurately by partitioning time during the day spent on specific activities, and using physical activity ratios (PAR; see ➲ Appendix 4, p. 871) it is possible to calculate a directly related PAL value for the day.

$$TEE = BMR \times [(PAR \times time\ for\ activity\ A) +$$

$$(PAR \times time\ for\ activity\ B) + \&\& ...]$$

SACN does not recommend this approach, but recognizes that currently no viable alternative is available

Energy intake
Energy is provided by the macronutrients and alcohol.
- Protein provides 4 kcal (17 kJ)/g.
- Carbohydrate provides 3.75 kcal (16 kJ)/g.
- Fat provides 9 kcal (37 kJ)/g.
- Alcohol provides 7 kcal (29 kJ)/g.

Polyols (e.g. sorbitol) and volatile fatty acids (produced by gut bacteria by fermentation of some fibre components) contribute small, negligible amounts of energy.

Energy consumption
The average daily energy intakes for adults in UK are 8.79 MJ (2100 kcal) for men and 6.87 MJ (1641 kcal) for women; these intakes are below estimated average requirements (EARs). The sources of energy are shown in Fig. 5.5.

❶ In the UK adults are not energy-deficient, as demonstrated by the rising prevalence of obesity. The low percentages of EARs may be a result of under-reporting. The level of PA is also important.

Energy requirements
The SACN recommendations are shown in Table 5.20 for babies and children aged up to 10 years. These are given as EARs. EARs for men and women grouped for age, height and weight at a BMI of 22.5 kg/m^2, and assuming a PAL of 1.63 are shown in Table 5.21.

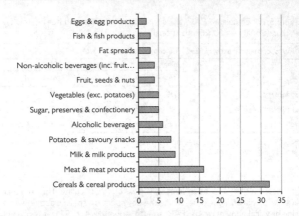

Fig. 5.5 Percentage contribution of food types to average daily total energy intake of UK adults. Source: data from Public Health England & Food Standards Agency (2014). *The National Diet and Nutrition Survey*: Results from Years 1, 2, 3 and 4 (combined) of the Rolling Programme (2008/2009 2011/2012). Public Health England, London.

Table 5.20 EARs for energy of children aged 0–18 years*

Age	EAR MJ/d (kcal/day)	
	Boys	Girls
0–3 months	2.6	2.4
4–6 months	2.7	2.5
7–9 months	2.9	2.7
10–12 months	3.2	3.0
1–3 years	4.1	3.8
4–6 years	6.2	5.8
7–10 years	7.6	7.1
11–14 years	9.9	9.1
15–18 years	12.6	10.2

*Source: data for EARs from SACN (2011). *Dietary reference values for energy*. TSO, London.

PA assessment

PA is the most variable component of TEE and most amenable to change. PA is a complex behaviour that includes any bodily movement produced by the contraction of skeletal muscles resulting in EE. It incorporates all daily activities and is not synonymous with exercise, which is a subcategory and tends to be structured leisure-time activity. Sedentary behaviour is

Table 5.21 EARs according to height and weight at BMI = 22.5 kg/m²
and assuming a PAL of 1.63*

	Height, cm	Weight, kg, BMI = 22.5 kg/m²	EAR, MJ/d
Males			
19–24	178	71.5	11.6
25–34	178	71.0	11.5
35–44	176	69.7	11.0
45–54	175	68.8	10.8
55–64	174	68.3	10.8
65–74	173	67.0	9.8
75+	170	65.1	9.6
Females			
19–24	163	29.9	9.1
25–34	163	59.7	9.1
35–44	163	59.9	8.8
45–54	162	59.0	8.8
55–64	161	58.0	8.7
65–74	159	57.2	8.0
75+	155	54.3	7.7

*Source: data from SACN (2011). *Dietary reference values for energy*. TSO, London.

independent from PA and should be considered as a separate component,
but can often be measured with the same instrument as PA. The choice
of measuring instrument is a balance between accuracy, reliability, detail,
and practical considerations. The timing of the assessment is important and
must include consideration of day-to-day variability in PA patterns, (e.g.
weekday vs. weekend day), and seasons and special occasions that could
influence habitual PA. The length of measurement period is dependent on
these factors and the aim of the assessment. If the aim is to assess habitual
PA, a longer measurement period is required and repeated measurement
periods (e.g. different times of year) should be considered (see Table 5.22).

PA assessment in children
There are additional challenges in assessing PA in children as their activity patterns are more varied and movement is more sporadic and
multi-dimensional than in adults and they have cognitive limitations in recalling their activity. With some of the objective instruments for PA assessment, changes in body size and energy efficiencies with growth also
need to be considered. Instruments can broadly be divided into subjective
and objective, and can be used in combination to provide complementary
measurements.

Table 5.22 Definitions in PA assessment

Measurement	Description
Intensity	Intensity of activity usually defined in terms of metabolic equivalents (MET), such as light (1.1–2.9 MET) moderate (3.0–5.9 MET), and vigorous (6.0+ MET) intensity*
Frequency	Frequency of time spent in specific activities or intensity levels over a set period of time
Duration	Time spent in specific activities or intensity levels including total time per day, proportion of waking hours, or length of bout of activity
Patterning	Occurrence of specific activities or intensity levels over set period of time, e.g. time of day or day of week
Types of activity	Specific activities of interest, e.g. walking or cycling
Domains of activity	Context of activities, e.g. home, work, leisure-time, or mode of transport
Sedentary behaviour	Time spent in activities involving being sedentary, e.g. watching television, reading, or on computer

*METS are used when describing PA intensity multiples of an individual's resting oxygen uptake, defined as the rate of oxygen (O_2) consumption of 3.5 mL of O_2/min/kg body weight in adults.

Subjective instruments
Diaries

PA recalls
Activity recalls are analogous to 24-hour diet recalls, but may cover a longer time period (1 day—1 month). Activities tend to be of moderate-vigorous intensity that are relatively easy to recall. Repeated recalls at intervals across a time period can be used to capture information on patterning or estimate habitual PA.

Questionnaires
Questionnaires are widely used, and there are many questionnaires used in different populations and age groups. Questionnaires vary from a few generic questions to detailed lists of questions on different activities. To assess total PA, questionnaires should include all domains and all common activities undertaken in the population of interest, taking into account culture-specific activities. It is important that a questionnaire is designed and validated against a criterion measure for use in the population group in which PA is being assessed (see Box 5.3).

Objective instruments
Pedometers
Pedometers are motion sensors worn on the hip or waist that measure locomotor activity as steps taken, walking or running. There is a large variation in the accuracy and reliability of different pedometer models. This, in part, reflects the different mechanics of the models and also variations in stride length. Some models allow a setting of the individual's walking stride length to improve estimation of the distance covered and steps taken (see Box 5.4).

Box 5.3 Good design features of questionnaires
- Good for use in large groups
- Assess patterns, frequency, duration, and type of PA
- Capture context of PA
- Measures of sedentary behaviour possible
- Limited in ability to assess EE
- Difficult for individual to quantify some activities
- Subject to recall bias or social desirability in reported activities
- Limited applicability in children due to cognitive stage
- Can require considerable data processing

Box 5.4 Pedometers
- A simple and inexpensive measure of walking activity
- Small and non-invasive for people to wear
- Only assesses locomotor activities, not activities of upper body, cycling, or water activities
- Unable to assess patterns, frequency, duration of activity, types of PA, or sedentary behaviour
- Measurement capability varies with body placement, e.g. hip or waist
- Limited application in groups of children as pedometer steps influenced by body size
- Limited applicability in those with restricted mobility
- Data not stored in memory of device
- Best for ranking individuals or assessing change in locomotor activities, e.g. to monitor adherence to a walking intervention
- Unable to estimate EE

Accelerometers

Accelerometers detect and record acceleration resulting from normal bodily movement (Box 5.5). Models can measure acceleration in one direction (usually vertical), two and three directions (triaxial; vertical, medio-lateral, and anterior-posterior), and are commonly expressed as a movement count value. The sampling period of current models vary from recording movement every second to every 60 seconds. The length of the measurement period depends on the sampling period and memory capacity of the accelerometer, but generally ranges from several days to weeks. Most models store the movement counts for downloading at the end of the measurement period into a PC via an interface. This allows the activity count data to be used to measure patterns, frequency, and duration of PA; estimate time spent in different intensities of activity with the use of appropriate cut points; and measure time spent sleeping and sleep quality.

HR monitors

HR provides an indirect measure of PA, as it measures the individual's physiological response to PA. Minute-by-minute HR data are recorded from a chest strap and can then be downloaded at the end of the measurement period into a PC via an interface for processing (see Box 5.6).

Box 5.5   Accelerometers

- Most commonly used objective instrument
- Small and non-invasive for people to wear
- Often used in children
- Limited applicability in those with restricted mobility
- Unable to assess types of PA
- Measurement capability varies with body placement, e.g. hip, ankle, or wrist, as does not capture all activity across the body, e.g. if worn on hip, upper body activity is not captured
- Most models are currently not waterproof so limited capability to measure water-based activities
- Time is required for processing output data. Many models have software provided for these analyses
- Some variation in the accuracy and reliability of different accelerometer models
- Estimation equations for EE have been developed for different accelerometer models and populations, but these have limited accuracy in estimating EE on an individual basis

Box 5.6   Heart monitors

- Can assess whole range of movements and activities (including water activities)
- Can measure patterns, frequency, and duration of PA
- Unable to assess types of PA or sedentary behaviour
- Can estimate time spent in different intensities of activity with the use of appropriate cut points
- At low levels of PA, HR is a less reliable measure of PA
- Can estimate EE and patterning of expenditure with an individualized calibration of the O_2/HR relationship
- HR responses reflect not only PA but are also affected by hydration, prandial status, body position, ambient temp., humidity, emotion stress, smoking, caffeine intake, and certain drugs e.g. β-blockers
- Relationship between individuals' HR and PA or EE can alter with changes in body weight, body composition, physical fitness, ageing, and illness
- Downloaded data require considerable processing to estimate PA or PA EE

Combined monitors

Instruments are increasingly becoming available that combine more than one objective method to overcome some of the limitations of the individual methods (e.g. combining HR monitoring with accelerometry). Some of these monitors can estimate EE, but may have limited accuracy in estimating on an individual basis.

Doubly labelled water

Doubly labelled water does not give a direct measure of PA EE. However, when combined with measured or estimated BMR, reasonable estimates of PA EE can be derived by subtraction of BMR and DIT, averaged over the period of isotope sampling (commonly 7–10 days; see Box 5.7). See previous section in this ➲ chapter for methodology (p. 87).

Box 5.7 Doubly labelled water
- Provides no measure of day-to-day PA EE
- Unable to assess patterns, frequency, duration, or types of PA or sedentary behaviour
- Most applicable in healthy groups, limitations in application in some illnesses
- Can be used in children and infants
- Application constrained by expense of method and specialist processing

Micronutrients

Micronutrients: introduction 100

Vitamins
Vitamins: introduction *101*
Vitamin A (retinol) and carotenoids *102*
Vitamin E *106*
Vitamin D (calciferols) *108*
Vitamin K *112*
Vitamin C (ascorbic acid) *114*
Riboflavin (vitamin B$_2$) *116*
Niacin (nicotinamide, nicotinic acid, vitamin B$_3$) *118*
Thiamin (vitamin B$_1$) *122*
Folate (folic acid) *126*
Vitamin B$_6$ *130*
Cobalamin B$_{12}$ *134*
Biotin (vitamin B$_7$) *136*
Pantothenic acid (vitamin B$_5$) *138*

Minerals and trace elements
Minerals and trace elements: introduction *140*
Calcium *142*
Phosphorus *146*
Iron *148*
Zinc *154*
Copper *156*
Iodine *160*
Selenium *162*
Magnesium *164*
Manganese *166*
Molybdenum *168*
Chromium *170*
Fluoride *172*

Micronutrients: introduction

The micronutrients are, by definition, required in small amounts. Many are essential as they cannot be made in the human body. They include vitamins, minerals, and trace elements.

Vitamins: introduction

Vitamins are a group of organic compounds that have a variety of functions in the body and that are chemically different from each other. To show that a compound is a vitamin it is necessary to show a deficiency in experimental subjects and that restoring the missing compound can reverse the effects of this deficiency. The name 'vitamin' is derived from 'vital amine'; as the name suggests, these essential compounds were initially thought to be amines. Vitamins can be divided into fat-soluble and water-soluble groups; vitamins A, E, D, and K are fat-soluble and may be stored in the body, the remainder being water-soluble and the body has limited or no stores.

Vitamin A (retinol) and carotenoids

Vitamin A is the term for the biologically active compound retinol and its provitamin (precursor) carotenoids. The most common provitamin A carotenoids are β-carotene, α-carotene, γ-carotene, and β-cryptoxanthin. Only 50 of approximately 600 naturally occurring carotenoids are converted into vitamin A. Carotenoids with no vitamin A activity include zeaxanthin, the pigment in sweet corn, and lycopene, the red pigment in tomatoes. The vitamin A activity of β-carotene is calculated as 6 μg being equivalent to 1 μg of retinol. Other carotenoids are considered to have lower activity; 12 μg is considered to be equivalent to 1 μg of retinol.

Function

- Vitamin A is essential for the production of rhodopsin in the rods of the retina. Exposure to light results in a series of changes in the configuration of rhodopsin, which leads to the adaptation of vision in the dark.
- Growth.
- Cell differentiation.
- Embryogenesis.
- Immune response.

Measurement

Biochemical assessment of vitamin A is controversial. Measurement of retinol concentration in serum or plasma is a useful and common measure of vitamin A status. Deficiency is indicated by values below 10 μg/dL (0.3 μmol/L) and values below 20 μg/dL (0.7 μmol/L) are marginal.

Deficiency

Deficiency of vitamin A is rare in the UK, but is common in Latin America, Africa, and Asia, especially amongst children.

- Eye changes: night blindness presents when vitamin A status is marginal and, with prolonged or severe deficiency, changes to the cornea and conjunctiva occur. These eye changes are known collectively as xerophthalmia, and consist of conjunctival xerosis, Bitot's spots, corneal xerosis, corneal ulceration, and corneal necrosis and scars.
- Epithelial tissues: skin keratinization occurs in vitamin A deficiency. Horny plugs block the sebaceous glands leading to follicular hyperkeratosis.
- Immunity: vitamin A deficiency results in ↑ susceptibility to infectious diseases, such as diarrhoea and respiratory infections.

A deficiency of vitamin A can contribute to nutritional deficiency anaemia.

Requirement and intake

See Tables 6.1 and 6.2, and Box 6.1. Fat is necessary for absorption of vitamin A; as retinol is found in foods of animal origin, some fat is usually consumed with it. Vitamin A absorption is impaired by mineral oils, neomycin, colestyramine, and commercial fat replacers, e.g. olestra. A low vitamin A intake is associated with lower socio-economic class and low consumption of cereals, milk, eggs, and vegetables.

Table 6.1 RNIs for all ages and average daily intakes for adult men and women for vitamin A provided by food (µg retinol equivalent/day)*

Age, years	RNI
0–1	350
1–6	400
7–10	500
11–14	600
Males 15+	700
Females 15+	600
Pregnancy	+100
Lactation	+350
	Mean daily intake for UK adults
Men	921
Women	825

*Source: for RNIs, Department of Health (1991). *Dietary reference values for food and nutrients for the United Kingdom*. HMSO. Source: for average daily intake of adults Public Health England & Food Standards Agency (2018). *The National Diet and Nutrition Survey: Results from Years 7 and 8 (combined) of the Rolling Programme (2014/2015–2015/2016)*. Public Health England, London.

Table 6.2 Contribution of foods to vitamin A intake*

Food group	% Daily intake
Meat and meat products	16
Liver and liver products	3
Vegetables and potatoes	28
Milk and milk products	15
Fat spreads	9

*Source: data from Public Health England & Food Standards Agency (2018). *The National Diet and Nutrition Survey: Results from Years 7 and 8 (combined) of the Rolling Programme (2014/2015–2015/2016)*. Public Health England, London.

Toxicity

The early reports of vitamin A toxicity are from polar explorers who ate the polar bears' livers, which are particularly rich in vitamin A. Acute toxicity occurs when more than 200 mg (0.7 mmol) is consumed by adults or more than 100 mg in children. The acute symptoms of vitamin A toxicity include vomiting, abdominal pain, anorexia, blurred vision, headache, and irritability. Chronic toxicity can occur when 10 mg is consumed over periods of a month or more. Symptoms include headache, muscle and bone pain, ataxia, skin disorders, alopecia, liver toxicity, and hyperlipidaemia. Not all the chronic symptoms are reversible. Vitamin A is teratogenic and

---

Box 6.1 Good food sources of vitamin A

Most concentrated sources of retinol in the diet
- Liver and liver products
- Kidney and offal
- Oily fish and fish liver oils
- Eggs

Most concentrated sources of β-carotene in the diet
- Carrots
- Red peppers
- Spinach
- Broccoli
- Tomatoes
- Sweet potatoes

---

pregnancy intakes should not exceed 3 mg/d. There is no risk of toxicity from carotenoids in foods, although large intakes can lead to yellow discoloration of the skin.

❶ Vitamin A supplements should not be taken during pregnancy (see ⮕ Chapter 2, 'Dietary reference values and food-based dietary guidelines', p. 21, and ⮕ Chapter 12, 'Diet before and during pregnancy', p. 237).

Consumption of liver is not recommended during pregnancy.

Vitamin E

Eight naturally occurring forms of vitamin E are synthesized in plants: four tocopherols (alpha, α-; beta, β-; delta, δ-; and gamma, γ-) and four tocotrienols (α, β, δ, and γ). α-tocopherol has the highest biological activity and is used as the standard against which the activity of other forms is measured. Synthetic vitamin E is a mixture of isomers and has biological activities ranging from 20% to 80%.

Function

- Antioxidant: vitamin E is a powerful antioxidant and protects cell membranes and lipoproteins from damage by free radicals.
- Maintenance of cell membrane integrity.
- Regulation of prostaglandin synthesis.
- DNA synthesis.

Measurement

Plasma concentration is the simplest measure and a direct indicator of status. Acceptable levels of intake are indicated by values of 5–20 μg/mL in adults and children aged 12 years and over, and 3–15 μg/mL for younger children.

Deficiency

Experimental, symptomatic vitamin E deficiency has not been induced in humans. Evidence for the essentiality of vitamin E in humans is provided by a genetically inherited disease familial isolated vitamin E (FIVE) deficiency. Sufferers develop reduced tendon reflexes by 3–4 years of age. By early adolescence they display symptoms of the nervous system including loss of touch and pain sensation, unsteady gait, loss of co-ordination, and impaired eye movement. In conditions that → chronic or severe fat malabsorption, cystic fibrosis, cholestatic liver disease, and abetalipoproteinaemia, similar symptoms may develop (especially in children) that can be corrected by vitamin E supplementation (5–25 IU/day).

Requirement and intake

See Tables 6.3 and 6.4, and Box 6.2. Vitamin E requirements are influenced by the amount of polyunsaturated fatty acids (PUFA); it is estimated that 0.4 mg α-tocopherol is required per gram dietary intake of PUFA. The average adult diet in the UK contains 7% energy from PUFA, which would mean a vitamin E requirement of 6 mg for women and 8 mg for men. Milk formulas should not be <0.3 mg α-tocopherol equivalents/100 mL reconstituted feed and not <0.4 mg α-tocopherol equivalents/g PUFA.

Toxicity

Vitamin E has low toxicity, but at very high doses it acts as an antagonist to vitamins A, D, and K. Symptoms of toxicity include headache, nausea, muscle weakness, double vision, and creatinuria, and gastrointestinal (GI) disturbances have been reported at intakes greater than 900 mg/kg.

Table 6.3 Average daily intakes of vitamin E (mg) for adult men and women provided by food (α-tocopherol equivalents)*

	Average daily intake UK
Men	9.9
Women	8.1

* Source: Public Health England & Food Standards Agency (2014). *The National Diet and Nutrition Survey*: Results from Years 1, 2, 3 and 4 (combined) of the Rolling Programme (2008/2009 – 2011/2012). Public Health England, London.

Table 6.4 Contribution of foods to vitamin E intake*

Food	% Daily intake
Fat spreads	11
PUFA spread	5
Cereals and cereal products	19
Vegetables (excluding potatoes)	15
Potatoes and savoury snacks	11
Meat and meat products	13

*Source: data from Public Health England & Food Standards Agency (2014). *The National Diet and Nutrition Survey*: Results from Years 1, 2, 3 and 4 (combined) of the Rolling Programme (2008/2009–2011/2012). Public Health England, London.

Box 6.2 Good food sources of vitamin E
- Wheat germ oil
- Almonds
- Sunflower seeds and oil
- Safflower oil
- Hazelnuts
- Peanuts and peanut butter
- Corn oil

Vitamin D (calciferols)

The term vitamin D refers to two molecules, ergocalciferol (D_2) and chole-calciferol (D_3). Cholecalciferol is the most effective form of vitamin D and is manufactured in the skin by the action of ultraviolet radiation on 7-dehydrocholesterol. Dietary ergocalciferol and cholecalciferol are biologically inactive and are activated to 25-hydroxyvitamin D in the liver (this has a limited amount of biological activity). Further conversion in the kidney results in the production of the more active form 1,25-dihydroxyvitamin D (calcitriol).

Function

- 1,25-dihydroxyvitamin D maintains plasma Ca by controlling Ca absorption and excretion. Vitamin D and its metabolites are also involved in bone mineralization.
- Children with vitamin D deficiency (rickets) often have impaired immune function that is corrected by the administration of vitamin D.
- It has recently been postulated that vitamin D may inhibit cell proliferation in some forms of cancer.
- SACN have recently reviewed the evidence for the role of vitamin D in musculoskeletal and non-musculoskeletal health.[1]

Measurement

Vitamin D status is assessed by measurement of plasma 25-hydroxy vitamin D, with normal values above 27.5 nmol/L. Plasma vitamin D levels vary with the seasons, being highest in the summer and lowest in winter. Plasma Ca and phosphate fall in severe deficiency and alkaline phosphatase is elevated in mild and severe deficiency states.

Deficiency

Severe deficiency results in rickets in children, which is characterized by reduced calcification of bone epiphyses. It results in skeletal deformities, bone pain, and muscle weakness. In adults, deficiency results in osteomalacia, which leads to bone pain, partial (Looser's zone) fractures, and muscle weakness. People who stay indoors and are fully covered or live at high altitudes are at risk of deficiency because of a lack of ultraviolet radiation from sunlight. It is recommended that people consider taking a supplement of 10 μg in autumn and winter in the UK. Housebound/care home residents, etc., those who cover their skin, and ethnic groups with dark skin should consider taking a supplement throughout the year. Malabsorption ↑ the risk of deficiency.

Requirement and intake

See Tables 6.5 and 6.6, and Box 6.3.

---

1 SACN (2016). *Vitamin D and health*. Available at: ℘https://assets.publishing.service.gov.uk/government/uploads/system/uploads/attachment_data/file/537616/SACN_Vitamin_D_and_Health_report.pdf

Table 6.5 RNIs for all ages and average daily intakes of vitamin D for adult men and women provided by food (µg/day)*

Age	RNI
Months	
0–12	8.5–10†
Years	
1–4	7.0†
4 and above	10.0
Average daily intake UK	
From food sources	
Men	2.9
Women	2.5
Total intake	
Men	4.5
Women	3.9

*Source: data for RNIs from Department of Health (1991). *Dietary reference values for food and nutrients for the United Kingdom*. HMSO, London. Source: data for average daily intakes for adults from Public Health England & Food Standards Agency (2018). *The National Diet and Nutrition Survey*: Results from Years 7 and 8 (combined) of the Rolling Programme (2014/2015–2015/2016).

† 'Safe intake'

Table 6.6 Contribution of foods to vitamin D intake*

Food group	% Daily intake
Meat and meat products	30
Fish and fish dishes	17
Oily fish	13
Cereals and cereal products	15
Fat spreads	11

*Source: data from Public Health England & Food Standards Agency (2018). *The National Diet and Nutrition Survey*: Results from Years 7 and 8 (combined) of the Rolling Programme (2014/2015–2015/2016). Public Health England, London.

Box 6.3 Good food sources of vitamin D
- Cod liver oil
- Oily fish (salmon, mackerel, etc.)
- Margarine
- Breakfast cereals
- Eggs
- Liver

Toxicity

Excessive exposure to sunlight does not → vitamin D toxicity as excess D_3 is converted to inert products. Overdose with supplements results in hypercalcaemia, which has symptoms of thirst and anorexia and is accompanied by the risk of soft tissue calcification and urinary Ca stones.

Vitamin K

Naturally occurring vitamin K can be classified into two groups. The major form of vitamin K_1 (phylloquinine) is found in plants while the vitamin K_2 group of compounds (menaquinones) is synthesized by intestinal bacteria.

Function

* Vitamin K promotes synthesis of γ-carboxyglutamic acid (Gla) in the liver. Gla is an essential part for prothrombin (factor II) and other coagulation factors (VII, IX, and X). Vitamin K is ∴ essential for blood coagulation.
* Other proteins contain Gla and require vitamin K for their synthesis. These include osteocalcin, a bone protein made by osteoblasts.

Measurement

Traditionally, vitamin K deficiency screening was based on coagulation assays of the levels of the active forms of coagulation proteins that require vitamin K. To entirely eliminate a diagnosis of congenital vitamin K deficiency, it is necessary to conduct individual factor assays. It is now possible to assay for undercarboxylated vitamin K-dependent proteins that are produced when vitamin K is in short supply or blocked by antagonists such as warfarin. A few specialist centres are now able to assay plasma and tissues levels directly by high performance liquid chromatography.

Deficiency

Vitamin K deficiency is characterized by poor blood clotting and results in low prothrombin activity. Newborn babies are given an injection of vitamin K at birth. Infants are born with very low stores and because of sterility of their intestines do not have bacteria producing vitamin K. Deficiency is rare in adults, but does occur in patients with obstructive jaundice as lack of bile can → poor absorption of vitamin K. The anticoagulants warfarin and dicoumarol can → a deficiency as their mode of action is to block some of the enzymes that recycle vitamin K in the liver.

Requirement and intake

See Box 6.4. Studies into vitamin K requirements are not entirely satisfactory as it is difficult to induce deficiency solely by dietary manipulation. It is suggested that the requirements are between 0.5 and 1.0 µg per kg/day. Determination of vitamin K levels in foods and unreliability of estimates of intake in the UK means that a consensus on usual intake is not available. Studies in the USA suggest that intakes vary between 30 and 100 µg/day.

Box 6.4 Good food sources of vitamin K

* Green leafy vegetables (spinach, broccoli, cabbage, and kale)
* Some vegetable oils especially soya bean oil. Corn or sunflower oils are not good sources
* Eggs
* Meat

Toxicity

Large intakes of naturally occurring vitamin K do not appear to be toxic. Synthetic preparation of vitamin K_3 (menadione) is used to treat intracranial and pulmonary haemorrhage in premature infants and overdosage can → liver overload and brain toxicity.

❶ Supplements containing vitamin K should not be taken when taking anticoagulant drugs, e.g. warfarin (see ➲ Chapter 38, 'Drug–nutrient interactions', p. 833).

Vitamin C (ascorbic acid)

Most animals can synthesize vitamin C from glucose or galactose; humans, primates, guinea-pigs, Indian fruit-eating bats, and some birds lack this ability and it is an essential nutrient in these species. L-ascorbic acid and L-dehydroascorbic acid are both biologically active forms of vitamin C.

Function

Vitamin C is a powerful reducing agent (antioxidant) and is essential for many oxidation-reduction reactions.

- Vitamin C is required for the synthesis of collagen, the main protein in connective tissue and ∴ essential for the maintenance of muscles, tendons, arteries, bone, and skin. It is essential for the normal functioning of enzymes involved in collagen synthesis.
- Hydroxylation of dopamine to the neurotransmitter noradrenaline requires vitamin C.
- Vitamin C is required for production of carnitine. Low levels of carnitine are associated with fatigue and muscle weakness.
- Various peptide hormones and releasing factors require activation by a vitamin C-dependent enzyme.
- Numerous other enzymes need vitamin C; these enzymes control many functions including the synthesis of bile and the metabolism of drugs and carcinogens by the liver.
- Vitamin C enhances the absorption of Fe when consumed in the same meal.

Measurement

Vitamin C status is assessed by measurement in plasma and leucocytes; plasma levels are the most practical measure of status. Plasma levels <11 μmol/L show deficiency, >17 μmol/L are adequate. Leucocyte levels of >2.8 pmol/10⁶ cells are adequate.

Deficiency

Vitamin C deficiency is uncommon except in populations where there is a prolonged lack of fruit and vegetables. Deficiency of vitamin C is characterized by abnormalities of the connective tissue including poor wound healing, which are described by the term scurvy. Weakness, fatigue, bleeding gums (gingival), hyperkeratosis, and skin haemorrhages are symptoms of scurvy.

Requirement and intake

See Tables 6.7 and 6.8, and Box 6.5. Regular smoking ↑ vitamin C turnover and it is estimated that smokers require 80 mg/day.

Toxicity

High doses (1–10 g/day) of vitamin C are sometimes taken in the belief that such doses can prevent the common cold. There is no evidence to support this hypothesis, although they may reduce the severity of symptoms to an extent. Sudden cessation of high-dose supplements may precipitate rebound scurvy. Intakes at such high levels have been associated with diarrhoea and ↑ risk of kidney oxalate stone formation.

Table 6.7 Reference nutrient intakes (RNI) for all ages and average daily intakes for adult men and women for vitamin C provided by food (mg/day)*

Age (years)	RNI
0–1	25
1–10	30
11–14	35
Males 15+	40
Females 15+	40
Pregnancy	+10[†]
Lactation	+30
Average daily intake UK	
Men	84
Women	82

* Source for RNIs, Department of Health (1991). *Dietary reference values for food and nutrients for the United Kingdom.* HMSO, London. Source for average daily intakes for adults, Public Health England & Food Standards Agency (2014). *The National Diet and Nutrition Survey: Results from Years 1, 2, 3 and 4 (combined) of the Rolling Programme (2008/2009–2011/2012).* Public Health England, London.

† Last trimester only.

Table 6.8 Contribution of foods to vitamin C intake*

Food group	% Daily intake
Non-alcoholic beverages	22
Fruit juice	12
Soft drinks, including low calorie	8
Vegetables excluding potatoes	23
Fruit	19
Potatoes and savoury snacks	15

* Source: data from Public Health England & Food Standards Agency (2014). *The National Diet and Nutrition Survey: Results from Years 1, 2, 3 and 4 (combined) of the Rolling Programme (2008/2009–2011/2012).* Public Health England, London.

Box 6.5 Good food sources of vitamin C

- Kiwi fruit
- Citrus fruit (oranges, lemons, satsumas, clementines, etc.)
- Blackcurrants
- Sweet potato
- Guava
- Mango
- Papaya
- Pepper

Riboflavin (vitamin B₂)

Function

Riboflavin is part of two coenzymes that are both oxidizing agents: flavin mononucleotide (FMN) and flavin adenine dinucleotide (FAD). FMN and FAD are contained in flavoproteins, which are involved in many oxidation-reduction reactions in many metabolic pathways. The functions of riboflavin include:

- promotion of normal growth;
- assisting synthesis of steroids, red blood cells, and glycogen;
- maintenance of mucous membranes, skin, eyes, and the nervous system;
- aiding Fe absorption.

Measurement

Riboflavin status can be assessed by measurement of urinary excretion or by measurement of erythrocyte glutathione reductase (EGR) activity co-efficient (EGRAC). FAD is a co-factor for EGR and its activity is directly correlated to riboflavin status. EGRAC is the method of choice as it reflects tissue saturation and long-term riboflavin status. Levels <1.3 are acceptable. Recently, doubts about the validity of EGRAC in pregnancy and exercise have been expressed.

Deficiency

- Symptoms of riboflavin deficiency include lesions of the mucosal surfaces of the mouth, angular stomatitis, cheilosis, glossitis, and magenta tongue, surface lesions of the genitalia, seborrhoeic skin lesions, and vascularization of the cornea.
- Deficiency is often accompanied by other nutrient deficiencies, e.g. pellagra (niacin deficiency).
- In animal studies, deficiency is associated with poor growth of the young and it is probable that similar effects occur in human neonates.
- Severe deficiency is unlikely in the UK, but the elderly, anorexia nervosa sufferers, and chronic 'dieters' are at risk.

Sources in the diet

Riboflavin is unstable when exposed to ultraviolet light and up to 70% will be lost from milk during 4 hour exposure to sunlight.

Requirement and intake

See Tables 6.9 and 6.10, and Box 6.6.

Toxicity

Toxicity is low because of the small amount that can be absorbed by the GI tract in a single dose. Harmless bright yellow urine is seen at high doses.

Table 6.9 RNIs for all ages and average daily intakes for adult men and women for riboflavin (mg/day)*

Age, years	RNI
0–1	0.4
1–10	0.6–1.0
Males 11–14	1.2
Males 15+	1.3
Females 11+	1.1
Pregnancy†	+0.3
Lactation	+0.5
Average daily intake UK	
Men	1.76
Women	1.42

*Source: data for RNIs from Department of Health (1991). *Dietary reference values for food and nutrients for the United Kingdom*. HMSO, London. Source: data for average daily intakes for adults from Public Health England & Food Standards Agency (2018). *The National Diet and Nutrition Survey: Results from Years 7 and 8 (combined) of the Rolling Programme (2014/2015–2015/2016)*. Public Health England, London.

†Last trimester only.

Table 6.10 Contribution of foods to riboflavin intake*

Food group	% Daily intake
Milk and milk products	27
Semi-skimmed milk	12
Cereals and cereal products	20
Meat and meat products	17
Vegetables including potatoes	7
Non-alcoholic beverages	6
Alcoholic beverages	4

*Source: data from Public Health England & Food Standards Agency (2018). *The National Diet and Nutrition Survey: Results from Years 7 and 8 (combined) of the Rolling Programme (2014/2015–2015/2016)*. Public Health England, London.

Box 6.6 Good food sources of riboflavin

- Eggs
- Milk and milk products
- Liver and kidney
- Yeast extracts
- Fortified breakfast cereals

Niacin (nicotinamide, nicotinic acid, vitamin B₃)

Niacin is the generic term for a group of compounds that prevent pellagra. Nicotinamide and nicotinic acid both occur in food, but have different physiological properties. Approximately 50% of niacin in the body is synthesized from the amino acid tryptophan. Sixty milligrams of tryptophan are equivalent to 1 mg of niacin or 1 niacin equivalents (NE).

Function

Nicotinamide is incorporated into the pyridine nucleotide coenzymes nicotinamide adenine dinucleotide (NAD) and nicotinamide adenine dinucleotide phosphate (NADP). The coenzymes are involved in numerous oxidoreductase reactions including glycolysis, fatty acid metabolism, tissue respiration, and detoxification.

Measurement

Niacin status is most often assessed by the measurement of its metabolites N^1-methylnicotinamide (NMN) and N^1-methyl-2-pyridone-5-carboxamide. These metabolites are ↓ in niacin deficiency. A deficiency should be considered when the NMN to creatinine ratio is <1.5 mmol/mol. This assay requires 24-hour urine collection, which may be problematical. Other measures of niacin status include red cell NAD concentration and fasting plasma tryptophan.

Deficiency

Deficiency of niacin is known as pellagra and classically it is characterized by the three Ds.

• Dermatitis: skin that is exposed to the sun becomes inflamed, which progresses to pigmentation, cracking, and peeling. The neck is frequently involved and the distinctive distribution of skin lesions is known as Casal's collar.
• Diarrhoea: this is often accompanied by an inflamed tongue.
• Dementia: symptoms range from mild confusion and disorientation to mania, occasionally psychoses may occur that require hospitalization.

Pellagra is rare in the UK, but still occurs in parts of Africa.

Requirement and intake

See Tables 6.11 and 6.12, and Box 6.7.

Table 6.11 RNIs for all ages and average daily intakes for adult men and women for niacin equivalents provided by food (mg/d)*

Age	RNI
Months	
0–6	3
7–9	4
10–12	5
Years	
1–3	8
4–6	11
7–10	12
Males	
11–14	15
15–18	18
19–50	17
50+	16
Females	
11–14	12
15–18	14
19–50	113
50+	14
Pregnancy†	
Lactation	+2
Average daily intake UK	
Men	42
Women	32

*Source: data for RNIs from Department of Health (1991). *Dietary reference values for food and nutrients for the United Kingdom.* HMSO, London. Source: data for average daily intakes for adults from Public Health England & Food Standards Agency (2014). *The National Diet and Nutrition Survey: Results from Years 1, 2, 3 and 4 (combined) of the Rolling Programme (2008/2009–2011/2012).* Public Health England, London.

†No increment is recommended during pregnancy.

Table 6.12 Contribution of foods to niacin intake*

Food group	% Daily intake
Meat and meat products	36
Chicken, turkey, and dishes including those coated	15
Cereals and cereal products†	25
White bread	6
Milk and milk products	7
Fish and fish dishes	7

*Source: data from Public Health England & Food Standards Agency (2014). *The National Diet and Nutrition Survey*: Results from Years 1, 2, 3 and 4 (combined) of the Rolling Programme (2008/2009–2011/2012). Public Health England, London.

†UK-produced wheat flour (except wholemeal) has niacin added by law.

Box 6.7 Good food sources of niacin
- Beef
- Pork
- Liver, kidney
- Chicken
- Wheat flour†
- Maize flour
- Yeast extract
- Milk (poor source of niacin but good source of tryptophan, which can be converted to niacin)

†UK-produced wheat flour (except wholemeal) has niacin added by law.

Toxicity

Nicotinic acid intakes of 50 mg/day → flushing as a result of vasodilatation, higher doses → dilatation of non-cutaneous vessels and can cause hypotension. Doses of 1–2 g/day are used in treatment of hypertriglyceridaemia and hypercholesterolaemia. Larger doses (3–6 g/day) cause reversible liver toxicity with changes in liver function, carbohydrate tolerance, and uric acid metabolism.

Thiamin (vitamin B₁)

Function
Thiamin forms part of the coenzyme thiamine pyrophosphate (TPP), which is involved in major decarboxylation steps in the following pathways.
- pyruvate → acetyl CoA at the entry to the citric acid cycle;
- α-ketoglutarate → succinyl CoA, halfway round the citric acid cycle;
- transketolase reactions in the hexose monophosphate shunt;
- catabolism of branched chain amino acids, leucine, isoleucine, methionine, and valine;
- thiamin is needed for the metabolism of fat, carbohydrate, and alcohol.

Measurement
Red cell transketolase assay is the most frequently used measure of thiamin status. It is essential to use fresh, heparinized whole blood. Thiamin deficiency is indicated by ↑ in transketolase activity after the addition of TPP. Higher values indicate greater deficiency; in Wernicke's encephalopathy, activity can be ↑ by 70–100%.

Deficiency
Thiamin deficiency manifests as beriberi and Wernicke–Korsakoff syndrome. Beriberi is usually classified as either 'wet' (cardiac) or 'dry' (neurological). They rarely occur together.
- Wet beriberi is the acute form of the disease and is characterized by high output cardiac failure, bounding pulse, warm extremities, peripheral oedema, and cardiac dilatation.
- Dry beriberi is the chronic form of the disease and is characterized by progressive, peripheral neuropathy. Foot drop is accompanied by loss of sensation in the feet and absent knee jerk reflexes.
- Wernicke–Korsakoff syndrome is seen in chronic alcoholics who have a poor diet. It is characterized by confusion, low levels of consciousness, and poor co-ordination (Wernicke's encephalopathy). Paralysis of one or more of the external movements of the eye is a diagnostic criterion. Memory loss (Korsakoff's psychosis) often follows the encephalopathy.

Requirement and intake
See Tables 6.13 and 6.14, and Box 6.8. Thiamin requirements are related to energy metabolism.

Sources in the diet
Thiamin is widely distributed in the diet. In the UK and many other industrialized countries, bread flour is fortified with thiamin by law and, in practice, it is added to many breakfast cereals.

Toxicity
Chronic intakes of more than 3 g/day are associated with symptoms of toxicity; these include headache, irritability, insomnia, weakness, tachycardia, and pruritus. Regular large intakes can → an allergic reaction.

Table 6.13 RNIs for all ages and average daily intakes for adult men and women for thiamin provided by food (mg/day)*

Age	RNI
Months	
0–9	0.2
10–12	0.3
Years	
1-3	0.5
4-10	0.7
Males	
11–14	0.9
15-18	1.1
19-50	1.0
50+	0.9
Females	
11–14	0.7
15-18	0.8
19-50	0.8
50+	0.8
Pregnancy†	+0.1
Lactation	+0.2
Average daily intake UK	
Men	1.59
Women	1.28

*Source: data for RNIs from Department of Health (1991). *Dietary reference values for food and nutrients for the United Kingdom.* HMSO, London. Source: data for average daily intakes for adults from Public Health England & Food Standards Agency (2014). *The National Diet and Nutrition Survey*: Results from Years 1, 2, 3 and 4 (combined) of the Rolling Programme (2008/2009–2011/2012). Public Health England, London.

†For last trimester only.

Table 6.14 Contribution of foods to thiamin intake*

Food group	% Daily intake
Cereals and cereal products†	35
White bread	9
Meat and meat products	22
Vegetables excluding potatoes	9
Potatoes and savoury snacks	13

*Source: data from Public Health England & Food Standards Agency (2014). *The National Diet and Nutrition Survey: Results from Years 1, 2, 3 and 4 (combined) of the Rolling Programme (2008/ 2009–2011/2012)*. Public Health England, London.

†UK-produced wheat flour (except wholemeal) has thiamin added by law.

Box 6.8 Good food sources of thiamin
- Cereal products (including fortified breakfast cereals and bread)†
- Yeast and yeast products
- Pulses
- Nuts
- Pork and other meats
- Vegetables
- Dried milk

†UK-produced wheat flour (except wholemeal) has thiamin added by law.

Folate (folic acid)

Folic acid (pteroyl glutamic acid) is the synthetic form of the vitamin and is the parent molecule for a number of derivatives known as folates. Folic acid is a very stable molecule with high biological activity. It is used in the fortification of foods and in supplements. Folates occur naturally as a number of tetrahydrofolates, which have variable biological activities.

Function

- Folates are involved in a number of single carbon transfer reactions particularly in the synthesis of purines, pyrimidines, glycine, and methionine. It is ∴ essential for the synthesis of DNA and RNA.
- The folate derivative 5-methyl tetrahydrofolate requires vitamin B_{12} to enable the use of methionine synthase in the synthesis of methionine and tetrahydrofolate.

Measurement

Recent intake is assessed by serum folate; normal levels are 2.0–11.0 g/dL. Cellular status is reflected by red cell folate; normal levels are 150–700 g/dL.

Deficiency

Dietary deficiency is seen occasionally, but secondary deficiency is fairly common. Secondary deficiency can result from malabsorption, the use of certain drugs, and in late pregnancy and some disease states including leukaemia. Deficiency results in megaloblastic anaemia with abnormal neutrophil nuclei and giant platelets. There may also be infertility and diarrhoea.

Benefits of extra folate

Folate supplements in early pregnancy (before the neural tube closes at 24–28 days) have been shown to reduce neural tube defects (NTD) (see → Chapter 12, 'Diet before and during pregnancy', p. 237). In many countries flour is supplemented with folate by law. SACN have recommended the supplementation of flour in the UK, but, to date, this has not had government approval.

Large doses (200 µg/day) reduce plasma levels of homocysteine. Raised plasma homocysteine is a risk factor for cardiovascular disease.

Requirement and intake

See Tables 6.15 and 6.16, and Box 6.9.

Toxicity

The toxicity of folates is low. Folate supplements given to patients with developing vitamin B_{12} deficiency may obscure diagnosis of pernicious anaemia.

Drug interactions

Chronic use of anticonvulsants has been associated with folate deficiency. Other drugs that interfere with folate metabolism include cytotoxic chemotherapy agents (methotrexate, aminopterin), and antimalarial (pyrimethamine) and antibacterial (co-trimoxazole) agents.

Table 6.15 RNIs and average daily intakes for adult men and women for folate provided by food (μg/day)*

Age, years	RNI
0–1	50
1–3	70
4–6	100
7–10	150
Males 11+	200
Females 11+	200
Pregnancy	+100†
Average daily intake UK	
Food sources only	
Men	267
Women	214
Total intake—all sources	
Men	300
Women	253

*Source: data for RNIs from Department of Health (1991). *Dietary reference values for food and nutrients for the United Kingdom.* HMSO, London. Source: data for average daily intakes for adults from Public Health England & Food Standards Agency (2018). *The National Diet and Nutrition Survey:* Results from Years 7 and 8 (combined) of the Rolling Programme (2014/2015–2015/2016). Public Health England, London.

†To prevent first occurrence of NTD: 400 μg during preconception and until the 12th week of pregnancy (on prescription or over the counter). 5 mg given to diabetic and obese women during pregnancy. To prevent recurrence of NTD: 5 mg during preconception and until the 12th week of pregnancy (on prescription only).

Table 6.16 Contribution of foods to folate intake*

Food group	% Daily intake
Cereals and cereal products	27
High-fibre breakfast cereals	5
Vegetables excluding potatoes	23
Potatoes and savoury snacks	13
Alcoholic beverages	6
Non-alcoholic beverages	5

*Source: data from Public Health England & Food Standards Agency (2018). *The National Diet and Nutrition Survey:* Results from Years 7 and 8 (combined) of the Rolling Programme (2014/2015–2015/2016). Public Health England, London.

Box 6.9 Good food sources of folate

- *Rich sources >100 μg per serving*: Brussel sprouts, kale, spinach
- *Good sources 50–100 μg per serving*: fortified bread and breakfast cereals, broccoli, cabbage, cauliflower, chickpeas, green beans, iceberg lettuce, kidneys, beans, peas, spring greens
- *Moderate sources 15–50 μg per serving*: potatoes, most other vegetables, most fruits, most nuts, brown rice, wholegrain pasta, oats, bran, some breakfast cereals, cheese, yoghurt, milk, eggs, salmon, beef, game

Vitamin B$_6$

There are three naturally occurring forms of vitamin B$_6$: pyridoxine, pyridoxal, and pyridoxamine. These three vitamers are interconvertible in the body.

Function

The three vitamers can be converted to the coenzyme pyridoxal-5-phosphate, which is involved in amino acid metabolism. These reactions include:

- transamination of amino acids to produce keto acids and synthesis of non-essential amino acids;
- decarboxylation to yield biologically active amines, e.g. neurotransmitters (adrenaline, noradrenaline, serotonin, and γ-amino butyric acid) and histamine;
- porphyrin synthesis, including haemoglobin.

Vitamin B$_6$ is also involved in the conversion of glycogen to glucose in muscles, the conversion of tryptophan to niacin, and in hormone metabolism.

Measurement

Vitamin B$_6$ status can be assessed by measurement of plasma concentrations of pyridoxal phosphate (normal values are above 30 nmol/L) or total vitamin B$_6$. Activation of erthyrocyte transaminases can be a useful measure. Metabolism of test doses of methionine can be used, but is technically difficult.

Deficiency

Severe deficiency of vitamin B$_6$ is rare. One outbreak was reported in 1954 caused by errors in the manufacture of infant's formula feed. The affected infants suffered seizures that responded to treatment with vitamin B$_6$. Patients suffering from malabsorption, receiving dialysis, or alcoholics are at risk of deficiency. Clinical signs include lesions of the lips and corners of the mouth, and inflammation of the tongue. Peripheral neuropathy may be a sign of vitamin B$_6$ deficiency, but as vitamin B$_6$ deficiency is usually associated with other vitamin deficiency the neuropathy may be the result of thiamin deficiency. Sideroblastic (microcytic, hypochromic) anaemia from poor haem synthesis is associated with vitamin B$_6$ deficiency.

Requirement and intake

See Tables 6.17 and 6.18, and Box 6.10. The importance of vitamin B$_6$ in amino acid metabolism mean that requirements are linked to protein intake.

Toxicity

Intakes of 50 mg/day and above have been associated with peripheral neuropathy and loss of sensation in the feet has been reported at higher doses (from supplements). The Department of Health recommends that the daily dose of vitamin B$_6$ should not exceed 10 mg/day.

Table 6.17 RNIs for all ages and average daily intakes for adult men and women for vitamin B$_6$ provided by food (µg/g protein)*

Age	RNI
Months	
0–6	0.2
7-9	0.3
10-12	0.4
Years	
1-3	0.7
4-6	0.9
7-10	1.0
Males	
11–14	1.2
15-18	1.5
19+	1.4
Females	
11–14	1.0
15-18	1.2
19+	1.2
Pregnancy†	
Lactation	
Average daily intake UK	
Men	2.5
Women	1.9

*Source: data for RNIs from Department of Health (1991). *Dietary reference values for food and nutrients for the United Kingdom*. HMSO, London. Source: data for average daily intakes for adults from Bates, B., Lennox, A., Swan, G. (2010). *The National Diet and Nutrition Survey: Headline results from Year 1 of the Rolling Programme (2008/2009)*. Food Standards Agency, London.

†No increment is recommended for pregnancy or lactation.

Drug interactions

Urinary excretion of vitamin B$_6$ is ↑ by isoniazid (used to treat tuberculosis). Penicillamine, levodopa, and cycloserine are vitamin B$_6$ antagonists.

Table 6.18 Contribution of foods to vitamin B$_6$ intake*

Food group	% Daily intake
Cereals and cereal products	17
Meat and meat products	24
Potatoes and savoury snacks	13
Fruit	6
Beer and lager	6

*Source: data for average daily intakes for adults from Henderson, L., Irving, K., Gregory, J. (2003). *The National Diet and Nutrition Survey: adults aged 19 to 64 years*. Vol. 3. *Vitamin and mineral intake and urinary analytes*. HMSO, London.

Box 6.10 Good food sources of vitamin B$_6$
- Meat
- Wholegrain cereals
- Fortified cereals
- Bananas
- Nuts
- Pulses

Cobalamin B$_{12}$

Cobalamin is a complex molecule that contains cobalt; it occurs naturally in usual forms. Cyanocobalamin is the commercially available form, which is converted to the natural forms. It requires salivary haptocorrin and 'intrinsic factor' to be absorbed. 'Intrinsic factor' is secreted by the parietal cells of the stomach.

Function

The functions of vitamin B$_{12}$ include:
- recycling of folate coenzymes;
- normal myelination of nerves;
- synthesis of methionine from homocysteine.

Measurement

Serum B$_{12}$ status is assessed by radioligand binding or microbiological assay. Levels 160-760 ng/L are considered normal. Absorption of B$_{12}$ is assessed by the Schilling test. Absorption of vitamin B$_{12}$ labelled with radioactive cobalt is measured with and without 'intrinsic factor'.

Deficiency

Vitamin B$_{12}$ does not occur in plant foods, and ∴ vegans and strict vegetarians are at risk of deficiency. Few exhibit deficiency symptoms as vitamin B$_{12}$ is also manufactured by intestinal bacteria. Children on macrobiotic or vegan diets are at particular risk. The most common cause of deficiency is malabsorption as a result of atrophy of the gastric mucosa or gastric bypass, which leads to inadequate production of 'intrinsic factor' or diseases of the ileum. Long-term metformin use increases the risk of deficiency. Deficiency results in pernicious anaemia (megaloblastic) and/or neurological problems. The anaemia is morphologically the same as that seen in folate deficiency and biochemical tests are necessary to establish the cause. The neuropathy is characterized by loss of sensation and motor power in the lower limbs resulting from degeneration of myelin. Deficiency is easily corrected by monthly injections (1 mg/m).

Sources in the diet

Vitamin B$_{12}$ is synthesized by bacteria and assimilated into the food chain. It occurs naturally in animal products, but can also be found in fortified foods such as breakfast cereals.

Requirement and intake

See Tables 6.19 and 6.20, and Box 6.11.

Toxicity

Toxicity has not been reported in humans.

Table 6.19 RNIs for all ages and average daily intakes for adult men and women for B$_{12}$ provided by food (μg/day)*

Age, years	RNI
0–1	0.3–0.4
1–3	0.5
4–6	0.8
7–10	1.0
11–14	1.2
Males 15+	1.5
Females 15+	1.5
Lactation	+0.5†
Average daily intake UK	
Men	5.7
Women	4.6

*Source: data for RNIs from Department of Health (1991). *Dietary reference values for food and nutrients for the United Kingdom*. HMSO, London. Source: data for average daily intakes for adults from Public Health England & Food Standards Agency (2014). *The National Diet and Nutrition Survey*: Results from Years 1, 2, 3 and 4 (combined) of the Rolling Programme (2008/2009–2011/2012). Public Health England, London.

†No increment is recommended during pregnancy.

Table 6.20 Contribution of foods to vitamin B$_{12}$ intake*

Food group	% Daily intake
Milk and milk products	33
Semi-skimmed milk	15
Meat and meat products	29
Fish and fish dishes	16
Oily fish	6

*Source: data for average daily intakes for adults from Henderson, L., Irving, K., Gregory, J. (2003). *The National Diet and Nutrition Survey: adults aged 19 to 64 years*. Vol. 3. *Vitamin and mineral intake and urinary analytes*. HMSO, London.

Box 6.11 Good food sources of vitamin B$_{12}$
- Meat and meat products
- Eggs
- Milk and dairy products
- Fish and fish products
- Yeast products and fortified vegetable extracts
- Breakfast cereals (fortified)

Biotin (vitamin B₇)

Of the eight isomers of biotin, only D-biotin is biologically active. Biotin is made by bacteria and yeasts. Biotin is obtained from the diet and synthesized by endogenous bacteria in the colon.

Function

Biotin is a coenzyme for several carboxylases involved in fatty acid synthesis and metabolism, gluconeogenesis, and the metabolism of branched chain amino acids.

Measurement

Microbiological assays are available to measure biotin in whole blood or urine. The normal range in whole blood is 0.22–0.75 μg/mL.

Deficiency

Biotin deficiency is rare, but has been reported in patients receiving total parenteral nutrition and should be added to the infusion solution. Deficiency is associated with scaly dermatitis, glossitis, hair loss, anorexia, depression, and hypercholesterolaemia. It is possible to induce biotin deficiency by the ingestion of large amounts of raw egg white. Egg whites contain the protein avidin, which binds biotin and prevents absorption. The effect is prevented by heating the egg whites.

Requirement and intake

See Table 6.21 and Box 6.12. No studies are available on which recommendations on intake can be based. It is believed that intakes of between 10 and 200 μg/day are safe and adequate.

Toxicity

There have been no reports of biotin toxicity.

Table 6.21 Average daily intakes for adult men and women for biotin (μg/day) in the UK*

Men	41
Women	29

*Source: data from Henderson, L., Irving, K., Gregory, J. (2003). *The National Diet and Nutrition Survey: adults aged 19 to 64 years*. Vol. 3. *Vitamin and mineral intake and urinary analytes*. HMSO, London. NB: Biotin is not reported in more recent NDNS surveys.

Box 6.12 Good food sources of biotin
- Liver
- Kidney
- Milk
- Eggs
- Dairy products

Pantothenic acid (vitamin B$_5$)

Function
- Pantothenic acid is part of coenzyme A (CoA) and as such is involved in the tricarboxylic acid cycle.
- The pantothenic acid derivative 4-phosphopantetheine is part of the acyl carrier protein.
- It is essential for reactions involved in carbohydrate and lipid metabolism.

Measurement
Pantothenic acid can be measured in blood and urine. Normal urinary excretion is 1–15 mg/day and normal blood values are >100 µg/dL.

Deficiency
Spontaneous deficiency of pantothenic acid has not been described. It is possible to induce a deficiency with experimental diets or by administration of the antagonist ω-methypantothenic acid. During World War II malnourished prisoners in the Far East developed 'burning feet' parathaesiae, which responded to treatment with pantothenic acid.

The symptoms of deficiency include a burning sensation in the feet, depression, fatigue, vomiting, and muscle weakness.

Requirement and intake
See Table 6.22 and Box 6.13. Information is not available to derive recommended intakes, but intake of 3–7 mg/day is considered adequate.

Sources in the diet
Pantothenic acid is widely distributed in food, but highly processed foods do not contain the vitamin.

Toxicity
There are no specific toxic effects, although large doses may cause GI symptoms such as diarrhoea.

Table 6.22 Average daily intakes of pantothenic acid provided by food (mg/day) in UK*

Men	7.2
Women	5.4

*Source: data from Henderson, L., Irving, K., Gregory, J. (2003). *The National Diet and Nutrition Survey: adults aged 19 to 64 years.* Vol. 3. *Vitamin and mineral intake and urinary analytes.* HMSO, London. NB: Pantothenic acid is not reported in more recent NDNS surveys.

Box 6.13 Good food sources of pantothenic acid
- Yeast
- Offal
- Peanuts
- Meat
- Eggs
- Green vegetables

Minerals and trace elements: introduction

Table 6.23 shows the minerals and trace elements known to be essential to humans. Fluoride is semi-essential in that no physiological requirement is known to exist, but there are known beneficial effects. Minerals are required in grams or milligrams, while trace elements are required in microgram amounts. Elements that are of biological importance, but are not currently considered essential include nickel, vanadium, cobalt, and boron.

Criteria for essentiality of minerals and trace elements

- Present in healthy tissues.
- Concentration must be relatively constant between different organisms.
- Deficiency induces specific biochemical changes.
- Deficiency changes are accompanied by equivalent abnormalities in different species.
- Supplementation corrects the abnormalities.

Table 6.23 Essential minerals and trace elements

Minerals	Trace elements
Calcium	Copper
Phosphorus	Chromium
Magnesium	Manganese
Sodium	Molybdenum
Potassium	Selenium
Iron	Iodine
Zinc	
Fluoride	

Calcium

Ca is the most abundant mineral in the human body (1.4 g/kg) and 99% is deposited, usually as hydroxyapatite, in bones and teeth where it provides structural rigidity. Ca plasma levels are tightly controlled by parathyroid hormone, 1,25 dihydroxycholecalciferol, and calcitonin. Plasma Ca levels are also controlled by the vitamin D metabolite $1,25(OH)_2D_3$, which controls the active absorption of calcium from the intestine and osteoclastic resorption of bone. Causes of abnormal Ca plasma concentrations are shown in Table 6.24.

Function
- Structural rigidity of bones and teeth, as hydroxyapatite.
- Intracellular signalling control of muscles and nerves.
- Blood clotting.
- Co-factor for enzymes, e.g. lipase.

Measurement
The normal plasma range for Ca is 2.15–2.55 mmol/L, and 50% of plasma Ca is bound to protein, principally albumin; ∴ the plasma value is frequently given as a corrected value. Plasma Ca levels are tightly controlled and are not usually affected by dietary insufficiency in healthy adults. Hypocalcaemia results in symptoms, such as tetany and cardiac arrhythmias. Bone mineral concentration can be measured by neutron activation analysis and dual energy x-ray absorptiometry can be used to directly measure bone mineral density.

Deficiency
In early adulthood, Ca deficiency can → stunted growth and failure to achieve peak bone mass. Peak bone mass is achieved in early adulthood and is determined by genetic factors, use of the skeleton, and nutritional factors including Ca intake. Failure to achieve peak bone mass is a risk factor for osteoporosis in later life. Poor Ca absorption from vitamin D deficiency leads to rickets in children (see ➲ this chapter, 'Vitamin D (calciferols)', p. 108).

Requirement and intake
See Table 6.25. The BDA recommend the calcium star system for the general public to check if they are getting enough calcium. Details are available at ♪ https://www.bda.uk.com/foodfacts/Calcium.pdf

Sources in the diet
See Table 6.26 and Box 6.14. Ca absorption is variable; Ca in milk and dairy foods is more readily absorbed than Ca in plants. The presence of phytates in cereals and oxalates in leafy green vegetables inhibits absorption. UK-produced wheat flour (except wholemeal) has Ca added by law.

Toxicity
Accumulation in blood and tissues from dietary excess is virtually unknown because of the tight homeostatic control of Ca. Hypercalcaemia is usually the result of an abnormality in this control, as shown in Table 6.24. Milk

Table 6.24 Causes of abnormal plasma Ca*

Hypercalcaemia	Hypocalcaemia
Malignant disease	Vitamin D deficiency
Primary hyperparathyroidism	Hypoparathyroidism (and pseu dohypoparathyroidism)
Sarcoidosis (and other granulomas)	
Vitamin D overdose	
Milk alkali syndrome	
Immobilization	
Thyrotoxicosis	
Hypercalcaemia of infancy	
Familial hypocalciuric hypercalcaemia	

*Reproduced from Garrow, JS., James, WPT., Ralph, A. (2000) *Human Nutrition and Dietetics*. Table 11.1, p. 169. With permission from Elsevier.

Table 6.25 Reference nutrient intakes for Ca (mg/day) for all ages and average daily intakes (mg) for adult men and women provided by food*

Age†	RNI
Months	
0–12	525
Years	
1–3	350
4–6	450
7–10	550
Men	
11–18	1000
19 +	700
Women	
11–18	800
19 +	700
Lactation	+ 550
Average daily intake UK	
Men	897
Women	746

*Source: data for RNIs from Department of Health (1991). *Dietary reference values for food and nutrients for the United Kingdom*. HMSO, London. Source: data from Public Health England & Food Standards Agency (2018). *The National Diet and Nutrition Survey*: Results from Years 7 and 8 (combined) of the Rolling Programme (2014/2015–2015/2016). Public Health England, London..

†There is no recommendation for an increase in Ca intake during pregnancy, Ca absorption ↓ during pregnancy.

alkali syndrome (MAS) results from excessive intake of Ca and alkali as ant-acid tablets, Ca supplements, and milk (which provides vitamin D and → ↑ absorption). MAS has been reported at Ca carbonate intakes of ≥4 g/day. A rare cause of MAS is excessive intake of Ca by the ingestion of betel nut paste containing oyster shells. Intakes of up to 2 g of Ca/day have been shown to be safe.

Table 6.26 Contribution of foods to Ca intake (NDNS)*

Food group	% Daily intake
Milk and milk products	34
Semi-skimmed milk	12
Cheese	10
Cereals and cereal products	31
White bread	10

*Source: data from Public Health England & Food Standards Agency (2018). *The National Diet and Nutrition Survey*: Results from Years 7 and 8 (combined) of the Rolling Programme (2014/2015–2015/2016). Public Health England, London.

Box 6.14 Food and portions that provide approximately 100 mg of Ca

- 85 mL milk
- 15 g cheddar cheese
- 50 g yoghurt
- 100 g cottage cheese
- 20 g sardines
- 200 g baked beans
- 3 large slices white bread
- 125 g pulses (e.g. chickpeas)
- 20 g tofu
- 15 g tahini

Phosphorus

Phosphate is present in every cell in the body, although 80–85% is found with Ca in hydroxyapatite.

Function
- Skeletal rigidity as the Ca compound hydroxyapatite.
- Energy for metabolism is derived from the phosphate bonds in adenosine triphosphate (ADP).
- Constituent of phospholipids and membranes.
- Constituent of nucleic acids.

Measurement
Serum total phosphate levels are measured by colorimetric methods. The normal adult range is 0.7–1.5 mmol/L.

Deficiency
P deficiency is unlikely to occur as it is present in all plant and animal foods. Hypophosphataemia does occur in poorly managed parenteral nutrition and re-feeding syndrome. Some studies have shown that P deficiency at birth is linked to rickets at a later age. Hypophosphataemia can occur in sepsis, liver disease, alcoholism, diabetic ketoacidosis, and excessive use of aluminium-containing antacids.

Requirement and intake
See Tables 6.27 and 6.28. Dietary requirements for P are equal to those for Ca, i.e. 1 mg P:1 mg Ca or 1 mmol P:1 mmol Ca.

Sources in the diet
Phosphate is present in all natural foods and is present in many additives. Good sources are shown in Box 6.15. Absorption is approximately 60% of intake; it is ↓ by non-starch polysaccharides (NSP). NSP rich diets are also rich in phosphate so compensating for the reduction in absorption.

Toxicity
Intakes above 70 mg/kg body weight may → high serum levels that are above any likely to be taken in foods. Generally, ↑ intakes are balanced by ↑ excretion in urine; this is disrupted in renal patients (see ➲ Chapter 29, 'Kidney disease', p. 703). The P:Ca ratio should not be above 2.2 mg P to 1 mg of Ca.

Box 6.15 Good food sources of P
- Milk and dairy products except butter
- Cereals and cereal products
- Meat and meat products
- Fish
- Nuts
- Fruits and vegetables

Table 6.27 Reference nutrient intakes for P (which are equivalent to those for Ca (mmol/d)) for all ages and average daily intakes (mg) for adult men and women provided by food*

Age	RNI
Months	
0–12	13.1
Years	
1–3	8.8
4–6	11.3
7–10	13.8
Men	
11–18	25.0
19 +	17.5
Women	
11–18	20.0
19 +	17.5
Pregnancy†	
Lactation	14.3
Average daily intake UK	
Men	1493
Women	1112

*Source: data for RNIs from Department of Health (1991). *Dietary reference values for food and nutrients for the United Kingdom.* HMSO, London. Source: data for average daily intakes for adults from Henderson, L., Irving, K., Gregory, J. (2003). *The National Diet and Nutrition Survey: adults aged 19 to 64 years.* Vol. 3. *Vitamin and mineral intake and urinary analytes.* HMSO, London. NB: Intake of P not reported in later NDNS surveys.

†No increment is recommended for pregnancy

Table 6.28 Contribution of foods to P intake (NDNS)*

Food group	% Daily intake
Milk and milk products	24
Semi-skimmed milk	9
Cereals and cereal products	23
White bread	5
Breakfast cereals	5
Meat and meat products	21

*Source: data from Henderson, L., Irving, K., Gregory, J. (2003). *The National Diet and Nutrition Survey: adults aged 19 to 64 years.* Vol. 3. *Vitamin and mineral intake and urinary analytes.* HMSO, London. NB: Intake of P not reported in later NDNS surveys.

Iron

There is approximately 4 g Fe in the body of an adult man, of which 2.4 g is present as haemoglobin; adult women have approximately 2.1 g, of which 1.6 g is haemoglobin. Haemoglobin consists of four units: each unit contains one haem group and one protein chain. Fe is also present in the non-haem form. Fe compounds in the body are shown in Table 6.29.

Transport and absorption

In the free state Fe is toxic; ∴ its transport and storage are closely controlled. Fe is actively absorbed in the duodenum. When the body needs Fe it passes directly through the mucosal cells and is transported by transferrin, with Fe released from old red blood cells, to the bone marrow (80%) and other tissues. If Fe is not required it is stored in the mucosal cells as transferrin. Fe will be lost in faeces when the mucosal cells are exfoliated. Excess Fe that is absorbed is stored as ferritin or haemosiderin in the liver, spleen, or bone marrow. Fe can be mobilized from these stores when demand is ↑. Haem Fe is absorbed directly into the mucosal cells where Fe is released by haem oxidase and then bound to transferrin. Haem Fe represents 10–15% of Fe intake, but contributes ≥40% of total Fe absorbed (Fig. 6.1). Non-haem Fe is poorly absorbed (1–20% of the total absorbed) and is influenced by dietary constituents (see Table 6.30).

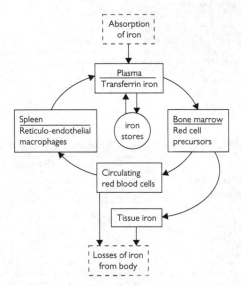

Fig. 6.1 Schematic representation of Fe metabolism.

Table 6.29 Fe compounds in the body (mg)

	Man (75 kg)	Woman (55 kg)
Functional Fe		
Haemoglobin	2400	1600
Myoglobin	350	230
Haem and non-haem enzymes	150	110
Transferrin-bound Fe	3	2
Total functional Fe	~2900	~1940
Storage Fe		
Ferritin and haemosiderin	500–1500	0–300
Total Fe	~4000	~2100

Table 6.30 Factors influencing Fe absorption

		Increased absorption	Decreased absorption
Haem	Physiological factors	Low Fe status	High Fe status
	Dietary factors	Low haem intake Meat	High haem intake Ca Tannins
Non-haem	Physiological factors	Depleted Fe stores Pregnancy Disease states (aplastic anaemia, haemolytic anaemia, haemochromatosis)	Replete Fe stores Achlorhydria
	Dietary factors	Vitamin C Meat, fish, seafood Organic acids: ascorbic, citric, lactic, malic, tartaric	Phytate Fe-binding phenolic compounds Inorganic elements: Ca, Mn, Cu, Cd, Co

Function

- As haemoglobin:
  - transport of oxygen;
  - cell respiration.
- As myoglobin:
  - oxygen storage in muscles.
- Other functions:
  - component of enzymes, including those involved in immune functions, and cytochromes, which are essential for energy production.

Measurement

Fe deficiency develops in three stages and measurements are appropriate to each stage.

- *Fe depletion*: Fe stores are depleted and serum ferritin levels will fall below 12 g/dL. Other measures of Fe status will be normal.
- *Fe deficient erythropoiesis*: Fe stores are depleted and supply does not meet needs for haemoglobin production. Serum ferritin levels will be low, serum Fe concentration is low, and transferrin saturation is <16%. Haemoglobin within normal range.
- *Fe deficiency anaemia*: haemoglobin levels <11.5 mg/L in women and <13 mg/L in men. Red cells are microcytic and hypochromic. Mean corpuscular volume (MCV) <77 fL and mean cell haemoglobin (MCH) <27 pg.

Requirement and intake

See Tables 6.31 and 6.32.

Table 6.31 Reference nutrient intakes for Fe (mg/day) for all ages and average daily intakes (mg) for adult men and women provided by food (NDNS)*

Age†	RNI
Months	
0–3	1.7
4–6	4.3
7–12	7.8
Years	
1–3	6.9
4–6	6.1
7–10	8.7
Men	
11–18	11.3
19–50 +	8.7
Women	
11–50	14.8
50 +	8.7
Average daily intake UK	
Men	11.6
Women	9.3

*Source: data for RNIs from Department of Health (1991). *Dietary reference values for food and nutrients of the United Kingdom*. HMSO, London. Source: data for average daily intakes for adults, Public Health England & Food Standards Agency (2018). *The National Diet and Nutrition Survey*: Results from Years 7 and 8 (combined) of the Rolling Programme (2014/2015–2015/2016). Public Health England, London.

†There is no recommendation for pregnancy and lactation as women should have enough Fe stores that will be enhanced by increased absorption and cessation of menstruation. Women with low Hb levels at the start of pregnancy may require supplementation.

Table 6.32 Contribution of foods to Fe intake (NDNS)*

Food group	% Daily intake
Cereals and cereal products†	38
High-fibre breakfast cereals	7
Meat and meat products	21
Vegetables including potatoes	15

*Source: data from Public Health England & Food Standards Agency (2018). *The National Diet and Nutrition Survey*: Results from Years 7 and 8 (combined) of the Rolling Programme (2014/2015–2015/2016). Public Health England, London.

†UK-produced wheat flour (except wholemeal) has Fe added by law

Deficiency

Fe deficiency anaemia (IDA) is the most common nutritional deficiency in the world. It is estimated that up to 30% of women have IDA, with prevalence of 78% in developed countries (see ➲ Chapter 13, 'Iron deficiency anaemia in infancy' (p. 284) and ➲ Chapter 20, 'Iron deficiency anaemia globally' (p. XX), and ➲ Chapter 16, 'Is a vegetarian diet a risk for health?' (p. 448). Up to 15% of pregnant women are Fe deficient (see ➲ Chapter 12, 'Dietary reference values and dietary guidelines during pregnancy', p. 242).

Physical signs include:
- pallor of fingernails and mucous membranes in the mouth and under eyelids;
- koilonychia (spoon-shaped nails);
- tachycardia, and in severe cases oedema;
- fatigue, breathlessness on exertion, insomnia, giddiness, anorexia;
- paraesthesia of fingers and toes.

Sources in the diet

See Table 6.33 and Box 6.16.

Toxicity

Because of tight metabolic control, dietary excess does not occur. Fe poisoning can occur from overdose of supplements: the lethal dose in children is 200–300 mg/kg body weight and approximately 100 g in adults. High doses of Fe supplements cause GI symptoms, especially constipation, although nausea, vomiting, and diarrhoea may occur. The absorption of other micronutrients, e.g. Zn, is reduced by high-dose Fe supplements.

The hereditary disease primary idiopathic haemochromatosis is characterized by high levels of Fe being absorbed. Fe deposits in the liver and heart and may → cirrhosis, liver cancer, congestive heart failure, and eventually death. Treatment requires regular blood removal.

Box 6.16 Dietary sources of Fe

Very good sources
- Meat, especially offal*
- Fish
- Eggs
- Meat extracts

Good sources
- Bread and flour
- Breakfast cereals
- Vegetables (dark green) and pulses
- Nuts and dried fruit—prunes, figs, apricots
- Yeast extract

*Liver is not recommended in pregnancy because of its high vitamin A content.

†UK-produced wheat flour (except wholemeal) has Fe added by law.

Table 6.33 Fe content of 50 g portions of foods

Food	Fe (mg)
Liver, cooked*	5
Liver pate	3
Roast or corned beef	1
Boiled egg	1
Sardines in tomato sauce	2
Wholemeal bread, 1 slice	1
Bran flakes, 30 g	6
Baked beans	1
Frozen peas	1
Lentils, cooked	1.5
Dark green leafy vegetables, cooked	0.5
Dried apricots	2
Tofu	0.5
Dry roasted peanuts	1

*Liver is not recommended in pregnancy because of its high vitamin A content.

Zinc

Function

- There are more than 200 Zn enzymes in plant and animal tissues including alcohol dehydrogenase, alkaline phosphatase, aldolase, and RNA polymerase. Zn is ∴ involved in digestion, carbohydrate metabolism, bone metabolism, and oxygen transport, and it is a powerful antioxidant.
- Zn is important in the immune response.
- It has other vital functions including structural properties in some proteins. Zn stabilizes the structure of DNA, RNA, and ribosomes; it has a vital role in gene expression.

Measurement

Less than 0.1% of the body's Zn is present in the blood and its measurement in plasma is not a good measure of Zn status. The measurement of thymulin activity is increasingly being used, although it is labour-intensive and ∴ not widely available. Thymulin promotes T-lymphocyte maturation and requires Zn for it to be active. Zn supplementation and observation of the subject's response is the most reliable method of diagnosing deficiency.

Deficiency

- Severe deficiency results in growth retardation, failure to thrive, delayed sexual maturation.
- Sore throat and immune defects.
- Circumoral and acro-dermatitis.
- Diarrhoea: Zn supplementation has been implemented in areas of the world where children are affected by persistent diarrhoea.
- Alopecia and neuropsychiatric symptoms.

Requirement and intake

See Tables 6.34 and 6.35.

Sources in the diet

See Table 6.36. Zn bioavailability is higher from animal sources than from cereals which contain phytate. Bioavailability is estimated to be 50–55% for an omnivorous diet in the UK; vegetarian and vegan diets have an estimated bioavailability of 30–35%.

Toxicity

Zn toxicity can occur following ingestion of water that has been stored in galvanized tanks or if this water is used for renal dialysis. Acute ingestion of 2 g or more of Zn results in nausea, vomiting, and fever. Intakes of 50 mg of Zn have been shown to interfere with Cu and Fe metabolism. Chronic intakes of 75–300 mg/day have been associated with symptoms of Cu deficiency including microcytic anaemia and neutropenia.

Table 6.34 RNIs for Zn (mg/day) for all ages and average daily intakes (mg) for adult men and women provided by food (NDNS)*

Age†	RNI
0–6 months	4.0
7 months–3 years	5.0
4–6 years	6.5
7–10 years	7.0
11–14 years	9.0
Males	
15+ years	9.5
Females	
15+ years	7.0
Lactation	
0–4 months	+6.0
4+ months	+2.5
Average daily intake UK	
Men	9.7
Women	.6

*Source: data for RNIs from Department of Health (1991). *Dietary reference values for food and nutrients for the United Kingdom.* HMSO, London. Source: data for average daily intakes for adults from Public Health England & Food Standards Agency (2018). *The National Diet and Nutrition Survey:* Results from Years 7 and 8 (combined) of the Rolling Programme (2014/2015–2015/2016). Public Health England, London.

†No increase is recommended in pregnancy.

Table 6.35 Contribution of foods to Zn intake (NDNS)*

Food group	% Daily intake
Meat and meat products	34
Beef, veal, and dishes	10
Turkey, chicken, and dishes	7
Cereals and cereal products	25
White bread	5
Breakfast cereals	3
Milk and milk products	14
Cheese	5
Semi-skimmed milk	4

*Source: data from Public Health England & Food Standards Agency (2018). *The National Diet and Nutrition Survey:* Results from Years 7 and 8 (combined) of the Rolling Programme (2014/2015–2015/2016). Public Health England, London.

Table 6.36 Food sources of Zn

Source	Food
Very rich	Lamb, leafy and root vegetables, crabs and shellfish, beef, offal
Rich	Wholegrains, pork, poultry, milk and milk products, eggs, nuts

Copper (Cu)

Adults have 80 mg of Cu in their bodies, 40% of which is present in muscle, 15% in the liver, 10% in the brain, and 6% in blood.

Function

Cu is incorporated into many metallo-enzymes, which are shown in Table 6.37.

Measurement

A totally reliable, sensitive method of assessing Cu status has yet to be established. Plasma Cu and caeruloplasmin (Cu-containing protein that normally binds 90% of the Cu present in plasma) are frequently used; they are both lowered in deficiency, but they plateau as levels of Cu ↑ and do not reflect high intakes. Neither is very specific. Normal serum Cu levels are 12–26 g/dL, but they are ↑ in late pregnancy and in women taking oestrogen-based contraceptives. Other methods include assessment of the activity of Cu enzymes in particular superoxide dismutase.

Deficiency

Cu deficiency is rare, although it can occur in premature infants and in patients receiving total parenteral nutrition. Cu is accumulated in the fetus during the late stages of pregnancy and full-term babies have large stores in the liver. ↑ Cu losses can occur in diseases such as cystic fibrosis, coeliac disease, and in children with chronic diarrhoea. Cu deficiency occurs in the hereditary condition Menkes disease, in which Cu transport is impaired.

The symptoms of Cu deficiency are:
- failure to thrive in babies;
- oedema with low serum albumin;
- Fe resistant anaemia;
- impaired immunity with low neutrophil count;
- skeletal changes including fractures and osteoporosis;
- abnormal blood vessels resulting from defects in collagen and elastin;
- hair and skin hypopigmentation with steely, uncrimped (kinky) hair;
- neurological abnormalities.

Cu deficiency may be a risk factor for coronary heart disease as it has been associated with raised plasma cholesterol levels and heart-related abnormalities.

Requirements and intake

See Tables 6.38 and 6.39. No increment for pregnancy is recommended as any ↑ in demand is met by the mother's adaptive responses. The average intake is ↑ to 1.48 mg/day in men and 1.07 mg/day in women by the use of supplements.

Sources in the diet

See Box 6.17. Bioavailability ranges from 35% to 70% and ↓ with age. The bioavailability of Cu in milk-based formulae is approximately 50%.

Table 6.37 Functions of Cu metallo-enzymes*

Enzyme	Functions
Blue proteins	Electron transfers
Cytochrome-c oxidase	Electron transport: reduction of O_2 to H_2O
Caeruloplasmin (ferroxidase I)	Fe oxidation and transport
Superoxidase dismutase	Antioxidant
Dopamine-hydroxylase	Hydroxylation of dopa in the brain
Diamine and monoamine oxidase	Removal of amines and diamines
Lysyl oxidase	Cross-linking in collagen and elastin, cardiovascular and bone integrity
Tyrosinase	Melanin formation
Chaperone proteins	Intracellular Cu transport
Chromatin scaffold proteins	Structural integrity of nuclear material
Clotting factors V, VIII	Thrombogenesis
Metallothionein	Metal sequestration
Nitrous oxide reductase	Reduction of NO_2 to NO

*Taken from Reilly, C. (2004). *The nutritional trace metals*, table 41, p. 120. Reproduced with permission from Blackwell Publishing.

Table 6.38 RNIs for Cu (mg/day) for all ages and average daily intakes (mg) for adult men and women provided by food*

Age†	RNI
Months	
0–12	0.3
Years	
1–3	0.4
4–6	0.6
7–10	0.7
11–14	0.8
15–16	1.0
18+	1.2
Pregnancy	+ 0.3
Average daily intake UK	
Men	1.24
Women	1.03

*Source: data for RNIs from Department of Health (1991). *Dietary reference values for food and nutrients for the United Kingdom*. HMSO, London. Source: data for average daily intakes for adults from Public Health England & Food Standards Agency (2014). *The National Diet and Nutrition Survey: Results from Years 1, 2, 3 and 4 (combined) of the Rolling Programme (2008/2009–2011/2012)*. Public Health England, London.

†No increase is recommended in pregnancy.

Table 6.39 Contribution of foods to Cu intake (NDNS)*

Food group	% Daily intake
Cereals and cereal products	33
White bread	7
Meat and meat products	1
Potatoes and savoury snacks	10
Salad, vegetables, and vegetable dishes	6
Fruits	6

*Source: data from Public Health England & Food Standards Agency (2014). *The National Diet and Nutrition Survey*: Results from Years 1, 2, 3 and 4 (combined) of the Rolling Programme (2008/ 2009–2011/2012). Public Health England, London.

Box 6.17 Good food sources of Cu
- Offal
- Nuts
- Cereals and cereal products
- Meat and meat products

Toxicity

Cu toxicity occurs either by the deliberate ingestion of Cu salts or by drinking contaminated water. The symptoms of acute toxicity are nausea, vomiting, and diarrhoea and may be fatal in extreme cases. Chronic Cu poisoning, from contamination by Cu water pipes or cooking utensils can → liver cirrhosis; infants and young children are particularly vulnerable. Wilson's disease is an inherited disease in which there is abnormal Cu transport that results in Cu accumulation in the liver, eyes, brain, and kidneys, and associated pathology.

Iodine (I)

Function

- Iodine is a component of the thyroid hormones thyroxine (T4) and tri-iodothyronine (T3).
- Thyroid hormones maintain the body's metabolic rate by controlling energy production and oxygen consumption in cells.
- They are required for normal growth and development.
- In the fetus and neonate normal protein metabolism in the brain and central nervous system (CNS) requires iodine.

Measurement

Levels of thyroid-stimulating hormone (TSH) are the most sensitive indicators of iodine status. It is raised in iodine deficiency. In severe deficiency serum T3 and T4 decline.

Deficiency

- Iodine deficiency disorder (IDD) in adults results in hypothyroidism and raised levels of TSH, which cause hyperplasia of thyroid tissues resulting in goitre. Hypothyroidism is characterized by lethargy, poor cold tolerance, bradycardia, and myxoedema.
- In the fetus IDD results in cretinism. This is characterized by mental retardation, hearing and speech defects, squint, disorders of stance and gait, and growth retardation. The degree of cretinism is variable and varying degrees of growth retardation and mental retardation are seen in infants and children with IDD.
- IDD is also linked to ↑ in the rates of stillbirth, miscarriage, and infertility.

It is estimated that 200–300 million people worldwide demonstrate some degree of IDD. Research in the UK has shown that pregnant women are at risk of deficiency, which may result in reduced intelligence.[2]

Intake

See Tables 6.40 and 6.41, and Box 6.18. The amount of iodine in the diet is affected by the geography of the areas of cultivation. Areas with poor soil content, e.g. mountainous areas such as the Himalayas, are often associated with endemic IDD. This is a result of iodine being washed from the soil. Supplementation of salt has been introduced in an attempt to reduce IDD. In the UK the iodine content of foods has gradually ↑ from supplements to cattle feeds, which are secreted in milk.

Absorption is reduced by the presence of goitrogens in some foods, e.g. brassica vegetables (cabbage, swede, Brussels sprouts, broccoli), cassava, maize, lima beans. Goitrogens are inactivated by heating.

Toxicity

High intakes can cause hyperthyroidism and toxic modular goitre; there is a weak relationship between persistently high intakes and thyroid cancer. The safe upper limit is 17 μg/kg/day.

2 Bath, S.C., et al. (2013). Effect of inadequate iodine status in UK pregnant women on cognitive outcomes in their children: results from the Avon Longitudinal Study of Parents and Children (ALSPAC). *Lancet*. **382**, 331–7.

Table 6.40 RNIs for iodine (μg/day) for all ages and average daily intakes (μg) for adult men and women provided by food*

Age	RNI
Months	
0–3	50
4–12	60
Years	
1–3	70
4–6	100
7–10	110
11–14	130
15+	140
Average daily intake UK	
Men	172
Women	140

*Source: data for RNIs from Department of Health (1991). *Dietary reference values for food and nutrients for the United Kingdom*. HMSO, London. Source: data for average daily intakes for adults from Public Health England & Food Standards Agency (2018). *The National Diet and Nutrition Survey*: Results from Years 7 and 8 (combined) of the Rolling Programme (2014/2015–2015/2016). Public Health England, London.

Table 6.41 Contribution of foods to iodine intake (NDNS)*

Food group	% Daily intake
Milk and milk products	34
Skimmed milk	15
Cereals and cereal products	12
Fish and fish products	10
Alcoholic beverages	8
Beer, lager, and perry	6

*Source: data from Public Health England & Food Standards Agency (2018). *The National Diet and Nutrition Survey*: Results from Years 7 and 8 (combined) of the Rolling Programme (2014/2015–2015/2016). Public Health England, London.

Box 6.18 Good food sources of iodine

- Milk and dairy products
- Sea fish, e.g. haddock, cod
- Shellfish
- Seaweed
- Iodized salt

Selenium

Function

Selenium (Se) is an integral part of over 30 selenoproteins; the most important of which are:

- glutathione peroxidases, which protect against oxidative damage;
- iodothyronine deiodinases, which are involved in the production of tri-iodothyronine from thyroxine;
- selenoprotein P, which is involved in antioxidant and transport functions.

Some studies suggest that higher Se intake/status may reduce the risk of some cancers, in particular prostate cancer. However, SACN (2013) have recently concluded that there are insufficient data to support a protective function of Se against any cancers.[3]

Measurement

Se levels are measured in plasma. There is considerable geographical variation in concentration: the range for the UK is 0.091–0.120 µg/mL.

Deficiency

Deficiency of Se is associated with two endemic causes: Keshan disease and Kashin–Beck disease.

- Keshan disease: outbreaks in Russia and several parts of Asia; it is characterized by a cardiomyopathy.
- Kashin–Beck disease: an endemic musculoskeletal disorder that has occurred in parts of Siberia and Asia.
- Iatrogenic causes of Se deficiency: include patients receiving total parenteral nutrition (TPN), phenylketonuric patients receiving a semi-synthetic diet. Patients exhibit symptoms of cardiomyopathy and/or musculoskeletal disorders.

Requirement and intake

See Tables 6.42 and 6.43. Se intake has ↓ over the last 20 years, because of ↑ consumption of European wheat that is low is Se, and the average intake is below the recommended intake. Epidemiological evidence suggests that this may contribute to ↓ risk of infection, cardiovascular disease, and the incidence of some cancers. Low Se levels have been reported in AIDS/HIV patients and ↓ SE levels appear to be correlated to ↑ mortality. Interventional studies are being conducted to establish the functional consequences of small supplements. Because of the potential risk of toxicity, self-administration of large supplements is not recommended.

Sources in the diet

See Box 6.19. Lacto-ovo vegetarians and vegans may be at risk of Se deficiency.

Toxicity

Acute Se poisoning is characterized by hypersalivation, nausea, vomiting, and garlic-smelling breath. This may be accompanied by diarrhoea, hair loss, restlessness, tachycardia, and fatigue. Chronic poisoning (selenosis) is associated with nail and hair changes, skin lesions, and neurological effects; numbness, pain, and paralysis may follow. Early nail changes have been observed at intakes of 450 µg/day and the recommended maximum safe intake is 6 µg/kg/day.

3 SACN Position Statement on Selenium And Health (2013). Available at: ℬ https://assets. publishing.service.gov.uk/government/uploads/system/uploads/attachment_data/file/339431/ SACN_Selenium_and_Health_2013.pdf

Table 6.42 RNIs for Se (mg/day) for all ages and average daily intakes (mg) for adult men and women provided by food*

Age	RNI
Months	
0–3	10
4–6	13
7–12	10
Years	
1–3	15
4–6	20
7–10	30
11–14	45
Men	
15–18	70
19+	75
Women	
15+	60
Lactation	+15
Average daily intake UK	
Men	55
Women	44

*Source: data for RNIs from Department of Health (1991). *Dietary reference values for food and nutrients for the United Kingdom*. HMSO, London. Source: data for average daily intakes for adults from Public Health England & Food Standards Agency (2018). *The National Diet and Nutrition Survey*: Results from Years 7 and 8 (combined) of the Rolling Programme (2014/2015–2015/2016). Public Health England, London.

Table 6.43 Contribution of foods to Se intake (NDNS 2018)*

Food	% Daily intake
Meat and meat products	32
Cereals and cereal products	27
Bread	11
Fish and fish dishes	15
Milk and milk products	6

*Source: data from Public Health England & Food Standards Agency (2018). *The National Diet and Nutrition Survey*: Results from Years 7 and 8 (combined) of the Rolling Programme (2014/2015–2015/2016). Public Health England, London..

Box 6.19 Food sources of Se

- Offal
- Fish
- Brazil nuts
- Eggs
- Poultry
- Meat and meat products

Magnesium (Mg)

Function
- Mg is an integral part of bones and teeth; 60% is found in the skeleton.
- Intracellular energy metabolism; a co-factor for enzymes requiring ATP, in the replication of DNA, and synthesis of protein and RNA.
- Essential for phosphate transferring systems.
- Muscle and nerve cell function.

Measurement
Serum Mg is the most frequently used index of status. The normal range is 0.7–1.0 mmol/L.

Deficiency
Mg is found in all animal and plant foods and its concentration in the blood is tightly controlled; a dietary deficiency is unlikely to occur. Low serum Mg levels occur when there are ↑ renal losses, malabsorption, or changes in tissue distribution because of disease or use of some drugs, e.g. diuretics, re-feeding syndrome. Hypomagnesaemia has been associated with cardiac arrhythmias and cardiac arrest. Very low levels of Mg are associated with hypocalcaemia.

Requirement and intake
See Tables 6.44 and 6.45

Sources in the diet
See Box 6.20. Hard drinking water may make a significant contribution to Mg intake.

Toxicity
If renal function is normal, hypermagnesaemia is virtually impossible to achieve by dietary means; it can occur in renal or adrenal disease. Large quantities of some Mg salts (Epsom salts) are used for their laxative effect.

> **Box 6.20 Good food sources of Mg**
> - Green vegetables
> - Pulses and wholegrain cereals
> - Meats

Table 6.44 RNIs for Mg (mg/day) for all ages and average daily intakes (mg) for adult men and women provided by food*

Age†	RNI
Months	
0–3	55
4–6	60
7–9	75
10–12	80
Years	
1–3	85
4–6	120
7–10	200
11–14	280
15–18	300
Men	
19+	300
Women	
19+	270
Lactation	+50
Average daily intake UK	
Men	302
Women	238

*Source: data for RNIs from Department of Health (1991). *Dietary reference values for food and nutrients for the United Kingdom*. HMSO, London. Source: data for average daily intakes for adults from Public Health England & Food Standards Agency (2018). *The National Diet and Nutrition Survey*: Results from Years 7 and 8 (combined) of the Rolling Programme (2014/2015–2015/2016). Public Health England, London.

† No increase recommended during pregnancy.

Table 6.45 Contribution of foods to Mg intake (NDNS)*

Food	% Daily intake
Cereals and cereal products	27
Breakfast cereals	5
Meat and meat products	15
Milk and milk products	9
Vegetables, excluding potatoes	16
Potatoes and savoury snacks	10

*Source: data from Public Health England & Food Standards Agency (2018). *The National Diet and Nutrition Survey*: Results from Years 7 and 8 (combined) of the Rolling Programme (2014/2015–2015/2016). Public Health England, London.

Manganese (Mn)

Function
- Mn is a component of several metallo-enzymes including arginase, pyruvate.
- It is needed for enzyme activity, including glutamine synthetase and various hydrolases, kinases, decarboxylases, and phosphotransferases.

Measurement
There is no accepted measurement of Mn status. Enzyme activity assays have been proposed, but none have been accepted into widespread practice.

Deficiency
Deficiency has only been observed in experimental studies: fingernail growth is slowed, black hair reddened, and a scaly dermatitis develops.

Requirement and intake
See Tables 6.46 and 6.47, and Box 6.21. No cases of nutritional Mn deficiency have been observed; ∴ no recommended nutrient intakes have been made in the UK. Safe levels are shown in Table 6.46.

Toxicity
Mn toxicity is low as absorption is ↓ when intake is high and any that is absorbed is excreted in bile and urine.

Table 6.46 Safe intakes for Mn for all ages and average daily intakes (µg) for adult men and women provided by food*

Age	RNI
Infants and children	>16 µg/kg/day
Adults	>1.4 mg/day
Average daily intake UK (mg/day)	
Men	3.32
Women	2.69

*Source: data for RNIs from Department of Health (1991). *Dietary reference values for food and nutrients for the United Kingdom.* HMSO, London. Source: data for average daily intakes for adults from Henderson, L., Irving, K., and Gregory, J. (2003). *The National Diet and Nutrition Survey: adults aged 19 to 64 years.* Vol. 3. *Vitamin and mineral intake and urinary analytes.* HMSO, London.

Table 6.47 Contribution of foods to Mn intake (NDNS)*

Food	% Daily intake
Cereals and cereal products	50
Bread	26
Breakfast cereals	11
Biscuits, cakes, etc.	5
Drinks	17
Tea	12
Vegetables excluding potatoes	10

*Source: data from Henderson, L., Irving, K., Gregory, J. (2003). *The National Diet and Nutrition Survey: adult aged 19 to 64 years.* Vol. 3. *Vitamin and mineral intake and urinary analytes.* HMSO, London.

Box 6.21 Good food sources of Mn

- Cereals and cereal products
- Tea
- Vegetables

Molybdenum

Function

Molybdenum is a co-factor in xanthine oxidase, sulphite oxidase, and aldehyde oxidase, and is ∴ involved in the metabolism of purines, pyrimidines, quinolines, and sulphites.

Measurement

Mo can be measured in whole blood and serum. Concentrations in whole blood vary widely, although the mean concentration is 0.5 g/dL.

Deficiency

Dietary deficiency of Mo has been reported in farm animals, but has not been observed in humans, although there is a single case reported following prolonged TPN. The symptoms included defects in sulphur metabolism, mental disturbance, and coma. An inborn error of metabolism results in abnormal production of the coenzyme. It is characterized by abnormal urinary metabolites, neurological and ocular problems, and failure to thrive. The genetic expression and symptoms are varied and in the most severe cases can be fatal at 2–3 years.

Requirement and intake

There are no reference nutrient intakes (RNIs), but safe intakes are believed to be between 50 and 400 μg/day in adults and 0.5 and 1.5 μg/day in children. Mean intakes in adults are reported as 0.12 mg/day.

Sources in the diet

Offal, nuts, cereals, bread, leafy vegetables, and peas are good sources.

Toxicity

Few data are available for dietary excess, although intakes >100 mg/kg/day have been reported to cause diarrhoea, anaemia, and high blood uric acid levels; this is associated with gout.

Chromium

The essentiality of Cr is widely accepted, although this is still challenged by some scientists. In nutrition the trivalent state appears to have physiological functions but it is interchangeable with hexavalent Cr.

Function

- Cr is believed to be part of an organic complex known as the 'glucose tolerance factor' (GTF), which potentiates the action of insulin. The evidence for essentiality of Cr comes from observations of patients receiving TPN who develop diabetic symptoms. The symptoms respond to Cr treatment, but not insulin. Studies on the use of Cr in management of type 2 diabetes are not conclusive.
- Cr may participate in lipoprotein metabolism.

Measurement

There is no totally reliable measure of Cr. Urinary excretion, expressed in terms of creatinine, has been suggested as a measure of chromium status. Hair Cr levels have been used as a measure of long-term exposure, although hair analysis is associated with several problems.

Deficiency

Deficiency in humans has only been observed in patients receiving long-term TPN. The symptoms include impaired glucose tolerance, weight loss, neuropathy, elevated plasma fatty acids, depressed respiratory quotient, and abnormal nitrogen metabolism.

Requirement and intake

There are no RNIs for Cr but the theoretical requirement extrapolated from balance studies is 25–30 µg/day in adults. In children the safe intake is believed to be 0.1–1.0 µg/kg/day. The average daily intake of Cr for adults is estimated as 0.1 mg.[4]

Sources in the diet

The richest sources of Cr in the diet are meat, wholegrains, legumes, and nuts.

Toxicity

The trivalent form is not associated with toxicity, but the hexavalent form is very toxic. Two fatalities have been reported following acute ingestion of very large doses of hexavalent Cr as dichromate (75 mg/kg) and chromic acid (4.1 mg/kg). Symptoms include gastrointestinal haemorrhages, renal and liver abnormalities. Chronic toxicity is associated with renal failure, liver failure, haemolysis, and anaemia.

---

4 Ysart, G., et al. (2000). 1997 UK Total Diet Study—dietary exposures to aluminum, arsenic, cadmium, chromium, copper, lead, mercury, nickel, selenium, tin and zinc. *Food Addit. Contam.* 17, 775–86.

Fluoride

Fluorine (F-) is considered semi-essential as it has biological functions, but its essentiality is still being debated.

Function

Fluoride has a role in bone mineralization and protects against dental caries.

Deficiency

Low intakes are associated with ↑ incidence of dental caries.

Requirement and intake

See Tables 6.48 and 6.49, and Box 6.22. There are no RNIs for Fl, although safe intakes are given in Table 6.48. Total intakes depend on the level of fluoridation in water consumed. In the UK, 10% of water is fluoridated or has a natural content above the recommended fluoridation rate of 1 ppm. A recent report (Ysart et al, 2018) by the FSA Iteland's report findings from the 2014–16 Total Diet Study on dietary exposure to fluoride.[5] Recent data is not available in the UK.

Toxicity

Intake three to five times the normal intake is mildly toxic. Tooth mottling occurs in mild toxicity and chronic excess (20-80 mg/d for 10-20 years) causes joint and bone abnormalities.

Table 6.48 Safe intakes of F- (mg/kg/day)

Age	Safe intake
0–6 months	0.22
6–12 months	0.12
>1 year	0.05

5 FSA! (2018). Total Diet Survey 2014-2016. Assessment of dietary exposure to fluoride in adults and children in Ireland. ℛ https://www.ifst.org/news/total-diet-study-dietary-exposure-fluoride-0 IRELAND.

Table 6.49 Mean adult intakes of F- (mg/day)

	Intake
Non-fluoridated water areas	1.82
Fluoridated water areas*	2.90

*Assumes an average daily intake of 1.1 L daily.

Box 6.22 Sources of 1 mg F-

- 1 l water (fluoridated at 1 ppm)
- 1 F- tablet
- 1 g F- toothpaste (accidental consumption)
- 5 ml F- mouthwash (accidental consumption)
- 2–3 cups of tea (depends on strength)
- 1400 g cooked spinach
- 250 g tinned sardines

Resource Zohoori V & Maguire A (2015) Database of the fluoride (FL) content of selected drinks and foods in the UK. Available at ℜ https://www.tees.ac.uk/docs/DocRepo/Research/FinalFluorideDatabase.pdf

Electrolytes and fluid balance

Electrolytes: introduction 176
Sodium 178
Potassium 180
Chloride 182
Fluid balance 184

Electrolytes: introduction

The monovalent electrolytes are sodium (Na), chlorine (Cl), and potassium (K).

Sodium

An adult male (70 kg) has total body Na of 4 mol (92 g); 2000 mmol is in extracellular fluid (ECF), 1500 mmol in bone, and 500 mmol in intracellular fluid (ICF).

Function
- Cation in ECF.
- Regulation of blood pressure and transmembrane gradients.
- Acid–base regulation.
- Electrophysiological control of muscles and nerves.

Measurement
Na is easily measurable in plasma, with a normal range of 135–150 mmol/L.

Deficiency
Hyponatraemia risk factors include lower body weight, increasing age, thiazide and thiazide-like diuretics, hypotonic intravenous fluids, and surgery. Na losses requiring repletion can result from excess sweating in extreme conditions of heat and exertion.

Requirement and intake
See Table 7.1.

Sources in the diet
Na is present in many food additives, e.g. monosodium glutamate, but most Na in the diet is present as salt (NaCl). Levels are comparatively low in unprocessed foods. Salt is added to food as a preservative and flavour enhancer; it can also be used as a fermentation control agent in bread making, and as a texturizer, binder, and colour developer. In the UK, cereals and meat and their respective products provide 31% and 26% of sodium in the diet: 3 g salt ≈ 1.2 g Na; 17.1 mmol Na =1 g NaCl.

Toxicity
It is a strong emetic, but excessive oral loads of Na are potentially fatal. Artificial intravenous load has severe and rapid effects.

Health implications of excess consumption
Excess Na intake has been linked to hypertension and heart disease. Scientific Advisory Committee on Nutrition has recommended that salt intake targets should be:
- 0–6 months, <1 g/day;
- 7–12 months, 1 g/day;
- 1–6 years, 2 g/day;
- 7–14 years, 5 g/day;
- >15 years, 6 g/day.

Table 7.2 shows foods high in salt. The Public Health Responsibility Deal in the UK encourages food manufacturers and retailers to reduce the amount of salt in a wide range of processed foods. Details can be found on the Action on Salt website (% http://www.actiononsalt.org.uk/about/).

Table 7.1 Reference nutrient intakes (RNI) for Na (mg/d (mmol/day)) for all ages and average daily intakes of NaCl (g/day) and Na (mg/d) for adult men and women provided by food (National Diet and Nutrition Survey, NDNS)*

Age	RNI
0–3 months	210 (9)
4–6 months	280 (12)
7–9 months	320 (14)
10–12 months	350 (15)
1–3 years	500 (22)
4–6 years	700 (30)
7–10 years	1200 (50)
11–14 years	1600 (70)
15–50+ years	1600 (70)

Average daily intakes UK		
	NaCl	Calculated Na intake
Men	9.1	3640
Women	6.8	2720

*Source: data for RNIs from Department of Health (1991). *Dietary reference values for food and nutrients for the United Kingdom*. HMSO, London. Source: data for average daily intakes for adults from Public Health England (2016). *National Diet and Nutrition Survey: assessment of dietary sodium. Adults (19 to 64 years) in England, 2014*. Public Health England, London.

Table 7.2 Foods high in salt*

Foods almost always high in salt	
Anchovies	Salami
Bacon	Salted and dry roasted nuts
Cheese	Salt fish
Gravy granules	Smoked meat and fish
Ham	Soy sauce
Olives	Stock cubes
Pickles	Yeast extract
Prawns	

Foods that can be high in salt	
Bread products, e.g. crumpets, bagels, ciabatta	Soup
Pasta sauces	Sandwiches
Crisps	Sausages
Pizza	Tomato ketchup, mayonnaise,
Ready meals	other sauces
	Breakfast cereals

* Source: data from NHS Choices. Available at: ℞ http://www.nhs.uk/livewell/goodfood/pages/salt.aspx.

Clinical restriction of Na

Some disease states, e.g. renal disease, require the restriction of Na. The level of restriction can be classified.

- *No added salt*: 80–100 mmol Na/day.
- *Low salt*: 40 mmol Na/day.
- *Low Na*: 22 mmol Na/day.

Potassium

Function

Intracellular cation is involved in acid–base regulation, electrophysiology of nerves and muscles, and is essential for the cellular uptake of molecules against concentration and electrochemical gradients.

Measurement

Normal plasma concentration is 3.5–5.0 mmol/L. Over 95% of total body K is found in cells; an adult male contains 40–50 mmol/kg (1.6–2.0 g/kg).

Deficiency

Lack of K alters the electrophysiology of cell membranes and causes muscle weakness. In cardiac muscle this leads to arrhythmias and cardiac arrest. Motility is lost in the intestine and mental depression and confusion can develop. Dietary deficiency of K is very unlikely as it is found in all foods. Causes of K depletion are shown in Box 7.1.

Requirement and intake

See Tables 7.3 and 7.4, and Box 7.2.

Toxicity

Toxicity as a result of dietary excess is unlikely. Acute intakes of supplements exceeding 17.6 g (450 mmol) may cause symptoms of hyperkalaemia. Hyperkalaemia causes paraesthesiae around the mouth and muscle weakness, although these symptoms may be absent. There is a risk of cardiac arrest.

Box 7.1 Causes of K depletion

Gastrointestinal causes
- Diarrhoea
- Vomiting
- Small bowel or gastric drainage
- Ureterocolic anastomosis
- Purgatives

Urinary losses
- Chronic acidosis or alkalosis
- Osmotic diuresis, e.g. uncontrolled diabetes
- Renal disease (tubular)
- Diuretic drugs
- Steroid excess (Cushing's disease, primary and secondary hyperaldosteronism)

Table 7.3 Reference nutrient intakes (RNI) for K (mg/day (mmol/day)) for all ages and average daily intakes (mg) for adult men and women provided by food*

Age	RNI
0–3 months	800 (20)
4–6 months	850 (22)
7–12 months	700 (18)
1–3 years	800 (20)
4–6 years	1100 (28)
7–10 years	2000 (50)
11–14 years	3100 (80)
15–50+ years	3500 (90)
Average daily intakes UK	
Men	3145
Women	2588

*Source: data for RNIs from Department of Health (1991). *Dietary reference value for food and nutrients for the United Kingdom.* HMSO, London. Source: data for average daily intakes for adults from Public Health England & Food Standards Agency (2018). The National Diet and Nutrition Survey: Results from Years 7 & 8 of the Rolling Programme (2014/2015–2015/2016). Public Health England, London.

Table 7.4 Contribution of foods to K intake (NDNS)*

Food group	% Daily intake
Cereals and cereal products	16
Meat and meat products	15
Potatoes and savoury snacks	15
Drinks	15
Milk and milk products	15
Vegetables (excluding potatoes)	9
Alcoholic beverages	2

*Source: data from Public Health England & Food Standards Agency (2018). *The National Diet and Nutrition Survey*: Results from Years 7 & 8 of the Rolling Programme (2014/2015–2015/2016). Public Health England, London.

Box 7.2 Rich food sources of K

- Fruit especially bananas, apricots, blackcurrant, rhubarb, fruit juices
- Vegetables especially potatoes and potato snacks
- Chocolate, cocoa, and chocolate products
- Coffee and coffee products
- Malted milk drinks
- Yeast extracts and spreads, tomato ketchup, stock cubes, bottled sauces
- Table salt substitutes

Chloride

Total body Cl is ~33 mmol (1.2 g)/kg; 70% is in ECF.

Function

Cl is the anion to the cations Na and K.

Measurement

Normal plasma concentration is 97–107 mmol/L.

Requirement and intake

There are no specific dietary reference values for Cl; it is recommended that Cl intake should equal Na intake in molar terms. The average intakes of Cl in foods are 4995 mg/day for men and 3481 mg/day for women.

Sources in the diet

Cl is usually consumed with Na as salt (NaCl).

Fluid balance

The human body is mainly water; a 70 kg man is composed of approximately 45 L water; ECF 15 L, ICF 30 L. Of fat free mass, 72% is water. ECF is composed of plasma and interstitial fluids. The monovalent electrolytes, Na, Cl, and K, determine the body's osmolality and their distribution determines the volume of ECF and ICF. ICF, plasma, and interstitial fluids are separated by semi-permeable membranes and are interdependent. Movement of fluid between the compartments is controlled by plasma osmolality and hydrostatic pressure gradients.

Regulation of fluid balance

Fluid balance is under tight homeostatic control and fluctuates by <1% per day despite large variations in fluid intake. Normally, the osmolalities of plasma and interstitial fluids are similar. Plasma osmolality reflects serum Na, which reflects total ECF. Hydration status can be assessed by many methods; plasma osmolality is frequently used. In free living individuals, urine colour has been calibrated against hydration status; a pale yellow colour or lighter is considered an indicator of being well hydrated.

Plasma osmolality

↑ in plasma osmolality → thirst and the hypothalamus will be stimulated to ↑ antidiuretic hormone (ADH). This leads to reabsorption of water by the distal tubules of the kidney, which corrects the osmolality. ↓ plasma volume can also → raised osmolality, which causes aldosterone to be released. This ↑ Na and water resorption.

Hydrostatic pressure

Plasma volume is also controlled by hydrostatic pressure. At the arterial end of the capillaries blood pressure is exerted, but less osmotic pressure is exerted by plasma proteins resulting in the movement of fluid out into the interstitial fluid. At the venous end of the capillary the process is reversed and fluid passes back into plasma.

Water balance

See Table 7.5.

Thirst

Thirst usually plays only a small role in fluid balance of normal subjects. Thirst receptors in the upper gastrointestinal tract are quenched after fluid intake; this is usually before the body's tissues are fully rehydrated. Thirst quenching is not a good marker of rehydration. Thirst in infants, children, and the elderly is not as sensitive as that of normal adults. Fluid is usually consumed for reasons other than thirst, e.g. habit and customs. Local drying of the mouth and throat will also cause thirst, e.g. public speakers often require water to lubricate the mouth and throat.

Fluid losses

Fluid output in urine is controlled by the kidneys but there are also insensible water losses through the skin and lungs and in faeces.
- Sweat glands secrete water in sweat, which evaporates from the skin. This evaporation cools the skin. Water is also lost directly through the

Table 7.5 People at risk of dehydration*

Reason	Cause
Increased fluid losses	Patients with tracheotomies or on ventilators
	Diarrhoea and/or vomiting
	Stomal losses
	Wound or burn exudates
	Pyrexia
	Diabetes insipidus
	Diabetic ketoacidosis
	Prolonged use of diuretics
	Patients receiving high protein high osmolar diets
Lack of awareness or inability to express the need for fluid	Patients who are unable to communicate, e.g. as a result of stroke
Low fluid intake	Poor food intake, e.g. anorexia, depression
	Apathy, chronic illness, physical immobility, etc.
	Eating difficulties
	Swallowing difficulties
	Deliberate fluid restriction to avoid incontinence
	'Nil by mouth' regimens

*Republished with permission of John Wiley and Sons Inc from Manual of Dietetic Practice 4th edition. B Thomas et al. Copyright © 2007 John Wiley and Sons Inc; permission conveyed through Copyright Clearance Center, Inc.

skin. 500–750 mL/day of fluid is lost through the skin and ↑ In fever and extreme temperatures or exertion. ↑ in 1°C in body temperature will ↑ fluid requirements by 500 mL/day.
• Healthy adults pass 50–400 g/day of faeces and approximately 75% of this will be fluid.
• Expired air contains 44 mg water/L and this will be ↑ in fever, with ↑ respiration rates, and by reduced water content of inspired air, e.g. at high altitudes.

Fluid requirements

The amount of fluid consumed is very variable. In normal conditions 30–35 mL/kg body weight is required daily. The European Food Safety Agency (2010)[1] has published a scientific opinion on adequate intake of water (Table 7.6). Note that >20% of daily water intake is consumed in food; this varies between cultures and countries. In some disease states, i.e. cardiac, hepatic, and renal disease, it may be necessary to restrict fluid intake to prevent fluid overload (see ➜ Chapter 23, 'Cardiovascular disease', p. 519, ➜ Chapter 28, 'Liver disease', p. 689, and ➜ Chapter 29, 'Kidney disease', p. 703).

1 European Food Safety Authority (2010). Scientific Opinion on Reference Values for Water. EFSA J. 8(3), 1459 [48 pp.]. doi·10,2903/j.efsa.2010.1459.

Table 7.6 Reference vales for adequate intake (AI) of water (European Food Safety Authority, EFSA, 2010)*

	Age	AI (mL/day)
Infants	0–6 months	680
	6–12 months	800–1000
Children	1–2 years	1100–1200
	2–3 years	1100–1200
	4–8 years	1600
	9–13 years	
	Boys	2100
	Girls	1900
	> 14 years	As adults
Adults (including elderly)	Men	2500
	Women	2000
Pregnant women		+ 300
Lactating women		+ 600–700

*Source: data from European Food Safety Authority (2010) Scientific Opinion on Reference Values for Water *EFSA Journal* 2010; 8(3):1459.

Food labelling, functional foods, nutrigenetics, and nutrigenomics and food supplements

Food labelling 188
Functional foods and nutraceuticals 196
Nutrigenetics and nutrigenomics 198
Food supplements 202

Food labelling

Many laws relating to food labelling in the UK are of European Union (EU) origin. How EU rules affect food labelling laws in the UK in the future will depend on the changes to the UK's membership of the EU.

Food labelling in the UK is mostly controlled by the Food Information for Consumers Regulation No. 1169/2011 (FIR). Its purpose is to ensure that people can make informed choices about food and to prevent misleading practices. It helps protect consumers by setting down rules to ensure food labels are easy to see, read and understand, and are honest.

Information required by law

Front of packet

Product name

This must be clearly stated and products with 'made up' names must give a description of the food. If the food has undergone processing, e.g. 'smoked', the process must be stated. The name must also distinguish between similar products. For example, 'orange drink' must contain oranges while 'orange flavoured drinks' can be made with artificial flavourings. Some foods have legal names that must be used if the product meets certain conditions.

Shelf life

Labels must give information on how long the product will last once it has been bought or opened. This information is intended to ensure the safety and quality of the food and to prevent food poisoning or food-borne illnesses. A lot number or 'use by date' must be shown. The 'use-by' date label must be present on perishable foods such as cooked meats, which deteriorate and can be dangerous to health after a relatively short period. 'Best before' must be expressed as a day, month, and year and is used to in-dicate that a food's flavour, colour, or texture may not be at its best beyond this period, although it is probably still safe to eat. For products with a shelf life longer than 3 months 'Best before end' is used. 'Display until' is used by some retailers to alert staff to the need to remove products from sale, although the practice is discouraged as consumers can find two date labels confusing. Wine and spirits do not have to be date marked.

Weight or volume

The volume or weight of the product must be shown on the label. This en-ables consumers to compare the value of different brands. The symbol 'e' shows that the weight complies with EU requirements in that the average pack is at least the declared weight. Some foods, e.g. butter, tea, are sold only in standard amounts. Products that weigh <5 g do not have to have a stated weight, except for herbs and spices. If a packaged food is sold instead by number, the number of items must be clearly seen and easily counted from the outside.

Any necessary warnings

The label should have an appropriate warning for certain ingredients (sweeteners or sugars, aspartame and colourings, liquorice, caffeine and polyols); the warnings are very specific and must confirm to guidance, e.g.

if polyols are present the label should have the following warning 'Excessive consumption may cause a laxative effect'.[1]

The following must be on the food label but not necessarily on the front.

Ingredient list and quantity

Ingredients are listed in descending order of weight if the product has two or more ingredients, including food additives. All ingredients including additives and water must be listed, and the ingredients that make up a compound ingredient, e.g. pepperoni on a pizza.

Quantitative ingredient declaration

An ingredient that is featured in a photograph or drawing on a pack or in the description of the product, e.g. potatoes in cheese and potato pie, must state the quantity of the ingredient declared as a percentage. This is required by EU labelling law and is known as quantitative ingredient declaration (QUID).

Name and address of manufacturer, packer, or seller

These details must be stated on the package so that the consumers have a point of contact if they want to make a complaint or need more information.

Storage instructions

Details must be given on the conditions needed to ensure freshness. Following the instructions should ensure that the product's appearance and taste are optimum and prevent spoiling too quickly, so minimizing the risk of food poisoning.

Country of origin

The label must clearly state where the food is from if it would be misleading not to show it, e.g. French onion soup made in Scotland.

Instructions for use

Instructions on how to prepare and cook the product must be printed on the packaging when necessary. Oven temperature and cooking time are stated if the product needs heating; instructions on microwave cooking may also be given. The instructions are given so that the food can be consumed at its best and to reduce the risk of food poisoning by usually heating to a core temperature of 75°C.

The label must also show any of the following that apply:
• a warning for drinks with an alcohol content >1.2%;
• a warning if the product contains genetically modified ingredients, unless their presence is accidental and ≤0.9%;
• a warning if the product has been irradiated;
• the words 'packaged in a protective atmosphere' if the food is packaged using a packaging gas.

Special rules

There are special rules about what the following products can be called and what must be shown on the label:
• bottled water;
• bread and flour;

1 Gov.uk. *Food labelling and packaging*. Available at: ℘ http://www.gov.uk/food-labelling-and-packaging.

- cocoa and chocolate products;
- fats and oils;
- fish;
- fruit juices and nectars;
- honey;
- jams and preserves;
- meat and meat products;
- milk and milk products;
- soluble coffee;
- sugar.

Allergenic ingredients

Food and drink labels must state clearly if they contain ingredients to which people may be allergic or intolerant. The list of allergens that must be labelled is set down in EU law (see Box 8.1). The manufacturer must also make it clear if ingredients are made-of or derived from the allergens, e.g. it is not enough to state 'glaze'; the label must state 'glaze made from eggs'. The exception arises for ingredients derived from allergens that have been processed and are no longer allergenic; these do not need to be labelled with reference to the parent allergen. For example, glucose syrup made from wheat can be labelled just as 'glucose syrup'. Only ingredients that have been assessed and deemed safe by the European Food Safety Authority (EFSA) are exempt.

There is a specific EU law covering composition and labelling of gluten containing foods. Set levels of gluten permitted in foods making gluten free claims are stipulated:

- gluten free—the gluten content of foods bearing this claim must not exceed 20 ppm;
- very low gluten—the gluten content of foods bearing this claim must not exceed 100 ppm (only foods with cereal ingredients that have been specially processed to remove the gluten may make this claim).

Box 8.1 Allergenic ingredients that must be listed

- Celery
- Cereals containing gluten—wheat, rye, oats, barley
- Crustaceans, e.g. lobster, crab
- Eggs
- Fish
- Lupin
- Milk (including lactose)
- Molluscs
- Mustard
- Nuts from trees—e.g. almonds, pistachios, brazil nuts, walnuts, hazelnuts, cashews, pecan, macadamia
- Peanuts
- Sesame seeds
- Soybeans
- Sulphur dioxide and sulphites at >10 mg/kg or L

Genetically modified ingredients

EU regulations stipulate that foods that contain genetically modified organisms (GMO) or ingredients made from GMOs must be indicated on the label. Foods produced using genetically modified (GM) technology and animal products from animals fed GM feed do not have to be labelled. Loose GM food must be displayed next to information that states that it is genetically modified. More information is available at ⅋ https://www.food.gov.uk/safety-hygiene/genetically-modified-foods.

Food additives

Additives in a product must be declared on the label in the ingredients list and must be listed by appropriate category, e.g. preservative followed by the specific name (e.g. sulphur dioxide) or E number (e.g. E220). See ➔ 'Food additives' in Chapter 9, p. 831.

Nutrition information labelling

Nutrition labelling is now required by law on the majority of pre-packed foods and must include the items shown below in bold. The nutrition information label can also, on a voluntary basis, include the amounts of monounsaturates, polyunsaturates, polyols, starch, fibre, and vitamins and minerals.

- **Energy** (kJ and kcal)
- **Fat** (g)
  - Of which:
  - Saturates (g)
  - Monounsaturates (g)
  - Polyunsaturates (g)
- **Carbohydrate** (g)
  - Of which:
  - Sugars (g)
  - Polyols (g)
  - Starch (g)
- **Fibre** (g)
- **Protein** (g)
- **Salt** (g)
- **Vitamins and minerals** (specific units are given in the regulation)

Salt is declared instead of sodium to aid consumer understanding. Values can be given per 100 g or per 100 mL, and per portion if the quantity and number of portions in the pack are shown. Vitamins and minerals can only be shown if the food will provide a significant amount of the nutrient reference value defined in the regulation.

Nutrition and health claims

In July 2006, an EU Regulation set out clear rules on nutrition and health claims to protect consumers from misleading or false claims. In 2011, the Department of Health published guidance on complying with this regulation.[2] Table 8.1 defines a 'nutrition claim' and a 'health claim'. This regulation not only covers claims made in words, e.g. 'high in fibre', but also claims

2 Department of Health. *Nutrition and health claims. Guidance to compliance with Regulation (EC) 1924/2006 on nutrition and health claims made on foods*, Version 2, November 2011. Available at: ⅋ http://www.gov.uk/government/uploads/system/uploads/attachment_data/file/204320/Nutrition_and_health_claims_guidance_November_2011.pdf.

Table 8.1 Definitions of nutrition and health claims

Claim	Definition	Example
Nutrition claim	'Any claim which states, suggests or implies that a food has particular beneficial nutritional properties from (a) the energy it provides at a reduced or increased rate, or does not provide, and/or (b) the nutrients or other substances it contains in reduced or increased proportions, or does not contain'	'High fibre, 'low energy', 'light', 'source of protein', 'high in vitamin D'
Health claim	'Any claim that states, suggests or implies that a relationship exists between a food category, a food or one of its constituents and health'	'Calcium helps build strong bones', 'good for you'

made as pictures, graphics, or symbols, e.g. a heart shape. It regulates claims made to consumers whether on food packets, websites, or leaflets.

Nutrition labelling must be given if a nutrition or health claim is made. Only authorized claims may be made. The list of nutrition claims is shown in Table 8.2. The EU maintains a searchable register of health claims, which can be found at ℞http://ec.europa.eu/food/safety/labelling_nutrition/claims/register/public/?event=register.home.

Organic
In the UK the Department for Environment, Food and Rural Affairs (DEFRA) regulates the bodies that can certify organic producers and manufacturers. The Soil Association administers 75% of certification. Organic food must contain at least 95% of organic ingredients by weight and can be labelled 'organic'. Organic food must use the EU's organic logo and display the code number and prefix of the certification body. Organic food cannot legally contain GM or irradiated foods.

Signposting
In addition to the nutrition labelling, some foods will have a display that signals to the consumer the % reference intake (RI), for energy, total fat, saturated fat, sugars, and salt consumed in a portion of the food. The actual amount in the portion is also displayed in kcal and kJ or g as appropriate. This is voluntary on the part of the manufacturers. In addition, a traffic light system can be used where red, amber, and green are used to indicate a 'high' content (red), amber 'medium' content, and green 'low' content. This is based on 100 g of the food unless the amount of the nutrient is >30% of the RI. Energy is not colour-coded. This type of labelling is often called 'front of pack' nutrition labelling, and serves to provide the consumer with 'at-a-glance' nutrition information.

Reference intakes
RIs, which replace guideline daily amounts (GDAs), are shown in Table 8.3. They are based on the requirements of a healthy, average woman without special dietary needs and an assumed energy intake of 8.4 MJ or 2000 kcal/d.

Table 8.2 Nutrition claims and the conditions applying to them

Nutrient	Claim	Conditions*
Energy	Low energy	≤40 kcal (170 kJ) per 100 g solids ≤20 kcal (80 kJ) per 100 mL liquids
	Energy reduced	≥30% reduction
	Energy free	≤4 kcal (17 kJ) per 100 mL
Fat	Low fat	≤3 g per 100 g solids ≤1.5 g per 100 mL liquids 1.8 g per 100 mL for semi-skimmed milk
	Fat free	≤0.5 g per 100 g or 100 mL 'X% fat free' prohibited
	Low saturated fat	≤1.5 g per 100 g solids ≤0.75 g per 100 mL liquids
	Saturated fat free	≤0.1 g per 100 g or 100 mL
	High unsaturated fat	≥70% of the fatty acids present derive from unsaturated fat under the condition that unsaturated fat provides >20% of energy of the product
	High polyunsaturated fat (PUFA)	≥45% of the fatty acids present derive from PUFA under the condition that PUFA provide >20% of energy of the product
	High monounsaturated fat (MUFA)	≥45% of the fatty acids present derive from MUFA under the condition that MUFA provide >20% of energy of the product
	Source of omega-3 fatty acids	≥0.3 g α-linolenic acid per 100 g and per 100 kcal, _or_ ≥40 mg of the sum of eicosapentaenoic acid (EPA) and docosahexaenoic acid (DHA) per 100 g and per 100 kcal
	High omega-3 fatty acids	≥0.6g α-linolenic acid per 100 g and per 100 kcal, _or_ ≥80 mg of the sum of EPA and DHA per 100 g and per 100 kcal
Sugar	Low sugar	≤5 g per 100 g solids 2.5 g per 100 mL liquids
	Sugar free	≤0.5 g per 100 g or 100 mL
	With no added sugar	Does not contain any added mono- or disaccharides or any other food used for its sweetening properties. If sugars are naturally present in the food, the following indication should also appear on the label: 'CONTAINS NATURALLY OCCURRING SUGARS'.

Table 8.2 (*Contd.*)

Nutrient	Claim	Conditions*
Sodium/salt	Low sodium/salt	≤0.12 g sodium or equivalent value for salt per 100 g or 100 mL
	Very low sodium/salt	≤0.04 g sodium or equivalent value for salt per 100 g or 100 mL
	Sodium or salt free	≤0.005 g sodium or equivalent value for salt per 100 g or 100 mL
	No added sodium/salt	Does not contain any added sodium/salt and product contains ≤0.12 g sodium or the equivalent value for salt per 100g or 100 mL
Fibre	Source of fibre	≥3 g per 100 g solids ≥1.5 g per 100 kcal
	High fibre	≥6 g per 100g ≥3 g per 100 kcal
Protein	Source of protein	≥12% energy from protein
	High protein	≥20% energy from protein
Vitamins/minerals	Source of (name of vitamin/s) or (name of mineral/s)	At least a significant amount (as a rule, significant amount means 15% of the recommended daily allowance provided by 100 g or 100 mL of the food, or per package if contains only a single portion)
	High (name of vitamin/s) or (name of mineral/s)	At least twice the value of 'source of' as above
Comparative claims	Increased	Meets the conditions for 'source of' and the increase is ≥30% compared with a similar product
	Reduced	≥30% compared with a similar product 10% for micronutrients 25% for sodium or salt
	Light/lite	As for 'reduced'
Naturally/natural	Where a food or drink naturally meets the conditions for the use of a nutrition claim, the term 'naturally/natural' may be used as a prefix to the claim	

*See Annex of Regulation (EC) No 1924/2006 for full details.

Table 8.3 Reference intakes (RI) for adults

Energy (kcal/kJ)	2000/8400
Fat (g)	70
Of which saturates (g)	20
Total carbohydrate (g)	260
Of which sugars (g)	90
Protein (g)	50
Salt (g)	6

Functional foods and nutraceuticals

- *Functional foods* are foods that when consumed regularly, as part of the usual diet, exert a specific health-beneficial effect beyond their basic nutritional value.
- *Nutraceuticals* (nutrition and pharmaceutical) are products isolated or purified from foods, generally sold in medicinal forms (such as a pill or capsule), and demonstrated to have a physiological benefit or provide protection against chronic disease.

Many nutrients and foods have nutrient or health claims as functional foods or nutraceuticals but the claims are not always proven. There is currently no law that controls these claims. It is generally accepted that health claims such as 'can help lower cholesterol as part of a low fat diet' can be made if the claim is supported by scientific research and is not misleading (➔ this Chapter, 'Food labelling', p. 188). Functional or 'novel' foods must go through a safety approval process before they are launched. Products that were on sale before 1997 do not have to undergo this process. In the UK, the Joint Health Claims Initiative has established guidance on a voluntary scheme for health.

A functional food may be:
- a natural food;
- a food to which a component has been added;
- a food from which a component has been removed;
- a food where one or more components has been modified;
- a food in which the bioavailability has been modified.

Categories of functional foods and nutraceuticals are shown in Table 8.4.

Functional food ingredients

The beneficial health effects of functional foods result from the presence of a variety of bioactive components that elicit their effects via a number of different mechanisms. These substances (bioactives) often originate from plant sources but some are also derived from animals and micro-organisms. Box 8.2 and Table 8.5 list examples of functional food ingredients.

Table 8.4 Categories of functional foods and nutraceuticals

Category	Example
Basic food	Tomatoes (rich in natural antioxidant lycopene)
Processed foods	Oat bran cereal
Processed food with added ingredients	Calcium-enriched fruit juice
Foods enhanced to have more of a functional component	Oat bran with higher levels β-glucan
Isolated, purified preparations of active food ingredients	Isoflavones from soya

Source: data from Arvanitoyannis, I.S., Van Houwelingen-Koukaliaroglou, M. (2005). Functional foods: A survey of health claims, pros and cons, and current legislation. *Crit. Rev. Food Sci. Nutr.*, 45, p. 390, table 3.

Regulation of functional foods

The effects of functional foods on health must be scientifically proven. In Europe, the assessment of the scientific evidence to support health claims is the responsibility of the EFSA (🔗 http://www.efsa.europa.eu). The process of assessment of claims is currently ongoing, but, to date, positive EFSA opinions on claims have included: plant sterol/stanols and cholesterol reduction, xylitol and caries reduction, α-linolenic acid (ALA) and brain development in children, and long-chain polyunsaturated fatty acids and visual development in children.

Box 8.2 Examples of functional foods

- Dairy spreads enriched with plant sterols/stanols
- Omega-3-enriched eggs and bread
- Yoghurts with probiotics and prebiotics
- Oat breakfast cereal rich in β-glucan

Table 8.5 Examples of bioactive functional food ingredients

Functional Ingredient	Food Source	Potential Effect on Health
β-glucan	Oats	↓ blood cholesterol; ↓ the postprandial glycaemic response; aid weight control
Conjugated linoleic acid (CLA)	Cheese, meat products	Improve body fat composition, enhance immune system; ↓ risk of cancer
Flavonoids (ex. catechins)	Tea, fruits, vegetables	Neutralize free radicals; ↓ risk of cancer
Lycopene (carotenoid)	Tomatoes	↓ risk of prostate cancer
Omega-3 fatty acids (α-linolenic acid, ALA, eicosapentaenoic acid, EPA, and docosahexaenoic acid, DHA)	Salmon and fish oils;	↓ risk of cardiovascular disease (CVD); may improve mental and visual functions
Phytoestrogens (e.g. isoflavones)	Soybeans and soy-based foods	Alleviate symptoms associated with the menopause; protect against heart disease and some cancers; ↓ low-density lipoprotein (LDL)- and total cholesterol; improve bone mineral density
Plant sterols/stanols/stanol esters	Corn, soy, wheat, wood oils	↓ absorption of cholesterol in the body and ∴ lower blood cholesterol levels (total and LDL-cholesterol by ~10%). ❶ May interfere with absorption of other fat-soluble components from the diet, data on effects of long-term consumption at levels >3 g/day are limited
Prebiotics (e.g. inulin, fructooligosaccharides)	Jerusalem artichokes, shallots, onion powder	Not digested by the gut and stimulate the growth of certain bacteria in the colon. Improve quality of intestinal microflora; gastrointestinal (GI) health
Probiotics ('live' bacteria e.g. *Lactobacillus acidophilus*)	Yoghurt and other dairy products	Improve quality of intestinal microflora; GI health

Nutrigenetics and nutrigenomics

Nutrigenetics is the influence of the genotype on nutritionally related disease; nutrigenomics is the effect of diet on whole-body metabolism (Fig. 8.1).

Nutri(epi)genetics refers to the study of heritable changes in gene expression that occur without a change in the primary DNA sequence. Epigenetic mechanisms of altering gene regulation are DNA methylation histone modifications and genetic imprinting (see Box 8.3).

Nutrigenomics refers to the study of interactions between dietary factors and genes that can promote health or cause disease. It involves the use of various molecular tools (genomics, transcriptomics, proteomics, metabolomics) to explore how dietary substances interact with the genome (see Box 8.4). Nutrigenomics views nutrients and bioactive food components as 'dietary signals' that can directly or indirectly alter the genomic structure or function and molecular events. The ultimate goal of nutrigenomics is to determine the dietary factors that are most compatible with health for a given individual (personalized nutrition).

Nutrigenomics adheres to the following precepts
- Poor nutrition can be a risk factor for diseases.
- Common dietary chemicals can act on the human genome (either directly or indirectly) to alter gene expression and/or gene structure.
- The degree to which diet influences the balance between health and disease depends on the individual's genetic makeup.
- Some diet-regulated genes (and their normal, common variants) are likely to play a role in the onset, incidence, progression, and/or severity of chronic diseases.
- Dietary intervention based on knowledge of nutritional requirement, nutritional status, and genotype can be used to prevent, mitigate or cure chronic disease.[3]

Practical applications of nutrigenomics
- Identify the genes and proteins expressed differentially in health and disease that are modifiable by nutrients.
- Identify which genes, proteins, and metabolites are influenced by specific nutrients that are known to be beneficial or harmful.
- Identify genetic variations that alter the nutrient-gene interactions in the applications above.[4]

Gastrointestinal microbiota

It is estimated that there are 10^{14} bacteria in the human gut. Some components of the gastrointestinal (GI) microbiota compete with enteropathogens, regulate innate and adaptive immune function, and ferment non-digestible carbohydrates to produce short chain fatty acids.[5] The GI microbiota can

---

3 Kaput, J., Rodrigues, R.L. (2004). Nutritional Genomics: the next frontier in the postgenomic era. *Physiol. Genom.* **16**, 166–77.

4 Kornman, K.S., *et al.* (2004). Genetic variations and inflammation: a practical nutrigenomics opportunity. *Nutr.* **20**, 44–9.

5 Neish, A.S. (2009). Microbes in gastrointestinal health and disease. *Gastroenterology* **136**, 65–80.

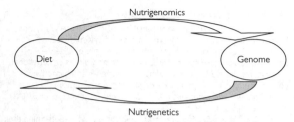

Fig. 8.1 The relationship between nutrigenomics and nutrigenetics.

Box 8.3 Nutrigenetics

- Aims to understand how the genetic makeup of an individual coordinates their response to diet.
- Characterizes gene variants associated with differential responses to nutrients and relates this variation to disease states.
- Typically characterizes single nucleotide polymorphisms (SNPs) with regards to their frequency in a given population and to their relevance for metabolic health disorders.

be modified using probiotics and prebiotics, and some studies have shown that this reduces the disease risk or severity.

Probiotics

Probiotics are defined as 'live microorganisms which when administered in adequate amounts confer a health benefit on the host'. The criteria for a probiotic include being safe for human use, able to survive transit through the GI tract, and having the physiological capacity to provide health benefits. Probiotics are usually acid-tolerant bacteria, such as lactobacilli and bifidobacteria, and are available in the form of functional foods (e.g. yogurts, fermented milks, juices) or as tablets, capsules, or powders.

The effect of probiotics has been investigated in numerous clinical settings. The results vary depending upon the strain and dose given, and therefore generic recommendations for probiotic use cannot be given. However, areas where evidence increasingly shows benefit for some probiotics include:

- symptoms of irritable bowel syndrome, e.g. *Lactobacillus plantarum* 299V, *Bifidobacterium animalis* DN-173 010;[6]
- treatment and maintenance of inflammatory bowel disease, e.g. *Escherichia coli* Nissle, *Saccharomyces boulardii*;[7]
- prevention of antibiotic-associated diarrhoea e.g. *Lactobacillus caseii* DN114 011;
- prevention of recurrent *Clostridium difficile* diarrhoea, e.g. *S. boulardii*.

6 Moayyedi, P., et al. (2010). The efficacy of probiotics in the treatment of irritable bowel syndrome: a systematic review. *Gut* **59**, 325–32.

7 Hedin, C., et al. (2007). Evidence for the use of probiotics and prebiotics in inflammatory bowel disease: a review of clinical trials. *Proc. Nutr. Soc.* **66**, 307–15.

Box 8.4 Nutrigenomic technologies

- *Transcriptomics:* The simultaneous analysis of the mRNA transcripts from a cell's genome, including modifications that may occur to the transcripts. It provides a comprehensive system-wide view of gene-expression patterns in states of health and disease. Nutritional transcriptomics studies the influence of nutrients and bioactive food components on global gene expression and transcription.
- *Transcriptome:* The complete collection of gene transcripts (mRNAs) in a cell or tissue at a given time.
- *Proteomics:* The study of proteomes which attempts to determine their role inside the cells and molecules with which they interact. Proteomics refers to techniques for measuring global protein expression.
- *Proteome:* The complement of expressed proteins in a biological system whether it be a cell, its organelles, or the entire organism at a given time.
- *Metabolomics:* The study of small molecules or metabolites present in biological samples (such as biofluids, tissues, and cellular extracts), which attempts to correlate the metabolomic profiles with known physiological or pathological states. The aim of metabolomics is to profile all the metabolites present in the samples to enhance the understanding of the effect of a particular stimulus on metabolic pathways. Metabolomics allows the analysis of hundreds of metabolites in a given biological sample.
- *Metabolome:* The full complement of metabolites in a sample at a given time (see Fig. 8.2).

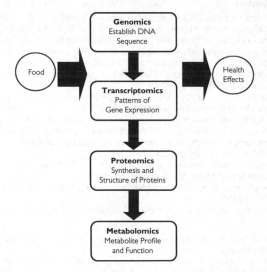

Fig. 8.2 Nutrigenomic technologies.

Prebiotics

Prebiotics are defined as non-digestible food components that 'selectively stimulate the growth and/or activity of one or a limited number of microbial genera, species or strains in the gut microbiota that confer health benefits to the host'. The major prebiotics are fructo-oligosaccharides (FOS), galacto-oligosaccharides (GOS), and lactulose. FOS are found naturally in chicory, wheat, and onions, and GOS are found in beans and pulses. Studies have shown that in their powdered supplement form (3.5–15 g/day), prebiotics can result in the increased growth of colonic bifidobacteria.

There is emerging evidence of the role of prebiotics in irritable bowel syndrome and inflammatory bowel disease.

Food fortification

Some foods are supplemented with nutrients for their benefits above normal health benefits. In the UK, flour is fortified with Ca, and margarine and spreads are fortified with vitamins A and D.

Folate fortification

Folate is frequently added to cereals, and there is considerable debate in the UK as to whether or not to fortify all flour and flour products. Flour is fortified with folate in the USA, Canada, and Chile. The arguments for and against folate fortification are as follows.

- Arguments for the fortification of flour with folate:
  - prevention of neural tube defects;
  - low folate status is associated with elevated homocysteine, which is a risk factor for cardiovascular disease and is linked to some cancers including colon and breast cancer.
- Arguments against the fortification of flour with folate:
  - there is uncertainty about the bioavailability of folate;
  - consumer choice;
  - high consumption of folic acid may mask the diagnosis of vitamin B_{12} deficiency in the elderly.

A recent Scientific Advisory Committee on Nutrition report recommended the supplementation of flour in the UK, although accompanied by some restrictions and a recommendation for careful monitoring of emerging evidence and dietary surveys of folate intake and status. However, in the UK this will require a change to the law and the government has not yet made a decision on folate fortification.

Food supplements

Food supplements

Food supplements are defined by EU law as 'foodstuffs the purpose of which is to supplement the normal diet and which are concentrated sources of nutrients (vitamins and minerals) or other substances with a nutritional or physiological effect, alone or in combination, marketed in dose form … designed to be taken in measured small unit quantities'.

The growing interest in diet and health has stimulated the market for dietary supplements. In 1991, the market for dietary supplements was £194 million and this had risen to £414 million in 2015. The range of supplements available in health food shops, chemists, and supermarkets is growing, but vitamins, minerals, and fish liver oils remain the most popular. In 2015/16, 65% of all adults reported taking supplements either daily or occasionally.

Health information

The average diet in the UK supplies adequate vitamins and minerals to prevent deficiency, and for the majority of people supplements are not necessary. Vulnerable groups, e.g. vegetarians, the elderly, and pregnant women, may benefit from supplements. There is little evidence to support the blanket use of supplements. However, there are a few well-established cases, e.g. additional folate in pregnancy (see ➦ Chapter 12, 'Diet before and during pregnancy', p. 237), additional calcium in osteoporosis. Most supplements are bought over the counter and are self-prescribed.

The range of nutrition supplements is vast and cannot be adequately covered in this format. Information on the health benefits of specific supplements can be obtained from the Health Supplements Information Service (🖱 http://www.hsis.org).

Micronutrient supplements

In 2003, the Expert Group on Vitamins and Minerals published its report on the safety of vitamins and minerals in food supplements and fortified foods. Safe upper limits were set for all vitamins and most minerals. The full report can be found at: 🖱https://cot.food.gov.uk/committee/committee-on-toxicity/cotreports/cotjointreps/evmreport.

Regulation

Food supplements fall between medicines and foods and it has been difficult to regulate their marketing. However, in 2002, the EU issued the Food Supplements Directive and the directive and regulations have applied since August 2005. The directive lists vitamins and minerals that can be used in supplements. Work was undertaken to permit additions to the originally listed vitamins and minerals, but at this time, tin, nickel, cobalt, and van-adium are excluded.

A second list gives details of the chemical forms that may be used. These forms are considered safe. Work on setting maximum and minimum dose levels for use in food supplements has never been progressed.

Labelling

Manufacturers must not make claims referring to the prevention, treatment, or curing of diseases or refer to such properties. The label must display:
- the words 'food supplement';
- names of the nutrients and substances;
- portion required for daily use;
- warning not to exceed stated dose;
- statement to the effect that supplements should not replace a varied diet;
- statement that the product should be stored away from children;
- it should not be implied that a balanced and varied diet cannot provide adequate amounts of nutrients;
- amounts of nutrients available in the recommended dose.

Oral nutritional supplements

A wide range of liquid, semi-solid, or powder supplement products are available that provide either one or more macronutrients or, more usually, a combination of macro and micronutrients. Oral nutritional supplements are regulated as foods for special medical purposes (No. 2016/128). In many cases oral nutritional supplements are nutritionally complete (nutrition-ally balanced), and, as such, they can be used as a sole source of nutrition if taken in sufficient quantities. See ➔ Chapter 25, 'Nutrition Support' (p. 555).

Non-nutrient components of food

Alcohol *206*
Biologically active dietary constituents *210*
Food additives *214*

Alcohol

The alcohol present in alcoholic drinks is ethanol (ethyl alcohol), C_2H_5OH. Ethanol is produced by fermentation of glucose in plants. Sugars in grapes and apples are fermented to produce wine and cider; barley starch is hydrolysed to glucose in the production of beer. Other fruits and cereals are used to produce alcoholic drinks, e.g. rice for sake and rye for some whisky. The resultant alcohol is diluted to produce the appropriate alcohol content of drinks. By law, drink labels must show the strength of alcohol present; this is expressed as the percentage alcohol by volume (abv). Note that 10% abv is equivalent to 7.9 g of alcohol per 100 mL (Box 9.1).

> **Box 9.1 Alcohol by volume in examples of alcoholic drinks**
>
> - *Ciders and beers:* 4–6% abv
> - *Wines:* 9–13% abv
> - *Fortified wines:* 18–25% abv
> - *Liqueurs:* 20–40% abv
> - *Spirits, e.g. gin:* 40% abv

Low alcohol and strong variations of some drinks are now produced. Other substances are added to provide flavour, such as juniper berries in gin and hops in beer. Alcoholic drinks may also contain sugars, small amounts of other alcohols, e.g. propyl alcohol, potassium, and small amounts of riboflavin and niacin. In the UK 1 unit of alcohol drink contains 8 g or 10 mL of pure alcohol (see Table 9.1). Other systems are used by other countries.

Alcohol metabolism

Ethanol is quickly absorbed in the stomach and jejunum and distributed throughout total body water including blood. Alcohol is distributed via the blood to the brain and the liver where it is metabolized by alcohol dehydrogenase (ADeH) to acetaldehyde, which is converted to acetate by the enzyme aldehyde dehydrogenase (ALDH). ADeH is the rate limiting step in the metabolism of alcohol and there is a great deal of variation between individuals in their ability to metabolize alcohol. On average, approximately 5–10 g of alcohol (1/2–1 unit of alcoholic drink) is metabolized per hour. The stages of alcohol intoxication are shown in Table 9.2. Alcohol absorption can be slowed by the presence of food in the stomach. Smaller people have smaller livers and ∴ metabolize alcohol more slowly; women have smaller livers than men and ∴ become intoxicated more quickly. Some alcohol is excreted in breath, which provides an easy monitor of alcohol intoxication. Disulfiram (Antabuse®) antagonizes ALDH and is a drug used to treat alcoholism. The build-up of acetaldehyde leads to headache, nausea, and vomiting. Alcoholics have an induced system of alcohol metabolism known as the microsomal ethanol-oxidizing system (MEOS); this system is thermogenic.

Table 9.1 Alcohol (units) in some popular drinks

Drink	Bar measure	mL	Units
Spirit, e.g. whisky, gin, vodka (abv 40%)	1 single optic measure	25	1
Wine (abv 12%)	1 small glass	125	1.5
Higher lager, beer, cider (abv 5.2%)	1 pint	573	3
Lower strength lager, beer, cider (abv 3.6%)	1 pint	573	2
Lager, beer, cider (abv 4.5%)	1 can	440	2
Lager, beer, cider (abv 5%)	1 bottle	330	1.7
Alcopop (abv 5.5%)	1 bottle	275	1.5

Table 9.2 Stages of acute alcohol intoxication

Blood alcohol concentration (mg/100 mL)	Stage	Effects
Up to 50	Feeling of wellbeing	Relaxed, talkative
50–80	Risky	Fine movements and judgement affected
50		Legal limit for drink driving prosecution in Scotland
80		Legal limit for drink driving prosecution in the rest of the UK
80–150	Dangerous	Slurred speech, balance affected, blurred vision, drowsiness, nausea and vomiting
200–400	Drunken stupor	Dead drunk, loss of bladder and bowel control, unconscious
450–600	Death	Shock and death

Nutritional value of alcohol

Alcohol is an energy source providing 29 kJ (7 kcal) per gram. Alcoholics do not obtain this level of energy from alcohol because of the thermogenic nature of MEOS.

Recommendation on alcohol intake

In the UK the Department of Health recommends that both men and women consume <14 units per week on a regular basis. If you drinking as much as 14 units/week, it is best to spread this out over 3–4 days. Standard measures of drinks providing 1 unit of alcohol are shown in Table 9.1.

A personal alcohol intake tracker is available at Drinkaware ($\mathcal{O}$ https://www.drinkaware.co.uk).

Alcohol consumption

It is difficult to estimate alcohol consumption because of the social stigma associated with excessive drinking and the effects of alcohol on mental capacity. The National Diet and Nutrition Survey[1] found that, on average, adult men consumed 3 units (31.7g)/day and women consumed nearly 2 units (17.5g)/day; this figure was calculated including non-drinkers.

Acute effects of alcohol

The response to alcohol is variable; this variation a result of the extent of stimulation of the sympathetic nervous system and the rate of production of acetaldehyde and acetate. The most common effects are ↑ in heart rate and peripheral vasodilatation. As a result of the peripheral vasodilation, some people feel excessively warm and some experience facial flushing. The psychological and physiological responses to acute alcohol excess are listed in Table 9.2

Alcohol is a central nervous system depressant and acts as an anaesthetic. Diuresis (increased urine production) results from the action of alcohol on the pituitary gland and leads to dehydration.

Effects of alcohol on health

Light to moderate consumption of alcohol has been shown to have beneficial health effects in reducing the risk of coronary heart disease in men and post-menopausal women. The most established mechanism is that this level of alcohol consumption ↑ plasma high-density lipoprotein. An additional proposed mechanism is that alcohol ↓ platelet aggregation and ∴ ↓ the risk of thrombosis. It has been proposed that polyphenolic compounds in wines have antioxidant properties that reduce the plasma levels of low-density lipoproteins.

Excessive alcohol consumption has been linked to ↑ risk of breast cancer in women and oesophageal and liver cancer in men and women. High intakes of alcohol are strongly associated with ↑ risk of liver disease. Hypertension risk is ↑ by high levels of alcohol intake.

The harmful physical effects of alcohol abuse are extensive and some are listed in Table 9.3. Thiamin deficiency can result from chronic, excessive alcohol intake as thiamin is required for ethanol metabolism and dietary intake may be poor. This can → Wernicke's encephalopathy and Korsakoff's psychosis. Other vitamin deficiencies are rare but do occur in alcoholics, e.g. folate and vitamin C. Alcohol is estimated to be a factor in 20–30% of accidents and has socio-economic consequences including domestic violence.

---

1 Public Health England & Food Standards Agency (2018). *The National Diet and Nutrition Survey: results from Years 7 and 8 (combined) of the Rolling Programme (2014/2015–2015/2016).* Public Health England, London.

Table 9.3 Physical health problems associated with excessive alcohol consumption

Body system	Effects
Nervous system	Acute intoxication, dementia, Wernicke-Korsakoff syndrome, cerebellar degeneration
Cerebrovascular system	Strokes, nerve and muscle damage
Liver	Fatty liver, cirrhosis, hepatitis, liver failure, cancer
Gastrointestinal system	Reflux, oesophageal rupture, oesophageal cancer, pancreatitis, gastritis, malabsorption
Nutrition	Reduced food intake and absorption leading to weight loss, obesity in early stages of heavy drinking
Heart and circulatory system	Arrhythmias, hypertension, heart muscle damage leading to heart failure
Respiratory system	Pneumonia from inhalation of vomit
Endocrine system	Overproduction of cortisol, hypoglycaemia, stimulation of the pituitary to cause diuresis
Reproductive system	Loss of libido, atrophy of testicles, reduced sperm count, menstrual abnormalities

Alcohol and vulnerable groups

Pregnant women: Alcohol may reduce the ability to conceive, and excessive consumption is associated with a greater risk of miscarriage. Pregnant women are advised not to drink at all, but, if they do, to consume no more than 1–2 units per week. Excessive alcohol consumption during pregnancy can → foetal alcohol syndrome, which may → facial deformities and growth problems (see ➲ Chapter 12, 'Diet before and during pregnancy', p. 237).

Diabetes: People with diabetes are advised not to drink excessively as this can → ↑ hypoglycaemic episodes.

Biologically active dietary constituents

Foods contain many chemicals that have no nutrient value but have physiological or pharmacological properties; these are often referred to as 'phytochemicals'. Some of these chemicals have protective properties, but some are toxic or may become toxic if taken in excess.

Antioxidants and anticarcinogenic phytochemicals

Epidemiological studies have shown that fruit and vegetables have positive effects on health, particularly the prevention of cancer and heart disease, as a result of the presence of the antioxidant vitamins, vitamin C, vitamin E, and β-carotene, and probably some as yet to be identified antioxidants or anticarcinogenic compounds. These chemicals prevent damage to body tissues by free radicals. This group of chemicals includes the carotenoids, polyphenols, glucosinolates, phytoestrogens, and sulphides.

Carotenoids

The carotenoids consist of approximately 100 compounds that occur naturally in plants; they often give fruits and vegetables a yellow or orange colour. Some can be converted into retinol (vitamin A) (see ➜ Chapter 6, 'Vitamin A (retinol)', p. 102); the most important of the carotenoids for retinol production is β-carotene. Carotenoids act as antioxidants by reacting with unpaired electrons in free radical and so neutralizing them. Another carotenoid that has received a lot of attention is lycopene; 85% of dietary lycopene is derived from tomatoes. Some studies have shown that lycopene may have anticarcinogenic properties and reduce the risk of heart disease.

Polyphenols

Phenolic compounds are found in many foods and beverages and act as a plant's defence system against animals and insects. Polyphenols are either antioxidants or potentiate the effects of other antioxidants. The following chemicals are types of polyphenols.
- Phytosterols are found in seeds and oils and inhibit cholesterol absorption.
- Over 4000 types of flavonoids have been identified. They are found in fruits, vegetables, nuts, and seeds. Onions, apples, and black tea are particular rich sources. Quercetin and catechins are examples of flavanoids.
- Tannins are present in red wines and tea, adding colour and flavour. They are antioxidants but bind to Fe and inhibit Fe absorption.
- Phytoestrogens are plant chemicals that are chemically similar to the animal hormone oestradiol. They compete for oestradiol receptors and can either ↑ or ↓ the effects of oestradiol. Isoflavones are phytoestrogens that are found in soya beans and soya products.
- Soya isoflavones have been shown to have hormonal effects and have been used to alleviate menopausal symptoms.
- Soya isoflavones have been shown to have anticarcinogenic properties in in vitro studies, but the effects are variable in humans. Some studies have suggested that excessive intakes of isoflavones may in fact be carcinogenic; ∴ concentrated supplements are not recommended.

- Sulphides are present in foods such as onion, leek, and garlic. They have been shown to have anticarcinogenic properties in animal studies. There is some epidemiological evidence to suggest that sulphides reduce the risk of colorectal and gastric cancers.
- Glucosinolates are present in plants of the brassica family such as cabbage, broccoli, kale, Brussels sprouts, and cauliflower. There is some evidence of anticarcinogenic properties of glucosinolates in experimental studies, but large intakes may actually be carcinogenic; more studies are required.

Caffeine and methylxanthines

Methylxanthines are a group of chemicals including caffeine, theophylline, and theobromine. They occur naturally in foods and drinks such as tea, coffee, cola drinks, and cocoa products (Box 9.2); they are also added to 'energy' drinks. Caffeine is a mild stimulant, although there is individual variation in this response. It is mildly addictive and abrupt cessation of caffeine intake can → mild withdrawal symptoms of headache, fatigue, and irritability. A daily intake of four to five cups of coffee is considered moderate; caffeine intake is dependent on the size of cup, the fineness of grinding, brewing method, roasting of beans, and type of coffee beans used. Arabica coffee beans contain less caffeine than Robusta beans. Tea has higher caffeine content than coffee on a dry weight basis but less tea is used to produce a drink.

By law, drinks containing caffeine in excess of 150 mg/L must carry a declaration in the same part of the label as the name of the food. Caffeine content, with the amount of caffeine expressed in mg per 100 mL, should be given to identify high levels of caffeine in some drinks (Box 9.2). This law does not apply to drinks based on tea or coffee, or coffee or tea extracts.

Box 9.2 Caffeine content of beverages

300 mg of caffeine is roughly equivalent to
- Four average cups or three average size mugs of instant coffee
- Three average cups of brewed coffee
- Six average cups of tea
- Eight cans of regular cola drinks
- Four cans of so-called 'energy' drinks
- 400 g (eight standard 50 g bars) of plain chocolate

Household measures of caffeine:
- Average cup of instant coffee—75 mg
- Average mug of coffee—100 mg
- Average cup of brewed coffee—100 mg
- Average cup of tea—50 mg
- Regular cola drink—up to 40 mg
- Regular energy drink—up to 80 mg
- 50 g bar of plain chocolate—50 mg. Caffeine in milk chocolate is about half that of plain chocolate

Caffeine is a mild diuretic if taken in quantities above that considered moderate. The evidence that caffeine reduces fertility is inconclusive. The Food Standards Agency (FSA) recommends that pregnant women should not have more than 200 mg of caffeine per day (see ➲ Chapter 12, 'Diet before and during pregnancy', p. 237). Some studies suggest that higher intakes are linked with miscarriage, low birth weight, and premature delivery. This is disputed by some researchers who have suggested that high caffeine intake is an indication of low hormone levels. Many women have a reduced desire for coffee during pregnancy, which is believed to result from high placental hormone levels, ∴ high coffee intake may be a marker of low hormone levels. The FSA recommends that coffee intake during breastfeeding should not be stopped, but that caffeine should only be taken occasionally as caffeine passes into breastmilk causing the baby to be restless and agitated (see ➲ Chapter 13, 'Breast versus bottle feeding', p. 262).

Decaffeinated brands are not totally free of caffeine, but usually contain <5 mg caffeine per cup; they contain smaller amounts of the other methylxanthines than normal brands.

Theobromine levels are low in beverages except chocolate products. High cocoa (70% cocoa beans) content brands have higher levels of caffeine and theobromine than average brands.

Vasoactive amines

Tyramine, histamine, tryptamine, and serotonin are all present in foods and are normally deactivated in the body. High intakes and intake in individuals with an impaired ability to deactivate them can → vasoconstrictive effects. Vasoactive amines can trigger migraine in susceptible people. People taking monoamine oxidase inhibitor type A drugs may experience a dangerous hypertensive interaction with vasoactive amine (see ➲ Chapter 38, 'Drug–nutrient interactions and prescription of nutritional products', p. 833).

Food additives

Food additives are substances added to food for technological reasons, which may be their organoleptic properties. They are classified into groups according to their purpose. The numbering system is being adapted for international use by the Codex Alimentarius Commission. The International Numbering System (INS) will use the same numbers used within the European Community but without the E prefix. The use of food additives is controlled by the Food Standards Agency in the UK and European Scientific Committee for Food (SCF) in Europe. Food additives must gain approval before their use in food manufacture is permitted at specified levels. The approval process is lengthy and detailed with most of the research being funded by the food manufacturer. Some additives are naturally occurring substances but they must also undergo safety testing and approval before they can be used in food manufacture. Approximately 3500 additives are in use today. Additives are used for the following reasons:

- the need to keep foods fresh until eaten so widening food choice and availability;
- convenience of packaging, storage, preparation, and use;
- attractive presentation;
- economic advantage, e.g. longer shelf life or reduced cost;
- nutritional supplementation.

E numbers

E numbers identify permitted food additives regarded as safe for use within the European Union. Some additives have a number but no E prefix as they are under consideration by the European Commission. All food labels must show the additive's name or E number in the list of ingredients. An up to date list of approved food additives and E numbers can be found at ✍ https://www.food.gov.uk/business-guidance/eu-approved-additives-and-e-numbers.

Additive groups

Colourings (E100–180)

Food is coloured to restore losses that occur in manufacture and storage, to meet consumer expectations, and to maintain uniformity of products. An example of this is that oranges have green patches when picked and are coloured orange before sale. Azo, coal tar-based, dyes are frequently linked to food allergy (see ➲ Chapter 37, 'Food hypersensitivity', p. 825). Lists of some natural and synthetic colours are shown in Tables 9.4 and 9.5.

Preservatives (E200–290)

Preservatives (E200-290)[2] are used to prevent food spoilage and enable consumers to have a wide range of goods that are available out of the usual season. Traditional preservatives include salt, vinegar, alcohol, and spices. Acetic acid is the major component of vinegar and may be considered as a natural additive but it has undergone extensive testing and has an E number

---

2 The preservative lysozyme has the E number, E1105.

Table 9.4 Examples of natural colours*

Name	E number	Food use
Riboflavin (yellow)	E101	Processed cheese
Chlorophyll (green)	E140	Fats, oils, canned and dried vegetables
Carbon (black)	E153	Jams, jellies
β Carotene (yellow/orange)	E160a	Margarine and cakes

*Source: data from Webster-Gandy, J. (2000). *Understanding Food and Nutrition*. Part of the Family Doctor Series Ltd in association with the British Medical Association.

Table 9.5 Examples of synthetic colours*

Name	E number	Food Use
Tartrazine (yellow)	E102	Soft drinks
Sunset (yellow)	E110	Orange drinks
Amaranth (red)	E123	Blackcurrant products
Erythrosine (red)	E127	Glace cherries
Indigo carmine (blue)	E132	Savoury food mixes
Green S	E142	Tinned peas, mint jelly and sauce

*Source: data from Webster-Gandy, J. (2000). *Understanding Food and Nutrition*. Part of the Family Doctor Series Ltd in association with the British Medical Association.

E260. Benzoic acid and benzoates occur widely in fresh foods, e.g. peas, bananas, and berries. Although rare, adverse reactions to benzoates have been seen. Some commonly used preservatives are listed in Table 9.6.

Sulphur dioxide destroys thiamin and ∴ is not permitted in foods that are significant sources of thiamine. Sulphur dioxide is used to destroy yeasts which can cause fermentation in food products.

Nitrates and nitrites kill the bacteria that cause botulism, a potentially lethal form of food poisoning. They preserve the red colour in meat and are ∴ used in meat products. A major source of these chemicals in the body is fertilizers that use these chemicals. Nitrites may react with other chemicals in the gut to form nitrosamines, which have been shown to cause cancer in experimental animals. There is no evidence to support the suggestion that these preservatives play a role in causing cancer in man.

Table 9.6 Commonly used preservatives*

Name	E number	Food use
Sorbic acid and derivatives	E200–E203	Cheese, yogurt, soft drinks
Acetic acid	E260	Pickles, sauces
Lactic acid	E270	Margarine, confectionery, sauces
Propionic acid and derivatives	E280–E283	Bread, cakes, flour
Benzoic acid and derivatives	E210–E219	Soft drinks, pickles, fruit products, jams
Sulphur dioxide	E220	Soft drinks, fruit products, beer, cider, wine
Nitrites	E249, E250	Cured meats, cooked meats, meat products
Nitrates	E251, E252	Bacon, ham, cheese (not cheddar or Cheshire)

*Source: data from Webster–Gandy, J. (2000). *Understanding Food and Nutrition*. Part of the Family Doctor Series Ltd in association with the British Medical Association.

Antioxidants (E300–322)
These additives (E300-322)[3,4] prevent the unpleasant taste and smell that occur when fats and oils go rancid. The most widely used antioxidants, butylated hydroxyanisole (BHA) and butylated hydroxytoluene (BHT), are used in a wide variety of foods. Table 9.7 lists the permitted antioxidants.

Emulsifiers, stabilizers, thickeners, and gelling agents (E400–495)
These additives are needed to ↑ the shelf life of some foods and are listed in Table 9.8. They affect the texture and constituency of products. This is the largest group of additives and many are natural substances, e.g. carrageenan, which is derived from seaweed. Polyphosphates have received a great deal of attention from consumer groups as they enable products to retain water so ↑ the product's weight. They are used in products such as frozen poultry and cured meats.

Sweeteners
Sweeteners can be divided into two groups:
- *Caloric sweeteners*: mannitol (E421), sorbitol and sorbitol syrup (E420), isomalt (E953), maltitol and maltitol syrup (E965), xylitol (E967), erythritol (968), and lactitol (E966). These additives add energy to the diet. Steviol glycoside (E960) is a high-intensity sweetener, being 250–300 × sweeter than sucrose ∴ virtually energy free;

---

3 The antioxidant 4-Hexylresorcinol is E586.

4 Agents with E numbers outside this grouping: lecithins E322, invertase E1103.

Table 9.7 Permitted antioxidants*

Name	E number	Food use
Ascorbic acid (vitamin C) and derivatives	E300–E305	Beer, soft drink, powdered milks, fruit, meat products
Tocopherols (vitamin A) and derivatives	E306–E309	Vegetable oils
Gallates	E310–E320	Vegetable oils and fats, margarine
BHA	E320	Margarine, fat in baked products, e.g. pies
BHT	E321	Crisps, margarine, vegetable oils, convenience foods

*Source: data from Webster-Gandy, J. (2000). *Understanding Food and Nutrition*. Part of the Family Doctor Series Ltd in association with the British Medical Association.

Table 9.8 Examples of emulsifiers, stabilizers, thickeners, and gelling agents

Name	E number	Food use
Lecithins (may be used as an antioxidant)	E322	Chocolate, margarine, potato snacks
Citric acid and derivatives	E472c	Pickles, dairy products, baked products
Tartaric acid and derivatives	E472d–f	Baking powder
Alginic acid	E400–E405	Ice cream, instant desserts, and puddings
Agar	E406	Tinned ham, ice cream
Carrageenan	E407	Ice cream
Gums	E410–E418	Ice cream, soups, confectionery
Pectin	E440	Preserves, jellies

- *Non-caloric sweeteners:* acesulfame K (E950), aspartame (E951), cyclamic acid and its salts (E952), saccharine and its salts (E954), thaumatin (E957), neohesperidine (E959), sucralose (E955) and the salt of aspartame-acesulfame (E962). Sucrose, glucose, fructose, and lactose are all classified as foods rather than as sweeteners or additives.

Other additives

These include:

- flavour enhancers, e.g. monosodium glutamate (E621);
- anti-foaming agents that prevent frothing during processing;
- propellant gases, e.g. in aerosol cream.

Nutrition and catering in institutions

Hospital catering 220
Schools 224
Prisons 228
The Armed Forces 230

Hospital catering

In the UK, NHS hospital catering provides ~150 million meals for inpatients each year as well as catering for outpatients, staff, and visitors. These meals are consumed by individuals who vary from those who are in good health to those who are very sick and may have highly specialized nutritional requirements; food may be provided in the form of a single meal or as an individual's exclusive intake for a long period (>3 months) or even indefinitely. The nutritional needs and preferences of such individuals vary considerably and yet the importance of providing optimum nutrition is imperative to promote healing and recovery, to minimize complications associated with poor nutrition, and to maintain and optimize health and quality of life. Provision of food is one important factor among many that influence the nutritional status of hospital patients (see Box 10.1, and ➡ Chapter 25, 'Nutrition support', p. 555). It can be challenging to provide food that people want to eat and to achieve a balance between under- and overnutrition in an environment of financial constraint, but addressing nutritional and hydration needs is mandated in UK law.[1]

Box 10.1 Factors influencing nutritional status

Missing meals contributes to inadequate intake (hypothetical case)
- Patient X, admitted for investigations prior to major surgery.
- Weight loss ±12 kg in last 3 months, now BMI = 18.1 kg/m².
- Misses breakfast for three consecutive mornings as nil by mouth prior to investigative procedures.
- Misses lunch on two of these days as off ward at mealtime and on third day as asleep following sedation.
- Early evening ward round followed by student teaching curtails time available to eat evening meal.
- Eats small amount of evening meal but unable to achieve adequate nutrient intake for whole day at one meal.

Optimizing nutritional intake through hospital food service
- *Ward kitchen services* mean hot beverages, toast, fruit juice, and cereals are available over 24 hours so that an early breakfast can be provided before nil by mouth restrictions start.
- *Out of hours meals and snacks* can be ordered so that a patient missing lunch because of visits to X-ray, physiotherapy, etc., can eat on their return, e.g. sandwiches, cheese and biscuits, fruit, and drink.
- *Protected mealtimes* require non-urgent clinical activity to stop so that patients can eat without interruptions and that ward staff can provide food-related assistance, e.g. feeding, when it is required. This includes ward rounds, teaching and visiting times.

---

1 UK Government (2014). *The Health and Social Care Act 2008 (Regulated Activities) Regulations 2014. Meeting nutrition and hydration needs.* Available at: ℛ https://www.legislation.gov.uk/ukdsi/2014/9780111117613/regulation/14.

10 key characteristics of good nutrition and hydration[2]

1. Screen all patients and service-users to identify malnutrition or risk of malnutrition and ensure actions are progressed and monitored.
2. Together with each patient or service user, create a personal care/support plan enabling them to have choice and control over their own nutritional care and fluid needs.
3. Care providers should include specific guidance on food and beverage services and other nutritional and hydration care in their service delivery and accountability arrangements.
4. People using care services are involved in the planning and monitoring arrangements for food service and drinks provision.
5. Food and drinks should be provided alone or with assistance in an environment conducive to patients being able to consume their food, i.e. protected mealtimes.
6. All healthcare professionals and volunteers receive regular training to ensure they have the skills, qualifications, and competency needed to meet the nutritional and fluid requirements of people using their services.
7. Facilities and services providing nutrition and hydration are designed to be flexible and centred on the needs of the people using them, 24 hours a day, every day.
8. All care providers to have a nutrition and hydration policy centred on the needs of users, and is performance managed in line with local governance, national standards, and regulatory frameworks.
9. Food, drinks, and other nutritional care are delivered safely.
10. Care providers should take a multi-disciplinary approach to nutrition and hydrational care, valuing the contribution of all staff, people using the service, carers, and volunteers working in partnership.

Initiatives addressing hospital food provision

Nutrition and Hydration Week

Nutrition and Hydration Week[3] focuses on highlighting and educating people about the value of food and drink in maintaining health and wellbeing in hospitals and other health and social care settings. Activities include promoting the 10 key characteristics of good nutrition and hydration, minimum standards of good nutrition, and sharing good practice.

Reduction of sugar sweetened beverages for sale

As part of action to reduce sugar intake to ↓ energy intake and improve dental health, NHS Trusts in England have restricted sales of sugar sweetened beverages (SSB).[4] Although this is helpful for most people with an adequate energy intake, there are concerns that this may adversely impact

---

2 NHS (2015). *10 key characteristics of 'good nutrition and hydration care'.* Available at: ℘ https://www.england.nhs.uk/commissioning/nut-hyd/10-key-characteristics/.

3 Nutrition and Hydration Week (2018). Available at: ℘ https://nutritionandhydrationweek.co.uk/.

4 NHS England (2018). *NHS Standard Contract 2017/18 and 2018/19 Technical guidance.* Available at: ℘ https://www.england.nhs.uk/wp-content/uploads/2018/05/8-nhs-standard-contract-technical-guidance-may-2018.pdf.

on those with poor appetites who might benefit from additional calories provided by SSB.

Better Hospital Food

Better Hospital Food (BHF) was introduced by the UK Department of Health to ensure consistent delivery of high-quality food and food services to patients. Although the BHF initiative has finished, elements introduced have been continued through the Hospital Caterers Association.[5] These include:

- flexible menus providing greater choice of meals;
- protected mealtimes to ↓ interruptions when patients are eating;
- 24-hour catering providing food at any time of the day or night;
- sustainability to help ↓ environmental impact of food production;
- nutrition that is adequate and appropriate.

Still Hungry to be Heard

The Still Hungry to be Heard campaign[6] was initiated by Age Concern (now part of Age UK) to address inadequate nutrition in older people in hospital.

Red tray / red jug initiative

Some UK hospitals have adopted a system where patients who are at nutritional risk are given their food on an easily identifiable tray (e.g. coloured red; see Box 10.2) so that their intake can be monitored and appropriate eating/nutritional support is given at mealtimes. Staff training is also provided. The introduction of red trays in one acute teaching hospital resulted in significant increases in energy and protein intakes in 64 patients at high nutritional risk and requiring assistance with feeding.[7] Some hospitals have introduced a similar approach using red jugs to ensure better hydration.

Types of hospital food production

- *Cook–serve*: food is prepared within the hospital site and served more or less immediately to patients, staff, and visitors.
- *Cook–chill*: food is prepared either within the hospital site or at another venue and rapidly chilled to ~0–4°C and stored for up to 5 days before

---

Box 10.2 Red tray education at Milton Keynes General Hospital NHS Trust

Remember the vulnerable patient in need of extra help at mealtimes
Encourage and assist patients where necessary
Dietary intake may be improved by extra attention at mealtimes
Tell patients and relatives about the benefits of the Red Tray Project
Remove red tray ONLY after recording food consumption
Assess and weigh patients regularly
You can improve the patients' mealtime experience!

---

5 Hospital Caterers Association. Available at: ℜ http://www.hospitalcaterers.org.

6 Age UK (2018). *Past Campaigns - Still Hungry to be Heard*. Available at: ℜ https://www.ageuk.org.uk/london/projects-campaigns/our-campaigns/info/still-hungry-to-be-heard/.

7 Duncan, A., *et al*. (2010). Few patients require one-to-one feeding assistance at meal times in an acute hospital. *J. Hum. Nutr. Dietet.* **23**, 446–7.

regeneration (reheating) either in the hospital kitchen or at ward level. Strict food hygiene procedures are required.
- *Cook–freeze*: food is prepared either within the hospital site or at another venue and rapidly frozen to approximately −18°C and stored for up to 3 months before regeneration (reheating) usually in the hospital kitchen. Again, strict procedures are required to maintain food safety and also to ensure food flavours, texture, and appearance are preserved.
- *Steamplicity*® (Compass Group, Uxbridge): a commercially developed meal delivery system that uses a patented micro-steaming system to cook a range of raw, semi-cooked, or fully cooked chilled foods. These are heated by micro-steaming at ward level for <5 minutes before serving. This process provides approximately 4.6 million patient meals per year.

Types of hospital food service
- *Plated meal service*: individual trays are served out for each patient in the main hospital kitchen and transported to the ward either in insulated trolleys (if hot and cold food) or chilled trolleys (if regeneration takes place at ward level).
- *Bulk service*: large containers of food are sent from the kitchen to each ward/dining area, where staff, e.g. nursing, care, or catering assistants or ward hostesses, serve out the meals for each patient. Food sent in bulk containers may be already hot, or still be chilled and regenerated at ward level.

Regulation and monitoring
The Care and Quality Commission (CQC) (℠http://www.cqc.org.uk) is charged with regulating nutrition in care provided by the NHS in England, and all care settings, including care homes, must be registered. CQC sets standards, holds organizations to account when they fail to meet these standards, and protects service users from malnutrition and dehydration. NHS and care setting regulations vary across the home countries. More information for Scotland can be found at The Scottish Commission for the Regulation of Care (℠http://www.healthcareimprovementscotland.org/home.aspx), for Northern Ireland at the Regulation and Quality Improvement Authority (RQIA) (℠http://www.rqia.org.uk), and for Wales at the Care Standards Inspectorate for Wales (℠http://www.cssiw.org.uk).

Resources
British Dietetic Association (2017) *The Nutrition and Hydration Digest*, 2nd edition. Available at: ℠ https://www.bda.uk.com/publications/professional/NutritionHydrationDigest.pdf.

Department of Health (2014) *Establishing food standards for NHS hospitals*. Available at: ℠https://www.gov.uk/government/publications/establishing-food-standards-for-nhs-hospitals.

Department of Health (2017) *Compliance with food standards 2017*. Available at: ℠ https://assets.publishing.service.gov.uk/government/uploads/system/uploads/attachment_data/file/586490/HFSP_Report.pdf

NHS (2016) *Hospital food standards*. Available at: ℠ https://www.nhs.uk/NHSEngland/AboutNHSservices/NHShospitals/Pages/hospital-food-standards.aspx.

Schools

Increasing levels of childhood obesity, and attempts to protect nutritionally vulnerable groups and children receiving free school meals have resulted in many government policies and initiatives in the UK, e.g. breakfast clubs, and other countries. In UK primary schools the take up rate for school lunches is approximately 46% in the primary sector and in secondary schools it is approximately 40%. School lunches represent a valuable opportunity to improve the nutritional intake of children and for nutrition education. In 2014, the UK government introduced free school lunches for children in reception, year 1 and 2. These initiatives also encompass children who receive their lunches outside of the school system. See ➔ Chapter 14, 'School-aged children and adolescents' (p. 303) for nutrition, food problems and factors that influence food choice in this age group.

The Healthy Schools Programme was launched in 1999, and since 2000 these initiatives have included:

• Food in Schools Programme (FSP) (2001);
• Education Act (2002) amended to widen the eligibility criteria for free school meals;
• in 2005 the FSP launched the 'Food in Schools Toolkit';
• the School Food Trust (SFT) was established in 2005 but is no longer functioning;
• the Independent School Food Plan was published by the Department for Education in 2013.

The School Food Plan

The SFP (🔗http://www.schoolfoodplan.com/the-plan/) is an agreed plan 'is about good food and happiness. It is about the pleasures of growing, cooking and eating proper food. It is also about improving the academic performance of our children and the health of our nation'. The plan includes food-based standards for school lunches (Table 10.1) and food provided outside lunch. The standards are mandatory in state schools and academies and free schools. A whole school approach is emphasized; headteachers, with the support of staff and governors, are responsible for ensuring that the plan is implemented. Ofsted school inspections now include a judgement on how successfully schools are supporting pupils to make informed healthy eating choices. SFP provide guidance for school headteachers and governors, provide resources (including training toolkits), portion sizes, recipes, examples of good practice, etc. Schools are expected to follow the government buying standards for food and catering services.

Table 10.1 School Food Plan food-based standards for school lunches*

Food	Standard
Starchy foods	≥1 portion every day
	≥3 different starchy foods each week
	≥1 wholegrain varieties each week
	Starchy food cooked in fat or oil no more than 2 days each week *(applies across the whole school day)*
	Bread—with no added fat or oil—must be available every day
Fruit and vegetables	≥1 portion of vegetables or salad as an accompaniment every day
	≥1 portion of fruit every day
	A dessert containing at least 50% fruit ≥2 times each week
	≥3 different fruits and 3 different vegetables each week
Meat, fish, eggs, beans, and other non-diary sources of protein	1 portion every day
	1 portion of meat or poultry on ≥3 days each week
	Oily fish ≥1 every 3 weeks
	For vegetarians, a portion of non-dairy protein on ≥3 days each week
	A meat or poultry product (manufactured or homemade, and meeting the legal requirements) no more than once each week in primary schools and twice each week in secondary schools *(applies across the whole school day)*
Milk and dairy	A portion every day
	Lower fat milk must be available for drinking at least once a day during school hours
Foods high in fat, sugar, and salt	≤2 portions of food that have been deep fried, batter-coated, or breadcrumb-coated, each week *(applies across the whole school day)*
	≤2 portions of food which include pastry each week *(applies across the whole school day)*
	No snacks, except nuts, seeds, vegetables, and fruit with no added salt, sugar, or fat *(applies across the whole school day)*
	Savoury crackers or breadsticks can be served at lunch with fruit or vegetables or dairy food
	No confectionery, chocolate, or chocolate-coated products *(applies across the whole school day)*
	Desserts, cakes, and biscuits are allowed at lunchtime. They must not contain any confectionery
	Salt must not be available to add to food after it has been cooked *(applies across the whole school day)*
	Any condiments must be limited to sachets or portions of ≤10 g or one teaspoonful *(applies across the whole school day)*

(continued)

Table 10.1 *Contd.*

Food	Standard
Healthier drinks	Free, fresh drinking water at all times
	The only drinks permitted are:
	Plain water (still or carbonated)
	Lower fat milk or lactose reduced milk
	Fruit or vegetable juice (max. 150 mL)
	Plain soya, rice, or oat drinks enriched with calcium; plain fermented milk (e.g. yoghurt) drinks
	Combinations of fruit or vegetable juice with plain water (still or carbonated, with no added sugars or honey)
	Combinations of fruit juice and lower fat milk or plain yoghurt, plain soya, rice or oat drinks enriched with calcium; cocoa and lower fat milk; flavoured lower fat milk, all with <5% added sugars or honey
	Tea, coffee, hot chocolate
	Combination drinks are limited to a portion size of 330 mL. They may contain added vitamins or minerals, and no more than 150 mL of fruit or vegetable juice. Fruit or vegetable juice combination drinks must be at least 45% fruit or vegetable juice

*Source: data from School Food Plan, School Food Standards, available at: ℘http://www.schoolfoodplan.com.

Prisons

The FSA (https://www.food.gov.uk/business-guidance/healthier-catering-guidance-for-different-types-of-businesses) produce nutrient- and food-based guidelines, which are based on the Eatwell Plate (see → Chapter 2, 'Dietary reference values and food-based dietary guidelines', p. 21) and guidance for food served in major institutions. These documents are aimed at caterers in all major institutions including prisons, and the guidance includes example menus compared with dietary reference values (DRVs). Unlike other institutions, prisons provide all the foods and drinks, apart from some snacks and soft drinks, consumed by prisoners. The provision of meals and food is seen as a key issue in helping to maintain order in prisons and to improving prisoners' health. In the UK, Her Majesty's Prison Service instruction PSI 44 (2010) details prison catering services. All prisons use a pre-select, multi-choice, cyclical menu for lunch and dinner, which covers a 2–5-week cycle. Where queuing is in operation, measures are taken to ensure that prisoners at the end of the queue are able to obtain their chosen meals; this reduces conflict and confrontation at the serving point. Portion sizes are tightly controlled to meet budgetary demands and for consistency.

The prison governor has overall responsibility for catering standards and daily inspection of the kitchens. The catering manager at each prison is responsible for implementing standards. Her Majesty's Inspectorate of Prisons and the Independent Monitoring Board are responsible for monitoring all aspects of prison life including catering. Health eating education is considered important during rehabilitation and re-integration phases

❶ Some studies have shown a link between poor diet and antisocial behaviour; however, this is equivocal. A large UK government-funded study is currently under way.

Dietetic practice in prisons

There is no guidance for dietitians working in prisons or how to deal with situations such as patients in restraints, lack of privacy, and the prison regimen. However the British Medical Association (BMA)'s (2009) guidance for providing medical care in hospitals (see Box 10.3) may be followed.

Box 10.3 Guidance for providing medical care to detained prisoners in hospitals (BMA, 2009)*

- Detained prisoners must have the same standards of care as the rest of society including patient's respect for dignity and privacy.
- Risk assessment must be carried out prior to a prisoner going into hospital to determine the degree of supervision. Risk assessment includes: the prisoner's condition, any medical objection to the use of restraints, nature of the prisoner's offence, security of the consulting room, and risk of violence to self or others.
- Where escape is unlikely, escort and bed watch by one prison officer, without restraints is sufficient.
- Hospitals should be informed in advance about levels of escort and restraint envisaged, and hospital staff should have the opportunity to discuss when level of restraint is clinically unacceptable.

*Source: data from BMA (2009). *Health care of detainees in police stations*. Available at: ⌖http://www.bma.org.uk.

The Armed Forces

Food is provided in three areas:
• non-operational (UK bases);
• operational (ration packs, overseas bases, and active theatres;
• civilian.

The Defence Catering Manual (Joint Services Publication 456) covers every aspect of food provision.

A system known as Pay as You Dine (PAYD) provides catering for non-operational food service. It is based on the provision of three core meals and personnel pay only for food that is taken. The system provides three core meals and must provide at least a six-item breakfast, lunch, and a three-course dinner. Most bases have self-catering facilities.

The Ministry of Defence (MoD) has developed Military Dietary Reference Values (2008) for macro- and micro-nutrients and all advice is centred around the FSA's Eatwell Guide. The Scientific Advisory Committee on Nutrition (SACN) produced a statement on recommendations for energy requirements for military personnel in 2016.[8] The MoD produce nutrition and hydration guidance for personnel that emphasizes increasing/maintaining performance, reducing the chance of injury, staying healthy and fit, and quick recovery from activity. The Armed Forces Nutrition Advisory Service offers expert advice and information on nutrition, diet, and military feeding; this is only available to UK military personnel and MOD civil servants.

Each unit commanding officer is ultimately responsible for standards of catering and the catering manager monitors provision of foods and patterns of consumption of high-fat foods, salt, and sugar. The DFS Quality Assurance team ensures the quality of food supplied and inspects all food premises.

Operational ration packs

All personnel are issued with ORP when operational, but the MoD provides field-catering facilities as soon as possible after deployment. ORPs are available for 10-man groups and individuals. They are the sole source of nutrition during these periods. The menus are varied and provide ethnic alternatives and choices for specific operations, e.g. jungle, cold climate.

---

8 SACN (2016). *Statement on military dietary reference values for energy.* Available at: ℘ https://assets.publishing.service.gov.uk/government/uploads/system/uploads/attachment_data/file/583321/SACN_military_DRVs_for_energy_position_statement.pdf.

Popular diets

Popular diets *232*

Popular diets

This section is included to help orientate healthcare professionals to diets that their patients may initiate or possibly seek advice about. It does not validate their efficacy. For many, evidence of benefit in the form of a randomized controlled trial is not available. However, the benefits and concerns, described below, are based on scientific principles. When thinking about following a popular diet, it is worth considering some key questions (Box 11.1).

- *5:2 diet:* is a modified form of intermittent fasting (◗ Chapter 21, p. 479 Intermittent fasting.) Energy intake is restricted to 400-600 kcal/day on 2 days and 5 days of healthy, not extravagant, eating based on the Mediterranian diet. There is evidence to support its use as a weight loss regiemn with potential health benefits.[1,2]
- *Alkaline diet:* advises ↓ intake of acidic foods and ↑ alkaline foods to promote health and reduce risk of cancer. There is no systematic evidence to support this.[3]
- *Atkins diet:* is a low carbohydrate, high protein diet for weight reduction (see ◗ Chapter 21, 'Weight management: dietary approaches, Low carbohydrate', p. 478).
- *Beverley Hills diet:* based on the belief that enzymes are required to break down specific foods and that certain foods provide these enzymes while undigested food in the gastrointestinal tract leads to the gain of fat. There is no scientific evidence to support this hypothesis.
- *Blood Group diet or Eat Right for Your Type:* this diet is based on the idea that blood groups evolved at different times during evolution and that a diet that reflects this period is optimum for health and weight control. There is no evidence to support health claims.[4]

Box 11.1 Key questions to ask before starting a popular diet

- Is there any scientific evidence that this diet will help or harm my health? If not, be careful.
- Who is promoting this diet and do they benefit financially from this? Commercial and scientific interests may conflict.
- Are dietitians (RD) or registered nutritionists (RNutr) supporting the use of this diet? If not, again, be careful.

Does it sound too good to be true? If so, it probably is.

---

1 Harvie, M.N., *et al.* The effects of intermittent or continuous energy restriction on weight loss and metabolic disease risk markers: a randomized trial in young overweight women. *Int. J. Obes.* **35**, 714–727.

2 Harvie, M.N. *et al.* The effect of intermittent energy and carbohydrate restriction v. daily energy restriction on weight loss and metabolic disease risk markers in overweight women. *Brit. J. Nutr.* **110**(8),1534–47.

3 Fenton, T.R., Huang, T. (2016). Systematic review of the association between dietary acid load, alkaline water and cancer. *BMJ Open.* **13**(6), e010438.

4 Cusack, L., *et al.* (2013) Blood type diets lack supporting evidence: a systematic review. *Am. J. Clin. Nutr.* **98**, 99–104.

- *Bristol Approach to Healthy Eating:* developed from the Bristol Diet, these nutritional guidelines are recommended by Penny Brohn Cancer Care for people living with cancer (see ➲ Chapter 24, 'Frequently asked questions, Alternative and complementary diets', p. 551).
- *Cabbage Soup diet:* encourages weight loss through consuming large quantities of home-made cabbage soup and few other foods. This restricts energy and nutrient intake. Although this regimen may lead to rapid weight loss, following the diet is not compatible with long-term health.
- *Clean eating:* avoids all processed foods and requires meals made from foods in their natural state. Reducing intake of processed foods that are high in fat, sugar, and salt is compatible with proven health benefits. However, concerns have been raised about obsessively following clean eating approaches using the term 'orthorexia'.[5]
- *Detox diets:* recommend strictly avoiding all perceived dietary 'toxins', e.g. wheat, dairy, alcohol, caffeine, colouring, and preservatives, as a means of reducing weight and/or promoting health. Short-term fasting is recommended on some regimes ± laxatives, diuretics, vitamins, and 'cleansing' foods, e.g. lemon juice, herbal tea. Few studies have evaluated efficacy; adverse effects have been reported. Overall, there is no evidence to support use of detox diets.[6]
- *Dukan diet:* aims at weight loss based on four phases, 'attack', 'cruise', 'consolidation', and 'stabilization', with emphasis on high protein. Evaluation of the diet is reported on the company's website but no good-quality clinical trials have been identified in peer-reviewed journals. Severe ketoacidosis has been reported.[7]
- *Food combining diets:* advise that food containing protein and carbohydrate should be consumed at different meals because they require different 'digestive secretions'. There is no scientific basis for this and no evidence that food combining leads to ↑ weight loss.[8]
- *Gerson diet:* a regime used in cancer (see ➲ Chapter 24, 'Frequently asked questions, Alternative and complementary diets', p. 551).
- *Glycaemic index (GI) diet:* is based on the principle that foods with a low GI are more satiating and have other health benefits compared to high GI foods (see ➲ Chapter 5, 'Glycaemic index', p. 81 and Chapter 21 'Low GI/GL', p. 478). A systematic review of six studies found significantly greater weight loss associated with low GI than with a control diet.[9]

---

5 McCartney, M. (2016). Clean eating and the cult of healthism *BMJ.* **354**, i4095.

6 Klein, A.V., Kiat, H. (2015). Detox diets for toxin elimination and weight management: a critical review of the evidence. *J. Hum. Nutr. Diet.* **28**, 675-86.

7 Freeman, T.F., *et al.* (2014). Acute intractable vomiting and severe ketoacidosis secondary to the Dukan Diet©. *J. Emerg. Med.* **47**(4), e109–12.

8 Golay, A., *et al.* (2001) Similar weight loss with low-energy food combining or balanced diets. *Int. J. Obes. Relat. Metab. Disord.* **24**, 492–6.

9 Thomas, D., *et al.* (2007). Low glycaemic index or low glycaemic load diets for overweight and obesity (review). *Cochrane Database Syst. Rev.* **3**, Art No: CD005105.

- *Grapefruit diet:* a low fat, very low energy diet to promote rapid weight loss in 1–2 weeks. Although grapefruits contain a number of biologically active compounds, systematic review indicates no evidence that grapefruits contribute to weight loss.[10]
- *Hay diet:* see 'Food combining diets' above.
- *Ketogenic diets:* are high fat and very low carbohydrate. They can be an effective treatment in epilepsy (see ➔ Chapter 33, 'Ketogenic therapy for epilepsy', p. 792). In weight management (usually <50 g/d carbohydrate), ketogenic diets are associated with greater short-term weight loss compared to low fat diets, but the long-term effect on health is unknown (see ➔ Chapter 21, 'Low carbohydrate', p. 478).
- *LighterLife:* is a commercial weight loss and health improvement programme providing total dietary replacement in the form of food packs and group talking therapy. Intake is ~ 600 kcal and 50 g protein/d (see ➔ Chapter 21, 'Meal replacements', p. 479 and 'Very low energy diets', p. 480). Although potentially expensive for individuals, economic evaluation found it cost-effective compared to no treatment.[11]
- *Meal replacements:* many commercial meal replacements, some for use in weight loss, are available in the form of milk shakes, soups, and bars, and also as ready-meals or complete food provision. Brand names include Diet Chef, Huel, Jenny Craig, and Slimfast (see ➔ Chapter 21, 'Meal replacements', p. 479).
- *Mediterranean diet:* is associated with many health benefits and reduction in mortality and supported by robust evidence[12] (see ➔ Box 23.2, 'A Mediterranean diet is not a single entity … ', p. 526).
- *Macrobiotics:* describes a philosophical approach to life that includes balancing yin and yang elements. The dietary element is based on predominantly vegetarian, high carbohydrate, low fat food, with regular consumption of soya and sea vegetables. Although some aspects of the diet follow healthy eating principles, more extreme versions are nutritionally inadequate and not recommended for health. The MaPi2 macrobiotic diet (12% protein, 18% fat, 70% carbohydrate) has been evaluated positively in type 2 diabetes.[13]
- *Paleo diet:* is based on the foods believed to have been consumed during the paleolithic era, i.e. before the cultivation of cereals. It is high in meat (preferably from grass-fed animals), fruit, vegetables, nuts and seeds, and avoids grains, legumes, potatoes, processed foods, and refined sugar. Although some aspects of the diet are compatible with health, it is potentially high in fat and low in dietary fibre. This diet is associated

10 Onakpoya, I., *et al.* (2017). The effect of grapefruits (Citrus paradisi) on body weight and cardiovascular risk factors: A systematic review and meta-analysis of randomized clinical trials. *Crit. Rev. Food Sci. Nutr.* **57**, 602–12.

11 Lewis, L. *et al.* (2014). The cost-effectiveness of the LighterLife weight management programme as an intervention for obesity in England. *Clin. Obes.* **4**, 180–8.

12 Sofi, F., *et al.* (2014). Mediterranean diet and health status: an updated meta-analysis and a proposal for a literature-based adherence score. *Public Health Nutr.* **17**, 2769–82.

13 Porrata-Maury, C., *et al.* (2014) Ma-Pi 2 macrobiotic diet and type 2 diabetes mellitus: pooled analysis of short-term intervention studies. *Diabetes Metab. Res. Rev.* **30**(Suppl 1), 55–66.

with short-term (<6 months) improvement in markers of metabolic syndrome,[14] but long-term effects have not been evaluated.

- *Pioppi diet*: a 21-day lifestyle plan that aims to reduce weight and risk of type 2 diabetes and heart disease. Although described as based on the Mediterranean diet, the plan differs by focusing on low carbohydrate and unrestricted saturated fat and protein intake, which is not compatible with current evidence-based dietary advice.[15]
- *Plant programme:* a non-dairy regime used in cancer (see ➲ Chapter 24, 'Alternative and complementary diets', p. 551).
- *Raw vegan:* combines eating uncooked and minimally processed food with avoiding all animal products. This practice requires planning and time-consuming preparation. Eating raw food can be associated with health benefits,[16] but raises concern over adequacy of vitamin B_{12} intake, which is also an issue in veganism (see ➲ Chapter 16, 'Types of vegetarian diets', p. 346). Intake of other nutrients may also be inadequate. Gastrointestinal obstruction has been reported.[17]
- *Slimming World*: provides group and online weight loss programmes, which include support for men and women, young people, during pregnancy, and via NHS referrals. It has been shown to be effective and compares well with similar weight loss programmes.[18]
- *South Beach diet:* was originally designed for heart health. It is now regarded as a weight loss diet, which is based on moderate carbohydrate restriction and GI advice. It has not been evaluated in trials.
- *Sugar Busters:* aims to 'cut sugar to trim fat' in obesity and diabetes. Although avoiding refined carbohydrate is compatible with a healthy, weight reducing diet, avoiding sugar on its own is insufficient to ensure long-term successful weight loss.
- *Weight Watchers:* provides a structured weight loss programme delivered either through local meetings or online. Energy restriction is achieved by using calorie-based points to construct a flexible intake, which is compatible with health eating guidelines and education about food and exercise. Systematic review of evidence shows this is effective in supporting weight loss.[19]

14 Manheimer, E.W., *et al.* (2015). Paleolithic nutrition for metabolic syndrome: systematic review and meta-analysis. *Am. J. Clin. Nutr.* 102, 922–32.

15 Public Health England (2017). *The Eatwell Guide*. Available at: https://www.gov.uk/government/publications/the-eatwell-guide.

16 Koebnick, C., *et al.* (2005). Long-term consumption of a raw food diet is associated with favorable serum LDL cholesterol and triglycerides but also with elevated plasma homocysteine and low serum HDL cholesterol in humans. *J. Nutr.* **135**, 2372–8.

17 Amoroso, S., *et al.* (2018). Acute small bowel obstruction in a child with a strict raw vegan diet. *Arch. Dis. Child.* **14**, pii: archdischild-2018-314910.

18 Madigan, C.D., *et al.* (2014). Which weight-loss programmes are as effective as Weight Watchers®? Non-inferiority analysis. *Br. J. Gen. Pract.* **64**, e128–36.

19 Gadzune, K.A., *et al.* (2015) Efficacy of commercial weight-loss programs: an updated systematic review. *Ann. Intern. Med.* **162**, 501–12.

- *Zone diet:* is a weight loss diet that aims to ↓ diet-associated inflammation. It requires each meal to comprise ⅓ plate of protein, ⅔ plate of carbohydrate derived from vegetables, legumes, and fruits and a dash of monounsaturated fat. Grains and starches are restricted so this is effectively a low carbohydrate diet and does not follow conventional healthy eating guidance.[15] Meta-analysis of studies shows comparable weight loss with similar interventions at 12 months.[20] No long-term follow up has been reported.

Further information

British Dietetic Association (2017). *Food fact sheet: Fad diets.* Available at: ✆ https://www.bda.uk.com/foodfacts/faddiets.pdf.

20 Johnson, B.C., *et al.* (2014) Comparison of weight loss among named diet programs in overweight and obese adults: a meta-analysis. *JAMA* **312**, 923–33.

Diet before and during pregnancy

Pre- and peri-conceptional nutrition *238*
Dietary reference values and dietary guidelines during
      pregnancy *242*
Vitamin and mineral supplements in pregnancy *244*
Food safety in pregnancy *246*
Maternal weight gain *248*
Dietary problems in pregnancy *250*
Vulnerable groups in pregnancy *254*
Useful websites *256*

Pre- and peri-conceptional nutrition

Why is nutrition important at preconception?

A mother's nutritional status is critical prior to conception (preconception is 3 months before conception), and immediately afterwards (peri-conception is 2–3 months after conception). The fetus is most vulnerable to nutritional deficiencies in the first trimester of pregnancy, often before a woman realizes that she is pregnant.

There is evidence that poor maternal nutrition has both immediate (e.g. low birth weight) and long-term consequences. Research on the 'fetal origins of adult disease' has found that fetal growth plays a major role in determining the risk of some nutrition-related non-communicable disease in adulthood, e.g. cardiovascular disease.

Dietary advice for preconception

What dietary changes can the mother make to increase the likelihood of conceiving and giving birth to a healthy infant?

Eat a varied diet. Refer to 'The Eatwell Guide' in Chapter 2, p. 27.

The main points are:

- include five portions of fruit and vegetables a day;
- eat a variety of different foods from all food groups;
- restrict foods containing too much saturated fat and sugar.

Folic acid and preconception

- Folic acid supplements should be taken to protect against neural tube defects (NTDs). In the UK, the recommendations are:[1]
  - *to prevent first occurrence of NTDs:* 400 µg during preconception and until 12th week of pregnancy (on prescription or over counter);
  - to prevent NTDs in high risk groups (previous pregnancy with NTD, one of parents or family history of NTD): 5 mg during preconception and until the 12th week of pregnancy (on prescription only);
  - *women with diabetes:*[2] 5 mg during preconception and until the 12th week of pregnancy (on prescription only).
  - ✍ *women taking anti-epileptic medication*: refer to their GP as may also need to take a higher dose of folic acid.

Foods rich in folic acid should be chosen (see Box 12.1).

Foods to avoid at preconception

Alcohol

- UK NHS recommendations are to advise women not to drink alcohol at all when pregnant.
- Alcohol intake may be associated with decreased fertility and can affect the growing fetus.
- Binge drinking in particular is dangerous. Advise women not to get drunk!

1 SACN (2009). *Folic acid and colorectal cancer risk: review of recommendation for mandatory folic acid fortification.* SACN, London.

2 NCC/WCH (2015). *Diabetes in pregnancy: management from preconception to the postnatal period. NICE guideline 3 Methods, evidence and recommendations.* Available at: ℳ https://www.nice.org.uk/guidance/ng3/evidence.

Box 12.1 Foods rich in folic acid

- *Rich sources:* >100 µg per serving: Brussels sprouts, kale, spinach
- *Good sources:* 50–100 µg per serving: fortified bread and breakfast cereals, broccoli, cabbage, cauliflower, chickpeas, green beans, iceberg lettuce, kidney beans, peas, spring greens
- *Moderate sources:* 15–15 µg per serving: potatoes, most other vegetables, most fruits, most nuts, brown rice, wholegrain pasta, oats, bran, some breakfast cereals, cheese, yogurt, milk, eggs, salmon, beef, game

Vitamin A supplements and liver

Avoid excessive intake of retinol/vitamin A (β-carotene is not toxic).

- Women should not take vitamin A supplements or fish liver oils, liver, liver pâté, haggis, or liver sausage as retinol is teratogenic at extreme intakes (8000–10000 µg).
- Avoid drugs that contain vitamin A or its analogues, such as cystic acne medications (isotretinoin; treinoin).

Certain fish

- Women can eat most types of white fish and smoked fish while they are trying to conceive; however, the NHS (UK) advice for pregnant women should be followed as a precautionary measure, advising women:
  - not to eat shark, swordfish, or marlin because of the mercury content which can affect neural development of the fetus;
  - to limit the amount of tuna they eat (high in mercury) to no more than two fresh tuna steaks a week (about 140 g cooked or 170 g raw each), or four medium size cans (drained weight of 140 g);
  - not to eat more than two portions a week of oily fish, e.g. salmon, trout, mackerel, and herring, as these may contain dioxins and polychlorinated biphenyls (1 portion = 140 g cooked weight), including fresh (but not canned) tuna.

Seafood

- Women can eat cooked shellfish (not raw because of the food poisoning risk), including cooked mussels, lobster, crab, prawns, scallops, and clams.
- Sushi can be eaten if the raw fish was either prefrozen or farmed (to reduce parasitic infection). If in doubt, women should avoid raw fish sushi and eat those with fully cooked eel (unagi) or shrimp (ebi) or vegetables, e.g. cucumber (kappa) maki, avocado California roll.

Food safety

Women should be encouraged to follow the food safety advice for pregnant women (see this ➐ Chapter, 'Food safety in pregnancy', p. 246 and 'Maternal weight gain', p. 248) as a precautionary measure for when conception occurs.

💣 Peanuts and preconception

Women trying to conceive are no longer advised to avoid peanuts because of a lack of evidence that this reduces likelihood of infant peanut allergy. Obviously, women who have peanut allergy should still avoid them! Previously in the UK (until 2009), it was recommended to avoid eating peanuts in pregnancy to reduce risk of allergy.

Healthy weight for conception

- Achieve and maintain ideal weight at preconception (BMI 18.5–24.9 kg/m²).
- Weight needs to be stabilized 3 months before attempting conception.
- Low body fat content of <22% of body weight can prevent ovulation (average body fat content of post-pubertal women is 28%).
- Obesity (BMI ≥30) can inhibit ovulation because of associated changes in insulin activity and its effect on hormone activity.
- Obesity at conception can influence the *pregnancy* (high blood pressure, impaired blood sugar metabolism, gestational diabetes; pre-eclampsia), *delivery* (preterm delivery; prolonged labour; unplanned caesarean), and *infant's health* (stillborn fetus; difficulty initiating and sustaining breastfeeding).
- Obese and overweight women should be advised to lose weight before conception (NICE guidance 2010[3]).
- Underweight (BMI <18.5) at conception can increase the risk of preterm delivery and of delivering a low birth weight infant.

3 NICE (2010). *Weight management before, during and after pregnancy*. NICE public health guidance 27. Available at: 🔗https://www.nice.org.uk/guidance/ph27.

Dietary reference values and dietary guidelines during pregnancy

Dietary recommendations are the same as for a normal healthy diet (see 'The Eatwell Guide', p. 27), except for additional requirements for six nutrients of protein, energy, folic acid, vitamins A, C, and D (see Table 12.1).

Caffeine and pregnancy

- Caffeine may contribute to low birth weight by increasing fetal heart rate and ↑ risk of miscarriage.
- Pregnant women do not need to completely cut out caffeine, but limit intake to <200 mg/day.
- Tea, coffee, cocoa, and cola-type drinks are advised in moderation (equivalent to <200 mg/day). Tea/coffee also reduce iron absorption.
- Suggest decaffeinated tea and coffee, fruit juice, or water.
- The FSA recommends drinking no more than four cups of herbal or green tea a day during pregnancy.

Box 12.2 Caffeine in drinks and chocolate

- One mug of brewed or filter coffee (140 mg each).
- One mug of instant coffee (100 mg each).
- One mug of tea (75 mg each).
- One can of cola (up to 40 mg each).
- One can of 'energy drink' (up to 80 mg each).
- 50 g bar of plain chocolate (up to 50 mg each).
- 50 g bar of milk chocolate (<10 mg each for UK brands).

Women should aim for <200 mg/day.

Alcohol in pregnancy

- Current UK NHS recommendations are to advise women not to drink alcohol at all when pregnant.
- Excessive binge drinking is most dangerous and can have teratogenic effects leading to fetal alcohol syndrome, which affects 1–2/1000 births/year. Risk is elevated in women drinking >8 units/day. Symptoms in the infant are: growth retardation, craniofacial, and central nervous system defects, cardiac and genitourinary abnormalities.

Eating fish in pregnancy

- Women can eat most types of white fish and smoked fish (e.g. smoked salmon/trout) while they are pregnant. But UK advice is complex on other types of fish, advising women:
  - not to eat shark, swordfish, or marlin because of the mercury content, which can affect neural development of fetus;
  - to limit the amount of tuna they eat (high in mercury) to no more than two fresh tuna steaks a week (about 140 g cooked or 170 g raw each), or four medium size cans (drained weight of 140 g).

Table 12.1 RNI for pregnant women*

Nutrient	Daily RNI (pre-pregnancy)	↑ in pregnancy
Energy, MJ/d	8.4	+0.8 (third trimester)
Folic acid, μg	200	+400 (first trimester) +5 mg if high risk group† (first trimester)
Protein, g	51	+6
Vitamin C, mg	40	+10 (third trimester)
Vitamin D, μg	0 (assumed gained from sun exposure)	+10
Vitamin A, μg	600	+100

*No increase recommended for intake of calcium and iron as evidence insufficient that this is needed above RNI. See Appendix 6 (p. 875) for RNI for adult women.

†See 'Pre- and peri-conceptional nutrition', p. 238 for high risk groups.

- not to eat more than two portions of oily fish a week, e.g. salmon, trout, mackerel, and herring, as these may contain dioxins and polychlorinated biphenyls (1 portion = 140 g cooked weight), including fresh (but not canned) tuna.

Eating seafood in pregnancy

- Women can eat cooked shellfish (not raw because of the food poisoning risk), including cooked mussels, lobster, crab, prawns, scallops, and clams.
- Sushi can be eaten if the raw fish was either prefrozen or farmed (to reduce parasitic infection). If in doubt, women should avoid raw fish sushi and eat those with fully cooked eel (unagi) or shrimp (ebi) or vegetables (e.g. cucumber (kappa) maki, avocado California roll).

Vitamin and mineral supplements in pregnancy

Women should try and obtain nutrients from a balanced diet (See 'The Eatwell Guide' in Chapter 2, p. 27), and should be advised against taking high dose multivitamin and mineral supplements (see Table 12.2).

Vitamin A (and liver products)

Vitamin A supplements and fish liver oils can quickly reach toxic levels, and may have teratogenic effects. Women in the UK should not use vitamin A supplements or fish liver oils. Liver, liver pâté, haggis, liver sausage, and other foods containing liver should not be eaten as they are a very rich source of vitamin A. However, in areas of the world where vitamin A deficiency is prevalent, supplementation may be beneficial for pregnant women.

Folic acid

Folic acid (400 µg/day) is the only supplement recommended for 'blanket' use by women until the 12th week of pregnancy. At-risk groups require a larger intake of 5 g/day (see 'Pre- and peri-conceptional nutrition in women', p. 238).

Iron tablets

In the UK, iron supplements are advised only if there is evidence of iron deficiency anaemia (see 'Iron', p. 148). Iron stores should be verified preconceptually and in pregnancy. Iron supplements can cause constipation and other gastrointestinal (GI) changes, and may interfere with zinc absorption.

Vitamin D supplements

The Department of Health (DH) recommends vitamin D supplements (10 µg/day) during pregnancy and breastfeeding in addition to sunlight between April and September (see 'Vitamin D (calciferols)', p. 108) and that only those on a restricted diet need extra vitamin D. Some Asian women could be at risk of vitamin D deficiency because of insufficient skin exposure (see 'Minority ethnic communities', p. 338) → neonatal hypocalcaemia and rickets, ∴ may need extra vitamin D supplements.

Table 12.2 Summary of nutrient supplements in pregnancy

Supplement	Recommendation
Vitamin A	Not advised in well-nourished populations
Folic acid	400 µg/day for most women until the 12th week of pregnancy Higher risk groups will require 5 mg/day until the 12th week of pregnancy
Iron	Only if there is evidence of iron deficiency anaemia
Vitamin D	10 µg/day during pregnancy and breastfeeding

Food safety in pregnancy

Box 12.3 Food items to avoid in pregnancy

Besides following normal safe food hygiene practices, pregnant women should be advised to avoid additional practices that have been linked to micro-organisms that can lead to fetal malformations.

Avoiding salmonellosis

In severe cases, this can cause premature labour and miscarriage. Pregnant women should avoid:

- raw or undercooked eggs because of the risk of salmonella. White and yolk should be solid/hard boiled. Raw egg may be found in home-made mayonnaise, ice-cream, mousse. Mayonnaise and salad cream made with cooked eggs is fine.
- raw/partially cooked meat, e.g. poultry, sausages, and burgers; they should be cooked thoroughly until brown on the inside.

Avoiding listeriosis

Caused by *Listeria monocytogenes*. Rare, but even mild infection can lead to miscarriage, still birth, or ill newborn. Pregnant women should avoid:

- all types of pâté (including vegetable);
- mould ripened soft cheese with white rind (unless cooked), e.g. brie, camembert;
- soft blue veined cheese (unless cooked), e.g. stilton, Roquefort, gorgonzola;
- soft cheeses made with unpasteurized milk, including cow, goat, and sheep's, and associated milk products (unpasteurized yogurts);
- eating uncooked or undercooked ready-prepared meals or leftovers >24 hours old.

Avoiding toxoplasmosis

Caused by *Toxoplasma gondii*—the mother will have flu symptoms and it can cause blindness and mental retardation in the infant. Pregnant women should:

- avoid cats as they can be carriers—wear gloves when gardening or changing cat litter and wash hands afterwards;
- cook poultry and all meat thoroughly so it is steaming hot and no trace of blood/pink meat;
- wash salads, fruit, and vegetables to remove all soil;
- thoroughly reheat ready-prepared meals and leftovers;
- freeze cured or fermented cold meats for 4 days at home before eating to kill parasites. Cooked deli meats, e.g. pepperoni on pizza, do not need freezing first;
- pre-packed meats such as ham and corned beef are safe to eat in pregnancy.

Reducing likelihood of developing peanut allergy

Pregnant women are no longer advised to avoid peanuts because of a lack of evidence that this reduces likelihood of infant peanut allergy. Obviously, women who have a peanut allergy should still avoid them.

Box 12.3 *Continued*

Avoiding food poisoning

Avoid raw shellfish. Cooked shellfish, including prawns, are fine. All beansprouts should be cooked until they are steaming hot throughout, before eating.

Avoiding toxins and other risks

❗ Advise caution about:
- herbal supplements (including liquorice root), as not evaluated for safety in pregnancy;
- eating game that has been shot with lead pellets. Venison and other large game sold in supermarkets is usually farmed and contains no/low levels of lead.

Maternal weight gain

How much weight should a woman gain during pregnancy? Weight gained in pregnancy is a combination of maternal/fetal tissues and fluid, as well as maternal fat stores. Rate of weight gain is not constant: around 2 kg (5 lbs) are gained in the first trimester and the rest in the second and third trimesters at a rate of ~ 0.4 kg (1 lb) per week.

To account for these ↑ energy demands, the DH (England) (see Table 12.1) makes a blanket recommendation for women to consume an extra 200 kcal/day in the last trimester, but the best advice is to encourage women to eat to appetite in pregnancy and monitor weight gain within the appropriate ranges.

An average weight gain of 10–12.5 kg (22–28 lbs) is recommended for women of normal BMI in the UK, but a higher average weight gain of 11.5–16 kg (25–35 lbs) is seen as acceptable in the USA.[4]

❶ Both too little and too much weight gain can adversely affect the fetus:
- *Too much maternal weight gain during pregnancy* can → post-partum maternal obesity; possibility of caesarean; infant macrosomia; and ↑ risk of gestational diabetes. See 'The Eatwell Guide', p. 27 for healthier eating to prevent weight gain.
- *Too little maternal weight gain* can → low birth weight baby with subsequent effects on long-term health (see 'Pre- and peri-conceptional nutrition', p. 238).

Weight gain in overweight and obese women

Women who are overweight or obese should not attempt to lose weight during pregnancy. NICE (2009)[5] makes no recommendation regarding acceptable weight gain for women who were overweight or obese pre-pregnancy, stating insufficient evidence. However, the US Institute of Medicine (IOM) recommends that, based on pre-pregnancy BMI, overweight women should limit weight gain to 7–11.5 kg (15–25 lbs) and obese women should limit weight gain to 5–9 kg (11–20 lbs).

Overweight and obese pregnant women need regular monitoring as there is ↑ risk of pre-eclampsia, gestational diabetes mellitus (DM), and hypertension (HT); the risk ↑ with BMI. At birth there is ↑ likelihood of caesarean section, post-operative complications, low Apgar score, excessive birth weight of newborn (macrosomia), ↑ perinatal mortality (3-fold), and neural tube defects (NTDs).

Weight gain with multiple pregnancies

Multiple births account for one in six of all births in the UK. Women carrying twins (or more!) will gain even more weight than women carrying one fetus.

---

4 IOM (Institute of Medicine) (2009). *Weight gain during pregnancy: Re-examining the guidelines*. The National Academies Press, Washington, DC. Available at: ℛhttp://www.nationalacademies.org/hmd/Reports/2009/Weight-Gain-During-Pregnancy-Reexamining-the-Guidelines.aspx.

5 NICE (2010). *Weight management before, during and after pregnancy*. NICE public health guidance 27. Available at:ℛ https://www.nice.org.uk/guidance/ph27.

In the absence of UK guidelines for multiple births, the IOM[4] recommendations are used that were revised in 2009. They advise that normal weight women carrying twins should gain 17–25 kg (37–54 lbs), overweight ♀ should gain 14–23 kg (31–20 lbs), and obese ♀ should gain 11–19 kg (25–42 lbs) during the pregnancy.

A healthy weight gain is particularly important in multiple pregnancies as they carry a higher risk of premature birth and low birth weight.

Dietary problems in pregnancy

Pregnancy sickness (also known as morning sickness)

During the first trimester, ~70% of women have pregnancy sickness (nausea and vomiting) as the woman adjusts to higher hormone levels, especially human chorionic gonadotrophin and high oestrogen levels. Although often referred to as 'morning sickness', vomiting can occur at any time of the day: it varies from slight nausea to frequent and severe vomiting. Most cases are mild, but it impacts on the pregnant woman's sense of wellbeing and daily activities. *Hyperemesis gravidarum* is the most severe form and is defined as persistent nausea and vomiting leading to dehydration, ketonuria, electrolyte imbalance, and weight loss greater than 5% of pre-pregnancy weight.

❷ *Advise the following:*

- Frequent small meals and snacks every 2 hours, avoiding large meals.
- High carbohydrates (CHO)/low fat foods are best tolerated, e.g. toast, dry biscuits, crackers, low sugar breakfast cereals.
- Avoid smells and foods that exacerbate nausea, e.g. high fat foods. However, these foods will depend on each woman.
- Taking food and drinks separately can help ↓ nausea.
- Encourage plenty of fluid, especially as water and other sugar-free fluids, as dehydration may occur in extreme cases. Recommend at least 35 ml/ kg body weight/daily; equivalent to nine mugs of fluid in a 65kg woman (1 mug = 250 ml).
- Avoid foods or smells that trigger symptoms. Eat cold meals, rather than hot ones because they do not smell as strong, which may provoke nausea.
- Eat plain biscuits before getting up.
- Avoid drinks that are cold, tart (sharp), or sweet.
- There is some evidence that ginger supplements may help reduce the symptoms of nausea and vomiting in some pregnant women. Ginger products are unlicensed in the UK, so advise purchase from a reputable source, such as a pharmacy or supermarket.
- Wear comfortable clothes without tight waistbands, which can sometimes cause discomfort.
- Take time to rest and relax; take fresh air.
- Reassure women that most cases resolve spontaneously in the first 16–20 weeks of pregnancy.
- When symptoms are persistent, severe, and prevent daily activities, drug treatment should be considered.[6]

Food aversions and cravings

Aversions are relatively common, especially for tea, coffee, fried food, and eggs. Food cravings can be strong but depend on the individual. There are no nutritional implications as long as a craving does not involve eating a lot of energy-dense foods that result in excessive weight gain.

6 Further information is available at: ⌘http://www.nhs.uk/conditions/pregnancy-and-baby/ pages/morning-sickness-nausea.aspx.

Pica

Pica is the persistent craving for non-food substances, ranging from coal, clay, candles, matchboxes, to soil. Pica can be harmful if the item craved and eaten is toxic or eaten in large enough quantities to have an impact on nutritional status. Eating soil could carry the risk of toxoplasmosis (see 'Food Safety in Pregnancy', p. 246). Evidence for a physiological basis of need is inconclusive. Pica is often associated with iron deficiency but it is uncertain whether iron deficiency causes pica, or conversely whether pica causes iron deficiency because of its effect on ↓ iron absorption.

Iron deficiency anaemia in pregnancy

Women with diets poor in iron prior to pregnancy and a history of anaemia require verification of haemoglobin and ferritin status to assess whether supplements are required. Anaemia is most likely to affect women on a low income (see 'Eating on a low income', p. 354), those with low BMI, or vegetarians with an unbalanced diet (see 'Vegetarians', p. 346). In the UK, iron supplements are advised only if there is evidence of iron deficiency anaemia (see diagnosis of anaemia in 'Iron', p. 148).

However, care should be taken not to 'blanket' prescribe iron supplements (can result in nausea and constipation), as in later pregnancy many women experience haemodilution and physiological changes that may resemble iron deficiency (↓ haemoglobin and ↓ ferritin). See 'Iron', p. 148, for good dietary sources of iron.

Gestational diabetes

Estimated prevalence is 3–5% of pregnancies in the UK. Abnormal glucose Intolerance occurs in pregnancy and usually disappears after birth, although there is evidence that it is a marker for development of type 2 diabetes in later life. Diagnosis is made at fasting blood glucose >7 mmol/L (see Table 22.1 for further information on diagnosis). Women who are obese/overweight, aged ≥30 years, and have a family history of type 2 diabetes are at greater risk of developing gestational diabetes, increased risk of macrosomia at birth, and increased likelihood of caesarean.

A meta-analysis of cohort studies[7] reported a 7.5-fold ↑ risk of developing type 2 diabetes for women who had been diagnosed with gestational diabetes. See 'Diabetes in pregnancy', p. 516 for advice on management.

Constipation in pregnancy

During pregnancy, 35–40% of women suffer from constipation as peristalsis is slower.

Encouraging fresh and dried fruit and vegetables for pectins, and wholemeal bread and breakfast cereals for cereal fibre will relieve symptoms, and plenty of fluid should be taken, preferably as water. Faecal bulking agents may help.

---

7 Bellamy, L., et al. (2009). Type 2 diabetes mellitus after gestational diabetes: a systematic review and meta-analysis. Lancet 373, 1773–9.

Women may intentionally restrict their fluid intake to reduce frequency of micturition; this could be a factor in them becoming constipated. See 'Constipation' (p. 672).

Heartburn in pregnancy

Heartburn is common and 30–50% of pregnant women experience symptoms. This can occur at any stage of pregnancy, but is common in the third trimester.

Suggestions for relief of heartburn

- Small, frequent meals.
- Eat earlier in the evening and avoid late night meals.
- Chew food thoroughly and slowly.
- Take fluids between meals, not at mealtimes.
- Dairy foods may relieve symptoms.
- Avoid spicy and acidic foods that may irritate GI mucosa. Food causing symptoms varies a lot in different women; examples include chilli, vinegar, pepper, acidic fruit juices.
- Avoid foods that relax oesophageal muscles before bedtime, e.g. chocolate, fatty foods, alcohol, and mint.
- Sleep propped up with cushions.
- Avoid bending after eating.

Vulnerable groups in pregnancy

Adolescents and pregnancy

Pregnancy in adolescence increases risk to the:
- *fetus* of low birth weight, perinatal mortality, and premature delivery;
- *mother* suffering anaemia, difficult labour, and hypertension.

As adolescents are still growing, optimal weight gain is unknown, but it is likely to be higher than for adult women (see 'Maternal weight gain', p. 248). They are less likely to eat healthily and have higher reference nutrient intakes (RNIs) for calcium and iron than women >18 years, ∴ they are less likely to meet requirements for calcium and iron (see 'Nutrient deficiencies in children', p. 312). Iron deficiency anaemia can result in low birth weight and preterm delivery.

Social problems may have an influence and will compound pregnancy outcome, including:
- reducing energy intake to try and hide pregnancy;
- low income;
- smoking;
- alcohol consumption;
- substance abuse;
- previous dieting leading to low nutrient stores;
- less knowledge and skills to eat a healthy diet.

Vegetarians

Being vegetarian should pose no problem in pregnancy if the woman is well informed and eating a balanced lacto-ovo and lacto-vegetarian diet. Pregnant vegan, fruitarian, and macrobiotic women should be seen by a dietitian to assess overall nutrient adequacy of their diets. They may require supplementation of vitamin B_{12}, iron, vitamin D, or calcium (if <600 mg/day consumed). Some fortified soya milks contain these nutrients. (see 'Vegetarians', p. 346).

Asian vegetarian women could be at risk of vitamin D deficiency if insufficient skin exposure → neonatal hypocalcaemia and rickets, ∴ may need additional vitamin D supplements (see 'Minority ethnic communities', p. 338).

Pregnant vegetarian adolescents are at particular risk of inadequate diet if they are the only 'veggie' in the house, as they may tend to eat the same as the rest of the family except 'remove' the protein aspect of the meal or replace it with cheese, ready-prepared vegetarian sausages, and burgers.

Low income and pregnancy

Although it is difficult to generalize, UK women on low incomes may find it harder to achieve an adequate diet (see 'The Eatwell Guide' p. 27 and 'Eating on a low income', p. 354). Key nutrients at risk of low intakes are: zinc and iron, and vitamins A, C, and E and essential fatty acids (EFAs) needed for fetal neural and vascular system development. EFAs are found in green vegetables, oily fish (e.g. tuna, sardines, mackerel, salmon, herring, pilchards, trout, and kippers), and certain vegetable oils (e.g. corn, sunflower, and soya oils). Cheaper blended vegetable oils and margarine are often consumed but they contain less EFAs.

Healthy Start scheme

In the UK, the welfare food scheme has been replaced by the Healthy Start scheme. The Healthy Start scheme allows beneficiaries to exchange tokens for fresh fruit and vegetables through general retail (see 'Healthy Start scheme', p. 276). For further information on Healthy Start, see ℘ http://www.healthystart.nhs.uk.

Closely spaced pregnancies

Women with closely spaced pregnancies may have low nutrient stores at conception and in early pregnancy, so taking a dietary history would be useful to assess previous and current diet for nutrient adequacy (including iron status).

Diabetic women

Regular glucose monitoring and good compliance will result in the same outcome as for non-diabetic mothers. However, poor control can ↑ risk of pre-eclampsia, ↑ fetal problems, and ↑ infant mortality.

Useful websites

ℙ UK NHS advice:
http://www.nhs.uk/conditions/pregnancy-and-baby/pages/pregnancy-and-baby-care.aspx

ℙ UK healthy eating advice:
http://www.nhs.uk/Livewell/healthy-eating/Pages/Healthyeating.aspx
https://www.gov.uk/government/publications/the-eatwell-guide

ℙ Healthy Start scheme:
https://www.healthystart.nhs.uk/

Infants and preschool children

Infant growth and development 258
Breast versus bottle feeding 262
Promoting and establishing breastfeeding 266
Dietary recommendations for lactation 272
Establishing bottle feeding 274
Weaning 278
Iron deficiency anaemia in infancy 284
Faltering growth 286
Obesity prevention in infancy 290
Constipation, toddler diarrhoea, and milk hypersensitivity 292
Nutritionally vulnerable infants 298
Fussy eaters 300

Infant growth and development

Dietary recommendations for infants and preschool children

In the first year of life, birth weight increases by 300%, doubling in the first 4–6 months; and height increases by 50%. This rapid growth involves tissue and organ maturation, so energy and nutrient requirements are high relative to body size, especially during the first year (see Table 13.1). In the first 3 months of life, 35% of energy requirements are utilized for growth, but by 12 months age, this has dropped to 3%. High protein synthesis rates in the newborn contribute to high energy and protein requirements.

Children aged <2 years need a higher fat and lower fibre diet than that proposed in the 'The Eatwell Guide' (see p. 27), as they need fat for growth and central nervous system (CNS) development. However, between the ages of 2 and 5 years, children should gradually move to eating the proportions shown in the Eatwell Guide, if they are growing normally.

Growth reference charts

Monitoring children's growth is essential to identify any faltering growth. Length/height, weight, and occipito-frontal head circumference (OFC) should be plotted on a growth reference curve. An infant's growth should follow the direction of the growth curves. Serial measurements are necessary to determine adequacy of growth; a one-off measurement is only a reflection of size. The chart (Box 13.1) can be a useful tool for communicating with parents so that they understand the importance of monitoring growth. Parents with naturally short children will need reassuring that s/he is growing well if they are progressing in parallel with the same centile throughout infancy and childhood.

Where growth is unimpaired, adult height can be estimated in children aged 2–4 years from the child's current height centile, using the adult height predictor for both boys and girls, in the 0–4-year UK-World Health Organization (WHO) growth charts (see Appendix 2, p. 861).

If there are any concerns that the child may be under- or overweight, it is recommended that from age of 2 years, body mass index (BMI) is calculated [weight (kg)/height (m²)], which should be adjusted for age and gender using BMI centile charts (see Appendix 2, p. 854). Alternatively, the BMI centile can be estimated using the weight-height to BMI conversion chart in the 0–4-year UK-WHO charts (see Appendix 2, p. 861).

Which growth charts should be used?

In April 2006, the WHO published Child Growth Standards for infants and children up to the age of 5 years. They are based on the growth of around 8500 healthy, non-deprived children from six different countries (USA, Norway, India, Ghana, Brazil, Oman), who were breastfed exclusively for the first 4 months, weaned by 6 months, by healthy mothers who did not smoke.[1] It is believed that all charts should be based on breastfed infants, as this is the biological norm and all infants should be compared to this whatever their ethnic origin and however they are fed in infancy. This standard was adopted by the UK for children under 4 years and used to construct the

1 De Onis, M., et al. (2004). The WHO Multicentre Growth Reference Study: planning, study design, and methodology. *Food Nutr. Bull.* **25**, S15–S26.

Table 13.1 Energy and RNI for infants and preschool children*

Nutrient	0–3 months	4–6 months	7–9 months	10–12 months	1–3 years	4–6 years
Energy, MJ/d Females	2.6	2.7	2.9	3.2	4.1	6.2
Energy, MJ/d Males	2.4	2.5	2.7	3.0	3.8	5.8
Energy, kcal/kg/day	100-115	95	95	95	95	90
Protein, g	12.5	12.7	13.7	14.9	14.5	19.7
Protein, g/kg/day	2.1	1.6	1.5	1.5	1.1	1.1
Fluid, ml/kg	150	130	120	110	95	85
Vitamin C, mg	25	25	25	25	30	30
Vitamin A, µg	350	350	350	350	400	400
Vitamin D, µg	8.5–10	8.5–10	8.5–10	8.5–10	10	10
Folic acid, µg	50	50	50	50	70	100
Thiamine, mg	0.2	0.2	0.2	0.3	0.5	0.7
Riboflavin, mg	0.4	0.4	0.4	0.4	0.6	0.8
Niacin, mg	3	3	4	5	8	11
Vitamin B_{12}, µg	0.3	0.3	0.4	0.4	0.5	0.8
Iron, mg	1.7	4.3	7.8	7.8	6.9	6.1
Calcium, mg	525	525	525	525	350	450
Phosphorus, mg	400	400	400	400	270	350
Magnesium, mg	55	60	75	80	85	120
Zinc, mg	4.0	4.0	5.0	5.0	5.0	6.5
Selenium, µg	10	13	10	10	15	20
Copper, mg	0.2	0.3	0.3	0.3	0.4	0.6

*Source: data on energy from SACN (2011). Dietary reference values for energy. ℘ https://www.gov.uk/government/publications/sacn-dietary-reference-values-for-energy Source: data on vitamin D from SACN (2016) Vitamin D and Health report. ℘ ttps://www.gov.uk/government/publications/sacn-vitamin-d-and-health-report Source: data on RNIs from DH(1991). Dietary reference values for food and nutrients for the UK. HMSO, London.

Box 13.1 Calculating adult height potential

Parental height plays a role in determining eventual height and mid-parental height (target centile range) is useful to estimate the genetic height potential of a child. To calculate adult height potential:

(a) = father's height
(b) = mother's height
(c) = sum of (a) + (b)
(d) = (c) ÷ 2
(e) = (d) −7 cm if girl or +7 cm if boy (mid-parental height)
(f) = (e) ±8.5 cm (target centile range)

UK-WHO charts[2] (🏶 www.rcpch.ac.uk/child-health/research-projects/uk-who-growth-charts/uk-who-growth-chart-resources-0-4-years/uk-who-0).

The existing UK90 growth reference charts were constructed using measurements from a large number of British children at different ages, collected in the late 1980s and were the main charts in use until 2009.[3] Because the WHO charts do not include preterm data, the UK 1990 data were used to make the birth section of the UK-WHO charts and low birth weight charts, as well as charts for use after the age of 4 years. They are a description of typical, but not necessarily healthy, growth in UK children from 1980 to 1990.

All charts have nine reference centiles of 0.4th, 2nd, 9th, 25th, 50th, 75th, 91st, 98th, and 99.6th that mean, for example:
- 98th centile curve, below which 98% of UK children lie (2 in 100 children will be as tall/heavy as this);
- 50th centile curve, below which 50% of UK children lie (average weight and height for a child of that age);
- 2nd centile curve, below which only 2% of UK children lie (2 in 100 children will be as small/light as this).

These are available at 🏶 http://www.healthforallchildren.com/hfac-support/.

UK-WHO growth charts are used in the UK, using appropriate girls' or boys' charts and are based on the following data:
- *Low birth weight:* 23 weeks gestation to 2 years (UK90 data).
- *Birth to 1 year* (WHO data + birth UK90 data).
- *0–4 years* (WHO data).
- *2–18 years* (UK90 data).

Six separate charts covering birth to 4 years are included in the UK Personal Child Health Record (PCHR) issued to each newborn (see 🏶 http://www.dchs.nhs.uk/assets/public/nhs_record_keeping/docs/Childrens%20red%20book.pdf). An addition to the growth charts (2013) is the childhood and puberty close monitoring chart, designed for use in children with growth or nutritional problems where close attention to underweight/overweight and pubertal status is required. There are also specific charts available to monitor growth for children with Downs's syndrome. See 🏶 http://www.rcpch.ac.uk/child-health/research-projects/uk-who-growth-charts/uk-growth-chart-resources-2-18-years/school-age#cpcm.

How often should infants be measured?

As part of the birth assessment, all babies should be weighed and OFC measured and plotted, and these measurements repeated at the 6–8 week

---

2 Department of Health (2007). *Application of the WHO Growth Standards in the UK*. Department of Health, London. Available at: 🏶http://www.sacn.gov.uk/.

3 Wright, C.M., *et al.* (2002). Growth reference charts for use in the United Kingdom. *Arch. Dis. Child* 86, 11–14.

check for healthy babies. Sick babies may need more frequent weighing.[4,5] Babies and young children can be further opportunistically weighed at immunization (8, 12, and 16 weeks, and 1 year age) and at surveillance contacts; new baby review at 10-14 days old, 12 month, and 2-2.5 year health review. As part of the Department of Health (DH) Healthy Child Programme 2-year review (2009),[6] both height and weight should be measured to calculate BMI. Previously it was not considered routine to measure length/height in healthy, term children until school entry at around 5 years of age.[4] Length, however, should be measured and plotted in any child whose health, growth, or feeding pattern is causing concern.[4]

Measuring too frequently may cause parental anxiety and it is recommended that babies should be weighed no more than monthly (aged <6 months), once every 2 months (aged 6–12 months), and quarterly (aged >1 year).

4 Hall, D.M.B., Elliman, D. (ed). (2006). Health for all children, 4th ed. OUP, Oxford.

5 NICE (2006). Postnatal care up to 8 weeks after birth (CG37). NICE clinical guideline 37. Available at: ℗ http://www.nice.org.uk/guidance/cg37.

6 DH (2009). Healthy Child Programme: review of children aged 2. Available at: ℗ https://www.gov.uk/government/publications/healthy-child-programme-review-of-children-aged-2.

Breast versus bottle feeding

Breastmilk is the best choice for infant feeding for many reasons (see Box 13.2). Infant formula has a different composition to breastmilk and does not provide all the same benefits, particularly the immunological active components, nor the same nutritional profile and bioavailability.

The composition of breastmilk is not homogeneous: colostrum is produced 1–3 days postpartum, eventually becoming mature milk after 3 weeks. The immunological factors are not only present in colostrum produced during the first few days of lactation, but continue throughout breastfeeding.

Box 13.2 Protective factors in breastmilk

- *Immunological active components*: lactoferrin; cytokines; T- and B-lymphocytes; neutrophils; macrophages; immunoglobulins; lysozymes; growth factors; thyroxin; antiviral lipids; antiprotozoan factors; and bifidus factor (promotes growth of protective *Lactobacillus bifidus* in infant's GI tract)
- *Essential long chain fatty acids (LCPs)*: amino acids (AA) and docosahexaenoic acid (DHA) important for cell membrane structure, especially CNS and retina development
- *Structured fats*: (palmitic acid) result in better fat and calcium absorption, producing softer stools, less constipation, and improved bone development
- *Proteins*: predominantly α-lactalbumin (rich source of essential amino acids) and free amino acids
- *Nucleotides*: supports development and maturation of the gut and immune system
- *Oligosaccharides (prebiotics)*: breastmilk contains >200 different oligosaccharides that help normal brain development, support the development of a healthy gut microbiome and produces softer stools, reducing constipation

---

Benefits of breastfeeding

For the mother
- Encourages bonding between mother and infant.
- Helps women lose excess weight gained during pregnancy.
- Breastfeeding stimulates uterine contractions that help return the uterus to normal size.
- Exclusive breastfeeding suppresses ovulation, helping iron stores return to normal.
- Breastmilk is free, except that the mother needs extra nourishment (see 'Dietary recommendations for lactation', p. 272).
- Convenience; no preparation required.
- Reduces mother's risk of developing premenopausal breast cancer.

For the infant
- Breastmilk offers complete nutrition for the first 6 months and high bioavailability of nutrients.

- Infants are less likely to experience gastrointestinal (GI) infections, as there is no need for access to clean water, which can be a problem in low-income countries in particular (may also be because of protective factors).
- Prevention of other infectious diseases, especially respiratory, ear, and urinary tract infections (greatest impact is for infants exclusively breastfed for first 6 months).
- Breastfed babies are less likely to be obese in later childhood.

Potential obstacles to breastfeeding

- Frequent myth of 'not enough milk': usually results from incorrect breastfeeding technique (see 'Promoting and establishing breastfeeding', p. 266). This is a common reason for women stopping breastfeeding.
- Freedom of the mother: she can feel exhausted as she takes complete responsibility for feeding ∴ she will need support of others with housework, especially in the first few weeks.
- Mother may be concerned that she cannot see how much milk the baby is taking.
- Engorged breasts and sore nipples can discourage some mothers; it should be ensured that the correct position is used for feeding and latching on.
- High stress levels: mother's mental state will affect the letdown reflex; anxiety → oxytocin ↓. She should be encouraged to rest more and relax when breastfeeding.
- Glamorous image of infant formula portraying healthy, beautiful babies via advertising.
- Social taboo of breastfeeding in public in some cultures, UK included.
- Lack of public facilities for breastfeeding, especially needed in colder months.
- Lack of employment legislation supporting breastfeeding mothers in some countries. Note: mothers are entitled to express breastmilk at work in the UK.
- May be perceived as offensive by some women, their partners, and older children.
- Breastfeeding of boys may be encouraged more in some cultures. It should be reinforced that breastfeeding is best for girls and boys.

Contraindications to breastfeeding

- HIV+ women: by vertical transmission from mother to infant, breastfeeding increases risk of transmission by up to 20%. The WHO states that health authorities should decide on the strategy that is most likely to give infants the greatest chance of HIV-free survival, i.e. whether health services will principally counsel and support mothers known to be HIV infected to either (i) breastfeed and receive antiretroviral (ARV) drugs for up to 12 months or (ii) avoid all breastfeeding.[7] In developed, well-resourced countries the latter is encouraged, e.g. HIV+ women living in the UK should not breastfeed.[8]

---

7 World Health Organization. (2016). *Maternal, newborn, child and adolescent health. Updates on HIV and infant feeding.* Available at: ℘ http://www.who.int/maternal_child_adolescent/documents/hiv-infant-feeding-2016/en/.

8 ℘ CHIVA Standards of Care for Infants, Children, and Young People with HIV (including infants born to mothers with HIV). Available at: ℘ https://www.chiva.org.uk/files/5215/3987/5455/CHIVA_STANDARDS_2017.pdf.

- Mothers with untreated tuberculosis should not breastfeed.
- Mothers with hepatitis C who have cracked or bleeding nipples should not breastfeed.
- Women who smoke or occasionally drink alcohol *can* still breastfeed; however, smoking will lower the vitamin C content of breastmilk. Even so, it is still preferable to infant formula.
- *Certain drugs:* illegal drugs will pass into breastmilk ∴ users should not breastfeed. Medicines should be checked for suitability in the *British National Formulary* (see ✒ https://bnfc.nice.org.uk/).
- Some types of breast surgery.
- Infants with galactosaemia (see Table 36.1, p. 817) as they cannot metabolize galactose present in breastmilk. Lactose-free infant formulae should be used.
- Phenylketonuria (PKU) infants should alternate breastmilk with phenylalanine-free formula.

Promoting and establishing breastfeeding

Promoting breastfeeding

Exclusive breastfeeding is recommended in the UK (nothing else but breastmilk, not even water) for the first 6 months (26 weeks) of life. However, the UK has some of the lowest exclusive breastfeeding rates globally. Breastfeeding initiation of ~74% is reported in England, based on data from electronic care records, which has remained steady (see ℜ https://www.england.nhs.uk/statistics/wp-content/uploads/sites/2/2014/03/Breastfeeding-1516Q11.pdf). In Scotland, breastfeeding data estimate that almost half of babies born in 2015/16 (49.3%) were being breastfed at around 10 days of age (see ℜ https://www.isdscotland.org/Health-Topics/Child-Health/Publications/2016-10-25/2016-10-25-Breastfeeding-Summary.pdf).

In low-income and middle-income countries (LMICs), only 37% of children < 6 months of age are exclusively breastfed for 6 months,[9] but this is much better than the UK context, e.g. in England only 1% of babies are exclusively breastfed for 6 months.[10] Breastfeeding duration is usually shorter in high-income countries than in LMICs. In the UK, breastfeeding rates vary greatly and are highest among mothers from managerial and professional occupations, those with highest educational levels, those aged 30 or over, those from ethnic minority groups and first time mothers. Young women in low-income areas with lower education levels are least likely to initiate and continue breastfeeding.

The DH in the UK has targeted increasing breastfeeding rates at 6–8 weeks and has undertaken to support the NHS by:

- supporting a National Helpline for breastfeeding mothers (see ℜ https://www.nationalbreastfeedinghelpline.org.uk/);
- encouraging adoption of UNICEF's Baby Friendly Initiative (see Box 13.3);
- developing a code of best practice for employers and businesses to support employees and customers who breastfeed (see ℜ http://www.nhs.uk/Conditions/pregnancy-and-baby/Pages/breastfeeding-back-to-work.aspx).

Promotion of breastfeeding is outlined in the Healthy Child Programme, which aims to bring together health, education, and other main partners to deliver an effective programme for prevention and support.[11] Training needs to target all health professionals to emphasize the benefits of breastfeeding and appropriate techniques, so that women receive consistent messages throughout their care.

9 Victora, C.G., *et al.* (2016) Breastfeeding in the 21st century: epidemiology, mechanisms, and lifelong effect. *Lancet* **387**, 491–504.

10 Available at: ℜ https://www.unicef.org.uk/babyfriendly/.

11 DH (2009). *Healthy Child Programme. Pregnancy and the first five years of life*. Available at: ℜ https://www.gov.uk/government/publications/healthy-child-programme-pregnancy-and-the-first-5-years-of-life.

Box 13.3 Baby Friendly Initiative standards*

- Building a firm foundation
  - Have written policies and guidelines to support standards.
  - Plan an education programme that will allow staff to implement standards according to their role.
  - Have processes for implementing, auditing, and evaluating standards.
  - Ensure that there is no promotion of breastmilk substitutes, bottles, teats, or dummies in any part of the facility or by any staff.
- An educated workforce
  - Educate staff to implement the standards according to their role and the service provided.
- Parents' experiences of maternity services
  - Support pregnant women to recognize importance of breastfeeding and early relationships for baby's health and wellbeing.
  - Support all mothers and babies to initiate a close relationship and feeding soon after birth.
  - Enable mothers to get breastfeeding off to a good start.
  - Support mothers to make informed decisions regarding the introduction of food or fluids other than breastmilk.
  - Support parents to have a close/loving relationship with their baby.
- Parents' experiences of health-visiting/public health nursing
  - Support pregnant women to recognize the importance of breastfeeding and early relationships for the health and wellbeing of their baby.
  - Enable mothers to continue breastfeeding for as long as they wish.
  - Support mothers to make informed decisions regarding the introduction of food or fluids other than breastmilk.
  - Support parents to have a close and loving relationship with their baby.

Full guidance available at ᵂ https://www.unicef.org.uk/babyfriendly/baby-friendly-resources/guidance-for-health-professionals/implementing-the-baby-friendly-standards/guide-to-the-baby-friendly-initiative-standards/.

The use of breastfeeding peer-support programmes is recommended, with joint working between health professionals and peer supporters.[12] In 2015, responsibility for children's public health commissioning transferred from NHS England to local authorities and as a result, guidance was produced to support local authorities in commissioning 'public health services for children and young people' including delivering the Healthy Child Programme for 0-5 years and 5-19 years.

Maternal education needs to begin antenatally with local healthcare services providing breastfeeding classes and written support, including leaflets. The father, family, and/or friends should be encouraged to participate

12 Public Health England. (2016). *Healthy child programme 0 to 19: health visitor and school nurse commissioning.* Available at: ᵂ https://www.gov.uk/government/publications/healthy-child-programme-0-to-19-health-visitor-and-school-nurse-commissioning.

so that the woman can be offered support. Focus should be on changing attitudes and knowledge of the technique and the recommended length of time to continue feeding. Many young mothers from lower income areas lack access to key sources of advice and information, such as antenatal classes, peer support programmes, friends, family, and other support networks. Support and education should be targeted at these groups.

Common reasons given by women in the UK for the choice of feeding method and reasons for stopping breastfeeding[13] are useful targets for public health measures (see Tables 13.2 and 13.3). Three-quarters of breastfeeding mothers who gave up said they would have liked to continue, suggesting that they are committed if obstacles can be overcome.

Table 13.2 Common reasons for feeding method in the UK

Breast	Bottle
Best for baby's health	Dislike idea of breastfeeding
Convenience	Lifestyle/convenience
Health benefits for mother	Others can feed baby
Closer bond between mother and baby	Previous feeding behaviour
Cheaper than infant formula	Embarrassed to breastfeed

Table 13.3 Common reasons for stopping breastfeeding in the UK

First 2 weeks	Later months
Rejecting the breast/baby not sucking	Returning to work
Painful breasts or nipples	
Mother feeling she has insufficient milk	
Too demanding/always hungry	

13 McAndrew, F., et al. (2012) Infant Feeding Survey 2010. Health and Social Care Information Centre. Available at: ℘ http://content.digital.nhs.uk/catalogue/PUB08694/Infant-Feeding-Survey-2010-Consolidated-Report.pdf.

Baby Friendly Initiative (BFI)

To improve breastfeeding rates, both maternity hospitals and community healthcare settings are seeking baby friendly accreditation (see Box 13.3).[14] New standards for the Baby Friendly Initiative, published by UNICEF in 2012 replace the former '10 steps to successful breastfeeding' (hospital) and the '7 point plan for protecting, promoting and supporting breastfeeding in community health care settings' (community). In addition, there are now Baby Friendly University Standard awards (usually for universities involved in training midwives), and work is under way for neonatal units. Infant Feeding Advisors are being employed to help achieve baby friendly accreditation.

Establishing breastfeeding (Box 13.4)

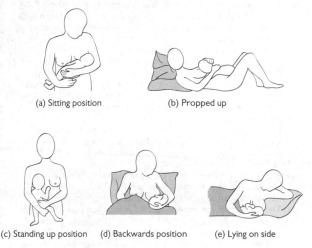

(a) Sitting position

(b) Propped up

(c) Standing up position   (d) Backwards position   (e) Lying on side

Fig. 13.1 Breastfeeding positions. Reproduced with permission from World Health Organization. *Breastfeeding: how to support success. A practical guide for health workers.* Geneva, Switzerland: World Health Organization. © World Health Organization 1997. ℘ http://www.euro.who.int/__data/assets/pdf_file/0019/118414/E57592.pdf.

14 Unicef UK. *The Baby Friendly Initiative.* Available at: ℘ www.babyfriendly.org.uk.

Box 13.4 Patients' FAQs for establishing breastfeeding

- How soon after the birth should I put my baby on the breast?
  - Start as soon after birth as possible (preferably within 1 hour) as suckling stimulates the letdown response.
- How often should I feed?
  - Feed as often as the infant wants; not restricting frequency or duration will help fully establish the milk supply initially. Infants usually feed 8–12 times a day, including at night. The first 3 weeks are crucial. Dummies should be avoided, as will ↓ baby sucking frequency.
- How long should I let my baby feed on each breast?
  - Always offer both breasts at each feed. Let the baby finish the first breast completely as incomplete emptying of the breasts means the baby may just drink 'foremilk' and not the fat dense 'hind milk'. If this is habitual practice, it may affect infant growth. Babies may seem sleepy but can often be coaxed awake to feed for longer. Start on a different breast from the one last emptied.
- Which position is best for feeding my baby?
  - The most comfortable and convenient position of the baby on the breast will depend on the mother (see Fig. 13.1 and see ℘ https://www.nhs.uk/start4life/breastfeeding#steps). If baby is restless at the breast and seems unsatisfied, it hurts to breastfeed, or the mother gets cracked nipples, adjust position of baby.
- How do I know if my baby is getting enough milk?
  - Plenty of wet nappies; bright yellow, regular stools (after the first week or two), contented baby after a feed; baby gains weight and looks well.
- Does my baby need extra drinks?
  - No. Foremilk is more watery and thirst quenching and in hot weather, babies tend to take shorter, more frequent feeds.
- My breasts are swollen, hard, and painful. Is this normal?
  - This is breast engorgement, which occurs when your milk comes in about day 3 and can occur if there has been a delay between feeds. Feeding on demand should prevent it. Lumps are likely to be blocked ducts. Feed from the breast and massage the lump towards the nipple. If there is a red, hot painful patch it may be mastitis. Keep feeding from the breast and avoid wearing a bra at night.
- I want to carry on breastfeeding, but I'm going back to work full-time when the baby is 3 months; what can I do?
  - If returning to work, exclusive breastfeeding will be challenging, unless the mother is extremely motivated and expresses and freezes breastmilk for use when at work. (Note: mothers are entitled to express breastmilk at work in the UK). A high quality breast pump is essential. Mixed bottle/breast may be a more realistic solution in this situation and the woman can continue with pre- and post-work breastfeeds. See 'Combining breast and bottle' in 'Establishing bottle feeding', p. 274.

Breastfeeding help and support further information

℘ Association of Breastfeeding Mothers (ABM). http://www.abm.me.uk.

Breastfeeding network supporter line (Tel. 0300 100 0210) or available at: ℘ http://www.breastfeedingnetwork.org.uk.

℘ DH *Start4Life*. https://www.nhs.uk/start4life/breastfeeding

℘ DH *Bump to Breastfeeding (Best Beginnings)* DVD, given during pregnancy or available at: https://www.bestbeginnings.org.uk/watch-from-bump-to-breastfeeding-online.

℘ DH Northern Ireland (2016). *The Pregnancy book*. http://www.publichealth.hscni.net/publications/pregnancy-book-0.

℘ NHS choices. http://www.nhs.uk/Conditions/pregnancy-and-baby/pages/pregnancy-and-baby-care.aspx.

℘ La Leche League (UK). http://www.laleche.org.uk.

℘ National Breastfeeding Helpline. http://www.nationalbreastfeedinghelpline.org.uk.

℘ National Childbirth Trust (NCT). http://www.nct.org.uk.

Dietary recommendations for lactation

Lactating women should follow the general healthy eating guidance in 'The Eatwell Guide' (see 'Food-based dietary guidelines', p. 26), but care should be taken to meet the extra requirements for energy, protein, two fat-soluble vitamins, five water-soluble vitamins, and six minerals (Table 13.4). On a practical level, this can be achieved by women eating larger quantities of a healthy diet. In addition, women should:

- Limit alcohol to 1–2 units once or twice a week, as alcohol will pass into breastmilk affecting its smell and potentially the baby's sleep patterns and digestion. Try to avoid breastfeeding for at least 2–3 hours per unit after drinking.
- Avoid too much caffeine as this will pass into breastmilk → infant hyperactivity and sleeplessness. Limit to 300 mg of caffeine/day. Tea, coffee, cocoa, energy drinks, and cola-type drinks need to be limited. Suggest decaffeinated tea/coffee. See 'Caffeine' p. 211.
- Consume at least 2 L of fluid a day to avoid dehydration (35 mL/kg body weight). See 'Fluid balance', p. 184.
- Avoid spicy foods that may alter the taste of breastmilk if the infant appears to reject milk as a result.
- Eat no more than two portions (140 g each) of oily fish/week (fresh mackerel, sardines, trout, and tuna). Limit shark, swordfish, or marlin to one portion/week.
- Can eat peanuts or foods containing peanuts as part of a balanced diet, even if a family history (siblings, mother, father) of allergy (asthma, eczema, hay fever) exists.
- Everyone, including those who are pregnant and breastfeeding, is advised to consider taking a vitamin D supplement to meet the reference nutrient intake (RNI) (10 μg).[15] Those eligible for the UK Healthy Start scheme[16] can obtain free vitamins (see 'Establishing bottle feeding,' 'Healthy Start Scheme', p. 276).
- Supplements of other vitamins and minerals are not usually necessary. Exceptions are vegan, macrobiotic, or fruitarian women who may need B_{12} supplements, and women following dietary restrictions, e.g. cows' milk-free diet. These, and women with poor dietary intakes should see a dietitian.
- When a woman is breastfeeding exclusively, her nutritional status will be compromised before that of the infant.

15 SACN (2016) *Vitamin D and health report*. Available at: ✍ https://www.gov.uk/government/publications/sacn-vitamin-d-and-health-report.

16 NICE (2008). *Improving the nutrition of pregnant and breastfeeding mothers and children in low-income households*. NICE Public Health Guidance 11.

Table 13.4 RNIs for lactating mothers*

	Daily RNI (15–50 years)	↑ in lactation
Energy, MJ/d	11.0–11.6	+1.38 MJ/d for first 6 months
Protein, g	51	+11 (0–4 months) +8 (>4 months)
Vitamin C, mg	40	+30
Vitamin A, µg	600	+350
Folic acid, µg	200	+60
Thiamine, mg	0.8	+0.2
Riboflavin, mg	1.4	+0.5
Niacin, mg	13–14	+2
Vitamin B$_{12}$, µg	1.5	+0.5
Calcium, mg	700–800	+550
Phosphorus, mg	550–625	+440
Magnesium, mg	270–300	+50
Zinc, mg	7.0	+6.0 (0–4 months) +2.5 (>4 months)
Selenium, µg	60	+15
Copper, mg	1.0–1.2	+0.3

Source: data on protein and zinc from SACN 2011 *Dietary reference values for energy*. TSO, London. Source: data on RNIs from Department of Health (1991). *Dietary reference values for food and nutrients for the United Kingdom*. HMSO, London.

Establishing bottle feeding

Care should be taken that women who choose to bottle feed are not made to feel guilty or inadequate as a result of their decision. Once their choice is made they need to be supported accordingly. Modified cows' milk infant formula will meet all nutrient requirements, but all protective immunological factors will be absent.

Combining breast and bottle

After breastmilk is well established (4–6 weeks), it may be possible to combine breast and bottle where circumstances dictate, e.g. woman returns to work; woman is exhausted (physically or mentally) from feeding continuously; or male partner needs to bond/help with the baby. Introducing one to two bottle feeds during the day, for example, and regularly continuing with breastmilk before and after returning from work should not affect the woman's ability to breastfeed.

🍼 This is preferable to stopping breastfeeding entirely, but is not the 'ideal' option as exclusive breastfeeding is recommended for the first 6 months of life.

Choice of infant formula

- In the UK, there are three main types of cows' milk formula:
- *Whey dominant* (most companies label as first milk, stage 1): ratio of whey to casein of ~60:40. Whey-based formula is recommended as it most closely resembles the protein structure of breastmilk. Formulas vary, with 'extras' added based on components in breastmilk (see Box 13.2 on protective factors of breastmilk, in breast versus bottle section); some have a higher ratio of α-lactalbumin, most contain added long chain polyunsaturated fats (docosahexaenoic acid and arachidonic acid), some have structured fats, many contain nucleotides and prebiotics, and some are organic. The wide choice can be confusing for parents.
- *Casein dominant* (most companies have removed this from their standard range). Whey to casein ratio of ~20:80; similar to doorstep cows' milk. They are marketed and perceived by parents as milks that can help fill up babies as they get 'hungrier' ~6–10 weeks (they contain the same energy, but more protein than whey dominant milks). Do not usually contain 'extras'.
- *Follow-on and toddler milks* (most companies now label follow-on formula as 'stage 2' and toddler milks as 'stage 3' upwards). In the UK, follow-on infant formula is widely used for infants aged >6 months. Some parents wish to change their infant's milk at 4–6 months as a symbolic 'developmental milestone'. In these cases, follow-on milk is preferable to introducing solids early or doorstep cows' milk. Follow-on formula is higher in iron, and toddler milks contain additional vitamins and minerals, with a lower protein and sodium content compared with doorstep cows' milk. There is no evidence of nutritional benefit from changing milks, compared with remaining on first stage whey-based infant formula during the first year of life, in infants and children who are following an otherwise well-balanced diet. However, 'follow-on' and

'toddler' milks may be useful in nutritionally at-risk infants, particularly because of their higher iron content.

Infant formula and energy

Although the energy content of breastmilk is reported to be 70 kcal/100 mL, this is based on the energy content of milk obtained by completely expressing the first breast. This is unlikely to be a true representation of suckled human milk, and doubly labelled water studies of suckled human milk have suggested values of 53–58 kcal/100 mL at 6 weeks and 3 months, respectively. The Scientific Committee for Food (SCF 2003) recommends a maximum energy content of 60–70 kcal/100 mL for both standard and follow-on infant formula.

Soya-based infant formula

Infant formula based on soya is not recommended for infants <6 months of age, because of both the phytoestrogen content which, may impact on future reproductive health, and risk of sensitization to soya protein. Soya formula should not be used in premature or low birth weight infants, or babies with impaired renal function. Soya formula should only be used in exceptional circumstances, e.g.
- vegan mothers who do not breastfeed;
- infants with cows' milk protein allergy, who consistently refuse elemental formula;
- galactosaemia.

If soya infant formula is used, it should be consumed as the main milk drink until ~2 years of age, when standard soya milk alternatives fortified with calcium, with energy content similar to semi-skimmed milk, can be used.

Goats' milk infant formula

Infant formula based on goats' milk protein is now considered suitable for infants, but it is *not* suitable for infants who are allergic to cows' milk formula or who are suffering from transient lactose intolerance post gastroenteritis. Goats' milk infant formula contains smaller fat globules and shorter chain fatty acids, e.g. caproic and caprilic acid (hence the taste difference) so is potentially easier to digest. However, it is significantly more expensive.

Preparation of infant formula

Powdered infant formula is not a sterile product and could contain bacteria such as *Cronobacter sakazakii*. Standard infant formula should be made up with water between 70°C and 80°C (equivalent to boiling a kettle and cooling for approximately 30 min). Higher temperatures will denature vitamin C. Microwaves should not be used. Bottles should ideally be made up one at a time, as storing bottles for any length of time increases risk of bacterial growth. A practical compromise would be to make up one bottle in advance and store in the back of a fridge (which should run between 2°C and 4°C according to DH advice) to facilitate on-demand feeding. Specialist formulae such as those designed to treat reflux or those containing probiotic bacteria have to be reconstituted at a lower temperature, otherwise the formula will be compromised.

Table 13.5 Nutrient content of free Healthy Start vitamin supplements

Nutrient	Pregnant and breastfeeding women	Infants and children
Vitamin D, μg	10	7.5
Vitamin C, mg	70	20
Vitamin A, μg	0	233
Folic acid, μg	400	0

Bottle feeding support literature for parents

ℙ NHS Choices. Bottle feeding http://www.nhs.uk/Conditions/pregnancy-and-baby/Pages/bottle-feeding-advice.aspx.

Healthy Start scheme

In the UK, the welfare food scheme, established in 1940 as a wartime measure, entitled pregnant women and children aged <5 years, receiving certain benefits, to tokens for either cows' milk or cows' milk-based infant formula per week and free supplements of vitamins A, C, and D. The NHS Plan 2000 reformed the welfare food scheme 'to use the resources more effectively to ensure that children in poverty have access to a healthy diet, with increased support for breastfeeding and parenting'. As a result, the welfare food scheme was replaced by 'Healthy Start' in 2006.

Healthy Start involves a broader range of foods; fresh fruit and vegetables, as well as cows' milk and infant formula. Fixed value vouchers are issued so they can be exchanged in a wide range of outlets and are of equal value for both breastfeeding and non-breastfeeding mothers. The age of children eligible has fallen from 5 to 4 years. Milk or fruit (not both) are available in nurseries. Free vitamin supplements continue to be available as part of the scheme, available in two versions: one for pregnant and breastfeeding women, and one for infants and children (Table 13.5).

The Scientific Advisory Committee on Nutrition (SACN) revised the recommendations for vitamin D and now encourages everyone, including all pregnant and breastfeeding women to consider taking 10 μg vitamin D (particularly during the autumn and winter months (October to March) when there is insufficient UV sunlight to synthesize vitamin D from skin. SACN has also introduced recommended safe intakes for children <4 years of age, with safe levels of 8.5-10 μg/day for infants aged 0-11 months and 10 μg/day for 1-3-year-olds. All breastfed infants should now be considered for a vitamin D supplement and as before, infants taking <500 mL infant formula should commence vitamins A, C, and D, and continue until they are 4–5 years old. Subsequently, a single vitamin D supplement should suffice.

Healthy Start is open to pregnant women and families with children aged <4 years who are in receipt of certain income support benefits or are <18 years (for further information see ℙ www.healthystart.nhs.uk).

Weaning

When to introduce solids

Introducing solids, also known as complementary feeding or weaning should start around 6 months of age,[17] whether infants are breastfed, fed solely on infant formula milk, or taking breast and infant formula combined. The choice of milk should continue >6 months, alongside complementary feeding.

The change in recommendation for introducing weaning from 4 months to 6 months of age in 2003 generated much debate, partly because of a lack of evidence to suggest that weaning after 4 months is detrimental to health in high income countries, such as the UK. However, it is accepted that introduction of solids should not commence until neuromuscular co-ordination is sufficiently developed to enable the infant to eat solid foods, i.e. i) the infant can stay in a sitting position and hold the head steady; ii) the infant can co-ordinate eyes, hands, and mouth to look at food, pick it up, and put it in the mouth; and iii) the infant can swallow food.

Babies who are not ready will push the food back out with the tongue. Weaning around 6 months is necessary to desensitize the mouth, and delayed weaning can result in food refusal, especially of lumpy foods. Some nutrient requirements also increase (see Table 13.1), especially for iron, B vitamins, energy, and protein, which cannot be met by milk alone.

◆ ESPGHAN (2008) state that exclusive or full breastfeeding for *about* 6 months is a desirable goal.[18] Complementary feeding should not be introduced before 17 weeks, and all infants should start solids by 26 weeks. EFSA (2009) support this more flexible approach, stating that starting complementary feeding between 4 and 6 months in the EU is safe and does not pose a risk for adverse health effects.[19]

Which foods to introduce

The overall aim of weaning is to introduce the infant gradually to a range of foods, textures, and flavours, so that normal family foods are taken by 12 months. The stages of weaning are summarized in Table 13.6.

If parents choose to start weaning before 6 months of age, foods should be introduced gradually, starting with pureed and mashed fruits, vegetables, rice, and potato (see Table 13.6). There is some evidence to suggest that commencing with a range of vegetables will result in a greater intake and liking for vegetables in the longer term.[20] If starting weaning from 6 months, babies will need to be exposed to a variety of foods from the outset, especially those containing iron. Foods can be offered two to three times a day, as thick purees or mashed textures and finger foods (see Box 13.5).

17 NHS. *Your baby's first solid foods.* Available at: ℛ http://www.nhs.uk/Conditions/pregnancy-and-baby/pages/solid-foods-weaning.aspx.

18 ESPGHAN-Society for Paediatric Gastroenterology, Hepatology and Nutrition (2008). Complementary feeding: a commentary by the ESPGHAN committee on nutrition. *J. Paed. Gastro. Nutr.* **46**, 99–110.

19 European Food Safety Authority (2009) Scientific opinion on the appropriate age for introduction of complementary feeding of infants. *EFSA J.* **7**(12), 1423–61.

20 Chambers, L. (2016). Complementary feeding: vegetables first, frequently and in variety *Nutr. Bull.* **41**, 142–6.

Table 13.6 Summary of guidance for weaning and feeding for under-5s

	6 months *	6–9 months	9–12 months	1–5 years
Milk	Breastmilk or 1 pint of infant formula. Introduce cup or beaker from 6 months			2–3 servings/day from full fat varieties, moving on to lower fat varieties > 2 years of: cheese (30 g), yogurt (pot), 1/3 pint milk
Dairy foods	Yogurt/custard	Cubed/grated hard cheese, cheese spread. Full fat yogurt, fromage frais, custard, full fat cows' milk in cooking		
	Goats' and sheep's milk should be avoided <12 months			
Fruit and vegetables	Smooth puree of softly cooked	2 servings/day. Mashed with fork/lightly cooked; soft peeled fruit and vegetables as finger foods	3–4 servings/day. No need to peel apple/pear. Raw/lightly cooked	≥ 4 servings/day. Same form as for adults
Meat, fish, and alternatives	After a few weeks: pureed meat, beans and lentils. No raw eggs, marlin, shark or swordfish, shellfish, nuts, or nut butter <6 months	1 serving/day. Mince/pure meat, beans and lentils; hard-boiled egg, fish, tofu	2 servings/day, e.g. mince/chopped red meat, chicken, fish, eggs, tofu	2 servings/day. As for 9–12 months. Aim to include oily fish (sardines, salmon, mackerel) up to twice weekly but no swordfish, shark or marlin. No whole nuts <5 years because of choking risk
Starchy foods	Baby rice/smooth potatoes Wheat/gluten-based cereal	2–3 servings/cay. Include gluten-containing foods, e.g. bread, breakfast cereals, toast, pasta	2–3 servings/day, e.g. toast, breadsticks, rice cakes	≥ 4 servings/day of bread, pasta, potatoes, rice, chapatti

Table 13.6 (contd.)

Sugary foods and drinks	No added sugar and no honey <12 months because of infant botulism risks	Drinks should be breast/formula milk or water. Fruit juices should be discouraged but if taken diluted 1 in 10. No sweet biscuits and rusks (including low sugar)	Limit sweet foods and drinks; especially between meals
	Herbal drinks, fizzy drinks, and squashes, including 'diet' drinks with artificial sweetener are not recommended. No tea/coffee		
Salty foods	Salt should not be added; kidneys not mature	Small amounts of gravy/ketchup	Limit crisps and savoury snacks
Vitamin drops	✓ If the infant is still breastfed > 6 months ✓ If a formula-fed infant is taking <1 pint of milk/day		✓ DH recommends for all 1–5-year-olds
Texture	Smooth purees, mashed foods	Mashed, soft lumps, soft finger foods, liquid in lidded beaker	Hard finger foods, chopped, minced family foods	Family foods

*But no earlier than 4 months (17 weeks) for parents deciding to wean their babies earlier.

Box 13.5 Healthier snack suggestions for 1–5-year-olds
- All fresh fruit
- Popcorn (unsweetened)
- Sticks of carrot, celery
- Plain biscuits
- Peppers, cucumber
- Cherry tomatoes
- Olives without stones
- Cubes or slices of cheese
- Yogurt/fromage frais (lower sugar varieties)
- Teacakes/scone
- Low sugar cereal and milk
- Fruit or malt loaf
- Pitta bread and hummus/cream cheese
- Oat cakes/crackers
- Sandwiches, tortilla wraps, toast
- Rice cakes, bread sticks
- Bagels

As breastfeeding is baby led, letting the baby choose when to wean is favoured by some. Emphasis is on the baby self-feeding and discourages the use of spo on-feeding. This approach may be extreme and many parents would find it difficult not to feed their baby, particularly as it is tends to result in low consumption until around 8-9 months.[21] A compromise might be to provide a meal containing a combination of finger foods such as vegetables and new potatoes or pasta and some mashed foods, so that the baby can feed him/herself and can also be fed by the parent/carer.

Which foods to avoid before 12 months

The UK NHS[22] recommends that infants <12 months should avoid:

For food safety reasons
- Raw or undercooked eggs (risk of salmonella).
- Some fish—swordfish, marlin, and shark (mercury affects CNS growth).
- Honey (risk of infant botulism—11 cases in the UK between 1980 and 2010).
- Whole nuts and raw jelly cubes (choking risk).
- Shellfish (risk of food poisoning).

For healthy diet reasons
- Salt (kidneys immature).
- Sugar (encourage sweet tooth).
- Foods high in saturated fat
- High fibre foods (risk of high bulk → low energy intake → faltering growth).
- Low fat/low energy foods (risk of → low energy intake → faltering growth).

21 Cameron, S.L., *et al.* (2012) How feasible is baby-led weaning as an approach to infant feeding. *Nutrients* 4, 1575–609.

22 NHS. *Foods to avoid giving babies and young children.* Available at: ◈ http://www.nhs.uk/Conditions/pregnancy-and-baby/Pages/foods-to-avoid-baby.aspx.

Weaning babies with risk of allergy
- Infants at risk have either an atopic parent or sibling (eczema, asthma, hay fever, food allergy).
- Ideally should breastfeed through weaning and introduce the key high allergen foods one at a time to assess effect within the first year of life.
- Delaying introduction of allergenic foods is now thought to potentially increase the risk of developing food allergies. 14 allergens have been identified that must be included on ingredients labels, according to the FSA (see Box 13.6).

❶ Nuts and nut allergy

Peanut allergy appears to be increasing in children (see 'Food hypersensitivity', p. 826). Advice used to be to delay introduction of peanuts to minimize the risk of developing peanut allergy. In 2009, the FSA reversed their advice, stating that there was no need for pregnant and breastfeeding mums to avoid peanuts. Subsequently, results from the LEAP studies in infants at high risk of peanut allergy convincingly demonstrated a significant reduction in the incidence of peanut allergy in those who began consuming peanuts between 4 and 11 months of age.[23] The EAT study involved breastfed infants and six food allergens, finding a benefit in reducing the incidence of food allergy for both peanut and egg if eaten in sufficient quantities from 3-4 months of age.[24]

Box 13.6 14 major allergens in foods*
- Milk
- Eggs
- Soya
- Peanuts
- Fish
- Oats
- Sesame seeds
- Lupins
- Mustard
- Celery and celeriac
- Sulphites/sulphur dioxide
- Nuts, e.g. almonds, hazelnuts, walnuts, pecan nuts, Brazil nuts, pistachios, cashews, and macadamia nuts
- Crustaceans, e.g. prawns, crabs, lobster, and crayfish
- Molluscs, e.g. clams, mussels, whelks, oysters, snails, and squid
- Cereals containing gluten (oats, wheat, rye, barley)

*Source: data from ℛ https://www.food.gov.uk/sites/default/files/media/document/top-allergy-types.pdf

---

23 Du Toit, G., et al. (2015). Randomised trial of peanut consumption in infants at risk for peanut allergy. New Engl. J.med. **372**, 803–13.

24 Perkin, M.R., et al. (2016). Randomized trial of the early introduction of allergenic foods in breastfed infants. New Engl. J.med. **374**, 1733–43.

The FSA advise that where a child already has another kind of allergy, e.g. diagnosed eczema or allergy to other foods, or if there is a history of allergy in the child's immediate family (parents, siblings), then parents/carers should talk to their GP, health visitor, or medical allergy specialist before giving peanut to the child for the first time, because these children are at higher risk of developing peanut allergy. Other infants can take peanuts and other nuts from 6 months of age. Whole nuts should be avoided generally until 5 years of age because of the risk of choking.

Weaning preterm infants

Advice on appropriate weaning age should be sought from the specialist paediatric medical and dietetic team caring for the infant. It is usually recommended that complementary feeding commences between 5 and 7 months actual birth age. Further information on feeding preterm infants is available at: ℔ http://www.bliss.org.uk.

Weaning support literature for parents

℔ https://www.nhs.uk/start4life/first-foods
℔ http://www.nhs.uk/Conditions/pregnancy-and-baby/pages/solid-foods-weaning.aspx

Common feeding problems

Prolonged use of feeder bottle and delayed weaning
The DH recommends that infants should be introduced to drinking from a cup at around 6 months of age, and actively discouraged from taking drinks in feeder bottles after 12 months. This is part of the natural progression for sipping and swallowing to replace sucking. Delayed weaning (>1 year) is more common in some deprived South Asian communities than for other ethnic groups.

Problems arising from prolonged use of the feeder bottle and delayed weaning include:
• Food refusal as the infant may be filling up on milk ∴ ↓ desire for food.
• Iron deficiency anaemia because increased iron requirements not being met from a mixed diet.
• Faltering growth.
• Speech development as child's ability to chew and the swallowing reflex may ↓.
• Dental caries if sugary/acidic drinks are given in a bottle.
• Obesity if sugary drinks are given in a bottle.

❶ Risk of choking

All babies have a sensitive gag reflex and it is normal for them to gag on exposure to increasing textures of food. This should not be a reason for avoiding such textures, and they soon adapt. However, babies should be supervised while eating, and given softer finger foods at first, such as banana, melon, or avocado. Once the child is able to chew well, s/he can be given non-dissolvable harder finger foods, e.g. apple. Infants do not need teeth to be able to chew solid foods. Whole nuts or olives containing stones should be avoided until 5 years of age because of the risk of choking.

Iron deficiency anaemia in infancy

Common causes:
- mother's diet was inadequate in iron during pregnancy;
- the baby is weaned late, i.e. >6 months;
- slow in progressing from weaning foods to family meals;
- early introduction of cows' milk as the main drink for children <1 year;
- heavy reliance on sweet baby foods (high in sugar, low in iron and protein), as avoiding savoury products that may have non-halal ingredients in some Muslim families.

A varied diet with a regular intake of red meat, fruit, green vegetables, fortified breakfast cereals, and beans and pulses should be encouraged. This is especially important for breastfed babies because, despite good absorption of iron from breastmilk, the iron content is insufficient after 6 months of age as infants' endogenous stores are depleted. Infant formula is higher in iron, but it should not be relied on as a sole source of iron in babies >6 months of age (see 'Iron,' for foods rich in iron, Chapter 6 p. 148).

Faltering growth

Weight faltering is defined as weight falling through centile spaces, low weight for height, or no catch-up from a low birth weight. Weight usually tracks within one centile, but an acute illness can cause a weight centile fall. Less than 2% of infants will show a sustained drop through ≥2 weight centile spaces on the WHO charts, compared with 5% using the UK90 charts.

Growth faltering is defined as crossing down through length/height centile(s) as well as weight, a low height centile, or a height <expected from parental heights (see Box 13.1).

Only 5% of young children whose weight or growth falters will have an organic root to the problem (see Box 13.7 for other causes). It is estimated that a further 5% will need the support of agencies involved in the safeguarding of children and young people. As a result, it is recommended that management for the majority of faltering growth should occur in primary care, rather than in hospitals.

Triggers for primary care assessment

- Weight or height below the 0.4th centile for the first time.
- A sustained fall through 2 centile spaces.

Managing faltering growth in primary care

In the UK, teams composed of health visitors, community paediatric nurses, and nursery nurses are best placed to identify and support infants because of their key responsibility for the health and wellbeing of children <5 years of age. It will depend on suspected cause as to whether a dietitian or paediatrician gets involved first (see Fig. 13.2).

Home visits to observe mealtimes are ideal and to collect data on:

- feeding and symptom history since birth;
- growth history since birth;
- any relevant medical or domestic details;
- food diary outlining food/drinks offered and taken and when;
- details of mealtime routines, including observation of food preparation and mealtime interactions;
- family's concerns/anxieties;
- interaction between parents/carers and child, with description of any behavioural problems.

The health visitor will need to identify areas where there is potential for change and offer appropriate advice and ongoing support. This is likely to include advice on:

- insufficient nutrient intake, e.g. faddy eating, excess drinking, poor parent–child interaction, strict adherence to a low fat-high fibre diet;
- insufficient nutrients offered, e.g. poor parent/carer nutrition knowledge or food skills, stressful social situations, including neglect/abuse;
- when a health visitor becomes concerned, s/he should discuss or refer to the most relevant member of the multidisciplinary team (see Fig. 13.2).

Box 13.7 Dietary and social causes of faltering growth
- Insufficient energy intake is major cause
- Formula milk too weak/too concentrated
- Late weaning >6 months
- Prolonged use of feeder bottle
- Fussy eating/behavioural problems at mealtimes
- Physical feeding problems, e.g. gastro-oesophageal reflux, oral motor dysfunction
- Over health-conscious parent/carer → diet low in fat and high in fibre
- Inadequacy of the nutritional content or frequency of meals
- Poor inherent feeding drive
- Developmental difficulties
- Illness—although it is rare for serious organic disease to present with weight and/or growth faltering alone
- Abuse and/or neglect (minority of cases)
- Unhealthy parent/carer–child relationship.

The dietitian's role is to use motivational interviewing and counselling techniques to address the following:
- positive food attitudes, value systems, and beliefs;
- appropriate parent/child interactions, particularly related to food and drink;
- drinking habits that discourage prolonged use of a bottle;
- age-appropriate structured mealtimes, snacks, and drinks;
- increasing nutrient density of meals using foods where possible;
- identifying and correcting for any micronutrient deficiencies;
- considering use of nutritional supplements if there is no improvement in growth as a result of the above interventions.

Also see this Chapter, 'Fussy eaters', p. 300.

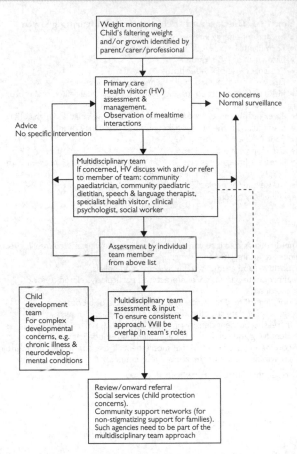

Fig. 13.2 Care pathway for young children's faltering growth/weight. Reproduced from the *Recommendations for best practice for growth faltering in young children* (Copyright 2002). With permission from the Children's Society.

Obesity prevention in infancy

The increase in number of children who are overweight or obese presents a major global public health challenge and hence the WHO have produced a number of documents including a commission report on ending childhood obesity (2016).[25]

Including guidance on preventing obesity in pregnancy and the first years of life. Making breastfeeding the norm is believed to reduce the risk of excess weight in later life; delay weaning until around 6 months when healthy foods and portion size control should be emphasized, and encourage an active lifestyle.

As a result, nutrition, active play and obesity prevention is one of the priorities. The UK government recently published guidance on childhood obesity, which includes involving industry with a soft drinks levy, reducing sugar in foods, improving food labelling and making healthier options available in public places, including nurseries and schools.[26]

The key age for identifying children who are overweight is 2 years, and for establishing life-long healthy eating and physical activity habits. Food that parents offer infants influences taste preferences and eating habits and therefore later health.

Factors influencing a child's weight include:
• parental attitudes to food, e.g. convenience foods;
• portion sizes;
• family eating behaviours, e.g. lack of family mealtimes;
• food choices, e.g. lack of healthy options;
• disincentives to physical activity;
• ease of sedentary entertainment, e.g. television and computers.

At 2 years, children at risk of obesity or causing concern should be measured for weight and height and a BMI centile obtained (see growth reference charts and Appendix 2, p. 861). A child with a BMI centile > 91st suggests overweight and BMI > 98th centile is very overweight (clinically obese).
Risk factors for obesity in infancy include:
• parental obesity;
• poverty;
• excessive weight gain in pregnancy;
• bottle feeding;
• rapid weight gain during infancy and early weaning.

If the child is confirmed as overweight or obese, the health visiting team should offer individual counselling and ongoing support of positive lifestyle changes and consider family-based as well as individual interventions, depending on the age and maturity of the child.

---

25 WHO. (2016). *Report of the Commission on ending childhood obesity*. Available at: ℘ http://apps. who.int/iris/bitstream/10665/204176/1/978924.

26 Department of Health and Social Care. *Childhood obesity: a plan for action*. Available at: ℘ https://www.gov.uk/government/publications/childhood-obesity-a-plan-for-action/ childhood-obesity-a-plan-for-action.

HENRY,[27] MEND,[28] and Trimtots[29] are projects aiming to optimize eating behaviours and physical activity for under-5s. HENRY's programme is based on training practitioners to work more effectively with parents of preschoolers around obesity and lifestyle issues. A 5-year Randomised Control Trial (RCT) is under way to determine whether it prevents obesity. Trimtots has been evaluated in two RCTs and shown to result in a significant reduction in obesity risk for overweight and obese children as BMIs were maintained in the long term (4-year) follow-up.[30]

Start4Life campaign

Start4Life (🖰 http://www.nhs.uk/start4life) is part of the UK government's social marketing Change4Life campaign, which is aimed at changing behaviour in relation to nutrition and physical activity in families with children aged 5–11 years. Start4Life is aimed at pregnant women and families with children from birth to 2 years. It provides healthcare and childcare professionals with up-to-date advice on breastfeeding, introducing solid foods and active play. The campaign supports existing activities to increase the levels of initiation and continuation of breastfeeding and educate on introducing solid foods, with the aim of reducing obesity levels (and related illnesses) in later life. Parent support literature has been developed on breastfeeding and weaning (see relevant sections in this Chapter).

Start4Life communicates six key messages designed to build healthy habits from day one:
- Mother's milk.
- Every day counts (continuation of breastmilk).
- No rush to mush (waiting to wean).
- Taste for life (variety of solids).
- Sweet as they are (avoid sweet tooth).
- Baby moves (active play).

27 Available at: 🖰 http://www.henry.org.uk.

28 Available at: 🖰 https://www.mendfoundation.org/.

29 Available at: 🖰 http://www.trimtots.com/.

30 Lanigan J., et al. (2013). The TrimTots programme for prevention and treatment of obesity in preschool children: evidence from two randomised controlled trials. *Lancet* **382**, S58. (13)62483-6.

Constipation, toddler diarrhoea, and milk hypersensitivity

Constipation in infants

Constipation is more common in babies fed infant formula compared with breastfed babies. Potential contributing factors include absence of structured fatty acids, LCPs, α-lactalbumin, and prebiotics in formula milk (see Box 13.2). The energy content of breastmilk may also be lower than originally thought, and hence fluid intake may differ.

In young infants who have not yet been weaned (<6 months of age), constipated bottle fed infants should be given extra water in between feeds and correct preparation of formula should be established. Bicycling the infant's legs, or an abdominal massage may also help. Prune juice is a particularly effective laxative. It can be given from a teaspoon from around 4-6 weeks, starting with 1 teaspoon daily and then doubling the amount as required.

Formula-fed infants may have constipation caused by an allergy to cows' milk. A trial of an extensively hydrolysed milk formula could be considered, particularly in children with a personal/family history of atopy who are not responding to first line medical management. Constipation in an exclusively breastfed child is unusual, and if physical causes have been ruled out (e.g. Hirschprungs disease), it may be appropriate for the mother to undertake a cows' milk-free diet in infants at risk of food allergy. Breastfeeding should be continued as long as practical.

In infants who have begun weaning or who are now taking solids, extra water or diluted juices should be offered that have high sorbitol content (e.g. apples, grapes, pears, prunes). Giving a high-fibre cereal such as Weetabix® or Shredded Wheat® may also help infants >6 months age.

Constipation from low fibre intake and sometimes low fluid intake is relatively common in UK infants. A higher fibre diet should be encouraged, containing foods that are acceptable to the child. Encouraging fresh and dried fruit and vegetables for pectins, and bread and high fibre 'brown' breakfast cereals for insoluble fibre will relieve symptoms along with plenty of fluid, preferably as water.

All constipated infants (weaned or not weaned) unresponsive to dietary measures should be prescribed an oral osmotic laxative[31] as first line treatment, starting with polyethylene glycol (macrogol 3550; Movicol® or Laxido®) or Lactulose is usually used in young infants but is a form of prebiotic and hence is fermented in the bowel and can cause abdominal discomfort.

Toddler diarrhoea

Symptoms: frequent, loose stools, containing undigested foodstuffs.
Usually a self-limiting problem, occurring in otherwise well infants <3 years, who are gaining weight and growing satisfactorily; commonly because of

---

31 NICE (2017) *Constipation in children and young people: diagnosis and management. Clinical guideline [CG99].* NICE clinical guideline 99. Available at: ℘ https://www.nice.org.uk/guidance/cg99.

immaturity of the GI tract. As well as reassuring parents that the condition will cease spontaneously, dietary treatment to recommend is:

- avoid large quantities of sucrose, fruit and fruit juice;
- reduce dietary fibre intake (choose white bread and avoid high fibre cereals, fibre-dense fruit and vegetables, such as peas and sweetcorn, and temporarily reduce consumption of fruit and vegetables in general);
- ensure sufficient fat in the diet. Where this is not possible, a fat-based nutritional supplement can be a useful addition.

If foodstuffs are observed in the stools within 12 hours of ingestion, however, this would be considered to be rapid gut transit, indicative of possible food allergy.

Milk hypersensitivity (see Chapter 37, p. 828)

Cows' milk hypersensitivity includes immediate (immunoglobulin E [IgE]-mediated) allergy, delayed symptoms (non-IgE mediated allergy), and lactose intolerance. IgE mediated reactions are relatively easy to diagnose because of the immediate response (<2 hours) following ingestion of cows' milk protein and can be confirmed by skin prick tests or specific IgE antibodies. These can subsequently be used to determine when to re-challenge with milk.

Often the diagnosis between lactose intolerance and non-IgE mediated cows' milk protein allergy (for which there are no tests) is confused and it is important to differentiate between them. This can be done by taking a detailed food allergy clinical history focusing on feeding history from birth, related symptoms pertaining to GI, cutaneous and respiratory systems, and family history of allergy.

Lactose intolerance

Symptoms of lactose intolerance[32] include diarrhoea, bloating, and cramping

- Developmental lactase deficiency is implicated in some cases of infantile colic (resolves around 4 months of age), associated with delayed production of lactase.
- Secondary lactose intolerance is associated with loss of lactase as a result of damage to gut, e.g. delayed recovery post-gastroenteritis (resolves in ~6 weeks).
- Primary lactose intolerance is associated with a gradual reduction in lactase activity over time, and generally does not affect infants and young children.

Treatment involves lactase drops (Colief®/Care Co-Lactase®) or a reduced or low lactose formula alongside a low/reduced lactose diet for as long as required.

Cows' milk protein allergy

Conditions associated with non-IgE mediated cows' milk protein allergy in infants, especially those unresponsive to first line medication include

---

32 Available at: ℘ https://nutrition2me.com/wp-content/uploads/2012/05/images_free-view-articles_free-downloads_Whatdoweknowaboutlactose.pdf.

gastro-oesophageal reflux (GOR), constipation, diarrhoea, mucus in stools, faltering growth, eczema, and aversive feeding behaviour.

Treatment involves use of an extensively hydrolysed or elemental infant formula alongside a strict cows' milk protein-free diet. The allergy is likely to be outgrown during childhood, and re-challenging at 6–12 monthly intervals will be required. For non-IgE mediated reactions, this can usually be done at home.

GOR in infants

GOR is the regurgitation of gastric contents into the oesophagus and reflux > twice/day and occurs in >40% of infants by 8 weeks old and resolves in 90% by 1 year of age. A minority will develop gastro-oesophageal reflux disease (GORD), defined as symptoms or complications of GOR such as:

- recurrent vomiting > 5 episodes/day (up to 2 hours after feeding);
- frequent and troublesome crying, irritability or back arching during or after feeding;
- feed refusal, frequent choking after feeds;
- sleeping difficulties, unable to lie down;
- apnoea, wheeze, cough, asthma, stridor, hoarseness;
- sinusitis and recurrent otitis media;
- anaemia and faltering growth.

Causes of GORD

Usually results from defective transient lower oesophageal sphincter tone. Reflux related to changes in pressure between oesophagus and stomach. GOR more likely to be triggered following straining, crying, coughing, eating, gastric distension, and delayed gastric emptying.

Diagnosis of GORD

History, physical examination, and empiric therapy is usually sufficient. Oesophageal bioimpedance/pH monitoring and endoscopy is only used in more severe cases.

Management of GORD

Step-wise approach, starting with parental reassurance and education, ensuring a calm environment. Initial advice should include:

- avoid bouncing after a feed;
- avoid pressure on abdomen;
- reduce volume of feeds in overfed babies (100-150 mL/kg);
- consider smaller, more frequent feeds;
- minimize air swallowing (aerophagia), check teat size and flow in bottle fed babies;
- careful winding during feeds;
- keep upright for 20-30 minutes after a feed (avoid slumped position);
- recognize child's cues and respond early to avoid excessive crying, increasing abdominal pressure;
- avoid constipation—aim for one stool motion a day, using a laxative/ prune juice if necessary;
- avoid giving your child other juices and acidic foods;
- consider weaning a little earlier, i.e. around 4-5 months of age, but never before 17 weeks of age.

Positioning adjustments can include placing the infant in the prone position while awake (SIDS awareness); elevating the head of the bed and supine position while sleeping; lying on the left lateral side (breastfeeding mums may find their baby feeds better from the right breast), although there is little evidence to support the benefits of changes to positioning.

Feed adjustments

For recurrent vomiting, NICE recommend feed thickeners before alginate therapy (Gaviscon Infant™).

Milk-thickening agents do not ↓ reflux, but ↓ no. episodes of vomiting. Pre-thickened feeds can be used or thickeners added to feeds. Some pre-thickened feeds use rice/corn starch and thicken on contact with the stomach. Adding a thickener to feed (carob seed flour in infants), which can also be used in breastfeeding, or using pre-thickened feed with carob bean gum requires a faster flow teat.

▶ Corn-based thickening agents are not generally recommended in children because of provision of significant additional energy risking reduction in intake of infant formula.

▶ Methods of formula preparation vary and use of antacids will compromise products requiring an acidic environment to thicken in the stomach.

Gaviscon Infant™ (alginic acid) thickens the stomach contents (should not be used with a thickened feed). The number of sachets is restricted because of its high sodium content (six doses/three dual sachets a day = 0.3g salt). Recommended intake is < 1 g salt/day in infants <1 year; standard formula provides about 0.3 g salt/day and therefore salt intake is doubled. If > 4.5 kg, two doses are required per feed, so it can only go in three feeds/day, which is not very practical. NICE suggest offering a trial for 1-2 weeks and if this works, to continue, but also to stop at regular intervals to see if beneficial.

Side effects—constipation is extremely common in practice but this is not recognized by NICE as it is not reported (yellow card).

The previous NICE Clinical Knowledge Summaries (CKS) guidelines recommended ruling out cow's milk allergy (CMA) before considering use of antacid medication (NICE CKS, 2011). NICE GORD guidelines[33] (2015) require more evidence to determine whether CMA mimics or aggravates GORD and have posed the following research question 'What is the effectiveness and cost effectiveness of a trial of hydrolysed formula in formula-fed infants with frequent regurgitation associated with marked distress?' However, given that there are potential risks from using antacids, such as effects on gut microbiome and absorption of minerals, taking an allergy-focused clinical history to rule out CMA before introducing antacids is advisable. Cows' milk allergy should be suspected if symptoms include loose stools with/without mucus or blood and/or personal or family history of atopic conditions, e.g. eczema, rhinitis. CMA has been linked with GOR in around 30-40% of infants in the first 2-3 years of life.

33 NICE, 2015. *Gastro-oesophageal reflux disease in children and young people: diagnosis and management.* Available at: ℅ http://www.nice.org.uk/guidance/ng1.

Medication for GORD

Do not use antacids to treat overt regurgitation as an isolated symptom (NICE, 2015[33]). Consider a 4-week trial of PPI or H2RA in infants with overt regurgitation, plus:

- feeding difficulties (food refusal, gagging/choking);
- distressed behaviour;
- faltering growth;
- children with epigastric pain etc.

⟶ Refer to a specialist for possible endoscopy if symptoms do not resolve. Consider age-appropriate preparations and preferences, and local procurement costs. Do not offer domperidone/metoclopramide/erythromycin to treat GORD without seeking specialist advice.

Further reading on GOR

Vandenplas Y, Rudolph CD, Di Lorenzo C, et al. (2009). Pediatric gastroesophageal reflux clinical practice guidelines: joint recommendations of NASPGHAN/ESPGHAN. *J Pediatr Gastro Nutr* **49**, 498–547.

Nutritionally vulnerable infants

Low income families

Children from families living on a low income are at a greater risk of having an unbalanced diet lacking diversity, developing micronutrient deficiency and faltering growth. See Chapter 16, 'Eating on a low income', p. 354.

The Family Nurse Partnership was introduced into the UK in 2008. It is a voluntary home visiting programme for first time young mums, aged 19 years or under. A specially trained family nurse visits the young mum regularly, from the early stages of pregnancy until the child is aged 2 years. The Family Nurse Partnership programme aims to enable young mums to:

- have a healthy pregnancy;
- improve their child's health and development;
- plan their own futures and achieve their aspiration.

Sure Start

Sure Start brings together childcare, early education, health and family-support services for families with children under 5 years old. It aims to tackle child poverty and social exclusion working with parents-to-be, parents, carers, and children to promote the physical, intellectual, and social development of babies and young children at home and when they get to school.

Children's centres are where children <5 years and their families can receive integrated services and information. Every community is served by a Sure Start Children's Centre, aiming to offer universal provision across the UK. For more information see ℘ https://www.gov.uk/find-sure-start-childrens-centre.

South Asian families

There is evidence that certain infant feeding practices in some South Asian families increase the risk of iron deficiency anaemia, faltering growth, and constipation. These include:

- late weaning, slow to move on to family foods;
- late progression from a bottle on to a feeder cup;
- adding honey/sugar to sweeten milk;
- adding solids to formula milk;
- choosing sweet commercially prepared baby foods so as to avoid running the risk of using non-halal meat products; ∴ lack of iron and protein in weaning foods;
- use of cows' milk as the main drink with infants <1 year.

The vegetarian baby

If infants consume a well-balanced vegetarian diet, there is no reason that they should not meet all requirements for growth. See Chapter 16, 'Vegetarians', p. 346.

ⓘ Diets that are unbalanced or more restrictive than this, e.g. vegan, strict macrobiotic, or fruitarian, are likely to result in nutrient deficiencies and need particular attention, especially in infants. Vegan diets do not easily give babies all the energy and nutrients they need and, therefore, referral to a dietitian is recommended.

Fussy eaters

Box 13.8 Parents' FAQs for fussy eaters for mealtimes

Every mealtime is like a battle of wills; how can I break the cycle?

Encourage parents to avoid arguments and try to keep calm. Mealtimes should actually be fun! The child is probably trying to either gain attention or show that s/he has control over parents. It is important not to give in and to ignore the behaviour. The child should not detect that his/her behaviour causes anxiety. Reassure parents that as long as a child is gaining weight overall there isn't too much cause for concern. Never force feed children.

Should I let my child have his/her dessert if the main course is not finished?

Advise parents to put the food on the table and if it is not eaten after 20–30 minutes, simply remove with no comment. Suggest not giving sweet foods if the savoury meal is rejected completely. Trying the savoury meal may be acceptable and deserve a dessert. This will help change behaviour long term. Cooking an alternative meal should be avoided, as this is just as likely to be refused.

I am worried about my 2-year-old daughter going hungry if she doesn't eat her meal, is it okay to let her have in-between snacks?

Children can go for days without eating, and if they are hungry their behaviour deteriorates. If they refuse their meal, having a small snack (see Box 13.6) a couple of hours later will not impact on mealtimes, and it is far enough off for them not to associate snacks with not eating meals. This helps relieve parental anxiety too, as the child is getting something to eat. Mealtimes are approximately 4 hours apart, and snacks (mid am, mid pm, and supper) fall between these, but should not be given any closer than 1½ hours before a meal. This applies to drinks too.

Is it okay to reward my child with sweets for eating his dinner?

Parents should avoid using sweet foods as a bribe to encourage children to eat their meals. Other non-food rewards could be used, like a cuddle, playing a game, or reading a story.

Could it help if he eats on his own, so that we can eat in peace later?

A young child should never be left alone while eating as there is a risk that s/he might choke. It is preferable if the whole family tries to sit down and eat together, ideally the same food, so that they are acting as role models and can share food. Inviting friends to eat can help as children often copy each other (as long as the guest is not a fussy eater too!). Parents need to try and create an enjoyable environment.

Box 13.8 (contd.)

Is it okay to feed him myself while he watches TV, because at least that way he eats his dinner?

Parents should not feed the child (when s/he is capable of doing so) as the attention will be enjoyed and there will be little incentive to self-feed. It is normal for children to make a mess when they feed, and they like to eat with their fingers. This should be encouraged and wiping the child's hands and mouth avoided until the end of the meal, as this can upset the child. The TV should be switched off during eating as this is distracting and the meal is a good opportunity for parent-child interaction.

School-aged children and adolescents

Nutrition and growth in childhood and adolescence *304*
Dietary recommendations for children and adolescents *306*
Children and adolescents' food habits *308*
Nutrient deficiencies in children *312*
Childhood obesity and weight problems *314*
Dental health and children *316*
Influences on children's food choices *318*
Promoting healthy eating in children *320*

Nutrition and growth in childhood and adolescence

- Children need a balanced diet to meet requirements for growth and development.
- Health-related behaviour and attitudes towards food are formed in childhood.
- The processes for some adult diseases may start early in life.

Growth and development

Each year of life from 1 year to adolescence, a child grows taller by 5–8 cm. Girls' growth spurt begins at 10–11 years. Boys' growth spurt begins at 12–13 years. About 25% of height is gained in adolescence. This requires increases of energy, protein, and several vitamins and minerals (see Table 14.1). If energy needs are not met this can result in stunting or delayed growth. Once the growth spurt is over, nutrient requirements become those of adults. During this period there is ↑ muscle growth in boys and adipose fat in girls. Genes have the strongest influence on onset of menarche.

See girls' and boys' growth charts in ➔ Appendix 2, p. 861. These have been endorsed by the Royal College of Paediatrics and Child Health and the Department of Health (DH). Also see discussion in ➔ Chapter 13, 'Infant growth and development', p. 258. BMI identification charts are on the back of growth charts and each centile represents 0.67 SD.

The charts have nine reference centiles of 0.4th, 2nd, 9th, 25th, 50th, 75th, 91st, 98th, and 99.9th, e.g.

- 98th centile curve, below which 98% of UK children lie (2 in 100 children will be as tall/ heavy as this);
- 50th centile curve, below which 50% of UK children lie (average weight and height for a child of that age);
- 2nd centile curve, below which only 2% of UK children lie (2 in 100 children will be as small/ light as this).

These are available from Harlow Healthcare (⌘ http://www.healthforallchildren.com).

Table 14.1 RNIs for school-aged children and adolescents*

Nutrient†	7–10 years		11–14 years		15–18 years	
	Boys	Girls	Boys	Girls	Boys	Girls
Energy, MJ/d	7.6	7.2	9.8	9.1	12.6	10.2
Fibre**	20	20	20-25	20-25	25-30	25-30
Protein, g	28.3	28.3	42.1	41.2	55.2	45.0
Fluid, mL/kg	75	75	55	55	50	50
Vitamin C, mg	30	30	35	35	40	40
Vitamin A, μg	500	500	600	600	700	600
Vitamin D, μg***	10	10	10	10	10	10
Folic acid, μg	150	150	200	200	200	200
Thiamine, mg	0.7	0.7	0.9	0.7	1.1	0.8
Riboflavin, mg	1.0	1.0	1.2	1.1	1.3	1.1
Niacin, mg	12	12	15	12	19	14
Vitamin B$_{12}$, μg	1.0	1.0	1.2	1.2	1.5	1.5
Iron, mg	8.7	8.7	11.3	14.8	11.3	14.8
Calcium, mg	550	550	1000	800	1000	800
Phosphorus, mg	450	450	775	625	775	625
Magnesium, mg	200	200	280	280	300	300
Zinc, mg	7.0	7.0	9.0	9.0	9.5	9.5
Selenium, μg	30	30	45	45	70	60
Copper, mg	0.7	0.7	0.8	0.8	1.0	1.0

*Source: data from Department of Health (1991). *Dietary reference values for food and nutrients for the United Kingdom.* HMSO, London.

**Source: data from SACN (2015). *Carbohydrates and Health.* ✆ https://www.gov.uk/government/publications/sacn-carbohydrates-and-health-report

***Source: data from SACN (2016). *Vitamin D and health report.* ✆ https://www.gov.uk/government/publications/sacn-vitamin-d-and-health-report

An RNI for Vitamin D of 10 μg (400 IU/day) is recommended for the UK population aged ≥4 years. This is the average amount needed by 97.5% of the population when UVB sunshine is minimal (October- March).

Dietary recommendations for children and adolescents

The 'Eatwell Guide' model (in ⊃ Chapter 2, p. 27) applies to older children (≥5 years) and adolescents, as there is evidence that early atherosclerotic plaques can develop from adolescence → cardiovascular disease (CVD) in later life.

In addition to a balanced diet, advise:

- Extra calcium requirements gained from drinking the equivalent of 1 pint of milk a day (see ⊃ Chapter 6, 'Calcium', p. 142 for equivalents).
- Regular meals if possible, healthy snack meals if not (see Box 14.1).
- Offering praise when a healthy food is eaten as this leads to ↑ consumption of the food in younger children.
- Parents to make healthy foods easily available and serve these foods in positive mealtime situations.
- As children prefer familiar foods, repeated exposure to new foods can alter the response from rejection to acceptance.
- Interventions promoting familiarity with foods, e.g. fruit and vegetable tasting, can increase consumption.
- Eating with peers can have a positive effect on eating behaviour.
- Eating together as a family is valued by children of all ages and it has been associated with lower levels of unhealthy weight-control behaviour and chronic dieting.
- Offering 'child sized' portions by starting meals with small servings and letting children ask for more.

Reference nutrient intakes (RNIs) vary for age and gender and are related to growth needs; ∴ they reflect differences in growth rates and body composition (Table 14.1).

Box 14.1 Healthy snack suggestions
- Fruit
- Vegetables: sticks of carrot, celery, cucumber, cherry tomatoes
- Toast, teacakes, scone, bagels
- Fruit or malt loaf
- Oat cakes, crackers or rice cakes
- Bread sticks
- Mixed nuts and raisins
- Popcorn (unsweetened)
- Plain biscuits
- Glass of milk
- Cubes or slices of cheese
- Yogurt/fromage frais (lower sugar varieties)
- Low sugar cereal and milk
- Sandwich

Children and adolescents' food habits

The UK National Diet and Nutrition Survey (NDNS) of 2012/13-2013/14 included data for 4- to 18-year-olds[1] and found the following:

- *Fruit and vegetable* intakes are low (~3 portions/day for boys and girls aged 11–18 years). Only 8% of children aged 11–18 years achieved the recommendation of at least five-a-day. During the time of the survey, portions of fruit and vegetables for the 'five-a-day' recommendation could include up to 150 mL of fruit juice and a portion of pulses, although this has now changed.
- *Non-milk extrinsic sugars (NMES)* intake of 4–18-year-olds exceeded the recommendation (≤ 11% of food energy from NMES). A new recommendation for sugar intake was set by SACN[2] in 2015. The new recommendation is that NMES should provide no more than 5% of total energy intake for adults and children aged > 2 years. NMES intake was high for children aged 4-10 years (13.4% of food energy) and 11-18 years (15.2% of food energy). Children's intakes are higher than those of adults in the NDNS. Mean daily consumption of sugar-sweetened soft drinks in children aged 4-10 years was significantly lower in 2012-14 (100 g/day) compared with 130 g/day in 2008-10. The SACN[3] report of nutritional wellbeing of the British population reported even higher intakes from NMES of 19% food energy, mainly from soft drinks (mean of 3 L/week in 7–10-year-olds).
- *Total fat* intake of 4–10-year-olds is at the top end of the recommendation (≤35% food energy from fat). Mean of ~33% energy from fat in those aged 4-18 years.
- *Saturated fat* intake of 4–18-year-olds is higher than the recommendation (≤11% food energy from saturated fat), with 4-10-year-olds (mean of 13.3% energy from saturated fat) reporting slightly higher intakes than 11-18-year-olds (mean of 12.6% energy from saturated fat).

Non-starch polysaccharides (aka dietary fibre) intakes are lower than the recommendation (mean intake of 18 g/day), with 4-10-year-olds (mean of 10.7 g/day) reporting lower intakes than 11-18-year-olds (mean of 12.2 g/day). Children's intakes are lower than those of adults in the NDNS (mean of 14 g/day). New UK recommendations were set by SACN for fibre intake in 2015 (see Table 14.1) based on a different definition of fibre, recommending a mean intake of 20 g/day for 5-11-year-olds, 25 g/day for 11-16-year-olds and 30 g/day for 16-18-year-olds.

1 Public Health England & Food Standards Agency (2016). *The National Diet and Nutrition Survey: Results from Years 5 and 6 (combined) of the Rolling Programme (2012/13–2013/14)*. Public Health England, London.

2 SACN (2015). *Carbohydrates and Health*. TSO, London

3 SACN (2008). *The Nutritional Wellbeing of the British Population*. TSO, London.

Missing breakfast

In the UK, around one in three children[4] aged 10–16 years miss breakfast on some or most days. More girls (38.6%) than boys (26.6%) skip breakfast some or all of the time, with girls motivated by controlling their weight and boys by lack of time. This has been linked to poor concentration and ↓ cognitive performance in the late morning.

Snacking

Adolescents eat at least three snacks/day, contributing ~25% of daily dietary energy. Snacking can have a negative effect on the nutritional value of the diet as snacks are often low in calcium and iron, and high in saturated fat and sugar. Most popular are crisps, sweets, biscuits, sandwiches, fruit, and milk chocolate. Box 14.1 lists some healthy alternatives.

Vegetarian children

Only 2% of children aged 4–10 years and 3% aged 11–18 years report being vegetarian in the UK's NDNS (2014). Vegetarian adolescents are at particular risk of inadequate diet if they are the only vegetarian in the house, as they may tend to eat the same as the rest of the family but 'remove' the animal protein aspect of the meal and replace it with too much cheese or vegetarian ready meals such as burgers, sausages, or pizza. They should replace it with suitable alternatives (see ➔ Chapter 16, 'Vegetarians', p. 346). They may have less knowledge of a balanced vegetarian diet than adults, resulting in low intakes of iron, zinc, protein, and vitamin B_{12}.

❶ Vegan children should be referred to see a dietitian as careful planning is needed to meet nutrient requirements.

Acne and diet

Young people and their parents often link acne with a diet high in fat and sugar. A systematic literature review has concluded that high glycaemic index diets may exacerbate acne. The link between dairy intake and acne is weaker. A healthy diet rich in fruit and vegetables has been shown to a protective effect, but further research is needed.[5]

Drinking alcohol

Binge drinking in adolescence is of particular concern. Although drinking by under-16s is still prevalent, there is evidence that this is falling.[6] The WHO[7] estimated that 55.9% of boys and 48.6% girls aged 15 years drink alcohol ≥once/week. Alcohol provides extra calories (can lead to weight gain) and can displace nutrient-rich foods in the diet. The SACN report (2008) found

---

4 Sandercock, G.J.M., et al. (2010). Associations between habitual school-day breakfast consumption, body mass index, physical activity and cardiorespiratory fitness in English schoolchildren. *Eur. J. Clin. Nutr.* 64, 1086–92.

5 Steventon, K., Cowell F. (2013). Acne and Diet: A review of the latest evidence. *Dermatolog. Nurs.* 12(2), 28–34.

6 Department of Health (2016). *Health Survey for England 2015*. The Health and Social Care Information Centre. TSO, London.

7 WHO (2014). *Global status report on alcohol 2014*. WHO, Geneva.

that boys and girls aged 15–18 years reported a mean alcohol consumption of 9 and 7 units of alcohol/week, respectively.

Sedentary behaviour

The Chief Medical Officer recommends that all young people aged 5–18 years should participate in moderate to vigorous intensity physical activity for 1 to several hours a day, with vigorous intensity activities on at least 3 days a week.[8] This can be accumulated throughout the day, e.g. four periods of 15 minutes, and through structured exercise, sport, or everyday physical activity as part of habits.

- Only about 23% of boys and 20% of girls (5–15 years old) meet this recommendation. For both boys and girls, activity levels decline with age and by 13-15 years 15% boys and only 9% girls achieve recommended levels of activity.[3]

- A sedentary way of life is similar for boys and girls and increases with age, e.g. TV or other sedentary time of >6 hours/day. High number of hours of television viewing is associated with ↑ risk of obesity.

8 Department of Health (2011). *Start Active. Stay Active. A report on physical activity for health from the four home countries*. CMO. London.

Nutrient deficiencies in children

The UK NDNS of 2008/9 included data for 4–18-year-olds (DH, 2010)[9] on nutrient intake and found that most children meet micronutrient recommendations, with some exceptions.

Iron

- Comparison of iron intake against dietary reference values (DRVs) for iron should be interpreted with caution because DRVs for iron are derived from uncertain data.[10]
- Iron is the most prevalent nutrient deficiency in the UK as 48% of 11–18-year-old girls do not meet the lower reference nutrient intake (LRNI), compared with only 9% of boys.
- Mean intakes of iron are <RNI (see Table 14.1) particularly for older girls (11–18 years), i.e. mean intake is 9.3 mg/day for girls and 11.4 mg/day for boys. See Box 14.2 for foods rich in iron.
- Failure to meet iron requirement in girls is mainly a result of iron requirement ↑ with onset of menstruation (from 8.7 to 14.8 mg/day at age 11 years).
- There is continued evidence of anaemia (indicated by low haemoglobin levels) and of low iron stores (indicated by low plasma ferritin), especially among females aged 11-18 years. Low iron intakes are associated with ↓ physical activity → ↓ peak bone mass.

Box 14.2 Foods rich in iron (see ➲ 'Iron' in Chapter 6, p. 148 for full list)

- Peanut butter sandwiches
- Fortified breakfast cereals
- Dried apricots and raisins
- Red meat, e.g. beef, pork, lamb, lean minced meat, ham
- Egg yolk
- Leafy green vegetables
- Peas, beans, and lentils
- Tinned tuna and salmon

Magnesium

Over a quarter of girls (27%) and 14% of boys did not meet the LRNI for magnesium. Mg is an integral part of bones and teeth and is a component of muscle and nerve cell function (see ➲ Chapter 6, 'Magnesium', p. 164 for further information; see also Box 14.3).

---

9 Department of Health/Food Standards Agency (2016). *National Diet and Nutrition Survey of 2015.* TSO, London.

10 SACN (2010). *Iron and Health Report.* TSO, London.

Box 14.3 Good food sources of magnesium
- Green vegetables
- Pulses and whole grain cereals
- Meat

Calcium

Adolescence is a critical period with ~25–40% of peak bone mass laid down at this time in females, while ~90–95% of peak bone mass is attained by 30 years of age. Adequate calcium and phosphate intake is necessary, combined with weight-bearing physical activity to maximize peak bone mass.

In the UK, more girls than boys do not achieve the LRNI for calcium; as 7% of 11–18-year-old girls and 4% of 11–18-year-old boys do not meet requirements. These estimates are lower than previously, suggesting that calcium content of diets is improving. However, mean intakes of 702 mg/day in 11–18-year-old girls are below RNI of 800–1000 mg/day. Boys fare better, with a mean intake of >919 mg/day.

Chronic dieting to lose weight in girls is also likely to contribute to suboptimal peak bone mass and osteoporosis in later life.

💧 Vitamin D also plays an important role in bone health as it is vital for calcium absorption. Use of sun creams that reduce access to vitamin D via sunlight may be one explanation for why requirements are not met.

Dietary fibre

Constipation as a result of low fibre intake, and sometimes low fluid intake, is relatively common in UK children. Encouraging fresh and dried fruit and vegetables for pectins, and bread and breakfast cereals for cereal fibre, will relieve symptoms along with plenty of fluid, preferably as water. Children's access to fluid may be restricted during the school day; if so, they should be encouraged to carry bottled water/sugar-free fluids with them. They may intentionally restrict their fluid intake to reduce frequency of micturition.

▶ Children from low income households

- Children living in households in receipt of benefits are more likely to have intakes of vitamins and minerals below LRNI and eat less fruit and vegetables than other children (<2 portions/day; boys < girls).[11]
- Children from low income households are more likely to eat sausages, coated chicken and turkey, burgers and kebabs than adults.
- Sweetened soft drinks contribute more to NMES intakes of children from low income households compared with the general population of children.

Also see ⭢ Chapter 16, 'Eating on a low income', p. 354.

11 Nelson, M., et al. (2007). Low income diet and nutrition survey. FSA. TSO, London.

Childhood obesity and weight problems

Obesity prevalence in children

↑ in childhood obesity worldwide because of a widespread transition to an energy dense diet and ↓ in physical activity, with an estimated 107.7 million children now classified as obese.[12] This is also the case in the UK, where approximately a sixth of boys (15%) and an eighth of girls (13%) aged 2–15 years are obese, and almost a third (28%) are either overweight or obese.[13] Prevalence of obesity increases with age, i.e. 18% of boys and 14.5% of girls aged 11–15 years are obese, and is higher in children from lower income families, with 18% of children from the lowest income quintile considered obese compared with 9% in the highest quintile.

▶Trends for obesity appear to be levelling off since 2006 in the UK.

Classification of childhood obesity

Assigning cut-off points for childhood obesity is more complex than for adults. The BMI percentile chart should be used to identify obesity and the UK 1990 chart is recommended for routine clinical diagnosis. Overweight is classified as ≥91st centile; and obesity ≥98th centile of the UK 1990 data.[14] For epidemiological studies, an internationally acceptable definition[15] to classify prevalence of child overweight (≥85th centile) and obesity (≥95th centile) of the 1990 data is recommended.[16]

Immediate effects on health

In extreme cases of childhood obesity, children can develop cardiomyopathy, pancreatitis, orthopaedic disorders, upper airway obstruction, or chest wall restriction.

Effects on wellbeing

Besides physical aspects, children also suffer from ↓ self-esteem, ↓ social interaction, and poorer academic achievement. Earlier puberty may also → emotional problems as a mismatch between physical and emotional development can → higher expectations from adults. However, obesity limited to childhood appears to have little impact on social, psychological, economic, and educational outcomes in adult life. Persistent child to adult obesity is associated with poorer employment and relationship outcomes particularly in females.

12 The GBD 2015 Obesity Collaborators (2017) Health Effects of Overweight and Obesity in 195 Countries over 25 Years. *N. Engl. J. Med.* **377**, 13–27. ℘ http://www.nejm.org/doi/full/10.1056/NEJMoa1614362.

13 Health and Social Care Centre (2016). Health Survey for England 2015. ℘ https://digital.nhs.uk/data-and-information/publications/statistical/health-survey-for-england/health-survey-for-england-2015

14 NICE (2014). Obesity: identification, assessment and management. Clinical Guidance CG189. ℘ https://www.nice.org.uk/guidance/cg189

15 Cole, T.J., et al. (2000). Establishing a standard definition for child overweight and obesity worldwide: international survey. *Br. Med. J.* **320**, 1240–3.

16 SIGN 115 (2010). Management of obesity: A national clinical guideline. Available at: ℘ http://www.sign ac.uk.

Long-term effect on health

The ↑ prevalence of obesity/overweight combined with a diet low in fruit and vegetables, high in saturated fat, and low in calcium and low physical activity means that it is likely that there will also be an ↑ risk of type 2 diabetes, CVD, suboptimal peak bone mass, osteoporosis, gallstones, and diet-related cancers in later life, especially if the increase in obesity is sustained in adult life. Older obese children are at a higher risk of becoming obese adults, 79% of obese children in their early teens are likely to remain obese as adults.[17]

Unnecessary dieting

An estimated fifth of UK female adolescents are dieting to lose weight at any time with little evidence of a structured weight-reducing plan. Inappropriate approaches are common, such as crash diets, binge eating, chaotic eating plans, missing meals, eating slimming products (alongside energy dense foods), replacing meals with high sugar and fat snacks. This can lead to low intakes of several nutrients, especially iron, calcium, vitamin B_6, and riboflavin, as well as ↑ risk of developing eating disorders. See ➡ Chapter 32, 'Eating disorders', p. 768.

Underweight

Prevalence of underweight in UK children is very low (<1.5%). Undernutrition in childhood and adolescence can result in stunting, i.e. inability to achieve inherited potential. Undernutrition may also impact on school achievement.
- *Diagnosis of stunting* in adolescents: height for age <2nd centile of WHO reference data or <−2 SD.
- *Diagnosis of thinness in adolescence*: BMI <2nd centile (UK National Child Measurement Programme). See ➡ Chapter 25, 'Malnutrition universal screening tool', p. 560 and 'Undernutrition', p. 564.

National child measurement programme

Beginning in 2006, this is part of the government's work programme on child obesity and is operated by Public Health England and the Department of Health. Every year, children in Reception (4-5 years) and Year 6 (10-11 years) are weighed and measured during the school year to inform local planning and delivery of services for children, and gather population-level surveillance data to allow analysis of trends in growth patterns and obesity. There has been a gradual shift from this being used to provide prevalence data to being used as a screening tool for childhood obesity, with each family receiving a letter informing them of the results of their child's BMI and signposting to local weight management and physical activity services.

For further information see: ℘ https://www.gov.uk/government/collections/national-child-measurement-programme.

Preventing childhood obesity

See ➡ this Chapter, 'Promoting healthy eating in children', p. 320.

17 NICE (2013) Weight management: lifestyle services for overweight or obese children and young people (Public Health Guidance ph47). https://www.nice.org.uk/guidance/ph47

Dental health and children

In the UK, dental health in young people is improving because of the introduction of fluoride toothpaste in the 1970s. However, it is still a public health concern, particularly in socially deprived groups, possibly because less preventive dentistry is practised; frequent consumption of sugary foods and ↓ regular brushing → ↓ fluoride intake.

Targeting for dental caries prevention is recommended as decay is unevenly distributed in the UK population: 27% of 5-year-olds.[18,19]

There is ongoing debate in the UK and the EU concerning introduction of fluoride in non-water-fluoridated areas.

Causes of dental caries
- Frequent consumption of NMES (glucose, sucrose, fructose) plays an unequivocal role in dental caries development as NMES act as a substrate for oral bacteria.
- Both quantity and stickiness of sugar affect the length of time it takes for surface pH to ↑ to normal. Sticky foods may become stuck in-between teeth and are in contact with teeth for longer.

For guidelines for good dental health, see Box 14.4.

18 Public Health England. (2016). *National Dental epidemiology programme for England, oral health survey of 5 year old children 2015*. TSO, London.

19 Further information is available from SIGN guideline '*Preventing dental caries in children at high caries risk*' 2000. Available at: ℘ http://www.sign.ac.uk.

Box 14.4 Guidelines for good dental health in children

- Decrease both quantity and frequency of sugar intake
- Avoid sugary foods in-between meals and just before bedtime
- Avoid drinks that are carbonated, acidic, or high in sugar in-between meals (→ dental erosion); water and milk are better choices
- Eat sweet foods (including dried fruit) with meals rather than in-between (↑ saliva at end of meal → buffer of low pH)
- Avoid eating sticky and chewy foods
- Choose sugar-free medicines
- Regular flossing and brushing with fluoride toothpaste, but not immediately after consuming sweet foods/acidic drinks as ↓ mineralization
- Regular dental visits

Influences on children's food choices

The key factors influencing the eating habits of children and adolescents are shown in Fig. 14.1.

Media and advertising
- Children spend on average 3–4hrs/day watching TV or a computer screen
- Food adverts during children's programmes are mainly for high fat and sugar food and drink.
- Unrealistic ideals of body image portrayed of 5 and subsequent desire for thinness.

Environmental issues
~2–3% of children are vegetarian and this increases in adolescence, often for concern over animal welfare.

Food choice in children and adolescents

School
- Influences food availability, e.g. school meals, vending machines, tuck shops, classroom rewards.
- School meals/whole school approach ncouraged.

Family-parents
- Parents influence the availability of food.
- Parents act as role models for their children and determine whether the family eats together: children eating dinner with their families ↓ with age and has ↓ over time. This ↑ likelihood for 'conven ience' foods and erratic eating patterns → diets higher in saturated fat.

Peer group
- Influence of peer pressure ↑ with age
- Adolescent girls more likely to see friend's support as key to maintaining dietary change.
- Eating with peers can have a positive effect on eating behaviour.

Available income
- 1 in 3 children in the UK live in poverty, which is associated with poor nutrition.
- Convincing evidence that parents make sacrifices so that children have similar foods/snacks as other children to avoid feeling excluded.

Fig. **14.1** Food choice in children and adolescents.

Promoting healthy eating in children

Implications from the various influences on children's food choice for nutrition education/health promotion are that a holistic approach should be used to tackle the multitude of influences on food choice. See ➲ Chapter 17, 'Influences on food intake', p. 366.

See ➲ Chapter 10, 'Schools', p. 224 for detailed information on catering standards for school meal provision.

Useful information

🕮 Children's food photograph resources at The Caroline Walker Trust (http://www.cwt.org.uk) for ages 5–11 years and 12–18 years.

🕮 The Government 'Change 4 Life Campaign' provides practical tips and resources for families. For more information, see http://www.nhs.uk/change4life.

🕮 Healthy eating for children: https://www.gov.uk/government/publications/the-eatwell-guide.

Chapter 15

Older people

An ageing population *322*
Dietary recommendations for older people *324*
Undernutrition in older people *326*
Other nutritional problems in older people *330*
Community strategies to promote a healthy diet for older people *332*
Model of a food policy for older people *334*

An ageing population

Globally, the older population (aged ≥65 years) is growing at a faster rate than any other age group. By 2050 the United Nations predicts that one in six of the global population will be ≥ 65 years (one in four in high income countries, one in seven in low and middle income countries).[1] In the UK, life expectancy at birth has increased steadily over the past 100 years. Life expectancy in England for a newborn baby boy is 79.5 years and for a newborn baby girl is 83.2 years.[2]

The 2011 census found that most older people in the UK live in the community with a partner, family, or in their own homes. Around 30% of older people live alone. Around 4% of older people live in communal settings, i.e. sheltered accommodation, nursing and residential care homes. Around 60% of residents in care homes are aged over 85 years.[3]

The ageing process

Ageing is associated with a physiological decline in most biological systems and is often accompanied by pathological changes, which collectively have significant nutritional implications. Low Basal Metabolism (LBM) ↓ and relative proportion of adipose tissue ↑ resulting in reduced basal metabolic rate (BMR). Bone density, immune function, taste, olfactory perception, nutrient absorption, and appetite all ↓. Physical activity typically declines with increasing age, which, together with reduced BMR, means that total energy requirements are lower and a nutrient dense diet is needed to achieve adequate intake of all nutrients.

What older people are eating

Older people are a heterogeneous group. The majority of older people are adequately nourished, and, in many respects, have a better diet than younger people. Institutionalized older people and the oldest old (>85 years) have poorer diets than the younger, free-living older adult population and ∴ have poorer nutritional status. The UK National Diet and Nutrition Survey[4] has shown that the reported energy intakes of older adults are below the estimated average requirements; however, a large proportion of the older adult population are overweight suggesting under-reporting of dietary intakes. Total fat intake in older adult women is within the reference nutrient intake (RNI) targets, but in men exceeds recommendations (≤35% total

---

1 Available at: ℘ https://www.un.org/en/sections/issues-depth/ageing/.

2 Office of National Statistics (2015). *Life expectancy at birth and at age 65 by local areas in England and Wales, 2012-2014.* Statistical Bulletin. Available at: ℘ https://www.ons.gov.uk/peoplepopulationandcommunity/birthsdeathsandmarriages/lifeexpectancies/bulletins/lifeexpectancyatbirthandatage65bylocalareasinenglandandwales/2015-11-04/pdf.

3 Office of National Statistics (2013). *What does the 2011 census tell us about older people?* Available at: ℘ http://www.ons.gov.uk/ons/dcp171776_325486.pdf.

4 *National Diet and Nutrition Survey: Results from Years 1, 2, 3 and 4 (combined) of the Rolling Programme (2008/2009–2011/2012).* Available at: ℘ https://www.gov.uk/government/statistics/national-diet-and-nutrition-survey-results-from-years-1-to-4-combined-of-the-rolling-programme-for-2008-and-2009-to-2011-and-2012.

energy). The average consumption of saturated fat exceeds the recommended 11% of total energy intake in both sexes. Consumption of free sugars also exceeds dietary reference values (DRVs). The majority of free-living older adults meet the RNI for vitamins and minerals as set out by COMA in 1991, with the exception of selenium and vitamin D intakes which are below recommendations. Compared to younger people, older adults eat more bread and biscuits.

In older adults in the UK living in private households:

- the average intake of fruit and vegetables is 4.6 portions/day, with 41% achieving the five portions of fruit and vegetables per day recommendation. Lower fruit and vegetable intakes in institutionalized older adults;
- the mean consumption of oily fish is below the recommended one portion per week;
- the average intake of dietary fibre is around 18 g/d and fails to meet the DRV (30 g/d);
- those who drink alcohol have an average consumption of 6.4% of total energy, which exceeds the 5% maximum recommendation;
- dietary supplement use is high: 35% of men and 47% of women aged ≥65 years report consumption of at least one dietary supplement per day;
- 17% of men and 24% of women have low vitamin D status (<25 nmol/L plasma 25(OH)D). A far higher prevalence exists in institutionalized older adults;
- 15% of men and 12% of women have low haemoglobin; however, the proportion with low haemoglobin and low plasma ferritin, indicative of iron deficiency is <4%. Iron deficiency anaemia is higher in institutionalized older adults;
- B vitamin status is a concern and has been associated with poor cognitive status. 6% of older adults have vitamin B_{12} concentrations below the lower threshold of normality and 8% are folate deficient (16% in institutionalized older adults).

There are categories of older people who are 'at risk' of malnutrition (see ➲ this Chapter 'Undernutrition in older people', p. 326).

Dietary recommendations for older people

Energy requirements ↓ with age. Per cent energy derived from fat, protein, and carbohydrate is unchanged. There is little difference between the RNIs for micronutrients of younger and older people, However because of the fall in energy requirements, older people need to consume a nutrient dense diet to meet micronutrient requirements. General healthy eating guidelines apply to healthy older people (see Chapter 2, 'The Eatwell Guide', p. 27). The healthy eating guidelines to reduce consumption of energy dense foods (from fat and sugar) do not apply to frail older people and those at risk of malnutrition. Full fat foods and sugar provide a useful calorie source, particularly in individuals with a poor appetite. However, a nutrient dense diet should always be promoted. Fruit and vegetable consumption should be encouraged (fresh, frozen, or canned).

The lack of specific recommendations for older people in the UK largely reflects the fact that dietary recommendations for older people have been derived from extrapolations from younger adult population data. Dietary recommendations differ around the globe, and the WHO and the USA have higher recommendations for a number of micronutrients of particular concern for older people including calcium, selenium, and the vitamins folate, B_{12}, B_6, C, and D. Calcium and vitamin D are important for musculoskeletal health and the prevention of falls and fractures. Vitamins folate, B_{12}, and B_6 have been implicated in cognitive function, and vitamin C is important for wound healing. In the UK a specific recommendation for people aged ≤65 years to consume 10 μg vitamin D/day has existed for some time.

Subgroups of older people do have specific dietary needs, particularly those who are living in institutions, who are frail or housebound, and those with non-communicable disease. Estimates of energy requirements can deviate significantly from predictions as a result of the health status and activity level of the older person. The existence of co-morbidities and infection can increase energy requirements, whereas immobility will reduce energy requirements.

People living in care homes are often frail and immobile. The desire to eat is often impaired, which presents challenges for maintaining a nutritionally adequate diet. There is also a high prevalence of dementia in care homes, which presents additional nutritional challenges.

Maintaining a good hydration status is important for older people as dehydration can lead to infection, mental confusion, and constipation. A non-alcoholic fluid intake of 1500-2000 mL/d is recommended (6–8 mugs, can include tea and coffee). A high fibre diet is also important to reduce constipation, but foods high in phytate (i.e. bran) should be avoided as phytate inhibits iron, calcium, and zinc absorption.

Undernutrition in older people

10% of older people in England are malnourished or at risk of malnutrition.[5] The causes of malnutrition are typically multifactorial.

Older people most at risk of malnutrition:

- oldest age groups (>75 years);
- people living in deprived or isolated circumstances;
- people living in care homes, nursing homes, or following admission to hospital;
- people who have difficulty eating, because of poor dentition or swallowing problems (dysphagia, often caused by stroke). Older people with dentures have a lower intake of fruit and vegetables and diet quality is poorer;
- people with long-term conditions (diabetes, kidney disease) or chronic progressive disease (cancer and dementia);
- people with a poor appetite—caused by the anorexia of ageing, and age-associated impairment of taste and smell;
- people reliant on others for shopping and preparing food;
- people on certain medications that alter appetite, taste, and gastrointestinal (GI) function (see ➲ Chapter 38, 'Drug–nutrient interactions', p. 834).

However, in most cases, the causes of undernutrition are multifactorial but an awareness of some specific contributory factors is a valuable first step in prevention. (see ➲ Chapter 25, 'Undernutrition', p. 564).

Nutrition screening for malnutrition risk factors in older people

More than 3 million people in the UK are at risk of malnutrition. Most people at risk of malnutrition live in the community, 5% are in care homes and 2% are in hospital.[6] Screening for risk of malnutrition allows early and effective intervention. Failure to recognize malnutrition or risk of malnutrition can have a wide-ranging impact on the health and wellbeing of the individual. NICE guidance[7] recommends that people in care settings should be screened for malnutrition by trained health and social care staff using a validated screening tool, e.g. MUST[8] (see ➲ Chapter 25, 'Malnutrition universal screening tool', p. 560). Patients admitted to hospital should be screened on admission and each week during the hospital stay. Outpatients and GP patients should be screened on initial clinic visit or GP registration

5 Elia, M., Stratton, R.J. (2005). Geographical inequalities in nutrient status and risk of malnutrition among English people aged 65 y and older. *Nutrition* **21**, 1100–6.

6 Public Health England (2017). *Helping older people maintain a healthy diet: A review of what works.* Available at: ℘ https://www.gov.uk/government/publications/helping-older-people-maintain-a-healthy-diet-a-review-of-what-works.

7 NICE (2012). *Nutrition support in adults.* Available at: ℘ https://www.nice.org.uk/guidance/QS24.

8 BAPEN (2016). Introducing 'MUST'. Available at: ℘ http://www.bapen.org.uk/screening-and-must/must/introducing-must.

and when there is clinical concern. People admitted to care homes should be screened on initial admission and at least once a month. Care needs to be taken to ensure continuity of care if a person is transferred between care settings, i.e. hospital to care home. Unintentional weight loss, loss of appetite, loose fitting clothes, altered bowel habit, and poor wound healing are all indicators of risk of malnutrition in older people and should raise clinical concern and prompt nutritional screening for malnutrition.

Consequences of malnutrition in older people

The impact of malnutrition on the health and wellbeing of older people is extensive. The effects vary from sub-clinical through to death, depending on the type, length, and degree of nutritional inadequacy, and the nutritional and health status of the individuals.

Malnourished older people are at increased risk of mortality and morbidity:

- loss of muscle tissue and strength: ↓ respiratory muscle leads to ↑ risk of chest infection, ↓ cardiac muscle leads to ↑ risk of heart failure, ↓ skeletal muscle leads to ↑ risk of sarcopenia and frailty, ↓ mobility, and ↑ risk of falls and fractures;
- reduced immune function: ↑ rates of infection, ↓ vaccine responsiveness;
- loss of mucosal integrity: ↓ nutrient absorption, ↑ GI and respiratory infections;
- impaired synthesis of new protein: poor wound healing;
- slower recovery from illness and ↑ length of hospital stay;
- psychological decline: ↑ apathy, ↑ depression.

See ➋ Chapter 25, 'Undernutrition', p. 564.

Treatment of malnutrition

The cause of malnutrition should be identified (e.g. infection) and addressed where possible, and nutrition support provided. Nutritional support in older people at risk of malnutrition improves both physical and mental health, reduces mortality and morbidity, reduces hospital admission, and reduces length of hospital stay. Nutritional support should aim to provide a nutritionally complete diet and not just increase calorie intake. A 'food first' approach should be considered and may be used in combination with oral nutritional supplements.

Treatment options could include:

- improving food access to nutrient rich foods, e.g. tackling barriers to eating, providing support through carers for shopping, cooking, and mealtime assistance in the community, or mealtime assistance in a care setting. Recommend consumption of cheese and full fat milk to increase protein and energy intake;
- oral nutritional supplements and fortified foods—available on prescription or over the counter, e.g. multivitamin and mineral supplements, milk or juice-based drinks, soups;
- artificial nutrition support (enteral feeding).

See ➋ Chapter 25, 'Enteral feeding', p. 574; see also Box 15.1.

Box 15.1 Tips for overcoming institutional factors contributing to malnutrition in care homes and hospitals

- Identify a named individual to be responsible for nutritional care.
- Monitor and promote fluid intake.
- Protect mealtimes to avoid medical rounds or investigations when food is served.
- Provide adequate staff or volunteers to assist patients/residents with eating at mealtimes.
- Food served should meet nutritional recommendations, i.e. average daily food intake, estimated over a week, should meet estimated average requirements and RNIs for nutrients.
- Offer patients/residents choice and variety of foods.
- Snacks and drinks should be available to residents/patients between meals.
- Food served should be the right temperature for eating.
- Make the environment conducive to eating, i.e. clean, light, comfortable, and attractive.
- A 10 μg/d vitamin D supplement is recommended, especially for the 'housebound' and during winter months.
- Consider individual food preferences and adjust portion sizes according to the individual.
- Encourage exercise/physical activity where appropriate.
- Provide storage facilities for patients'/residents' own food.

Other nutritional problems in older people

Arthritis

See ➲ Chapter 34 'Osteoarthritis', p. 796 and ➲ 'Rheumatoid arthritis', p. 798.

Bone loss

Osteoporosis and osteopenia increase the risk of falls and fractures (typically of the wrist and hip) and are associated with a high risk of mortality in older people. Calcium and vitamin D are important nutrients for maintaining bone health. Vitamin D supplements are recommended to all people.

Chronic disease

Older people often have a number of diet-related non-communicable diseases that can impact on dietary intake and nutritional status, e.g. type 2 diabetes, cardiovascular disease (CVD), cancer, and chronic obstructive pulmonary disease (COPD).

Dehydration

Thirst sensation declines with age, making older people, particularly those in long-term care and with cognitive impairments, susceptible to dehydration. Dehydration leads to urinary tract infections, constipation, mental confusion, and increased mortality and morbidity.

Dementia

Alzheimer's disease and vascular dementia are common in older people. Eating and drinking can become a challenge as dementia progresses. See ➲ Chapter 32, Dementia, p. 774.

GI problems

Atrophic gastritis leads to impaired secretion of intrinsic factor and ↓ secretion of vitamin B_{12}, which can lead to pernicious anaemia and peripheral neuropathy. Constipation is common in older people probably because of declining intestinal motility, reduced physical activity, dehydration, low fibre intake, and drug regimens. Constipation contributes to diverticular disease. Fibre and fluid intake, alongside regular physical activity should be encouraged. (see ➲ Chapter 26, 'Disorders of the colon', p. 672).

Obesity

The change in body composition coupled with reduced physical activity, leads to reduced energy requirements and makes older people particularly susceptible to excess energy intake and obesity. Of those aged ≥65 years, 28% of men and 30% of women were classified as obese in the UK National Diet and Nutrition Survey.[4] Obesity increases the risk of age-related chronic diseases, e.g. type 2 diabetes, CVD, and cancer (see ➡ Chapter 21, 'Obesity', p. 469).

Community strategies to promote a healthy diet for older people

Barriers to a healthy diet in older people include poor access to healthy food, food poverty, difficulties with food preparation and eating, social isolation, and physical and cognitive impairments.[6]

Community strategies to promote a healthy diet include:

- *Lunch clubs:* run through day centres, churches, and other voluntary organizations provide a hot meal for older people in a social setting. Provide nutritious food and help combat social isolation.
- *Meals on wheels and frozen meal home delivery services:* provided through the local authority, voluntary organizations, i.e. Age UK, WRVS, or the private sector.
- *Community transport:* provide transport for older people to get to and from food shops. Often run by local authorities or supermarkets.
- *Home delivery services:* delivery of groceries by supermarkets and smaller local retailers/farmers (often fruit and vegetable box schemes) and doorstep delivery of milk.
- *Community-based nutrition support:* typically involve health and social care staff in the detection, early prevention, and treatment of malnutrition in the community.
- *Cooking clubs/shopping trips:* provide practical support to improve cooking skills, menu planning, and knowledge of nutrition.
- *Food banks:* provide emergency food supplies for all ages of people in severe financial difficulty. Run by charities, churches, and community groups. Vouchers to access the food banks are provided by GPs, social workers, and charitable organizations.
- *Grow your own:* food grown at home in gardens and in private and community allotments.
- *Food policy:* develop a food policy for older people including guidelines for care homes (see Fig. 15.1 and Box 15.1).

Model of a food policy for older people

See Fig. 15.1. The composition of a working party could be as follows:
- dietitians working with older people;
- GPs, hospital doctors;
- social services; social worker;
- community dental health service;
- community nurses;
- older people's hospital nurses;
- non-governmental organisation (NGO) representative working with older people, e.g. Age UK;
- representative of residents/patients;
- residential care home representative;
- occupational therapist.

Further information

& Caroline Walker Trust (2004) Eating well for older people—nutritional and practical guidelines. CWT, Abbots Langley, Herts WD5 0DQ. http://www.cwt.org.uk

& http://www.ageuk.org.uk

& http://www.bapen.org.uk

& http://www.malnutritionpathway.co.uk/

& http://www.malnutritiontaskforce.org.uk/

& https://www.nutrition.org.uk/healthyliving/healthyageing.html

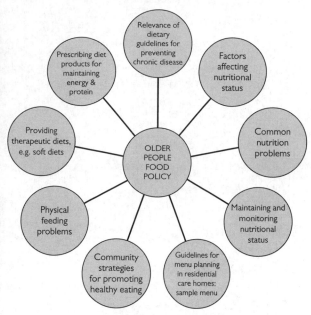

Fig. 15.1 A suggested format for a joint community–hospital-based food policy for older people.

Nutrition in vulnerable population groups

Minority ethnic communities *338*
Vegetarians *346*
Eating on a low income *354*
Refugees and asylum seekers *358*
Homeless people *360*
Local food projects for reducing food poverty *362*
Useful websites *364*

Minority ethnic communities

Traditional dietary habits and food restrictions

Data on the diets of UK minority ethnic populations are limited because of a lack of nationally representative datasets that encompass all groups in sufficient numbers. However, according to the Health Survey for England, there is some evidence that diets are healthier, as minority ethnic groups (both males and females and all ages) tend to eat more fruit and vegetables and eat less fat, sugar, and salt than the majority white population.[1]

Traditional food restrictions for ethnic minority communities that are predominant in the UK are shown in Tables 16.1–16.3. There is a great deal of variety in dietary habits within all communities, including those of minority ethnic and religious groups and this has implications for nutrition education (Box 16.1); it is essential to find out the nature of an individual's diet as one cannot assume anything. However, it is important to be aware of these orthodox food restrictions, even though there is great diversity in following them within UK minority ethnic communities. Younger generations of some ethnic groups are more likely to adopt a mixed diet incorporating that of the mainstream food culture (known as dietary acculturation).

Influences on dietary behaviours in ethnic minority populations

Just as in the majority population, a broad range of different factors influence food choice in minority ethnic communities. For example, in Europe, some ethnic minority populations have a higher risk of non-communicable diseases than the majority population. Diet contributes to this risk, shaped by a range of factors. The factors that have the strongest influence across all ethnic minority populations are summarized in Fig 16.1. There is much commonality between the factors influencing dietary behaviours in different ethnic minority groups and the majority population. However even if factors are shared, their importance and focus might differ, e.g. the social role of food might be stronger in more collective cultures. Migration context and the social and material resources that individuals and families experience are particularly important to account for in developing interventions.

1 Leung, G., Stanner, S. (2011). Diets of minority ethnic groups in the UK: Influence on chronic disease risk and implications for prevention. *Nutr. Bull.* **36**(2), 161–98.

Table 16.1 Traditional food restrictions of Chinese and Jewish communities living in Great Britain*

	Chinese	Jewish
Religion	Include Taoism, Confucianism, Buddhism, Christianity, Islam	Judaism
Origin	Hong Kong, Malaysia, Singapore, China, Taiwan, Vietnam	Europe, Middle East
Language (besides English)	Written Chinese is common to all. Cantonese or Hakka are often spoken	Hebrew, Yiddish
Fasting	✗	✓ 1 day for Yom Kippur and Tish'ah B'av
Staple cereals	Rice	–
Eggs	✓	✓
Dairy	✓ But not frequently. Warm milk may be taken	✓ Some, but no cheese with rennet. Dairy foods not consumed at a meal with meat. Separate dishes and pans may be used for meat and dairy foods
Fish and shellfish	✓ Also salted fish	✓ If fins and scales. No shellfish
Poultry	✓	✓ Chicken, turkey, goose, and duck. No birds of prey. Do not eat fish and meat at the same meal
Red meat	✓ Mostly; except some religions	✓ Kosher† only meat, but pork and its products prohibited
Alcohol	✓ Mainly for celebrations	✓ Wine (ideally approved by the rabbi)
Caffeine	✓ But coffee not commonly drunk	✓
Nutritional implications	Low calcium intake could result from low consumption of dairy foods. High sodium intake could be a problem (from mono-sodium glutamate in soy sauce). Note. Food is seen as contributing to the body's balance, i.e. yang (foods that have a hot effect on body) and yin (cold effect). Cold food is often avoided	Traditional diet is high in total fat, saturated fat, and salt. ↑ Risk of obesity, type 2 diabetes, and cardiovascular disease

*There is great diversity in following food restrictions as they should be used as a guide and not a substitute for discussing individual dietary patterns.

†Kosher, slaughtered in a prescribed way.

Table 16.2 Traditional food restrictions of Asians living in Great Britain (4% of population census 2001, Office National Statistics)*

	Indian	Indian	Pakistani	Bangladeshi
Religion	Hindu	Sikh	Muslim	Muslim
Origin	Gujarat	Punjab	Pakistan	Bangladesh
Language (besides English)	Hindi/Kutchi	Punjabi, Hindi	Urdu, Punjabi	Bengali/Sylheti
Fasting	✓ Certain holy days, especially month of Shravan	No religious obligation to fast	Especially month of Ramadan: no food during daylight. Pregnant, lactating, and menstruating women, prepubescent children, diabetics, and those needing regular medication are exempt	
Staple cereals	Chapatti, rice	Chapatti, rice	Chapatti, rice	Rice
Eggs	✗ If strict	✓ Probably; not if strict	✓	✓
Dairy	✓ Milk, yogurt (may be home-made), but no cheese with rennet			
Fish and shellfish	✗ If strict	✓ Possibly	✓ Possibly	✓ Often eaten
Poultry	✗	✓ But not if strict	✓ Halal†	✓ Halal†
Red meat	✗	✓ Except no beef. May be lacto-vegetarian. Not if strict.	✓ Halal† only, but pork and pork products prohibited	

Alcohol	✗ If strict	✓ If strict	✓
Caffeine	✗ If strict	✓	✓
Nutritional implications	If unbalanced vegetarian diet, possible deficiencies in protein and energy (faltering growth in infants), B₁₂ and iron (anaemia), calcium and vitamin D (rickets/osteomalacia). See ⊙ 'Vegetarians', this chapter, p. 346 and ⊙ 'Nutritionally vulnerable infants', Chapter 13, p. 298	If curry cooked for a long time → ↓ folic acid, vitamins B₁₂ and C	Attention for infant feeding: commercially prepared baby foods with non-halal meat may be replaced with sweet baby foods, low in iron and protein. See ⊙ 'Nutritionally vulnerable infants', Chapter 13, p. 298

↑ Risk of developing obesity, type 2 diabetes, and coronary heart disease in later life; ∴ advice ↓ in fried foods (e.g. samosa, sev, bhaji, ganthia, puri, chevda, chips, crisps) and sweets (e.g. Indian sweets, including jelabi, burfi, gulab jamen, kulfi and laddo, and gur, jaggery, honey, chocolate, cakes, and biscuits)

---

*There is great diversity in following food restrictions; they should be used as a guide and not a substitute for discussing individual dietary patterns.

†Halal, slaughtered in a prescribed way.

Table 16.3 Traditional food restrictions of African-Caribbeans and Black Africans living in Great Britain (2% of population census 2001, Office National Statistics)*

	African-Caribbean			Black African
Religion	Christian	Rastafarian	Seventh Day Adventist	Muslim, Christian
Origin	West Indian Islands, especially Jamaica (60%), Dominica, Barbados, Trinidad			Mainly Nigeria, Ghana, Somalia
Language (besides English)	Patois			Nigeria: Hausa, Yoruba, Ibo Ghana: Twi. Somalia: Somali
Fasting	–	–	✗	✓ Especially month of Ramadan: no food during daylight Pregnant, lactating, and menstruating women, prepubescent children, diabetics, and those needing regular medication are exempt
Staple cereals	Rice, plantain, yam, potato, pasta			Cassava, yam, plantain
Eggs	✓	✗	✓	✓
Dairy	✓ But condensed and evaporated milk may be used instead of fresh milk	✓ Unless vegan	✓	✓ Milk, yogurt but possibly no cheese with rennet

Fish and shellfish	✓ Including salt fish	✓ If fins and scales. No shellfish	✓ If fins and scales. No shellfish	✓ Possibly
Poultry	✓	✗	✓	✓ Halal† if Muslim
Red meat	✓	✗ Mostly vegetarian; some are vegans	✓ Mostly vegetarian, but some may eat meat but no pork	✓ If Muslim, possibly halal †only, but pork and pork products prohibited
Alcohol	✓	✗ If strict	✗	✗ If strict Muslim
Caffeine		✗ If strict	✓	✓
Nutritional implications	Can be high in fat, sugar and salt. ↑ risk of developing hypertension, CVD, and type 2 diabetes later	B$_{12}$ deficiency seen in strict adherence to ital diet	Attention for infant feeding Commercially prepared baby foods with non-halal meat may be replaced with sweet baby foods, low in iron and protein. See ⊕ 'Nutritionally vulnerable infants', Chapter 13, p. 298	
	Possibly higher prevalence of lactose intolerance (see ⊕ Chapter 26, p. 650)			

*There is great diversity in following food restrictions; they should be used as a guide and not a substitute for discussing individual dietary patterns.

†Halal, slaughtered in a prescribed way.

Developing interventions to promote healthier diets

'Mainstream' interventions targeting the general population could address many factors identified as there is much in common between minority and majority populations. Two different ways to develop interventions reaching ethnic minority populations are proposed[2]:

- *'Diversity sensitive'*: adapting mainstream interventions for the majority population, so that they can be equally effective for all citizens regardless of ethnicity, religion or culture.
- *'Migrant-specific'*: culturally adapting services and interventions to individual backgrounds of specific minority ethnic groups. As for the case for 'majority' populations, a needs assessment will remain a necessary part of the process.

2 Razum, O., Spallek, J. (2014). Addressing health-related interventions to immigrants: migrant-specific or diversity-sensitive. *Int. J. Public Health* **59**(6), 893–5.

Vegetarians

Trends in vegetarianism

In the UK, the number of vegetarians is estimated at 2–3% of the population in the National Nutrition and Diet Survey.[3] Vegetarianism is most prevalent in females, young people and adolescents, black and minority ethnic groups, and higher socio-economic groups. The same surveys report that a further 5–7% of adults describe themselves as 'partly vegetarian' (avoiding red meat or fish). It is important to respect the individual's choice when giving dietary advice.

Common reasons for choosing a vegetarian diet include:

- religion (e.g. strict Hindus, Buddhists, and 7th Day Adventists);
- cultural;
- ethical, moral, or political beliefs;
- environmental concerns for use of global resources;
- animal welfare;
- perceived health benefits;
- food safety scares;
- limited availability of halal or kosher meat;
- financial constraints.

Types of vegetarian diets

One cannot always categorize individuals along these lines, as there is a large variation, so health professionals should avoid making assumptions about which foods are acceptable, but generally vegetarians fall into the groups shown in Table 16.4.

Is a vegetarian diet a risk for health?

A well-planned vegetarian diet is more likely to comply with food-based dietary guidelines for reducing long-term risk of certain nutrition-related non-communicable diseases (NR-NCDs). There is evidence that vegetarians suffer fewer NR-NCDs than non-vegetarians, with better BMI, waist circumference, or blood pressure than people who consume meat.[4] However, this may be partly a result of vegetarians adopting other health-promoting behaviours, e.g. being physically active, avoiding smoking, or drinking less alcohol.

A well-balanced vegetarian diet can be nutritionally adequate for all age groups, *but* life stages of extra nutritional requirements need specific attention, i.e. pregnancy, lactation, infancy, childhood, and adolescence. Children consuming a well-balanced vegetarian diet should meet all requirements for growth. Those who rely heavily on full fat cheese and dairy foods could have a high saturated fat diet.

❶ Diets that are unbalanced or more restrictive, e.g. strict macrobiotic or fruitarian, are likely to result in nutrient deficiencies and need particular attention, especially in infants, children, and pregnant and lactating women. Referral to a dietitian for assessment is essential (Box 16.2).

---

3 Public Health England. *National Diet and Nutrition Survey*. Available at: ℘ https://www.gov.uk/government/collections/national-diet-and-nutrition-survey.

4 Chiu, Y.-F., et al. (2015). Cross-sectional and longitudinal comparisons of metabolic profiles between vegetarian and non-vegetarian subjects: a matched cohort study. *Br. J. Nutr.* 114, 1313–20.

Table 16.4 Types of vegetarian diet

Type of vegetarian	Eggs*	Dairy	Fish and shellfish	Poultry	Red meat†
Vegan	✗	✗	✗	✗	✗
Lacto-vegetarian	✗	✓	✗	✗	✗
Lacto-ovo-vegetarian	✓	✓	✗	✗	✗
Demi-vegetarian	✓	✓	✓	✓	✗
Pescatarian	✓	✓	✓	✗	✗
Macrobiotic	✗	✗	✓‡	✗	✗
Fruitarian	✗	✗	✗	✗	✗

*Possibly free-range only.

†Beef, lamb, pork; also sometimes their derivatives, e.g. gelatine, rennet.

‡Eaten at certain lower 'levels' of macrobiotic diet. Highest level eliminates everything except brown rice and water.

Box 16.1 Implications for nutrition interventions targeting ethnic minority populations

- Do not assume anything: drivers of dietary behaviours are not the same in all ethnic minority populations. There is a need to acknowledge this heterogeneity in nutrition education interventions.
- Promote positive aspects of traditional diets and eating patterns.
- Encourage use of readily available fruit and vegetables to incorporate into traditional eating patterns.
- Encourage cooking and food preparation methods that reduce fat and sugar consumption of some traditional practices, e.g. oil/ghee/butter in curry or spread on chapattis.
- Respect and take into account religious and cultural food restrictions (see Tables 16.1–16.3).
- Take account of the diverse patterns of responsibility for food shopping and cooking, e.g. men in some communities may be responsible for buying food.
- Promote healthy eating within the whole family, not just centred on individuals.
- Identify target groups that may be nutritionally at risk—low income groups, pregnant and lactating women, young children, older people.
- There is a need to have good knowledge of health issues for each community to conduct evidence-based interventions.
- Members of the local minority ethnic community should be employed as community or health workers where possible.
- Information as leaflets, video, and audio should be available in the mother tongue, and recognize the diversity of food consumption in a given community, wherever possible.
- For interventions using one-to-one communication, use interpreters where possible and necessary.
- People from African, African-Caribbean, and South Asian backgrounds may not get enough vitamin D from sunlight in the summer in the UK. The UK government therefore recommends that they consider taking a vitamin D supplement of 10 μg/day all year.

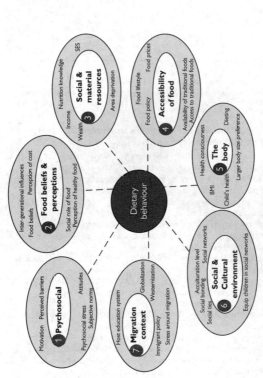

Fig. 16.1 A framework of the main factors influencing dietary behaviour in ethnic minority populations living in Europe. Reproduced from Holdsworth, M., et al. Developing a systems-based framework of the factors influencing dietary and physical activity behaviours in ethnic minority populations living in Europe – a DEDIPAC study, *Int. J. Behav. Nutr. Phys. Act.* 14(1). 154. Copyright © 2017 Holdsworth et al. This article is distributed under the terms of the Creative Commons Attribution 4.0 International License (ℜ http://creativecommons.org/licenses/by/4.0/).

Possible nutrients needing special attention for vegetarians

The main nutrients to keep an eye on are: protein, energy, vitamin B_{12}, vitamin D, calcium, and iron. Zinc intakes should also be verified. There is a high prevalence of inadequacy for dietary vitamin B_{12} and iodine in vegans.[5]

Energy

Energy intake is usually lower in vegan diets,[6] but this is only an issue of concern if BMI is <18.5 in adults. Those with more restrictive macrobiotic and fruitarian diets may also have low energy diets. They need to avoid a low energy diet that is too bulky and rich in fibre for infants and children as this could restrict growth; vegan children tend to be leaner than omnivores. See ⊋ Chapter 13, 'Nutritionally vulnerable infants', p. 298.

Protein

Plant protein can meet protein requirements if a wide variety of plant foods are consumed and energy needs are met, i.e. in well-balanced vegetarian diets. Protein is usually adequate if the diet contains a variety of the following (two to three servings/day):
• nuts and seeds, peanut butter;
• beans and pulses, e.g. baked beans, red kidney beans, soya beans, chick peas, lentils, hummus;
• soya products, e.g. bean curd (tofu), textured vegetable protein (TVP);
• eggs;
• dairy products: milk, cheese, yogurt, fromage frais.

For vegans, high quality protein (see ⊋ Chapter 5, 'Protein', p. 64) can be achieved by 'protein complementing', but energy intakes need to be adequate; otherwise protein is used for energy. Protein complementing foods must be consumed on the same day, but not necessarily at the same meal:

$$\text{High quality protein} = \text{grain (insufficient lysine)} +$$
$$\text{pulse (insufficient methionine)}$$

e.g. rice and dhal, baked beans on toast, or rice and peas.

Vitamin B_{12}

Animal foods are the main source of vitamin B_{12} (see ⊋ Chapter 6, 'Cobalamin B_{12}', p. 134). Deficiency is rare, but vegans and those following stricter macrobiotic and fruitarian diets need to be advised to consume suitably fortified foods:
• yeast extracts/fortified vegetable stocks;
• fortified rice and soya milks;
• breakfast cereal fortified with B_{12};
• fortified blackcurrant cordial;
• fortified tinned spaghetti;
• almonds.

5 Sobiecki, J.G., *et al.* (2016). High compliance with dietary recommendations in a cohort of meat eaters, fish eaters, vegetarians, and vegans: results from the European Prospective Investigation into Cancer and Nutrition-Oxford study. *Nutr. Res.* **36**(5), 464–77.

6 Tong, T.Y.N., *et al.* (2018). Anthropometric and physiologic characteristics in white and British Indian vegetarians and nonvegetarians in the UK Biobank. *Am. J. Clin. Nutr.* **107**(6), 909–20.

> **Box 16.2 Vegetarian groups at risk of an unbalanced diet**
> - Vegans
> - Macrobiotics
> - Fruitarians
> - Strict Asian vegetarians
> - Pregnant and lactating vegans
> - Vegan infants and children
> - Adolescent vegetarians
> - 'New' vegetarians
> - Vegetarians with an erratic eating pattern

If vitamin B_{12} supplements are recommended, these should not exceed the reference nutrient intakes (RNIs). See DRV tables (➔ Appendix 6, p. 875).

NB. Vitamin B_{12} analogues in seaweed and algae are not well absorbed.

Vitamin D

New advice on vitamin D from Public Health England was issued in 2016, recommending that adults and children aged >1 year should have 10 µg/d (400 IU/d) of vitamin D every day. This means that some people will need to take a supplement. The new advice is based on recommendations from the UK government's Scientific Advisory Committee on Nutrition (SACN) following its review of evidence on vitamin D.[7]

People who have a higher risk of vitamin D deficiency are being advised to take a supplement all year round. Vegetarians are no exception to this. At-risk vegetarian groups are:
- Asian vegetarian children, adolescents, and women (see ➔ Chapter 12, p. 242 'Dietary reference values and dietary guidelines during pregnancy');
- children on strict vegan diets, especially African-Caribbean infants;
- older vegetarians who are housebound or live in residential care.

Calcium

Vegetarians who consume dairy products regularly are not at risk of calcium deficiency. However, vegans, fruitarians, and macrobiotics may be at risk. Three servings should be eaten daily from a variety of sources:
- dairy products: milk, cheese, yogurt (if lacto-vegetarian);
- tofu;
- nuts: almonds, brazil, hazelnuts;
- fortified soya or rice milks;
- fortified bread;
- green leafy vegetables, e.g. broccoli, spinach, rocket, watercress;
- peas, beans and pulses, e.g. baked beans, red kidney beans, soya beans, chickpeas, broad beans;
- sesame seeds, tahini;
- dried fruit, e.g. apricots, figs;
- white bread and white flour products.

---

7 Scientific Advisory Committee on Nutrition. (2016). *Vitamin D and Health*. Available at: ℘ https://assets.publishing.service.gov.uk/government/uploads/system/uploads/attachment_data/file/537616/SACN_Vitamin_D_and_Health_report.pdf.

As vitamin D enhances calcium absorption, vegetarians at risk of poor vitamin D status in particular need to be encouraged to eat a variety of the above foods regularly and follow government advice on vitamin D supplementation. Vegan children and pregnant women should be referred to a dietitian who may recommend calcium supplements if dietary sources are insufficient.

Iron

UK vegetarians generally consume similar intakes of dietary iron to UK non-vegetarians. However, non-haem iron (plant sources) is absorbed less readily than haem iron (animal sources). Vegetarians should be encouraged to consume a good source of vitamin C to help absorption, e.g. citrus fruits and juices, and avoid drinking tea at the same meal (↓ absorption). See ➔ Chapter 6, 'Iron', p. 148 and 'Vitamin C (ascorbic acid)', p. 114.

Good vegetarian sources of iron:
- eggs;
- wholemeal flour and bread;
- breakfast cereals fortified with iron;
- dark green leafy vegetables;
- beans and pulses;
- dried prunes, figs, and apricots;
- yeast extract.

Iodine

As milk is an important source of iodine in the UK, vegans, fruitarians, and macrobiotics are at risk of low intakes → ↑ levels of thyroid-stimulating hormone. Encourage vegans to use iodized salt, sea vegetables, or take iodine supplements.

n-3 fatty acids

Vegetarian diets are often low in n-3 fatty acids. Diets that do not include fish, eggs, or large amounts of algae are low in n-3 fatty acids, eicosapentaenoic acid (EPA) and docosahexaenoic acid (DHA). n-3 fatty acids are important for cardiovascular health, eye, and brain development. Encourage vegetarians to include good sources of α-linolenic acid in their diets, e.g. flaxseed, walnuts, canola oil, and soya. Linolenic acid converts to EPA, but bioconversion is only about 10%.

Zinc

Intakes of zinc by vegetarians and vegans are not lower than for omnivores. However, there is low bioavailability from plant sources as a result of phytates inhibiting zinc absorption; therefore intakes of at least the RNI should be encouraged (7–9.5 mg/day in adults, depending on age and gender; see dietary reference values (DRV) tables, ➔ Appendix 6, p. 875).

Dietary guidelines for a balanced vegetarian diet

See ➔ Chapter 2, 'The Eatwell Guide', p. 27.

Vegetarians and pregnancy

Being vegetarian should pose no problem in pregnancy if the woman is well informed and eating a balanced lacto-ovo and lacto-vegetarian diet. Pregnant vegan, fruitarian, and macrobiotic women should be seen by a dietitian to assess the overall nutrient adequacy of their diets. They may require supplementation of vitamin B_{12}, iron, vitamin D, or calcium (if <600 mg/day consumed). Some fortified soya milks contain these nutrients. DHA-rich microalgae may be needed by pregnant and lactating vegetarian women to meet n-3 fatty acid requirements.

Asian vegetarian women could be at risk of vitamin D deficiency if there is insufficient skin exposure → neonatal hypocalcaemia and rickets, therefore may need vitamin D supplements.

Vegetarianism in childhood and adolescence

See ➋ Chapter 14, 'Vegetarian children', p. 309.

The vegetarian baby

See ➋ Chapter 13, 'Nutritionally vulnerable infants', p. 298.

Further information

℘ Further information on vegetarianism at the Vegetarian Society is available at: ℘ https://www. vegsoc.org/.

Position of the American Dietetic Association. Vegetarian diets (2016). *J. Acad. Nutr. Diet.* **116**, 1970–80.

Eating on a low income

Scale of poverty in the UK

In 2017, nearly a quarter of the UK population was considered to be in either income poverty (22.8%) or expenditure poverty (21.8%).[8] Unsurprisingly, households in expenditure poverty spend the highest proportion of their total expenditure on food-related items. Nearly a fifth (17.7%) of all children were reported as living in families experiencing both income and expenditure poverty. Almost a third (31.7%) of all lone parents were considered to be in both income and expenditure poverty. The poor are not a homogeneous group and people can move in and out of poverty with changing employment, relationships, or other circumstances. This impacts on financial resources, and therefore reduces opportunities for eating a healthy diet.

Food poverty

Food poverty is widely defined as 'the inability to acquire or consume an adequate quality or quantity of food in socially acceptable ways, or the uncertainty that one will be able to do so'.

Data from the UN using the Food Insecurity Experience Scale show that in 2014 over 10% of people living in UK households reported having insufficient food, which was ranked in the bottom range of European countries.[9] There have been calls for government to introduce regular monitoring of household food security using a reliable tool to guide policy.[10]

Causes of food poverty are multifactorial, but poverty is strongly related to income, social exclusion, and physical access to food (proximity of shops selling healthy foods of good quality at affordable prices). This may be because people lack shops in their area (known as 'food deserts') or have trouble reaching them. Other factors are transport, fear of crime, knowledge about what constitutes a healthy diet, and the skills to create healthy meals.

Mean weekly spending on food and non-alcoholic beverages in the general UK population has been estimated at £56.80 per household/per week (in 2016) and this is roughly the same for low income households. Lower income UK households spend more of their food budget on basic groceries (milk, bread), unlike higher income households, who spend a higher proportion on vegetables. In 2016, lower income households spent a higher proportion of their total expenditure on food and non-alcoholic drinks; with the lowest income groups spending 17% of total expenditure on food and

8 Office for National Statistics. *Income and wealth*. Available at: ℘ https://www.ons.gov.uk/peoplepopulationandcommunity/personalandhouseholdfinances/incomeandwealth/articles/anexpenditurebasedapproachtopovertyintheuk/financialyearending2017.

9 Loopstra, R., *et al*. (2015). Rising Food Insecurity in Europe. *Lancet* 385(9982), 2041.

10 Time to count the hungry (2016). *The case for a standard measure of household food insecurity in the UK*. Available at: ℘ https://foodfoundation.org.uk/wp-content/uploads/2016/07/Food-Poverty-workshop-report-1-05-04-16.pdf.

non-alcoholic drinks. In comparison, households with the highest income spent around 8% of total expenditure on this category.[11]

In the UK, the provision of food parcels by charitable food banks has increased rapidly (by over 350%) since the introduction of austerity measures and welfare reform.[12] Most food bank users are young, have low paid, sporadic employment or are unemployed, and experience some degree of food insecurity.[13]

Nutritional problems that are associated with food poverty do not usually arise because money is spent poorly on food, but because there is not enough money to spend. Several studies have shown that spending is often based on maximizing value for money in terms of energy intake and therefore compromising micronutrient intake. Several key influences in food choice take prominence to influence behaviour: particularly access to shops, cost of food, budgeting strategies, and the need for cultural and social acceptability (see ➲ Chapter 17, 'Influences on food intake', p. 366).

Dietary and nutritional consequences of poverty

The National Diet and Nutrition Survey reports differences in nutrient intake between the poorest 20% and richest 20% of the UK population. The poorest eat less fish, fruit and vegetables, and therefore have diets that are lower in fibre, protein, and saturated fat than the richest, but higher in sugar.

A previous survey specific for low income groups has not been recommissioned by the UK government since 2007. The UK Low income Diet and Nutrition Survey (LIDNS) of almost 2500 households[14] (representing the poorest 15% of the population) found that lower income households eat a diet that fails to meet recommended intakes, but it is only marginally worse than the diet of the rest of the population. There is convincing evidence that parents make sacrifices so that children have similar foods/snacks as other children, to avoid being teased or ostracized by their peers.

Children aged <5 years from low income families are also at greater risk of having an unbalanced diet, developing micronutrient deficiency, such as iron deficiency anaemia and faltering growth. Poverty is also associated with how tall older children grow. Data from England illustrate that by age 10 years, the least deprived white children were on average >1 cm taller than the most deprived children.[15]

11 Office for National Statistics. (2017). *Family spending 2016*. Available at: ◌https://www.ons.gov.uk/peoplepopulationandcommunity/personalandhouseholdfinances/expenditure/bulletins/familyspendingintheuk/financialyearendingmarch2016.

12 Lambie-Mumford, H., Green, M. (2015). Austerity, welfare reform and the rising use of food banks by children in England and Wales. *Area* **49**(3), 273–9.

13 Middleton, G., et al. (2018). The experiences and perceptions of food banks amongst users in high-income countries: An international scoping review. *Appetite* **120**, 698–708.

14 Nelson, M., et al. (2007). *Low income diet and nutrition survey*. Food Standards Agency TSO, London. Available at: ◌ https://discover.ukdataservice.ac.uk/catalogue/?sn=5808&type=data%20catalogue.

15 Hancock, C., et al. (2015). Socioeconomic variation in height: analysis of National Child Measurement Programme data for England. *Arch. Dis. Child.* **101**(5), 422-6.

The short- and long-term consequences of poor diet in childhood include: reduced immune status, increased dental caries, reduced cognitive function and learning ability, and increased risk of developing obesity and overweight. The long-term consequences for adults include increased prevalence of central obesity and of overweight/obesity in lower social economic groups (62% of men and 63% of women were obese or overweight in LIDNS), and reduced life expectancy for men and women.

Older adults and low income

There is evidence that intakes of a range of nutrients are lower in older people living on a low income. Poor access to shops may be one contributing factor and more than half of poorer older adults >65 years do not have their natural teeth (>general population of >65-year-olds), which may → ↓ fruit and vegetable intake.

Older people are not a homogeneous group and, although the majority are adequately nourished and meet the RNI for most vitamins and minerals, those living in institutions and in lower socio-economic groups are most at nutritional risk. See ➜ Chapter 15, 'An ageing population', p. 326.

Box 16.3 Terminology

Food poverty

Widely defined as 'the inability to acquire or consume an adequate quality or quantity of food in socially acceptable ways, or the uncertainty that one will be able to do so'.[16]

Food security

Widely defined by the Food & Agriculture Organization as meaning that 'people at all times should have physical and economic access to sufficient, affordable, safe and nutritious food necessary and appropriate for a healthy life, and the security of knowing that this access is sustainable in the future'. See ➲ Chapter 19, 'Food security', p. 429.

Refugee

A refugee is a person who 'owing to a well-founded fear of being persecuted for reasons of race, religion, nationality, membership of a particular social group or political opinion is outside the country of his nationality and is unable, or owing to such fear, is unwilling to avail himself of the protection of that country; or who, not having a nationality and being outside the country of his former habitual residence, as a result of such events, is unable to or, owing to such fear, is unwilling to return to it'.[17]

Asylum seeker

An asylum seeker is someone who has applied for refugee status to be recognized as a refugee in the UK.

Statutorily homeless

After local authority assessment, the statutorily homeless qualify for permanent council/housing association housing. Includes people with children, pregnant women, and vulnerable single people, who often wait in temporary accommodation, e.g. bed and breakfast, and hostels with limited cooking and storage facilities.

Non-statutorily homeless

The non-statutorily homeless do not qualify for permanent housing; and are usually single men. They often live in temporary accommodation, e.g. bed and breakfast/hostels with limited cooking and storage facilities, but many 'sleep rough' on the streets.

16 Dowler, E., O'Connor, D. (2012). Rights-based approaches to addressing food poverty and food insecurity in Ireland and the UK. *Soc. Sci. Med.* **74**, 44e51.

17 United Nations (1951). *Convention relating to the status of refugees.* Available at: ℘ http://www.unhcr.org/uk/1951-refugee-convention.html.

Refugees and asylum seekers

Refugees' health and nutritional status varies widely, and they should be treated on an individual basis as they are not a homogeneous group. Children may be well nourished or they may suffer from chronic undernutrition with growth stunting. The UK centiles have been complied using data from Caucasian children (see ➔ Chapter 13, 'Infant growth and development', p. 258) and therefore some ethnic groups, e.g. Ethiopians, may appear unusually tall, whereas others may appear unusually short. It is important to refer children where there is more than a two centile discrepancy between height and weight, or where serial measurements of growth fail to show adequate weight or height gain.

However, there are a number of factors indicating nutritional risk.

- *Nutritional status on arrival in the UK*: depends on the nature of their departure from their country of origin, whether time was spent in refugee camps, and exposure to communicable disease, which could all ↓ nutritional status and weight.
- *Poverty*: after arrival in the UK, many refugees live in poor housing, receive limited financial support, and have difficulty obtaining paid work → low income and poor diet. Professional skills may not be recognized.
- *Cultural factors*: foods eaten, preparation methods, and the social context of eating help define cultural identity. For refugees displaced from their own culture, friends, and family, the symbolic value of food can grow. Certain foods may not be available locally and familiar cooking implements or facilities unavailable. Although many refugees adapt, food intake will change by necessity, which may ↑ risk of a nutritionally inadequate diet compared with a traditional diet. Some refugees may have poor cooking skills as they are not used to preparing food, e.g. young men.
- *Communication*: refugees who do not speak English may have difficulty shopping for food, which is compounded when foods are unfamiliar and ingredients or cooking instructions cannot be read.
- *Psychological issues*: many have experienced violence, loss, or separation in their country of origin and two-thirds of adult refugees in the UK report anxiety or depression. This could ↓ appetite and interest in eating. Cooking and sharing food has been used as therapy with some refugees.

Homeless people

There are two main groups of homeless people: statutory and non-statutory homeless (see Box 16.3); these include those living in hostels and bed and breakfast accommodation, and those sleeping rough on the streets. Most homeless people have few or no means of buying, storing, or preparing fresh food. A number of studies have shown that the health of homeless people is severely compromised because of inadequate diets, and those who do have usually received a free meal at a day centre. There is evidence of a high level of alcohol use among people sleeping rough, often co-existing with a mental health problem.

Some of the short-term consequences of a poor diet are:
• iron deficiency anaemia resulting from low intakes of meat, fruit, and vegetables;
• ↑ susceptibility to infection because of micro- and macronutrient deficiencies;
• constipation because of low dietary fibre intake from fruit and vegetables, and higher fibre cereals.

Some of the long-term consequences are:
• An increased risk of premature mortality from cardiovascular disease and cancer. The average mortality rate of a homeless man is at ~42 years compared with the national average of 76 years.
• Dental caries and gum disease as a result of poor oral hygiene and eating patterns. If untreated, could → difficulty eating certain 'hard' foods; therefore ↑ chance of malnutrition.

Strategies to improve nutritional status of the homeless

Partnership working between staff and residents at hostels/bed and breakfasts, dietitians, city and borough councils, and health improvement officers can lead to improvements in the nutritional quality of meals provided by:
• developing nutrition education, e.g. practical nutrition resources and running cooking classes for residents on preparing healthy, affordable meals with limited cooking and storage facilities;
• lobbying for funding for 'mini-fridges' and microwaves in residents' rooms, locked food storage facilities, and better communal cooking facilities;
• producing a nutrition information pack for catering staff and home leaders that includes nutritional standards for meals provided.

See Box 16.4.

Box 16.4 Nutritional standards for meals provided in hostels, bed and breakfast accommodation, and day centres for homeless people

- Involve residents in menu planning.
- Encourage the social and pleasurable aspects of eating.
- Staff and volunteers need to be fully trained in food hygiene procedures.
- Plan meals around a healthy eating food model (see ➲ Chapter 2, 'The Eatwell Guide', 27).
- Use less salt and saturated fat in foods provided, e.g. ↓ processed foods used with low nutritional value, such as processed meat products, soups, and sauces.
- Provide fortified breakfast cereals with a choice of full and lower fat milk.
- Provide fruit and vegetables with every meal.
- Provide plenty of foods rich in non-starch polysaccharides.
- Provide water with meals.
- Offer special diets where appropriate, i.e. therapeutic diets, and take into account dietary needs of people from different cultural groups (see ➲ this Chapter, 'Minority ethnic communities', p. 338).

Local food projects for reducing food poverty

The UK Low income Diet and Nutrition Survey of almost 2500 house-holds[18] found that lower income households eat a diet that fails to meet re-commended intakes, but it is only marginally worse than the diet of the rest of the population. It has led to recommendations that health promotion campaigns on a national level should target the whole population, rather than low income groups. Cross-cutting policy initiatives that move beyond simple targeting and local action should be encouraged, that encompass a life-course approach and also recognize the diversity of 'low income' households.[19]

Ideas for local food projects

- *Community shops*: not-for-profit shop serving isolated shoppers, usually grocery produce. Also adds a social focus to communities.
- *Community cafés*: where people can eat a cheap meal in a sociable setting, e.g. at pensioners clubs, community centres.
- *Food co-operatives*: a group of people organizing to buy food in bulk direct from wholesalers or farmers to save money.
- *Community transport*: to help bring shops nearer to the isolated. Could be run by a local supermarket or local authority funded. Especially useful for older people and people with disabilities.
- *Links with local shops*: to stock and promote healthier food produce, encouraging people to use their local shops.
- *Food vouchers and coupons*: e.g. provided by local authorities by distributing 'money-off' coupons to local people or national government 'Healthy Start' vouchers for parents on a low income.
- *Farmers' markets*: where farmers and growers make up the majority of vendors.
- *Cooking club*: practical group cooking sessions to improve food skills working with a health professional. Members of the group will cook and taste different recipes.
- *Breakfast clubs*: providing healthy breakfast choices at school.
- *Box schemes*: customers receive a weekly box of fresh fruit and vegetables from a farmer that is distributed to a central place in the community. A group of people have to buy food regularly. Prices are more affordable as produce is bought directly from the farmer.
- *Lunch clubs and meals on wheels*: provide hot meals for older and disabled people; may be run by the local authority or a voluntary organization such as Age UK or the Women's Royal Voluntary Services (WRVS) (largest provider).

18 Nelson, M., *et al.* (2007). *Low income diet and nutrition survey*. Food Standards Agency TSO, London. Available at: ℒ http://www.food.gov.uk.

19 Dowler, E. (2008). Policy initiatives to address low-income households' nutritional needs in the UK. *Proc. Nutr. Soc.* **67**, 289–300.

- *Food redistribution:* surplus food is moved from shops and supermarkets to day centres and homeless facilities to provide free meals.
- *Grow your own:* e.g. growing food in allotments, on wasteland, schools, parks, and in back gardens.
- *School nutrition groups:* multidisciplinary groups that develop a whole school approach to better nutrition.
- *Food banks:* emergency food banking has become more common in the UK, Europe, and North America in response to concerns about rising food poverty. Food banks are usually run by non-profit, charitable organizations that distribute food to food insecure households.

Using a community development approach

The above local policy options need to be developed using a community development approach, i.e.

- community-based, involving genuine partnerships between local residents, local workers, and professionals;
- reaffirms community identity and meets local needs;
- promotes active citizenship;
- combats age, gender, and discrimination based on ethnicity;
- encourages community participation;
- addresses other social and cultural issues, as well as eating behaviour;
- is flexible and responsive.

Useful websites

⌖ http://www.cpag.org.uk (Child Poverty Action Group)
⌖ http://www.endchildpoverty.org.uk
⌖ http://www.actionforchildren.org.uk
⌖ http://www.ukfg.org.uk (The UK Food Group is a network of NGOs working on global food and agriculture issues)
⌖ http://www.sustainweb.org (food and farming)
⌖ http://www.fareshare.org.uk (food waste and hunger reduction projects)
⌖ http://www.refugeecouncil.org.uk
⌖ http://www.foodfoundation.org.uk (independent analysis of UK food system)
⌖ https://www.trusselltrust.org/ (food banks)

Resources

Press, V. (2004). *Nutrition and food poverty. A toolkit for those involved in developing or implementing a local nutrition and food poverty strategy.* National Heart Forum/Faculty of Public Health. ⌖ www.fph.org.uk/uploads/section_c.pdf.

Nutrition interventions with patients and individuals

Influences on food intake *366*
Developing effective nutrition education messages *370*
Planning and delivering nutrition education sessions *372*
Designing nutrition education materials *376*
Communication and counselling skills *378*
Health behaviour models *382*
Further information on behaviour change *390*

Influences on food intake

This chapter will outline factors affecting food related behaviour and how you can consider these when working to promote health related behaviour change with patients and individuals. A range of different models have been developed to summarize the factors influencing food intake;[1,2] most have several facets in common, i.e. that many factors interact to influence the foods individuals eat, besides a basic physiological need to eat. These factors act at many inter-related levels on an individual's food intake, including societal/community, national/international levels (see Fig 17.1).

Within public health, professionals may work at a local, national, or international level to know what the local and national policies are to consider these influences on food intake when planning interventions. They need to

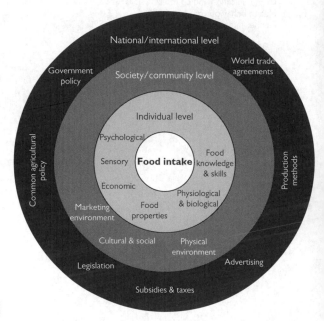

Fig. 17.1 Influences on food intake: individual, societal, and national/international levels.

1 Story, M., *et al*. Creating healthy food and eating environments: policy and environmental approaches. *Annu. Rev. Public Health* **29**, 253–72. Available at: ℜ http://publhealth.annualreviews.org.

2 Stok, F.M., *et al*. (2017). The DONE framework: Creation, evaluation, and updating of an interdisciplinary, dynamic framework 2.0 of determinants of nutrition and eating. *PLoS One*. **12**(2), e0171077.

be fully aware of the wider influences on food choice such as legislation, subsidies and taxes, world trade agreements, government policy, production methods, and agricultural policy and advertising. They need to be informed in relation to global public health policy from organizations such as the World Health Organization (WHO) and the Food and Agricultural Organization of the United Nations (FAO) and United Nations International Children's Emergency Fund (UNICEF). Professionals need to be mindful of the global economic bodies such as the World Bank, International Monetary Fund (IMF), and World Trade Organization and intergovernmental agreements. It is important to be aware that global public health policy, regional and country policies are linked by the same underlying principles such as partnership working, reducing inequality, and creating and using the current evidence. These are then translated into specific plans relevant to the population needs at the local level.

Health professionals working at the local level are able to influence some of the individual and societal/community influences on food choice (see Fig. 17.2). This could be during one-to-one consultations with patients, with group education or when developing appropriate public health nutrition programmes. It is not just important to understand 'what' is eaten, but also 'why' and in which context, to help people eat more healthily. Health professionals working locally will also need to have a wider vision of the public health context to be able to promote health. An example is the rapid increase in obesity, which is related to factors that are much wider than those that are modifiable locally and is illustrated in the Foresight Obesity systems map (see Chapter 18, 'Systems approaches to public health', p. 396).[3]

See Chapter 18, p. 391 for nutrition policy.

3 Butland, B., et al. (2007). *Reducing obesity: future choices*. Project report. Available at: ℜ https://www.gov.uk/government/publications/reducing-obesity-future-choices.

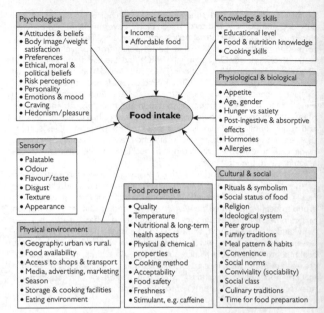

Fig. 17.2 Individual and societal/community influences on food choice.

Developing effective nutrition education messages

Nutrition education[4] is a component of promoting healthier eating and is the process of applying scientific knowledge about nutrition and health to individuals' dietary behaviour to improve health literacy (nutrition and health related knowledge, attitudes, motivation, behavioural intentions, personal skills, and self-efficacy).

Nutrition education messages are most effective if they are:
- clear, simple, avoiding technical jargon;
- use foods rather than nutrients to communicate;
- consistent with other sources;
- personally relevant to the audience;
- sensitive to how consumers perceive the risk of unhealthy eating;
- positive (eat more fruit), rather than negative (eat less fat);
- emphasize the benefits of change;
- acknowledge barriers to change;
- avoid messages that stigmatize individuals;
- use persuasion, prompts, and reminders.

The breadth of opportunities to share evidence-based nutrition messages must be considered, including the use of media, social marketing, written information, policy, educational events, and social media. Appropriately qualified individuals must engage with different media, and health professionals at a local level need to be trained to ensure consistent messages are given.

4 Contento, I.R. (2015). *Nutrition education—linking research, theory and practice.* Jones and Bartlett, Sudbury. 3rd edition.

Planning and delivering nutrition education sessions

Nutrition education sessions can be for a variety of audiences, including other health professionals and patients. Group education can be a good use of resources, providing detailed information to a larger number of people but this must be effective and evaluated.[5]

Where to start

- Identify the priorities for nutrition education in terms of information and participants. Consider relevant policy and funding. You may need to undertake a needs assessment to support prioritization because of limited resources.
- Identify the most suitable way to recruit participants.
- Find appropriate venues, e.g. do you need food preparation facilities, is the venue accessible?
- Ascertain current knowledge of participants and identify the gaps that the education will need to fill.

Planning the session: aims, objectives, and learning outcomes

- Define the overall *aim* for the session, i.e. the result that the education is aiming to achieve.
- Decide on your *objectives*, i.e. what you plan to do to meet your aim. You may have three to four specific and precise objectives to support the overall aim.
- Specify the desired endpoint for the participants, i.e. what you want them to be able to do after attending the session to achieve the aim. These are the *learning outcomes* and there may be several. The key word is *do*; so include active verbs such as define, explain, demonstrate, analyse, design, and/or evaluate. The level of complexity will relate to the participant group being targeted, e.g. adults or children, professionals or patients. Learning outcomes should be measurable and have a timescale. The number of learning outcomes will vary and may relate to the length of the education session. Longer sessions can be used to deliver more learning outcomes, but for an hour three to five outcomes would be appropriate.

Learning outcomes

Learning outcomes make it clear what the participants can expect to gain from attending a particular teaching session (which may help them to decide whether to attend or not). They also help practitioners to design the education session more effectively by acting as a template and focus for them. See Table 17.1 for examples of active verbs and how they relate to different levels of learning. This is hierarchical, with 'knowledge' as the lowest level of learning and 'evaluation' as the highest level.

---

5 Avery A.J., et al. (2016). *How to facilitate lifestyle change: Applying group education in healthcare.* Wiley Blackwell, Chichester.

Table 17.1 Possible active verbs for defining learning outcomes

Knowledge	Comprehension	Application	Analysis	Synthesis	Evaluation
Arrange	Classify	Apply	Analyse	Arrange	Appraise
Order	Locate	Operate	Differentiate	Formulate	Judge
Define	Describe	Choose	Appraise	Assemble	Argue
Recognize	Recognize	Practice	Discriminate	Manage	Predict
Duplicate	Discuss	Demonstrate	Calculate	Collect	Assess
Label	Report	Schedule	Distinguish	Organize	Rate
Recall	Explain	Sketch	Categorize	Compose	Attach
List	Express	Employ	Examine	Plan	Score
Repeat	Review	Solve	Compare	Construct	Choose
Memorize	Identify	Illustrate	Experiment	Prepare	Select
Name	Select	Use	Contrast	Create	Compare
State	Indicate	Interpret	Question	Propose	Support
Relate	Translate	Write	Criticize	Design	Estimate
Reproduce			Test	Write	Evaluate
Lowest learning level					Highest learning level

Example learning outcomes at the end of educational sessions

- *Knowledge*: recalling appropriate previously learned information
  - e.g. participants will be able to list all food groups in the Eatwell Guide;
- *Comprehension*: understanding the meaning
  - e.g. participants will be able to identify foods that may contain gluten on a restaurant menu;
- *Application*: using previously learned information in new situations to solve problems that have single or best answers
  - e.g. participants will be able to interpret their blood sugar readings and adjust insulin dose appropriately;
- *Analysis*: breaking down information into its component parts, examining and trying to understand the organizational structure of such information to develop divergent conclusions by identifying causes, making inferences
  - e.g. participants will be able to calculate patients' MUST scores and identify patients at nutritional risk;
- *Synthesis*: creatively applying prior knowledge and skills to produce a new or original whole
  - e.g. with extra reading, participants will be able to create a nutrition information leaflet appropriate for a specified patient group;
- *Evaluation*: judging the value of material based on personal values/ opinions, resulting in an end product, with a given purpose, without right or wrong answers;
  - e.g. participants will be able to appraise the quality of nutrition information presented in media articles.

Learning theories

Any group of participants will have a variety of preferred learning styles and good group education will include a variety of teaching methods to help participants stay engaged.[6]

There are many learning styles, e.g. surface and deep learning, Honey and Mumford learning styles, and VARK (℘ http://vark-learn.com/).

Some examples of methods and tools using VARK include:

- *Visual*-diagrams, flow charts, Eatwell Guide;
- *Aural/auditory*-spoken word, talk from group facilitator, opportunities for discussion and sharing ideas;
- *Read/wRite*-written information, presentations, opportunities to write such as action plans, food diaries;
- *Kinaesthetic*-role play, obtaining information from food labels, completing case studies.

Lesson plans

Lesson plans should be sufficiently detailed for a suitably qualified colleague to pick up and be able to deliver the session. In practice, many group education sessions are delivered by a variety of people and on a regular basis, e.g. cardiac rehabilitation. The lesson plan should include the aim, objectives, learning outcomes, target group, teaching methods, timings, and evaluation methods. See Table 17.2 for a sample lesson plan. It will *identify resources needed*, such as food and cooking equipment, information leaflets, computer and projector, refreshments.

Evaluating teaching

Evaluation is an essential part of developing group education and needs to be planned in advance and clearly linked to the aim and learning outcomes. It is important to consider what needs evaluation and how it is going to be undertaken. The following should be considered:

- formative evaluation: this is part of the development process;
- process evaluation: how things were done and if it worked as planned;
- impact evaluation: the immediate changes in knowledge and skills (or whatever the learning outcomes are designed to achieve);
- outcome evaluation: the effect or consequences that can be measured and are related to the aim of the session.

Evaluation methods need to be realistic in terms of the time required and appropriate for the group participants in terms of literacy required, language used, accessibility, culture and age appropriate.

Once all of this process is complete you are ready to deliver and evaluate your group education and then revise it in light of the evaluation.

---

6 More information on teaching skills: Rogers, A., Horrocks, N. (2010). *Teaching Adults* 4th Edition. OUP, Oxford.

Table 17.2 Sample lesson plan—Current healthy eating recommendations

Audience: Practice nurses; *Number expected* = 20; *Duration of session*: 2 hours

Aim: to enable practice nurses to deliver appropriate healthy eating advice to their adult patients

Objectives:

- To inform nurses of healthy eating guidelines using the Eatwell Guide
- To demonstrate how to explain the Eatwell Guide in simple terms

Learning outcomes: at the end of the session participants will be able to:

- Describe the Eatwell Guide in layman's terms
- List the five food groups in the Eatwell Guide
- Describe the core functions and nutritional content of each food group
- List at least five foods from each food group.
- Describe what an appropriate fluid intake is for adults
- Teach a member of the public to read a food label
- Suggest at least five healthier food alternatives

Time	Activity	Resources
5 mins	Introduction, housekeeping, plan for the session and learning outcomes	Verbal/flip chart
10 mins	Introduce the Eatwell Guide and briefly explain its purpose	Poster
20 mins	Split into groups and allocate each a food group, ask participants to write a script to explain key points about their food group in everyday words. Share examples with group	Paper and pens, Eatwell guide online
20 mins	Provide group with a variety of foods. Get them to place the foods in the right group. Facilitator to discuss if correct. Include composite foods which do not fit neatly into one group and foods high in fat and sugar	Food models and packets, floor mat of Eatwell Guide outline
20 mins	Short presentation about fluid intake. Ask participants to identify healthy and unhealthy sources of fluid. Include discussion about alcohol, fruit juices/smoothies, sugar free alternatives and sweeteners	Flip chart, pens, leaflets about alcohol recommendations
20 mins	Food label exercise. Split into five groups. Introduce traffic light system. Give each group a selection of food packets to identify whether food is healthy and whether they would recommend it to patients with hypertension and/or needing to lose weight	Empty food packets with traffic light labels, handout to complete
15 mins	Food diary exercise. Give participants a completed food diary. Ask them to identify sources of excess fat, salt, and sugar and suggest alternatives. Discuss responses	Food diary
5 mins	Summarize key points to take away, referring to learning outcomes	Flip chart
5 mins	Evaluation, participants to complete form	Evaluation form

Designing nutrition education materials

Writing skills are an important part of practice and can include dietary information such as diet sheets, reports, guidelines, policies, research papers, articles, and patient records. The most common target audiences will be peers, other health professionals, patients, carers, and the general public. The purpose is to transmit relevant evidence-based information in a format that is accessible and appropriate for the reader. How well the practitioner succeeds will depend on several factors, including the readability of the text, format of the information and accessibility of the resource for the target audience.

Developing patient literature

Some key points to consider when developing new patient literature

- Check that appropriate materials do not already exist! Resource-production is very time-consuming.
- Where might you get funding? This will impact on use of colour and how the resource can be printed.
- Check if your organization has a policy or standard template that you need to follow.
- Review the current literature on the subject.
- Share a first draft with peers for feedback.
- Follow guidance from the Plain English Campaign.
  ℬ http://www.plainenglish.co.uk/
- Proofread, review, and edit. There may be patient groups who can read the resource and comment from the patient's perspective.

See Box 17.1 for a checklist for evaluation of educational materials.

Readability of materials

Readability is concerned with matching the readability of the text with the average patient's reading ability. An accomplished reader is likely to be bored by simple repetitive texts. A poor reader will soon become discouraged by texts that s/he finds too difficult to read fluently.

A typical readability index uses an average sentence length and average number of words of three to four syllables per sample used, but they do not account for the order of words in a sentence. A suitable diet sheet/patient information leaflet needs to match the reading age of the general public (average range of 9–11 years). About 16% of adults in England have literacy levels ≤ that expected of 11 year olds. Access the Literacy Trust for guidance and access to online tools.[7]

There are many readability tests available, including the SMOG (simplified measure of gobbledygook) and online Gunning Fog Index at ℬ http://gunning-fog-index.com/.

---

7 ℬ National Literacy Trust. *Adult literacy*. Available at: http://www.literacytrust.org.uk/adult_literacy/illiterate_adults_in_england.

Box 17.1 Suggested checklist for evaluating the quality of educational materials for patients and the general public

Content
- Is there a clear description of the purpose and structure of the text?
- Are headings present? If so, are they appropriate?
- Are the facts correct and up to date?
- Is the quality and strength of the evidence discussed?
- Does the material take account of current government policy?
- Are nutrition messages clear, unambiguous, and consistent throughout?
- Are any statements about nutrition placed within the context of a healthy lifestyle and based on the Eatwell Guide (if appropriate)?
- Is the source of information given (e.g. nutrition and dietetic service)?
- If the use of a branded product can be justified in terms of helping users to identify types of products, is the use sparing and in a relevant context?
- Are references to product names used as examples only, so that single products are not favoured over others?
- Where there is reference to particular foods, are generic groupings used?
- Have contact numbers, addresses, or websites been given for further information, e.g. self-help groups?
- For commercial literature, are logos and brand names used sparingly and in context?
- Is the date of production included?

Appropriateness for the intended audience
- How technical is the vocabulary in the text? Are all acronyms and jargon explained?
- How readable is the text?
- Is it clear who the writer and intended audience are?
- Have users been consulted?
- Have materials been pretested for comprehension?
- Is the visual layout satisfactory, e.g. layout, font size, large enough for intended audience, white space, visual appeal?
- Is the information adapted for the socio-cultural characteristics of target audience in terms of language and food habits?
- Are foods suggested affordable, acceptable, and appropriate for the target group?

Communication and counselling skills

Communicating effectively is a core skill for nutrition and dietetic professionals as they interact with peers, colleagues, and patients to inform, educate, and facilitate behaviour change.[8] The importance of the communication skills of healthcare staff has been explicitly linked with a patient-centred approach.[9] Healthcare staff should treat each patient as an individual, considering psychological and emotional support, and enable patients to actively participate in their care and treatment decisions. Active listening has been emphasized as essential in the development and maintenance of successful caring relationships.[10] All healthcare professionals should be trained in reflective listening, demonstrating empathy, building rapport, developing motivation, and delivering behaviour change techniques.[11]

Essential practitioner characteristics and skills

A number of qualities need to be developed to improve the practitioner's patient relationship:

- *Unconditional acceptance:* accepting and respecting patients, not judging.
- *Congruence:* genuine, being sincere and not defensive.
- *Empathy:* understanding the patient's perspective, what it is like to be in their world.

As well as these qualities, the practitioner needs to develop an appropriate skill set:

- An open questioning style (see Table 17.3).
- Good listening skills (see Table 17.4): appropriate use of active versus passive listening.
- Awareness of the effect of *non-verbal communication*: posture, gestures, appearance, voice, eye contact, and facial expressions.
- A *patient-centred approach* to give more control to the patient, rather than the practitioner; build on the patient's expertise about him or herself.
- Recognize that the patient has the *right to decide* if s/he wants to change behaviour or not, i.e. patient autonomy.

8 Gable, J., Herrmann, T. (2016). *Counselling skills for dietitians*, third edition. Wiley Blackwell, Chichester.

9 Department of Health (2010). *Essence of care benchmarks for communication.* The Stationery Office Limited, London.

10 National Institute for Health and Care Excellence (2012). *Patient experience in adult NHS services (CG138)*. National Institute for Health and Care Excellence, London.

11 National Institute of Health and Care Excellence (2014). *Behaviour change: Individual approaches. Public health guidance No. 49.* National Institute of Health and Care Excellence, London.

Table 17.3 Asking questions: open vs. closed questioning

Open questions	Closed questions
Include 'what', 'how', 'where', and 'when', and invite more extensive answers e.g. *Tell me about where you do your food shopping?*	Invite a monosyllabic response, such as 'yes or 'no' e.g. *Have you been to the supermarket this week?*
Encourage patients to talk in more depth and demonstrate interest in the patient e.g. *Could you explain a bit more about how food fits into your day?*	Hard to establish empathy. Can be useful for clarifying information. Many closed questions can lead to the consultation feeling like an interrogation. This can destroy rapport and needs to be considered, in particular during diet histories e.g. *Do you take sugar in your tea?*
Help the patient keep the control, rather than the dietitian	The dietitian retains control over the interview

Note. Avoid 'why' questions as they can sound judgemental and cause patients to become defensive.

Table 17.4 The process of listening

Active	Passive
Dynamic process includes using: Minimal encouragers (e.g. 'go on', 'mm', 'uh-huh', and allowing silence) Verbal following (a word, phrase, or sentence using the patient's own words) Paraphrasing (repeating back the general content of what was said) Reflection of feelings (feeding back to show patients that they have been understood emotionally) Summarizing (condense the substance of what was said including content and emotions)	Sit back while the patient talks
Giving full attention (attending): face the patient squarely; adopt open posture; lean towards patient; maintain eye contact	Full attention is not given; may start to think about something else
Boredom less likely for practitioner	Practitioner can feel bored or irritated
The patient feels valued	The patient feels undervalued

Value of counselling skills for motivating dietary change

Good communication skills have been shown to demonstrate empathy, lead to higher levels of patient satisfaction, greater agreement between the patient and practitioner about what has been discussed and more extensive dietary changes being made.[12] These skills are helpful in ensuring that the patient has the opportunity to tell their story, set appropriate goals for themselves, and feel supported. Patients are more likely to feel empowered and talk about their feelings. Extra consideration may be required with limited English and/or minority ethnic groups with different cultural background and foods eaten.

12 Whitehead, K. (2015). Changing dietary behaviour: the role and development of practitioner communication *Proc. Nutr. Soc.* **74**, 177–84. doi:10.1017/S0029665114001724.

Health behaviour models

Interventions that help people change their unhealthy behaviours to healthier ones have the potential to improve health and decrease healthcare costs. NICE guidance has outlined how best to undertake interventions.[11] NICE conclude that the evidence does not support any specific model of behaviour change over others, but that interventions should be based on behaviour change theory.

A behaviour change model is a hypothetical description of a complex process, in this case relating to behaviour change. Models can help us understand and explain how things function and are particularly useful when planning interventions and deciding on what outcomes to measure. Although there is no one model that fits all people and all situations, whatever is used should incorporate the range of mechanisms that may be involved with change (see Fig. 17.3). Some approaches will embrace many elements from different models.

Most models of behaviour change have been highly criticized for not being comprehensive and not encompassing a complete understanding of human behaviour. For example, food related issues such as habit, self-control, or emotional processes are missing from the Theory of Planned Behaviour/Theory of Reasoned Action and Health Belief Model, which are highly relevant for food related behaviour change.[13] The Transtheoretical Model 'Stages of Change'[14] has commonly been used in dietetics, but there is little evidence for its use in eating and activity behaviours and there is now widespread agreement that it should not be used to categorise patients into a particular stage. Indeed, one of the functions of consultations is to support behaviour change and help patients towards action.

The behaviour change wheel

The behaviour change wheel was developed from 19 frameworks of behaviour change identified in a systematic review,[15,16] providing a summary of factors that influence health related behaviour to support the design of appropriate interventions.

It uses the COM-B model ('capability', 'opportunity', 'motivation' and 'behaviour'), which recognizes that behaviour is part of a system involving all these components.

Capability relates to the individual's psychological (understanding, reasoning, etc.) and physical ability to engage with the behaviour change concerned. It includes having the necessary skills and knowledge. This is an area

---

13 Michie, S., *et al.* (2011). The behaviour change wheel: A new method for characterising and designing behaviour change interventions. *Implementation Sci.* 6, 42.

14 Norcross, J.C., *et al.* (2010). *Changing for good: a revolutionary six-stage program for overcoming bad habits and moving your life positively forward.* Kindle edn, New York.

15 Michie, S., *et al.* (2011). The behaviour change wheel: A new method for characterising and designing behaviour change interventions. *Implementation Sci*, 6, 42. Available at: ℘ https://www.ncbi.nlm.nih.gov/pmc/articles/PMC3096582/pdf/1748-5908-6-42.pdf.

16 Available at: ℘ http://www.behaviourchangewheel.com/.

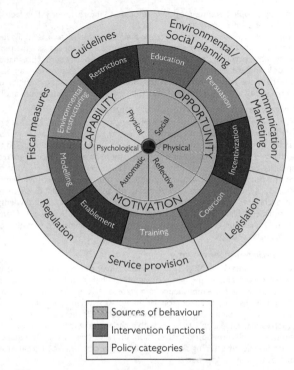

Fig. 17.3 The behaviour change wheel.

Reproduced from Michie S et al. (2011). The behaviour change wheel: A new method for characterising and designing behaviour change interventions. *Implementation Sci.*, 6, 42. Copyright © 2011 Michie et al.; licensee BioMed Central Ltd. This is an Open Access article distributed under the terms of the Creative Commons Attribution License (♒ http://creativecommons.org/licenses/by/2.0).

where dietetic practice is key, as we can provide knowledge and facilitate skill development to improve capability, e.g. by delivering group education for diabetes management. Increased capability can improve motivation as the change becomes more realistic for the individual and they have increased self-efficacy.

Motivation refers to the brain processes that direct our behaviour and give us drive to undertake activities. This is not just the goals and conscious decision making but includes aspects patients may be less aware of such as habits, emotions, and how they make decisions. Motivational interviewing may help people become more aware of these internal motivating factors and also of barriers to change.

Opportunities are all of the factors that are external to the individual person and that make the change in behaviour possible or act as a prompt, for example, providing a new service for managing obesity during pregnancy or cook and eat sessions for new mums. Public health practice can also work to make appropriate resources more accessible to communities or change wider practice. Greater opportunities can also increase motivation.

Planning interventions with the behaviour change wheel

COM-B can be used to support the planning of interventions. Once a priority for an intervention has been identified, the behavioural target can be clarified. It is then important to ascertain what components would need to be changed to achieve that. For example, is there a need to support greater capability or create more opportunities? These principles are relevant to both population and individual interventions but are delivered differently. Traditionally, dietetic practice was based on an educational/advice giving approach, but it has been acknowledged that providing dietary knowledge is insufficient. Dietitians need to consider this more holistic way of supporting behaviour change, whether they work in clinical, community, or public health settings.

Motivational interviewing

Motivational interviewing (MI) is a collaborative, person-centred form of guiding to elicit and strengthen motivation to change by exploring and resolving ambivalence. Ambivalence is a state of having simultaneous, conflicting feelings toward a person or thing. Ambivalent patients may be uncertain or unable to decide about what course to follow and health professionals may have a role to work with a patient, provide information, and help them decide on appropriate action. MI relies heavily on a foundation of good reflective listening skills. The following process makes a counselling approach into a MI approach:

Engage

This is about listening, demonstrating empathy, and attempting to understand the patient's perspective and to see the world through the patient's eyes. This person-centred approach and communication style has been described as the 'spirit' of MI. It can sometimes be lost in healthcare communication when there are time and workload pressures on health professionals who may perceive it is too time-consuming.

Focus

There needs to be a particular identified target for change that is the topic of conversation. The practitioner can help the patient to focus on an area that is important to them that they are struggling to change.

Evoke

The health professional attempts to help the patient draw on their own ideas and motivations for change using the 'elicit-provide-elicit' information exchange process, which begins and ends with exploring the client's own experience to frame whatever information is provided to the client. Advice can be given but the professional should gain permission, e.g. 'Would you

Table 17.5 Examples of change talk

Type of change talk	Examples of statements
Desire	I want to lose weight
	I would like to be fitter
	I wish I could walk upstairs more easily
Ability	I could try using a sweetener
	I can change to a low fat spread
	I might be able to do some short walks
Reasons	It would probably be better if I lost some weight
	I need to get back to work
	I have to be fitter if I am going to complete this sponsored walk
Need (feel obliged)	I ought to be a better example to my children
	I have to lose weight before I can get surgery
	I really should take better care of my diabetes
Commitment	I am going to start walking to work
	I intend to start eating more regularly
	I will start planning my meals
Taking steps (Action)	I actually went for a swim
	I have changed to 1% fat milk
	I've halved the amount of sugar I use in my tea and coffee
	I'm using a smaller plate for my dinner

mind if I gave you some information?'. They will need to ascertain what the patient made of that information before moving on.

Plan

Putting a change plan in place, i.e. a specific scheme to implement a change goal for the desired behaviour change. An existing change plan can also be reviewed to determine what is working or not. See Box 17.2 for an example change plan.

Throughout these four steps, the health professional must support self-efficacy of the patient, by helping them believe that change is possible, and respect patient autonomy, i.e. the patient has a choice about their action. Additionally the health professional must roll with resistance and avoid trying to persuade the patient to do something they do not wish to do. They need to avoid arguing with the patient to try and get them to change as this leads to discord in the consultation.

Change occurs when patient perceives a difference between where they are and where they want to be. Change talk is when the patient is talking about possible change (see Table 17.5 for examples). Health professionals need to listen for change talk, and when they hear it, reflect it back verbally.

They may be able to work with the patient to explore these statements so they can move from desire, ability and reasons to commitment and actions.

Whereas health professionals can support change, sometimes their actions are unhelpful. Examples of what can get in the way of patients talking about change include:

- Ordering, directing, commanding
- Warning, threatening
- Giving advice when it is not asked for
- Persuading
- Questioning
- Criticising and judging
- Agreeing
- Ridiculing and shaming
- Sympathising (as opposed to demonstrating empathy)
- Changing the subject

These types of health professional behaviour can lead to so called 'sustain' talk, where the patient indicates that they prefer the status quo rather than moving towards the change goal, e.g. 'I don't think I can do that' or 'It's the best I can do at the moment'. It can also lead to discord within the relationship. The combination of sustain talk and discord were previously described as 'resistance' in MI. Patients who are ambivalent may have both change talk and sustain talk in the same conversation and the MI approach can help resolve the ambivalence and reduce sustain talk.

There have been positive trials of MI with a variety of diet related conditions such as CVD and diabetes. However some poor quality studies led to NICE[11] not recommending the use of MI in healthcare. How MI has been delivered should therefore be well documented in future studies using reliable observational codes.[17] There is some recent evidence of MI use in dietetics, which indicated that training and ongoing coaching led to some improvement in MI skills (but not to a proficient level) and more change talk from patients.[18] Although becoming proficient in MI requires training and practice, all health professionals should develop the foundations of reflective listening, use open questions and decrease the amount of unhelpful actions to ensure they do not cause sustain talk or discord.

🕭 More information can be found at the Motivational Interviewing Network of Trainers: www.motivationalinterviewing.org

Planning change

Once a patient has reached the stage of committing to change, they will need help with setting goals and creating a change plan.

17 Miller, W., Rollnick, S. (2102). *Motivational Interviewing: Helping People Change.* London: Guilford Press.

18 Britt, E., Blampied, N.M. (2014). Training Dietitians in Motivational Interviewing A Pilot Study of the Effects on Dietitian and Patient Behaviour. *Motivational Interviewing: Training, Research, Implementation, Practice* 1(3), 7–12. DOI 10.5195/mitrip.2014.55

Goal setting

In healthcare, collaborative goal setting is seen as a process by which professional and patient agree on a health-related goal with a concrete course of action to move the patient toward the goal.[19] Goal setting has been described as a 4 step process:

- Recognising the need for change
- Establishing a goal
- Monitoring goal related activity
- Rewarding yourself for goal attainment

Goals need to be patient-centred and have been found to be motivational, particularly when the patient freely makes the decision and feels responsible for it.[20] Goals have to be important and related to the overall behaviour change but the patient also needs to believe that they are achievable. An action plan or change plan is a course of action that will lead to the goal: there may be several actions that lead to the same goal. It is also helpful to include a start date and timescale. What people consider a reward is highly individual and should be decided by the patient. Ideally if the change is nutrition-related then the reward should not be food! See Box 17.2 for a change plan for a patient wanting to lose weight.

19 Bodenheimer, T., Handley, M. A. (2009). Goal-setting for behavior change in primary care: An exploration and status report. *Patient Educ. Couns.* **76**, 174–80.

20 Cullen, K.W., *et al.* (2001). Using goal setting as a strategy for dietary behavior change. *J Am. Diet. Assoc.* **101**, 562–6.

Box 17.2 A change plan for a patient wanting to lose weight

Recognizing the need for change
- Weight has been gradually increasing and clothes no longer fit.
- Have just been diagnosed with high blood pressure and do not want to go on medication.

Goal
- Gradual weight loss, to lose 2 kg in the next 4 weeks.

Goal related activity
  This week:
- Plan meals for the week and develop shopping list to decrease risk of buying other foods and resorting to takeaways.
- Keep a food and activity diary.
- Check if my swimming costume still fits. Research local swimming facilities and times.
- Cut alcohol consumption to within recommended limits.
  Next week:
- Go swimming twice a week.
- Based on food diary, identify unhealthy snacks consumed and ensure healthy alternatives are available.

I will know that my plan is working if
- I have a healthy meal plan and stick to it.
- I have been swimming.
- I haven't eaten more than one takeaway meal in a week.
- I lose 2 kg in 4 weeks.

Rewards for goal attainment
- I will buy my favourite magazine and allow myself time to read it.
- I will have a leisurely bath with my favourite bubble bath.

Some things that could interfere with my plan
- I can't fit into my swimming costume.
- I can't find a time that suits me to go swimming.
- I don't make time to prepare the meal plan.
- Lack of support from my partner.

Further information on behaviour change

Avery A.J., Whitehead K.A., Halliday V. (2016). *How to facilitate lifestyle change: Applying group education in healthcare*. Wiley Blackwell, Chichester.

Contento, I.R. (2015). *Nutrition education—linking research, theory and practice*. Jones and Bartlett, Sudbury. 3rd edition.

Holli B.B., Beto J.A. (2014). *Nutrition counseling and education skills for dietetics professionals (6th ed.)*. Wolters Kluwer/Lippincott Williams and Wilkins, Baltimore/Philadelphia.

Michie S., Atkins L., West R. (2014). *The Behaviour Change Wheel; a guide to designing interventions*. Silverback Publishing, Great Britain. Available at: ℜ http://www.behaviourchangewheel.com/.

Miller, C.H., Bauman, J. (2014). Goal setting: an integral component of effective diabetes care. *Curr. Diab. Rep.* **14**, 509.

Pearson D., Grace C. (2012). *Weight management: A practitioner's guide*. Wiley-Blackwell, Chichester.

Rogers, A., Horrocks, N. (2010). *Teaching Adults 4th Edition*. OUP, Oxford.

Nutrition policy

National bodies influencing UK nutrition policy 392
Conceptual models in public health 396
Obesity prevention 398
UK national level nutrition strategies and policies 406
National nutrition programmes, initiatives, and campaigns 408
Surveys to monitor diet, nutrient intake, and nutritional
    status in the UK 414
Local nutrition policy and action 416
Evaluation of local diet and weight management
    interventions 420

National bodies influencing UK nutrition policy

Major causes of mortality and morbidity in the UK are cardiovascular disease (CVD), type 2 diabetes, and cancer. CVD, type 2 diabetes, and some cancers, such as bowel, mouth and throat cancers, have a nutritional aetiology. Public policy that includes population-level interventions and direct contact with the public presents opportunities to reduce risk factors (poor diet, physical inactivity, smoking, and obesity) associated with the major non-communicable diseases (NCDs). Policies for preventing NCDs are influenced, developed, and implemented by a number of different national bodies.

Health departments

Since 2010, the Department of Health (DH) has been responsible for nutrition policy in England. The DH is responsible for health protection, health improvement, and health inequalities issues in England. It is a ministerial department, supported by 27 agencies and public bodies including National Health Service (NHS) England, Public Health England (PHE), and the National Institute for Health and Care Excellence (NICE).

In the devolved administrations of Scotland and Northern Ireland, nutrition policy is the responsibility of Food Standards Scotland and the Food Standards Agency (FSA), who are accountable to the Northern Ireland Assembly and Scottish government. In Wales, the Health Improvement Division of the Welsh Government is responsible for nutrition policy and is advised by the Food Standards Agency.

The Department for Environment, Food and Rural Affairs (DEFRA)

From 2010, three key areas of food policy moved from the FSA to the Department for Environment, Food and Rural Affairs (DEFRA) in England:
• policy on food labelling, where this does not relate to food safety or nutrition;
• policy on food composition standards and labelling, where unrelated to food safety;
• leading on EU negotiations for all non-safety or nutrition aspects of food labelling.

The Department of Education (DfE)

In England, the DfE currently supports and is responsible for overseeing the actions within the 'School Food Plan' (see p. 407).

Public Health England (PHE)

The Health and Social Care Act 2012 led to an extensive reorganization of the structure of the NHS. This reorganization included abolishing NHS Primary Care Trusts and Strategic Health Authorities, and transferred associated healthcare funds to Clinical Commissioning Groups (CCGs). A new executive agency of the DH, PHE was established under the Act in April

2013. PHE's mandate is to 'protect and improve the nation's health and wellbeing, and reduce health inequalities', and its responsibilities include:

- helping to make the public healthier by encouraging discussions, advising government, and supporting action by local government, the NHS, and other organizations;
- supporting the public so they can protect and improve their own health;
- protecting the nation's health through the national health protection service, and preparing for public health emergencies;
- sharing information and expertise with local authorities, industry, and the NHS, to help them make improvements in the public's health;
- undertaking research to improve understanding of health;
- reporting on improvements in the public's health (monitoring/ surveillance);
- helping local authorities and the NHS to develop the public health system and its specialist workforce;
- further information is available at: ℘ http://www.phe.gov.uk.

NHS England

NHS England is an executive non-departmental public body of the DH and leads the NHS in England as set out in the Health and Social Care Act 2012. This includes commissioning health services such as GPs, pharmacists, dentists and supporting local health services led by CCGs.

Food Standards Authority (FSA)

FSA is a non-ministerial government department. It is accountable to parliament via health ministers, and to the devolved administrations of Wales and Northern Ireland for its activities within these areas. In 2010, the DH became responsible for nutrition policy in England, and DEFRA for food labelling which is unrelated to food safety or food composition policies in England. Since 2010, the main roles of the FSA in England are to:

- reduce food-borne illness by improving food safety throughout the food chain;
- improve the enforcement of food law.

The FSA Strategy 2015-2020 pledges to ensure that consumers have access to food that is safe, affordable, and healthy, and can make informed choices about what they eat.

Further information is available at: ℘ www.food.gov.uk.

Scientific Advisory Committee on Nutrition (SACN)

From 1963 to 2000, the UK government relied on expert nutrition advice from the Committee on Medical Aspects of Food and Nutrition (COMA), which produced a series of reports that were used to inform nutrition policy. Since the establishment of the FSA in 2000, the Government replaced COMA with the Scientific Advisory Committee on Nutrition (SACN). SACN's remit includes advising UK health ministers, PHE, and other governmental departments on:

- nutrient content of individual foods and on diet as a whole, including defining a balanced diet;
- nutritional status in the UK and how it may be monitored;

- nutritional issues that affect wider public health policy issues including where nutritional status is one of a number of risk factors, e.g. CVD, cancer, osteoporosis, and/or obesity;
- nutrition of vulnerable groups, e.g. infants and nutrition issues relating to inequalities;
- research needs arising from these areas.

Further information on SACN is available at: ℘ https://www.gov.uk/government/groups/scientific-advisory-committee-on-nutrition.

National Institute for Health and Care Excellence (NICE)

NICE is a non-departmental government body, accountable to the DH, but operationally independent of government. NICE provides the following through independent committees:

- evidence-based guidance and advice for health, public health, and social care practitioners;
- quality standards and performance metrics for those providing and commissioning health, public health, and social care services;
- a range of information services for commissioners, practitioners, and managers across the spectrum of health and social care.

Further information is available at ℘ http://www.nice.org.uk.

Conceptual models in public health

Socio-ecological models of public health

In recent years, national and local level policy and action have been driven by approaches that assess the evidence base and address public health nutrition need across the life-course from prenatal to older populations. This approach is viewed within a socio-ecological model of health. This model was advocated by the 1986 Ottawa Charter for Health Promotion and emphasizes the reciprocal relationship between the individual and the social environment and the interaction between and interdependence of factors within and across all levels of health behaviours. This concept recognizes that most public health issues are complex and cannot be adequately understood or tackled by a single-level explanation or solution.

Social inequalities in public health

Two key reports reflect the above concepts and have shaped policy and research to enhance the evidence base in the last decade. The 2010 Marmot Review,[1] highlighted the influence of social determinants on health and tackling patterns of inequalities and has been a key driver for policy and action. Evidence of the socio-economic gradient in dietary behaviours and diet-related health in populations is well established and drives much national and local level action.

Systems approaches to public health

Systems thinking can simply be defined as 'looking at things in terms of the bigger picture'.[2] Linked with social determinants of health, it is a conceptual framework of inter-related, complex, and adaptive systems in relation to health. A system-based approach is now widely acknowledged as a fundamental basis for thinking about population-level health,[3,4] and is a holistic way of developing interventions, because it accounts for the interrelationship of the individual and their social and physical environments. This concept is used practically in relation to tackling obesity in the UK.[5]

1 Institute of Health Equity (2010). *Fairer Society, Healthy Lives.* Available at: Ⅾ http://www.instituteofhealthequity.org/resources-reports/fair-society-healthy-lives-the-marmot-review.

2 Homer, J., Hirsch, G. (2006). Opportunities and demands in public health systems. *Am. J. Public Health* 96(3), 452–8.

3 Carey, G., *et al.* (2015). Systems science and systems thinking for public health: a systematic review of the field. *BMJ Open* 30(5), 12.

4 Rutter, H., *et al.* (2017). The need for complex systems model of evidence for public health. *Lancet.* doi:10.1016/S0140-6736(17)31267-9.

5 Government Office for Science/DH (2007). *Foresight Tackling Obesities.* Available at: Ⅾ https://www.gov.uk/government/uploads/system/uploads/attachment_data/file/287937/07-1184x-tackling-obesities-future-choices-report.pdf.

Obesity prevention

Although it is by no means the only priority for public health nutrition in the UK and England, obesity has emerged as a public health problem of an unprecedented scale. Around one-third of adults and one-fifth of Year 6 children in England are classified as obese, putting them at a greater risk of NCDs. The cost to the health service of treating obesity related disease is estimated to be £5.1 billion per annum.[6] Obesity has ∴ been a key focus for national and local nutrition policy over the past decade.

Systems approaches to obesity prevention

It is widely acknowledged that preventing obesity requires more than a health or medical perspective and needs to be viewed from a wider societal and economic context and with a holistic approach. The Foresight report on 'Tackling Obesities: Future Choices'[5] describes obesity as a complex, adaptive system with a variety of causal pathways. See the Foresight 'Obesity system map' in Fig 18.1, which illustrates the multi-factorial and complex nature of the aetiology of obesity, clustering positive and negative influencing variables into the following themes related to each side of the energy balance equation:

• individual psychology,
• social psychology
• individual physical activity,
• physical activity environment,
• physiology,
• food consumption,
• food production.

This 'whole systems approach' to obesity prevention and treatment is a current driver for government policy on obesity at national and local levels. At the local level, a range of complementary strategies are needed that address the individual, social, and environmental determinants of obesity and consider the complex, adaptive nature of the obesity 'system'. The UK government's 'Child Obesity Plan'[7] lists national and locally delivered actions to reduce England's rate of child obesity. It includes 12 actions related to nutrition (see 'Child Obesity Plan (DH)', p. 406).

In 2016, the WHO published the report of the 'Ad hoc Working Group on Science and Evidence for Ending Childhood Obesity',[8] which highlighted two overlapping conceptual models for child obesity: the 'life-course model' and the 'total environmental assessment' model. These models reflect a

---

6 Scarborough, P., et al. (2011). The economic burden of ill health due to diet, physical inactivity, smoking, alcohol and obesity in the UK: an update to 2006/07 NHS costs. *J Public Health* 33(4), 527–35.

7 HM Government (2016). *Childhood obesity: a plan for action.* Available at: ℘ https://www.gov.uk/government/publications/childhood-obesity-a-plan-for-action.

8 WHO (2016). Consideration of the evidence on childhood obesity for the Commission on Ending Childhood Obesity: report of the ad hoc working group on science and evidence for ending childhood obesity'. Available at: ℘ http://apps.who.int/iris/bitstream/10665/206549/1/9789241565332_eng.pdf?ua=1.

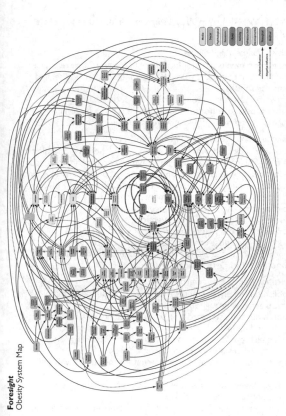

Foresight
Obesity System Map

Fig 18.1 The Foresight 'Obesity system map'. Reproduced from Government Office for Science/DH. Foresight Tackling Obesities. London, UK: Government Office for Science/DH. © Crown Copyright 2007. Contains public sector information licensed under the Open Government Licence v3.0. ℗ https://assets.publishing.service.gov.uk/government/uploads/system/uploads/attachment_data/file/296290/obesity-map-full-hi-res.pdf.

holistic conceptual framework for public health and in particular, public health nutrition related policy and action. On the basis of current evidence available, the report makes policy recommendations relating to preventing child obesity across several sectors. Many of these recommendations are reflected in policies and actions in the UK. These recommendations are summarized in Box 18.1

Box 18.1 WHO key policy recommendations for child obesity*

1. Built environment and food
- Increase community geographic access to healthy foods retailers, through a variety of policies, such as tax incentives, land use, and zoning regulations.
- Improve transportation routes to healthy food retailers.
- Restrict access to unhealthy foods around schools by zoning regulations, and make drinking water available in school.

2. Education (over-arching recommendation)
- Adopt a coordinated 'whole-school approach' including assessing the entire school environment and implementing policies and practices to support healthy weights, diet, and the promotion of physical activity.
- Integrate teaching on physical activity and healthy eating with changes to the physical and food environments.
- Use community and parental engagement to amplify the impact of childcare and school-based interventions.
- Address the whole school, regardless of weight status.
- Include pre- and post-care, and extracurricular activities.
- Support/train teachers and other staff to implement health promotion strategies and activities.

3. Education (school environment)
- Establish school environments that support healthy eating choices and physical activity throughout the school day.
- Establish nutrition standards for schools that include a healthy diet with limited fat intake.
- Provide high-quality school meals and healthy, appealing food/beverage choices outside school programmes.
- Create a pleasant, sociable environment for mealtimes with staff supervision.
- Ban sugar-sweetened beverages (includes flavoured/sweetened milk) and limit portion size of 100% juice.
- Make drinking water freely available to students in dining areas and throughout the day.
- Create and support school gardens.
- Plan building layout, recreational spaces.

4. Education (programmatic)
- 'Hands-on' activities that encourage touching and tasting foods.
- Gardening programmes are promising for increasing children's fruit and vegetable consumption.

- Schools should offer opportunities to be physically active throughout the day and there should be at least one hour daily of school-based physical activity.
- Schools should try to increase the amount of time students spend doing moderate to vigorous physical activity, either by increasing the duration, or intensity, of activity in physical education classes.
- Teacher training in physical education modules is recommended.
- Children should be encouraged to develop movement skills by having appropriate opportunities, equipment, and classes.

5. *Agriculture*

- Strengthen and improve local and regional food systems, through agricultural policies/incentives that promote local food production and processing, e.g. forming grower cooperatives, instituting revolving loan funds, and building markets for local farm products through economic development.
- Use of incentives to promote the production of fruit and vegetables for local markets.
- Adoption of programmes to protect fruit and vegetable farmers from natural disasters.
- Review national policies and investments and integrate nutrition objectives into food and agriculture policy, programme design and implementation, to enhance nutrition sensitive agriculture, ensure food security, and enable healthy diets.
- Support urban agriculture to improve access to fresh and healthy foods, in a way that minimizes risks to the environment.
- Improve food supply chains (traditional and modern) to increase the local availability, affordability, diversity, and nutritional quality of foods.
- Develop local solutions to reduce post-harvest food losses.
- Preserve and promote agricultural biodiversity/promote the diversification of crops, including underutilized traditional crops.

6. *Trade (applicable for all countries)*

- Promote 'policy coherence' between health policies and trade agreements and strengthen capacity to undertake rigorous health impact assessments in relation to free trade agreements.
- Adopt safeguards on the level of foreign ownership of agricultural land and of local food production and for trade agreements to protect national and local food sovereignty in more general terms.
- Explore trade agreements in relation to food and obesity prevention for excluding some foods from tariff reduction based on health/financial implications of their inclusion.
- Conduct research to identify policy instruments and measures that can be used to support local food systems and obesity prevention strategies triggering trade disputes.
- The right to nutritionally adequate food should be part of the overall goal and policy of all institutions regulating or deregulating international trade, investments, development loans, and external debt relief.

(Continued)

Box 18.1 (Contd.)

- Provisions could be made to exclude health and social security from trade and investment agreements, as a form of safeguard to protect the right of democratically elected governments to maintain policy space for regulation, licensing, cost-containment, and limiting or reversing commercialization, where this is in the public interest.
- The Codex Alimentarius can be an appropriate mechanism to promote healthier diets worldwide and fair practices in food trade through its role in setting standards on labelling, and, to a lesser extent, food composition.
- Research could inform the development of future Codex standards, e.g. on food labelling.

7. *Labelling*
- Front-of-package labelling with simple (e.g. traffic light scheme), consistent format and placement.
- Mandated nutrition fact panels or front-of-pack labels/icons.
- Front-of-package labelling should include key components of: calories, saturated and trans fats, sodium, and added sugars.
- Clear information on portion size with nutritional information per portion.
- Endorsement schemes (such as a healthy choice symbols) identifying products on front of package that meet specific standards.
- Point of purchase schemes identifying and promoting healthy food options.
- Regulate nutrient and health claims that can be made on packages or to promote food items (e.g. permissible fat content to market food as 'low in fat').
- Quick service restaurant menu labelling.
- Aggregate nutritional content information on food purchased, and traffic light labels provided at checkout.
- Use menu labelling alongside other interventions to influence healthier menu choices.
- Monitor real-life menu labelling experiments to expand the evidence base.

8. *Quality of food supply*
- Improve access to healthy foods, including fruit and vegetables.
- Introduce voluntary, or regulated, reformulation of food products to reduce specific nutrients (e.g. reduce salt, fat, trans fats, energy density, sugar content).
- Reduce portion size of processed meals, dishes, snacks, foods, and drinks.
- Reduce number of calories served to children in quick service restaurants.

9. *Informed choice and public information campaigns*
- Long-term campaigns with simple targeted messages and frequent exposure to messaging.

Box 18.1 (*Contd.*)

- Comprehensive public health campaigns promoting healthy eating habits across various media, such as television, radio, and social media.
- Implement public information campaigns in conjunction with other measures within a comprehensive obesity prevention strategy, including increasing availability, labelling, or reformulation.

10. Dietary guidelines

- Evidence-based national guidelines on healthy eating that are updated regularly, adapted for specific populations, and effectively communicated to the population.
- Develop and implement national food-based dietary guidelines.
- Educate the public on food-based guidelines.
- Efforts should be made to keep recommendations evidence-based and to grade evidence in a way that is easy for guideline users to understand.

11. Fiscal measures

- The introduction of fiscal measures to shift consumption away from unhealthy foods and beverages should be considered. The most important criterion for considering a policy is the potential for harm it might cause, rather than the extent of its impact on obesity.
- The introduction of a tax on sugar-sweetened beverages and unhealthy food. Conduct context-specific studies (e.g. price and cross-price elasticity of demand) to establish feasibility, risks, and potential impact.
- Subsidies on healthy foods, especially fruit and vegetable subsidies, primarily targeting children and low-income households.
- Flexible financing or tax credits to support health-promoting food and beverage retailing and distribution policies.
- Financial incentives to promote physical activity.
- Combined or multipronged fiscal measures.
- Combined or multipronged approach, especially for children and adolescents, of changing relative prices by both taxing less healthy, energy dense foods and subsidizing healthier, less energy dense foods.
- The acceptable level of tax/subsidy and the most effective fiscal policy, or combination of policies, is likely to be context-dependent.
- Health impact assessments recommended to determine the unintended effects of new and/or existing fiscal measures designed to target other sectors.
- Removal of subsidies to unhealthy foods.

12. Built environment and physical activity

- Locating schools within easy walking distance of residential areas.
- Create safe routes to schools by improving the built environment.
- Ensure open spaces and public paths can be reached on foot, by bicycle, and using other modes of transport involving physical activity. They should also be accessible by public transport.

(Continued)

Box 18.1 (Contd.)

- Improve access to outdoor recreational facilities such as parks and green spaces.
- Ensure public open spaces and public paths are maintained to a high standard. They should be safe, attractive, and welcoming to everyone.
- Enhance personal and traffic safety in areas where people are, or could be, physically active.
- Creation of, or enhanced access to, places for physical activity (e.g. trails or facilities) by reducing barriers to access, combined with informational outreach activities: strongly recommended.
- Communities, transportation officials, community planners, health professionals, and governments should make promotion of physical activity a priority, by substantially increasing access to places and opportunities for such activity.
- Improve access to public transportation.
- Point-of-decision prompts are recommended, for health benefits or weight loss.

Further information

Blackshaw, J. (2016). Public Health Nutrition in the civil service (England): approaches to tackling obesity. *Proc. Nutr. Soc.* **75**, 356–66.

Brown, T., Moore, T.H.M., Hooper, L., et al. (2019) Interventions for preventing obesity in children. *Cochrane Database Syst. Rev.* Available at: ♚ https://www.cochranelibrary.com/cdsr/doi/10.1002/14651858.CD001871.pub4/full.

European Union: Diet, Physical Activity and Health—EU Platform for Action. Available at: ♚ http://ec.europa.eu/health/nutrition_physical_activity/platform/index_en.htm.

INFORMAS Benchmarking food environments. Available at: ♚ https://www.informas.org/.

Kremers, S., Reubsaet, A., Martens, M., et al. (2009). Systematic prevention of overweight and obesity in adults: a qualitative and quantitative literature analysis. *Obes. Rev.* **11**, 371–9.

NOURISHING database. Available at: ♚ https://www.wcrf.org/int/policy/nourishing-framework

Swinburn, B.A, Sacks, G, Hall, K.D, et al. (2011). The global obesity pandemic: shaped by global drivers and local environments. *Lancet* **378**(9793), 804–14.

UK national level nutrition strategies and policies

NHS Five Year Forward View

The NHS 'Five Year Forward View' was published in 2014 and sets out new models of working that prioritize the needs of local communities and focus on preventative approaches to health.

The strategy is available here: ⅒ https://www.england.nhs.uk/five-year-forward-view/.

Evidence into Action (PHE)

The 'Evidence into Action' strategy was published by PHE in 2014 alongside the NHS 'Five Year Forward View' and makes the case for action across seven public health priorities, including tackling obesity in children.

The strategy is available here: ⅒ https://www.gov.uk/government/uploads/system/uploads/attachment_data/file/366852/PHE_Priorities.pdf.

Child Obesity Plan (DH)

The Child Obesity Plan was published in August 2016. The plan outlines the government's aim to significantly reduce England's rate of childhood obesity within 10 years. The plan includes these actions:

- introducing a soft drinks industry levy;
- taking out 20% of sugar in products;
- helping businesses to make their products healthier;
- updating the Nutrient Profiling Model to align restrictions on food and drink advertising to children with the most recent dietary recommendations;
- making healthier options available in the public sector;
- continuing to provide support with the cost of healthy food for those who need it most, such as through the Healthy Start scheme (see pp. 276 and 409);
- creating a new healthy rating scheme for primary schools to recognize and encourage their contribution to preventing obesity by helping children to eat better and move more;
- undertaking a thematic review, through Ofsted, on obesity, healthy eating and physical activity in schools;
- making school food healthier;
- making food labelling clearer;
- supporting early years settings (including providing resources on how to meet dietary recommendations for early years developed by the Children's Food Trust);
- harnessing the best new technology such as through the use of apps in the Change4Life campaign (see 'Change4Life' p. 408);
- enabling health professionals to support families, e.g. through PHE resources for the wider public health workforce on influencing behaviour change;
- helping all children to have an hour of physical activity every day;
- improving the co-ordination of quality sport and physical activity programmes for schools.

The full plan is available at: ✆https://www.gov.uk/government/uploads/system/uploads/attachment_data/file/546588/Childhood_obesity_2016__2__acc.pdf.

The School Food Plan (DfE)

The School Food Plan was published by the Department of Education (DfE) in 2013 and sets out 17 cross-governmental actions to transform children's diets in schools and how they learn about food. The actions within the plan are part of the Child Obesity Plan (see 'Child Obesity Plan', p. 406). Actions include:

- mandatory standards for all food served in maintained schools and academies since 2015;
- work directly with schools to increase take up of universal infant free school meals;
- increase financially self-sufficient breakfast clubs;
- support local authorities to deliver food teaching and healthy catering and the implementation of nutrition criteria in the 'Government Buying Standards for Food and Catering Services';
- train teachers to foster a positive food culture within schools;
- assess how 'children and learners keep themselves healthy, including healthy eating' as part of Ofsted inspections.

Further information is available at:
✆www.gov.uk/government/publications/the-school-food-plan
✆www.schoolfoodplan.com
✆https://www.gov.uk/government/uploads/system/uploads/attachment_data/file/418072/gbs-food-catering-march2015.pdf
✆ PHE/Town and Country Planning Association/Local Government Association (2016) Building the foundations: Tackling obesity through planning and development: ✆https://www.local.gov.uk/sites/default/files/documents/building-foundations-tack-f8d.pdf

National nutrition programmes, initiatives, and campaigns

National Child Measurement Programme

The National Child Measurement Programme (NCMP) is an important element of the UK Government's work programme on child obesity and is operated by PHE and the DH. The NCMP was established in 2006. Every year, as part of the NCMP, children in Reception (aged 4-5 years) and in Year 6 (aged 10-11 years) are weighed and their height measured. The NCMP measures the height and weight of around 1 million school children in England every year, providing a detailed picture of the prevalence of childhood obesity. In 2015/2016, 19.8% of children aged 10-11 years were obese and a further 14.3% were overweight. Of children aged 4-5 years, 9.3% were obese and another 12.8% were overweight.

For further information see: ℘ www.gov.uk/government/collections/national-child-measurement-programme.

See Chapter 14, 'National Child Measurement Programme', p. 315.

Change4Life

Change4Life is PHE's flagship programme for preventing child obesity in England and Wales. It is a social marketing campaign with clearly recognizable branding that has been used to launch a number of initiatives such as the 2016 'Sugar Smart' and '10 minute shake up' campaigns. The branding has been applied to other PHE programmes and initiatives relating to obesity, physical activity, and eating well such as the '5 A Day' logo. The branding can also be used by local authorities and schools.

For further information see: ℘https://www.nhs.uk/change4life.

One You

One You is a campaign by PHE that aims to inform and engage with adults, especially in the 40-60 years age group to make small changes to improve their own health by eating well, moving more, drinking less, and stopping smoking.

For further information see: ℘ https://www.nhs.uk/oneyou/.

5 A Day Programme

The 5 A Day Programme is a government campaign to encourage adults and children to eat more fruit and vegetables and aim for five portions of fruit and vegetables daily. Resources such as a '5 A Day' logo and tools to help families increase their fruit and vegetables intake have been developed through the Change4Life campaign. The '5 A Day' message is also embedded in the 'Eatwell Guide' (see Chapter 2, p. 27).

For further information see: ℘ https://www.nhs.uk/live-well/eat-well/why-5-a-day/.

The School Fruit and Vegetable scheme

The School Fruit and Vegetable Scheme is part of the 5 A Day Programme to increase fruit and vegetable consumption. Under the scheme, all 4–6-year-olds in state-funded infant, primary, and special schools are entitled to a free piece of fruit or vegetable each school day, if schools have 'chosen' to participate in the scheme.

Further information is available at: ℘ https://www.nhs.uk/live-well/eat-well/school-fruit-and-vegetable-scheme/.

Healthy Start scheme

Healthy Start is a UK-wide statutory scheme providing a nutritional safety net to pregnant women, women with an infant <1 year or children in early years (aged 6 months to 5 years) in low income families in receipt of certain benefits or tax credits. All pregnant women <18 years old qualify, whether or not they are in receipt of benefits. The Healthy Start scheme provides vouchers to eligible families that can be exchanged for fresh or frozen fruit or vegetables, milk and infant formula milk. The scheme also provides free vitamins to women during pregnancy, with an infant <1 year and for children in early years (aged 6 months to 5 years). Heathy Start vitamins for women contain: folic acid, vitamin C, and vitamin D. Healthy Start vitamins for children contain: vitamins A, C, and D. See Chapter 13, p. 276.

Further information is available at: ℘ www.healthystart.nhs.uk.

Sugar Reduction programme

Following the publication of the SACN 'Carbohydrates and Health' report,[9] which provided new dietary recommendations for intake of 'free sugars' and fibre, PHE published 'Sugar Reduction: the evidence for action'.[10] This report outlined eight actions to reduce population sugar consumption, including a structured programme of reformulation to reduce levels of sugar in everyday food and drink, which was embedded in the Child Obesity Plan (see p. 406). PHE identified where the food industry needed to focus efforts on sugar reduction by identifying the main foods and drinks that contribute to children's consumption of sugar using National Diet and Nutrition Survey (NDNS) data. These data demonstrated that the nine product categories that contribute most of the sugar that children eat are: breakfast cereals, confectionary, ice-cream, yoghurt and fromage frais, morning goods, spreads, biscuits, cakes, and puddings. In 2017, PHE published technical guidance for all sectors of the food industry on how to achieve a 20% sugar reduction across these nine categories of food.[11]

---

9 SACN (2015). *Carbohydrates and Health.* Available at: ℘ https://www.gov.uk/government/publications/sacn-carbohydrates-and-health-report.

10 PHE. (2015). *Sugar Reduction: the evidence for action.* Available at: ℘ https://www.gov.uk/government/uploads/system/uploads/attachment_data/file/470179/Sugar_reduction_The_evidence_for_action.pdf.

11 PHE. (2017). *Sugar reduction: achieving the 20%.* Available at: ℘ https://www.gov.uk/government/uploads/system/uploads/attachment_data/file/604336/Sugar_reduction_achieving_the_20_.pdf.

Soft drinks industry levy

The UK government introduced a levy on soft drinks that contain added sugar to help tackle childhood obesity in April 2018.[12] The aim of the levy is to encourage producers of added sugar soft drinks to reformulate their products to reduce the sugar content and to reduce portion sizes for added sugar drinks, and for importers to import reformulated drinks with low added sugar to encourage consumers of soft drinks to move to healthier choices. The levy is paid by producers and importers of soft drinks that contain added sugar. The levy is charged on volumes according to total sugar content, with a standard rate of 18 pence per litre charged for drinks >5 g sugar/100 mL and a higher rate of 24 pence per litre for drinks with >8 g sugar/100 mL. The levy does not apply to pure fruit juices or any other drink with no added sugar. Milk-based drinks are excluded as a source of calcium and other nutrients. See https://www.gov.uk/topic/business-tax/soft-drinks-industry-levy.

Regulation of food and drink advertising to children

Regulation of food and drink advertising to children is a recognized measure contributing to a whole systems approach to tackling child obesity and protecting children from exposure to marketing of less healthy foods. The UK currently employs a combination of statutory and government approved private sector self-regulation techniques to control commercial promotion of food to children. Statutory rules apply to child-targeted TV advertisements for high fat, sugar, or salt foods (HFSS), as defined by the nutrient profiling model.[13] The PHE Sugar Reduction evidence package published in 2015 (see 'Sugar Reduction programme' section) stated that a clear definition for high sugar foods was needed to help significantly reduce opportunities to market and advertise high sugar food and drink products to children and adults. The regulatory framework for doing this is via the FSA and Ofcom nutrient profiling model (NPM), which, it suggested, would benefit from being reviewed and strengthened. This work is being taken forward as part of the Child Obesity Plan published in 2016 (see 'Child Obesity Plan' p. 406) to reflect new SACN dietary recommendations for consumption of free sugars and fibre.[9]

'Child-targeted' marketing is defined as marketing during preschool children's programmes, during programmes made for children <16 years in children's airtime, and youth-orientated programming that attracts a significantly higher-than-average proportion of viewers <16 years (i.e. the proportion of viewers <16 years is 20% higher than the general viewing population). The rules apply to commercial and public service broadcast channels, and all cable and satellite channels. The rules also include additional measures that ban the use of licensed characters, celebrities, health claims, and free gifts in HFSS food advertisements directed at young children. The debate also concerns non-broadcast media, such as print and digital media, including the Internet (see Box 18.2).

12 Available at: ℗ https://www.gov.uk/government/publications/soft-drinks-industry-levy/soft-drinks-industry-levy.

13 Further information regarding the nutrient profiling model is available at: ℗www.gov.uk/government/publications/the-nutrient-profiling-model.

Box 18.2 International recommendations on marketing of foods and non-alcoholic beverages to children

Agreement was reached by member states at the Sixtieth World Health Assembly in 2007 for the World Health Organization (WHO) to 'develop a set of recommendations on marketing of foods and non-alcoholic beverages to children' as part of the implementation of the Global Strategy on the prevention and control of non-communicable diseases (NCDs).

Subsequently, the WHO published a set of recommendations in 2010 on the marketing of foods and non-alcoholic beverages to children to reduce the impact of foods high in saturated fats, trans-fatty acids, free sugars, and salt. The recommendations complement objective 3 of the action plan for the global strategy for the prevention of non-communicable diseases, which identifies as a proposed key action for member states to 'prepare and put in place, as appropriate, and with all relevant stakeholders, a framework and/or mechanisms for promoting the responsible marketing of foods and non-alcoholic beverages to children, in order to reduce the impact of foods high in saturated fats, trans-fatty acids'.

Further information on WHO recommendations on the marketing of foods and non-alcoholic beverages to children: ℜ http://www.who.int/dietphysicalactivity/marketing-food-to-children/en/

Nutrition labelling

Nutrition labelling has been mandatory under EU law for the majority of pre-packed foods since December 2016. It is mandatory for nutrition labelling to declare: energy value (in kilojoules and kilocalories), grams of fat, saturated fat, carbohydrates, sugars, protein, and salt. Nutrients from a specified 'supplementary' list can be declared on a voluntary basis. If vitamins and minerals are declared, percentage reference intakes must be provided as well as absolute amounts. Additional technical guidelines exist regarding the declaration of other aspects of the nutrient content of the product.[14]

From 2010 responsibility for food labelling shifted from the FSA to DH in the UK. In addition to the EU-mandated labelling regulations described above, the UK government recommends standardized 'traffic light', colour coded, front of pack labelling. Revised 'front of pack' nutrition labelling guidance was published in 2016[15] (see Chapter 8, 'Food labelling', p. 188).

---

14 Technical guidance on nutrition labelling (Department of Health, 2017) is available at: ℜ https://www.gov.uk/government/uploads/system/uploads/attachment_data/file/595961/Nutrition_Technical_Guidance.pdf.

15 'Guide to creating a front of pack (FoP) nutrition label for pre-packed products sold through retail outlets' (Department of Health, Food Standards Agency, Welsh Government, Food Standards Scotland, 2016) available at: ℜ https://www.food.gov.uk/sites/default/files/media/document/fop-guidance_0.pdf.

The Eatwell Guide

The 'Eatwell Guide' was published in 2016 and provides a visual aid and additional written information summarizing the government's recommendations for a healthy diet for the UK population. The guide shows the different types of foods and drinks we should consume and in what proportions for a healthy diet, and is intended to apply to most people regardless of weight, dietary restrictions/preferences, or ethnic origin. (Chapter 2 on the Eatwell Guide, p. 27).

The 'Eatwell Guide' updates the 'Eatwell Plate' in light of new dietary recommendations relating to the SACN 'Carbohydrates and Health' report published in 2015 (Chapter 5, p. 81). The 'Eatwell Plate', published by the Food Standards Agency in 2007, was developed from the 'Balance of Good Health', published in 1994, which was based on the existing UK dietary recommendations including the COMA 'Diet and Cardiovascular disease' report published in 1994.

Further information on the 'Eatwell Guide' and its historical and methodological development is available here: ℬ https://www.gov.uk/government/publications/the-eatwell-guide

'The Eatwell Guide—how does it differ from the Eatwell Plate and Why' (PHE, 2016): ℬhttps://www.gov.uk/government/uploads/system/uploads/attachment_data/file/528201/Eatwell_guide_whats_changed_and_why.pdf

'From plate to guide: what, why and how for the Eatwell model' (PHE, 2016): ℬhttps://www.gov.uk/government/uploads/system/uploads/attachment_data/file/579388/eatwell_model_guide_report.pdf

Surveys to monitor diet, nutrient intake, and nutritional status in the UK

Household food purchase surveys

An example of a household food purchase survey (as opposed to a survey of food consumed by individuals) is 'Family Food' (formerly called the National Food Survey, Expenditure and Food Survey and the Living Costs and Food Survey). The survey was established in the 1940s to monitor the diet of the urban 'working class' population during the war years. It was extended to cover all households in the general population in the 1950s and to collect data on food expenditure and consumption. It is a continuous survey run by the Office for National Statistics (ONS).

One element of the survey collects detailed information on quantity and expenditure of food and drinks purchases for households and eating out consumption from around 8000 households. Information collected on eating out is less detailed than on household purchases. The household member who does most of the food shopping is asked some questions about the household and its food purchasing. They are then asked to keep a diary for 7 days, recording food coming into the household, including quantities and expenditure and some detail of the household meals (including snacks and picnics prepared from household supplies). Energy and nutrient content are derived from the data on purchases using standard profiles for around 500 types of foods and are used as a proxy for intake. 'Family Food' reports based on the survey analysis are published annually by DEFRA. The survey provides long term trend data of food purchases and the nutrient content of purchases at household level.

Further information is available here: 'Family Food' reports: ℘ www.gov.uk/government/collections/family-food-statistics.

Data from the Living Costs and Food Survey (and Expenditure and Food Survey): ℘ https://discover.ukdataservice.ac.uk/series/?sn=2000028.

Individual dietary surveys

The first national survey of diet and nutrition in individuals was the Dietary and Nutritional Survey of British Adults in 1986/7. Following this, the National Diet and Nutrition Survey (NDNS) programme was set up in 1992 as a series of cross-sectional surveys, each covering a different age group: pre-school children (aged 1.5-4.5 years); young people (aged 4-18 years); adults (aged 19-64 years); and older adults (aged 65 years and over). Since 2008, the NDNS has been a rolling programme covering adults and children aged 1.5 years and over with a representative UK sample of 1000 (500 adults, 500 children) each year plus additional recruitment in the devolved countries. ℘ Further information is available at: https://www.gov.uk/government/statistics/ndns-time-trend-and-income-analyses-for-years-1-to-9

The NDNS is the only source of high quality nationally representative data on the types and quantities of foods consumed by individuals, from which estimates of nutrient intake for the population are derived. The NDNS is jointly funded by PHE and the UK FSA and carried out by the

National Centre for Social Research (NatCen) working with the Medical Research Council Elsie Widdowson Laboratory.

Dietary intake data are collected using a 4-day diary with estimated weights, accompanied by a face-to-face interview, including physical measurements and blood and urine samples (from a sub-sample). Nutrient intakes in the NDNS are derived from food consumption data combined with a databank of the nutrient content of food. This is based on data from the government's long running nutrient analysis programme supplemented by data from product labels and data calculated from recipes. These data also form the basis of the UK food composition tables: McCance and Widdowson's *The Composition of Foods* and the online version *Composition of Foods Integrated Dataset*. Available at: ℘ https://www.gov.uk/government/ publications/composition-of-foods-integrated-dataset-cofid.

The published reports from the NDNS focus on food consumption and nutrient intakes for adults aged 19–64 years and 65 years and over and for children aged 1.5–3 years, 4–10 years, and 11–18 years. Intakes are compared with government recommendations and comparisons with findings from previous surveys are also made. The results of the survey are used to develop nutrition policy and to contribute to the evidence base for government advice on healthy eating.

Health Survey for England

The Health Survey for England comprises a series of annual surveys beginning in 1991.[16] The series is part of an overall programme of surveys commissioned by the DH and designed to provide regular information on various health topics in England for adults >16 years and children since 1995, including infant feeding practices A number of core questions are included every year, but each year's survey also has a particular focus on a disease or condition or population group. Topics are brought back at appropriate intervals to monitor change. The survey combines questionnaire-based answers with physical measurements and the analysis of blood samples. Blood pressure, height and weight, smoking, drinking, and general health are covered every year. An interview Is conducted with each eligible person in the household. Information is obtained directly from persons aged ≥13 years. But, information about children aged <13 years is obtained from a parent, with the child present.

Since 2001 the survey has usually included a number of 24-hour dietary recall questions relating to fruit and vegetable consumption. These data are used to derive estimates of the number of portions of fruit and vegetables consumed on average by adults and children. Data are available for each year for adults and children from 2001 apart from for 2012 and 2014 in adults and 2012 in children (when this question was not asked). The estimates of average portions of fruit and vegetable consumed are not directly comparable with those reported from the NDNS because of the different dietary assessment and data collection methods used for each survey.

---

16 Available at: ℘ https://data.gov.uk/dataset/health_survey_for_england.

Local nutrition policy and action

The organization and delivery of local level services

The Health and Social Care Act 2012 had a significant impact on the organization and delivery of health services in the UK, including those relating to nutrition at local level. The Act abolished NHS Primary Care Trusts and Strategic Health Authorities and transferred associated healthcare funds and associated statutory responsibilities to CCGs and local authorities.

PHE centres

At a regional level, PHE centres were established to transfer and translate national level policy, guidance, and knowledge to support local level delivery of public health services. There are nine PHE centres in England, covering four regions (including London, which is an integrated region and centre).

CCGs

CCGs are clinically led statutory NHS bodies responsible for the planning and commissioning of healthcare services for their local area. There are over 200 CCGs in England. CCGs are responsible for the delivery of community, mental health, and hospital services, including clinical nutrition and dietetics services and Tiers 3 and 4 obesity services, (see Box 18.3 for the NHS England care pathway for obesity services). Many CCGs also have delegated responsibilities (from NHS England) for primary care and specialist services commissioning.

Health and Wellbeing Boards (HWBs)

Under the Health and Social Care Act, Health and Wellbeing Boards (HWBs) were established to act as a forum in which key leaders from the local health and care system could work together to identify local need, improve the health and wellbeing of their local population, and reduce inequalities including those related to nutrition and diet related health. HWBs operate in all 152 upper tier local authorities and have adult and social care responsibilities. The boards must include a representative of each relevant CCG, a local Healthwatch representative, a local councillor, a director of adult social care, a director of children's services and a director of public health. HWBs are a key forum for encouraging commissioners from the NHS and local authority to work together and central to achieving this is the production of a Joint Strategic Needs Assessment (JSNA) and Joint Health and Wellbeing Strategy (JHWS) through which the HWB can monitor performance.

Local authorities

Since April 2013, local authorities, upper tier and unitary authorities have had responsibility for improving the health of their local populations. Local authorities fulfil this responsibility through:
- a 'ring-fenced' public health budget;
- a specialist public health team, led by a Director of Public Health;
- joint working with the CCGs and other parts of the local health and care system (including a statutory function to provide public health advice to CCGs) through the HWB;

population health needs assessment and performance monitoring through the Joint Strategic Needs Assessment and Health and Wellbeing Strategy;

• taking 'whole systems' and 'place-based' approaches to tackling complex public health issues at a local level.

Included within the provision of public health services more widely, local authorities are responsible for Tier 1 and 2 obesity services and delivery of the NCMP (through schools and school nursing teams). See Chapter 14, National Child Measurement Programme, p. 135.

Box 18.3. 'Joined Up Clinical Pathways for Obesity' (NHS England, 2016)*

Tier 1: Preventative programmes: public health interventions aimed at prevention and reinforcement of healthy eating and physical activity messages.

Tier 2: Weight management services: lifestyle weight management advice. This may be given in primary care as part of ongoing personalized care. Weight management services delivered in the community led by a healthcare professional (e.g. dietician) trained in obesity. This may also include additional support by commercial weight management services. These commercial programmes will be well defined, with scientific leadership and with clear protocols.

Tier 3: Specialist care: 1:1 management by a medically qualified specialist in obesity. This may be community or hospital based ± outreach and delivered by a team led by a specialist obesity physician. Patient management will also include specialist dietetic, psychological, and physical activity input. This will include group work and access to leisure services. There will be access to a full range of medical specialists as required for co-morbidity management.

Tier 4: Specialist care: 1:1 management provided by specialist obesity medical and surgical multidisciplinary teams with full access to a full range of medical specialists as required. All patients will be referred to Tier 4 by a Tier 3 service. The difference between the medical specialty at tiers 3 and 4 will be a qualitative level of experience in complex patient management. All surgical procedures will take place in Tier 4.

*Source: data from 'Joined Up Clinical Pathways for Obesity' (NHS England, 2016), available at ℔ https://www.england.nhs.uk/wp-content/uploads/2014/03/owg-join-clinc-path.pdf.

Translating government policy and national guidelines on nutrition and obesity into local delivery

Many national policies and plans contain guidance and recommendations for local level delivery. PHE, NHS England, and other organizations such as the Local Government Association (LGA), also provide specific guidance for local authorities regarding particular aspects of local service provision relating to food, nutrition, and obesity. Implementation of national level public health policy and guidance at local level is also supported by the PHE centres (see above).

Tackling obesity locally

Local authorities are uniquely well-placed to drive population-level changes to tackle obesity in a way that addresses the specific needs and characteristics of their local communities. Driven by national-level strategies such as the NHS 'Five Year Forward View', the PHE 'Child Obesity Plan', and evidence-based guidance such as the 'Foresight' report (see p. 406), local authorities can ensure a holistic approach is taken by fully involving all other statutory agencies and council departments such as planning, transport, education, leisure, schools, and social care. They are also well-placed to engage with the private sector, such as local food businesses and employers, to encourage action to address a range of aspects of the environment that may contribute to obesity. Further guidance and case studies for such actions can be found in the LGA's 'Tackling Obesity' report and the LGA/PHE 'Building the foundations: Tackling obesity through planning and development' report, detailed in Further information).

Some examples of how local authority departments can work together to tackle obesity can be found on the archived National Obesity Observatory web pages here: ℘ http://webarchive.nationalarchives.gov.uk/20170210161227/http://www.noo.org.uk/LA/tackling.

'Place-based' local public health

The NHS 'Five year forward view' (2014) and the subsequent 'Delivering the forward view: NHS Planning Guidance' (2015) focused on 'place' as the direction of travel for the delivery of the NHS, local government, and ultimately, a sustainable health system for the future.

'Place-based' service delivery focuses on the blurring of institutional boundaries across a geographical location to provide integrated care for individuals, families, and communities. This new method of collaborative service delivery goes beyond the boundaries of NHS and social care services, with the management of common available resources based on the needs of local populations. This shift in the nature and organization of local service delivery also reflects the concept of 'complex adaptive systems' (as described in the 'Foresight' report) and relies on a commitment to prevention and early intervention and services that are integrated through investment in workforce planning and collaborative performance and outcome frameworks.

Further information

'Commissioning Guidance to support devolution to CCGs of Adult Obesity surgical services in 2016/17' (NHS England, 2016) available here: ℘ https://www.england.nhs.uk/wp-content/uploads/2016/05/devolved-services-ccg-guid-obesity.pdf.

'Five Year Forward View' (NHS, 2014) available here: ℘https://www.england.nhs.uk/wp-content/uploads/2014/10/5yfv-web.pdf.

'Delivering the Forward View: NHS Planning Guidance 2016/17-2020/21', (NHS, 2015) available here: ℘ https://www.england.nhs.uk/wp-content/uploads/2015/12/planning-guid-16-17-20-21.pdf.

'Place-based systems of care—a way forward for the NHS in England' (The King's Fund, 2015) available here: ℘https://www.kingsfund.org.uk/sites/files/kf/field/field_publication_file/Place-based-systems-of-care-Kings-Fund-Nov-2015_0.pdf.

'Strategies for encouraging healthier 'out of home' food provision' (PHE/LGA, 2017) available here: ℘https://www.gov.uk/government/publications/encouraging-healthier-out-of-home-food-provision.

'Planning the foundations: Tackling obesity through planning and development' (2016, PHE/Town and Country Planning Association/Local Government Association') available here: ℘ https://www.tcpa.org.uk/Handlers/Download.ashx?IDMF=7cfb9952-700b-419a-b1d5-d4bb23272a1e.

'The new NHS: how providers are regulated and commissioned' available here: ℘ https://www.kingsfund.org.uk/sites/files/kf/media/NHS%20Structure_2016.pdf.

Evaluation of local diet and weight management interventions

Evaluation is about judging the value of an activity and assessing whether or not it has achieved what it set out to do. An evaluation determines the extent to which a programme has achieved its objectives and will assess how different processes contributed to achieving these objectives. Evaluation is an essential part of public health delivery, regardless of whether what is being delivered is a national-level social marketing campaign or a local community public health nutrition intervention. Evaluation is particularly vital for developing a robust evidence base for complex, holistic public health interventions that focus on prevention, where we know that 'gold standard' evidence in the form of randomized controlled trials is lacking and challenging to conduct. Developing an evidence base on which to base commissioning decisions is even more important in the context of restricted public finances. There are many different approaches that can be taken to an evaluation including different theoretical bases, research designs, methods of data collection (e.g. questionnaires, interviews, assessment tools), analysis, and reporting. Box 18.4 contains some practical tips for conducting an evaluation and a number of resources for further information and guidance.

Box 18.4 Tips and resources for conducting evaluations

- Plan the evaluation from the beginning of the development of the intervention or service.
- Allocate a realistic part of the budget for the intervention to evaluation (WHO recommendations are for at least 10% of budget).
- Identify the aim of the intervention or service, what are its intended outcomes, and the rationale for the intervention. For example, is there existing evidence to support the intervention? Logic models can help to focus on an intervention's likely impact and identify primary and secondary or short, medium and long term outcomes.
- Be clear about who the evaluation is for and the different expectations that different stakeholders may have in the evaluation, e.g. commissioners, community members, local councillors. Take this into consideration when setting objectives, identifying outcome indicators, and planning reporting.
- Think carefully about the data that you need and that you can collect. Do not collect data that are not related to the intervention objectives or outcome indicators.
- Consider ethical issues and whether the evaluation needs approval from an ethics committee.
- Plan data collection carefully and think about the resources needed, e.g. time, specialist staff, equipment, analysis software.

Further information and reading

Nutbeam, D., Bauman, A. (2006). *Evaluation in a Nutshell*. McGraw Hill, NSW Australia.
Pawson, R., Tilly, N. (1997). *Realistic Evaluation*. Sage Publications.
Weight management interventions: standard evaluation framework. Available at: ✍ https://www.gov.
    uk/government/publications/weight-management-interventions-standard-evaluation-framework

Healthy and sustainable diets

Sustainability and nutrition *424*
Environmental impacts of diets *425*
Sustainable nutrition policy in the UK *426*
Sustainable development goals *428*
Food security *429*
Climate change and obesity *430*
Useful websites and further reading *434*

Sustainability and nutrition

The public health nutrition field[1] has identified a need to integrate nutrition and environmental sustainability, placing nutrition within its wider structural settings including the political, physical, socio-cultural, and economic environment, which influence individual behaviour and health. As a consequence, the impact of what is eaten on the natural environment as well as the impact of environmental and climate change on all components of food security, must be addressed, i.e. on what food is available, accessible, utilizable, and stable.[2]

The concept of incorporating sustainability into the human diet, from the perspectives of both environmental capabilities in food production terms, and the provision of nutritional guidance to inform citizens, was first addressed over 30 years ago.[3] Despite this, there is still some uncertainty about exactly what constitutes a sustainable diet. The first attempt to define a sustainable diet for intergovernmental policy development was in 2010 at a scientific symposium in Rome hosted by United Nations Food and Agricultural Organization and Biodiversity International.[4] Here the first broad definition of sustainable diets was proposed:

'Sustainable Diets are those diets with low environmental impacts which contribute to food and nutrition security and to healthy life for present and future generations. Sustainable diets are protective and respectful of biodiversity and ecosystems, culturally acceptable, accessible, economically fair and affordable; nutritionally adequate, safe and healthy; while optimizing natural and human resources.'

This broad definition has been criticised for suggesting that these multiple elements of sustainability are synergistic when there will inevitably be trade-offs. For example, fish is good for health but many species are depleted and overfishing of specific species damages ecosystems. Furthermore, there will also be trade-offs within the different sustainability parameters. For example, fruit and vegetables are good for health and are generally low in greenhouse gas emissions (GHGE) but some horticultural practices require large amounts of water for irrigation thus there is potential conflict between GHGE mitigation and water use objectives.[5]

1 Lawrence, M., *et al.* (2015). Public health nutrition and sustainability. *Public Health Nutr.* **18**(13), 2287–92.

2 Schmidhuber, J., Tubiello, F.N. (2007). Global food security under climate change. *Proc. Natl Acad. Sci.* **104**, 19703–8.

3 Gussow, J.D., Clancy, K.L. (1986). Dietary guidelines for sustainability. *J. Nutr. Educ.* **18**(1), 1–5.

4 Biodiversity and Sustainable Diets—United against Hunger, 3–5 November 2010, FAO Headquarters, Rome, Italy. Food and Agriculture Organization, Rome.

5 Garnett, T. (2014). What is a sustainable diet? Food and Climate Research Network. https://www.fcrn.org. uk/sites/default/files/ fcrn_what_is_a_sus-tainable_healthy_ diet_final.pdf

Environmental impacts of diets

Food production and consumption is linked with various environmental impacts, including: biodiversity loss, land use change, water use, and GHGE. Livestock production is associated with the greatest environmental impacts because of the larger quantities of resources (land, feed, water) required for rearing the animals and processing the meat.[6] Ruminant animals are associated with the greatest GHGE because of enteric fermentation. Diets that are rich in red and processed meat, animal products, and energy dense foods are associated with the greatest environmental impacts. Mediterranean, pescatarian and vegetarian diets,[7] and diets with minimal or no animal products are associated with the lowest GHGE.[8]

Modelling studies have shown that adhering to UK healthy eating guidelines and moderating the consumption of meat and dairy consumption could reduce GHGE by around 25%.[9] Furthermore, the adoption of plant-based diets that contain minimal amounts of red and processed meat, has been predicted to reduce food-related GHGE by 30% and diet-related mortality by 5 million people compared to a reference diet by 2050.[10]

6 Steinfeld, H., et al. (2006). *Livestock's Long Shadow. Environmental issues and options.* FAO, Rome.

7 Tilman, D., Clark, M. (2014). Global diets link environmental sustainability and human health. *Nature* 515, 518–22.

8 Scarborough, P., et al. (2014). Dietary greenhouse gas emissions of meat-eaters, fish-eaters, vegetarians and vegans in the UK. *Clim. Change* 125(2), 179–92

9 Macdiarmid, J., et al. (2012). Sustainable diets for the future: can we contribute to reducing greenhouse gas emissions by eating a healthy diet? *Am. J. Clin. Nutr.* 96, 632–9

10 Springmann, M., et al. (2016). Analysis and valuation of the health and climate change co-benefits of dietary change. *Proc. Natl. Acad. Sci.* 113(15), 4146–51.

Sustainable nutrition policy in the UK

Between 2007 and 2010, much progress was made in incorporating environmental sustainability into government nutrition policy in the UK. This was largely a result of the Sustainable Development Commission's work,[11] which included a shift towards providing sustainable hospital food,[12] the introduction of the Healthier Food Mark Scheme for public sector caterers, and a campaign to reduce household waste (WRAP).

This work informed the development of a national food policy strategy Food 2030,[13] which was published by the government in 2010. This strategy committed the government to encouraging sustainable diets and linked ecological public health with food supply chain resilience.[14]

Following the 2010 general election under the new government, the Department for Environment, Food and Rural Affairs (DEFRA) set up the Green Food Project initiative comprising stakeholders from across the food and farming sector, government, and academia. As part of this work, key principles of healthy sustainable eating were published by the Government Global Food Security Programme[15] in 2014 (Box 19.1). However, there is still currently (2020) no government advice in the UK on what a sustainable, healthy diet should be.

In 2016, Public Health England revised the national dietary guidance, *The Eatwell Guide* Chapter 2 'The Eatwell Guide', p. 27, recommending that consumers reduce red and processed meat consumption for both health and climate reasons.[16] Other countries around the world have incorporated environmental sustainability into their official national dietary guidelines, including Brazil, Germany, Sweden, and Qatar.[17]

11 Department of Health (2009). *Sustainable food—a guide for hospitals.* Department of Health, London.

12 Sustainable Development Commission (2009). *Setting the Table. Advice to Government on priority elements of sustainable diets.* SDC, London.

13 DEFRA (2010). *Food 2030 strategy.* Department for Food, Rural Affairs and Environment, London.

14 Lang, T., Mason, P. (2018). Sustainable diet policy development: implications of multi-criteria and other approaches, 2008–2017. *Proc. Nutr. Soc.* **77**(3), 331-46..

15 Garnett, T., Strong, M. (2015). *The principles of healthy and sustainable eating patterns.* UK Government Global Food Security Programme, London.

16 Public Health England (2016). *The Eatwell Guide: helping you eat a healthy, balanced diet.* Public Health England, London.

17 Fischer, C.G., Garnett, T. (2016). *Plates, pyramids and planets - developments in national healthy and sustainable dietary guidelines: a state of play assessment.* Food and Agriculture Organization of the United Nations and Food Climate Research Network (FCRN), University of Oxford.

Box 19.1 Principles of healthy and environmentally sustainable eating patterns

- Eat a varied balanced diet to maintain a healthy body weight.
- Eat more plant-based foods, including at least five portions of fruit and vegetables a day.
- Value your food. Ask about where it comes from and how it is produced. Don't waste it.
- Choose fish sourced from sustainable stocks, taking seasonality and capture methods into consideration.
- Moderate your meat consumption and enjoy more peas, beans and pulses, tofu, nuts, and other plant sources of protein.
- Include milk and dairy products in your diet and/or seek out plant-based alternatives, including those that are fortified with additional vitamins and minerals.
- Drink tap water.
- Eat fewer foods high in fat, sugar, and salt.

Source: Garnett, T., Strong, M. (2015). *The principles of healthy and sustainable eating patterns*. UK Government Global Food Security Programme, London.

Sustainable development goals

Sustainable development was first defined as 'Development that meets the needs of the present without compromising the ability of future generations to meet their own needs' (World Commission on Environment and Development, 1987). In 2015, the 193 member states of the United Nations adopted the 17 sustainable development goals of the 2030 Agenda for Sustainable Development, global objectives expected to guide the actions of international community over the next 15 years.[18] Below are nine of these goals that have targets relating to action on food. The FAO considers healthy environmentally sustainable diets a key part of SDG12, stating that 'consumers must be encouraged to shift to nutritious safe diets with a lower environmental footprint'.[19]

- SDG1—End poverty
- SDG2—Zero hunger
- SDG3—Health and Wellbeing
- SDG6—Water
- SDG7—Energy
- SDG12—Sustainable production and consumption
- SDG13—Combat climate change
- SDG14—Oceans, seas, and marine resources
- SDG15—Life on land

The Paris Climate Agreement,[20] a global treaty to limit climate change, was also held in 2015 in which 200 nations agreed to aim to limit the global average temperature rise to <2°C above pre-industrial levels and to try to limit the temperature increase even further to 1.5°C. To meet these targets will require mitigation efforts across every sector, including food and agriculture. There is growing evidence to suggest that improvements and technological advances in food production alone will not be sufficient to meet these climate change mitigation targets, therefore dietary changes will be necessary.[21]

18 United Nations (2017). *Sustainable Development Goals*. Available at: ℜ http://www.un.org/sustainabledevelopment/sustainable-development-goals/.

19 Food and Agricultural Organization (2015). *FAO and the 17 sustainable development goals*. Food and Agricultural Organization of the United Nations, Rome. Available at: ℜ http://www.fao.org/3/a-i4997e.pdf.

20 United Nations Framework Convention on Climate Change. Available at: ℜ http://unfccc.int/paris_agreement/items/9485.php.

21 Bryngelsson, D., et al. (2016). How can the EU climate targets be met? A combined analysis of technological and demand-side changes in food and agriculture. *Food Policy* **59**, 152–64.

Food security

The idea of food security was developed in 1974 at the World Food Summit in response to concerns about rapidly rising food prices that threatened the world food system. Since then many definitions of food security have emerged (>100 different possibilities!). Food security definitions have become broader, shifting from focusing on availability, to access; ↑ importance given to quality, not just quantity; incorporation of the notion of wellbeing in its broadest sense and not just related to food; changing scale from global/national to households/individuals.

Widely defined as meaning that 'people at all times should have physical and economic access to sufficient, affordable, safe and nutritious food necessary and appropriate for a healthy life, and the security of knowing that this access is sustainable in the future' by the Food and Agriculture Organization (FAO). This definition of food security incorporates four dimensions of whether food is:

• available (production, distribution, trade);
• accessible (affordable, quality and quantity);
• utilizable (nutritional value, social value, food safety);
• stable.

See ➲ Chapter 16, 'Eating on a low income' in relation to household food security, p. 354.

Climate change and obesity

Relationship of obesity and climate change

How does food consumption have an impact on climate change? Around 15% of the global population is now obese or overweight (2010) and carbon emissions have ↑ from 250 ppm (50 years ago) to 380 ppm in 2007.[22] Some have suggested that it is no coincidence that countries with higher obesity rates tend to have higher carbon emissions, such as the USA.

The cost of obesity and overweight is now starting to be felt and the cost to the UK economy alone is an estimated £10 billion annually, which is projected to ↑ 5-fold in the next 40 years as a result of ↑ obesity rates. Many of the costs from ↑ obesity worldwide will be carbon-intensive, e.g. ↑ reliance on medical services and drugs for 'managing' obesity, as well as managing its health consequences, e.g. cardiovascular disease, type 2 diabetes, and cancers.

Causes of obesity and climate change

↑ consumption of food, especially energy dense processed foods, accompanied by ↓ physical activity contribute to both obesity and climate change. The relationship between obesity/diet-related non-communicable diseases (NCDs) and GHGE is shown in Box 19.2 and Fig. 19.1.

Box 19.2 Greenhouse gases

- Methane (CH_4), carbon dioxide (CO_2), and nitrous oxide (N_2O), are the main contributors to a rise in the global temperature of 0.4°C since the 1970s.
- Twenty-two per cent of global greenhouse gases come from agriculture[23] and livestock production accounts for about 80% of this.
- Methane and N_2O are closely related to livestock production and a greater byproduct of this sector than CO_2. These are mainly produced by the digestive system of ruminants (enteric fermentation).
- Food production makes a significant contribution to carbon emissions, equally split between food production, distribution and retailing; energy used in buildings; transport/travel; consumption of other goods and services than food.[24]
- Although low-income countries produce only 20% of CO_2 emissions, they produce more than half of N_2O and nearly two-thirds of CH_4.

---

22 Egger, G. (2008). Dousing our inflammatory environment(s): is personal carbon trading an option for reducing obesity – and climate change? *Obesity Rev.* **9**(5), 456–63.

23 McMichael, A.J., et al. (2007). Food, livestock production, energy, climate change, and health. *Lancet.* **370**(9594), 1253–63.

24 Griffiths, J., et al. (2008). Ten practical actions for doctors to combat climate change *Br. Med. J.* **336**, 1507.

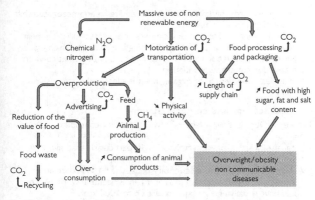

Fig. 19.1 How obesity/NCDs and greenhouse gas emissions are linked.

Source: Holdsworth M, Bricas N (2016). Impact of Climate Change on Food Consumption and Nutrition. In: Torquebiau Emmanuel (ed.). *Climate Change and Agriculture Worldwide*, pp. 227-38. Springer. ☞http://www.springer.com/gb/book/9789401774604#aboutBook.

Diet and climate change

The food chain contributes ~1/5th of UK greenhouse gases emissions and is a major source of waste.

- ↑ demand for convenience food → ↑ CO_2 emissions from production and processing, carbon-intensive packaging, as many prepared foods use plastic packaging, which is oil-dependent.[25]
- ↑ in demand for convenience foods has contributed to a diet that is more energy dense.
- Populations need to ↓ consumption of energy dense foods to ↓ CO_2 emissions.
- Diets of obese people have been linked to climate change because they need to eat more calories and larger portions to meet their basal metabolic rate to maintain body weight → producing more organic waste, including CH_4 production when the waste decomposes!
- World meat consumption varies greatly between lower (47g/day) and higher income countries (224 g/day).[26] Meat consumption is ↑, especially in countries in rapid economic and nutritional transition, e.g. S. and E. Asia. This has obvious implications for GHGE, as well as for obesity.
- Lowering meat consumption in high income countries to 90 g/day (of which no more than 50 g/day should come from red meat from ruminant animals), which would allow lower income countries to

25 Stern, N. (2006). *Stern Review on the economics of climate change*. Bodley Head, Reading.

26 McMichael, A.J., *et al.* (2007). Food, livestock production, energy, climate change, and health. *Lancet* **370**(9594), 1253–63.

converge towards this level. This would require an unprecedented shift in the eating habits for many.

- The British Meat and Livestock Commission suggest that eating meat can be made more sustainable by choosing British meat, which would have less transportation carbon costs, and by changing what cows are fed to reduce methane production.
- It is unclear whether eating organic meat is a less carbon-intensive option.

Physical activity and climate change

The key drivers in how a lack of physical activity contributes to climate change are:

- ↑ car use, which ↓ physical activity levels, particularly that involving travel to and from work and → ↑ carbon emissions.
- At work, people are more sedentary because of ↑ in service and commercial sector sedentary jobs and ↓ in agricultural work, which could have ↓ daily energy expenditure up to 1000 kcals.[27]
- Host of labour saving household appliances, such as the washing machine, dishwasher, vacuum cleaner, that ↓ energy expenditure and ↑ carbon emissions.
- It is estimated that ~ 40% of car journeys in the UK are <2 miles, which could be walked in less than 30 min.
- Car drivers walk less than adults who do not own cars, leading to almost 1 hour less walking every week.
- Heavier individuals use more fuel when using transport.
- Watching TV or computers → to CO_2 emissions and weight gain.
- Redesigning the built environment to make it easier to walk and cycle, would help ↓ obesity and climate change.

Policy options for obesity and climate change

Some of the policies mentioned in ➔ Chapter 18, 'Obesity prevention', p. 398 could also reduce GHGE. The UK government's 'Foresight report'[28] also focused on how a sustainable response to obesity could be delivered. Other suggestions are:

- >50% of global population live in cities; therefore, changes in urban design are fundamental to making physical activity easier and the norm, benefiting both carbon emissions and body mass index.
- A low carbon transport system involving walking/cycling will help to ↓ obesity and national/local governments can provide safe cycle lanes, footpaths, and wide public transport routes.
- Ensuring sustainable catering and food procurement policies so that local foods are sourced wherever possible, particularly for basic foods produced with minimal processing. Low energy dense foods are more environmentally sustainable, as they are less carbon-intensive.

27 Egger, G. (2008). Dousing our inflammatory environment(s): is personal carbon trading an option for reducing obesity—and climate change? *Obesity Rev.* **9**(5), 456–63.

28 Department of Health (2007). *Tackling obesities: future choices.* Available at: ✍ www.foresight. gov.uk/OurWork/ActiveProjects/Obesity/Obesity.asp.

- Supermarkets can influence GHGE by resolving existing tensions between how diets can be both healthy and sustainable (including sustainably sourced fish, meat, and dairy). A policy that encourages supermarkets and food manufacturers to demand reformulated products, shift marketing to healthier products, and introduce front of pack food labelling based on the traffic light system, will help ↓ obesity, and direct consumers away from more carbon-intensive foods.
- Educating the public to change their attitudes to both obesity and behaving in a more sustainable manner can be part of the solution, but alone this is not enough. Changes in attitude may be more successful if carbon-intensive behaviours become taboo.

Useful websites and further reading

Bere, E., Brug, J. (2008). Towards health-promoting and environmentally friendly regional diets- a Nordic example. *Publ. Health Nutr.* 12(1), 91–6.

Clonan, A., Roberts, K.E., Holdsworth, M. (2016). Socioeconomic and demographic drivers of red and processed meat consumption: implications for health and environmental sustainability. *Proc. Nutr. Soc.*75(3), 367–73.

Clonan, A., Wilson, P., Swift, J.A., Leibovici, D.G., Holdsworth, M. (2015). Red and processed meat consumption and purchasing behaviours and attitudes: impacts for human health, animal welfare and environmental sustainability. *Public Health Nutr.* 13, 1–11.

Delpeuch, F., Maire, B., Monnier, E., Holdsworth, M. (2009). *Globesity—a planet out of control*. Routledge.

FAO (2016). *FAO and the 17 Sustainable Development Goals*. Food and Agricultural Organization of the United Nations, Rome. Available at: ℘ http://www.fao.org/3/a-i4997e.pdf.

Garnett, T., Mathewson, S., Angelies, P., Borthwick, F. (2015). Policies and actions to shift eating patterns: what works? *Food Climate Research Network*. Chatham House.

Gill M, Feliciano D, Macdiarmid J *et al.*, (2015) The environmental impact of nutrition transition in three case study countries. *Food Security* 7:493–504.

Holdsworth, M., Bricas, N. (2016). Impact of climate change on food consumption and nutrition. In: Torquebiau Emmanuel (ed.). *Climate change and agriculture worldwide*, pp. 227–38. Springer. Available at: ℘ http://www.springer.com/gb/book/9789401774604#aboutBook.

Lancet series (2019) Food in the Anthropocene: the EAT–Lancet Commission on healthy diets from sustainable food systems. https://www.thelancet.com/commissions/EAT

Lang, T., Barling, D., Caraher, M. (2009). *Food policy: integrating health, environment and society*. Oxford University Press, Oxford.

Macdiarmid, J., Kyle, J., Horgan, G., Loe, J., Fyfe, C., Johnstone, A., McNeill, G. (2012). Sustainable diets for the future: can we contribute to reducing greenhouse gas emissions by eating a healthy diet? *Am. J. Clin. Nutr.* 96, 632–9.

McMichael, A.J., Powles, J.W., Butler, C.D., Uauy, R. (2007). Food, livestock production, energy, climate change, and health. *Lancet*. 370(9594), 1253–63 Tilman D and Clark M (2014) Global diets link environmental sustainability and human health. *Nature* 515: 518–522.

Tilman D., and Clark M. (2014). Global diets link environmental sustainability and human health. *Nature* 515: 518–522.

Food Climate Research Network: ℘ http://www.fcrn.org.uk

Food Climate Research Network: ℘ http://Foodsource.org.uk

Sustain: ℘ http://www.sustainweb.org

UN (2017) *Sustainable Diets for Healthy People and a Healthy Planet*. Rome, Italy. https://www.unscn.org/uploads/web/news/document/Climate-Nutrition-Paper-EN-WEB.pdf

United Nations Framework Convention on Climate Change: J℘ http://unfccc.int/paris_agreement/items/9485.php

℘ http://www.wwf.org.uk/what-we-do/area-of-work/food

℘ https://www.cieh.org/

℘ http://www.environment-agency.gov.uk

℘ http://www.defra.gov.uk

℘ http://www.fao.org

Global nutrition

Global nutrition problems 436
Types of childhood 'malnutrition' 438
Consequences of undernutrition in low and middle income
    countries 440
Infant feeding 441
Causes of global undernutrition 442
Millennium Development Goals 444
World Health Assembly targets 445
Sustainable Development Goals 446
Iron deficiency anaemia globally 448
Iodine deficiency disorders globally 450
Vitamin A deficiency globally 452
Nutrition transition 454
Nutrition in emergencies 456
Common types of malnutrition seen in humanitarian
    emergencies 458
Anthropometric surveys to assess for acute undernutrition 462
Food security 463
Tackling undernutrition in low income countries 464

Global nutrition problems

Problems that persist despite much effort

- *Chronic undernourishment (hunger):* 815 million people (11%) in 2016.
  The highest prevalence of hunger is in Sub-Saharan Africa, closely linked
  with poverty, but most of the world's undernourished are in Asia;
  absolute numbers of undernourished people are largest in Asia (SOFI
  2017).[1]
- *Low birth weight (2014):* 20 million (15%) (*Global Nutrition Report*- GNR
  2017[2]).
- *Chronic undernutrition or stunting in infants under 5 in 2016:* 155 million
  (23%) (GNR 2017).
- *Micronutrient deficiency (hidden hunger):* > 2 billion:
  - vitamin A deficiency—responsible for almost 6% and 8% of all deaths
    of <5s in Africa and South Asia, respectively;
  - iron deficiency anaemia —responsible for 18% of maternal deaths
    in Low and Middle Income Countries (LMICs).
- *Global acute malnutrition (GAM) or wasting in infants under 5 in
  2016:* 52 million cases (8%) globally, of which 16.9 million (2.5%) have
  severe acute malnutrition (SAM) (GNR 2017).

Most cases are found in South Asia and Sub-Saharan Africa.

Problems that are increasing in low and middle income countries

- *Obesity (worldwide epidemic according to WHO):* 641 million adults (13%)
  in 2014 (11% in males vs. 15% in females) (GNR 2017).
- *Overweight:* 1,929 million adults (39%) in 2014 (38% in males vs. 39%
  in females); ↑ in children under 5 years of age (41 million [6%] in
  2014) (GNR 2017).
- Predictions are that overweight/obese prevalence will affect > 50% of
  the world's population by 2030.[3]
- Dietary-related chronic disease (cardiovascular disease, diabetes,
  cancers). 422 million of adults have diabetes.

Age groups affected

Newborn and infants
- Low birth weight <2,500 g (intrauterine growth retardation).
- Problems of physical and psychomotor development.

Children and adolescents
- Faltering growth.
- Underweight, chronic hunger (chronic low energy intake).
- Overweight and obesity.

---

1 Available at: https://www.wfp.org/content/2017-state-food-security-and-nutrition-world-sofi-report.

2 GNR-Global Nutrition Report (2017). Available at: http://www.globalnutritionreport.org/.

3 Kelly, T., *et al.* (2008). Global burden of obesity in 2005 and projections to 2030, *Int. J. Obes.*
32(9), 1431–7.

Adults
- Underweight, chronic hunger (chronic low energy intake).
- Overweight, obesity, and nutrition-related chronic disease.

All ages
- Micronutrient deficiencies.
- 88% of countries globally face a serious burden of either two or three forms of malnutrition (GNR 2017).

Types of childhood 'malnutrition'

- Weight-for-height/length < -2 standard deviations (SD) of the WHO Child Growth Standards median = *wasting* (also known as 'global acute malnutrition').
- Height/length-for-age < -2SD of the WHO Child Growth Standards median = *faltering linear growth or stunting* (also known as 'chronic malnutrition').
- Weight-for-age < -2SD of the WHO Child Growth Standards median = *underweight* (this can reflect wasting, stunting, or both).

See Chapter 25, 'Malnutrition universal screening tool', p. 560 and 'Undernutrition', p. 564 and Chapter 13, 'Infant growth and development', p. 258 and 'Faltering growth', p. 286.

Consequences of undernutrition in low and middle income countries

The consequences of undernutrition are significant in terms of

- ↑*Mortality rates in children:* Half of deaths of under-5s, i.e. 6 million each year, are linked to poor nutrition. 19.1% of deaths of under-5s are attributable to wasting; 3.2% of deaths of under-5s are attributable to stunting, and 6.3% of deaths of under-5s are attributable to underweight. 54.3% of deaths of under-5s are attributable to poor maternal and child nutrition (GBD 2016[4]).
- Long-term illness.
- Infection.
- Deficiency disease.
- Impaired development → impact on local and national economy.
- Poor physical development.
- Short stature.
- Poor mental development and school achievement.

Consequences of short stature for individuals/populations

Being small in itself is not a problem, but there is a relationship between maximal physical work capacity and the capacity to maintain physical effort and lean body mass. There is also an inter-generational effect because a stunted mother increases the risk of giving birth to a newborn with faltering linear growth.

Impaired linear growth can be a symptom of a poor diet and underlying health problems. It is indicative of an increased risk to health (morbidity, mortality, poor physical and psychomotor development). Observation of problems of stunting (when adult) or faltering growth (when a child) is important on a population level and suggests the need for public health interventions but also the development of programmes to fight social and economic deprivation.

For further information see ACC/SCN, UNICEF, 1989; *Lancet* 2008 Maternal and Child Undernutrition series.

4 Wang, H., *et al.* (2016). Global, regional, and national life expectancy, all-cause mortality, and cause-specific mortality for 249 causes of death, 1980–2015: a systematic analysis for the Global Burden of Disease Study 2015. *Lancet* **388**(10053), 1459–544.

Infant feeding

See Chapter 13, 'Infant growth and development', p. 258; ➜ 'Breast versus bottle feeding', p. 262; 'Promoting and establishing breastfeeding', p. 266, and 'Weaning', p. 278.

Causes of global undernutrition

Undernutrition is caused by a range of factors and is rarely because of a simple lack of food. People vulnerable to undernutrition are those who depend on others, especially children, adolescent girls and women, and the elderly. Risk factors for undernutrition include:

- low food intakes;
- low levels of female schooling, education, and empowerment/ autonomy;
- poor access to sanitation and clean water;
- low national expenditure on health and education;
- poor food supply;
- unequal world trade, food distribution;
- drought;
- war/conflicts;
- introduction of formula feed instead of breast;
- weaning onto poor quality foods/sub-optimal complementary feeding regime (e.g. timing of complementary feeding, low dietary diversity, inadequate meal frequency);
- in large families with a high number of children under 5, mothers feeding children before themselves/inadequate intra-household distribution of food;
- infection → ↓ appetite, ↑ diarrhoea, malabsorption, basal metabolic rate → ↓ food intake and ↑ nutrient losses and requirements.

A conceptual framework of the causes of undernutrition presents different levels of causative factors. Without a clear understanding of the multiple causes of undernutrition, it is very difficult to successfully reduce the prevalence of undernutrition.

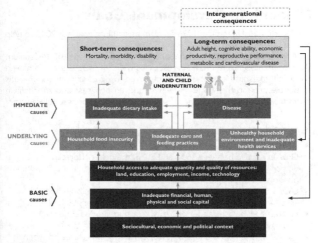

The black arrows show that the consequences of undernutrition can feed back to the underlying and basic causes of undernutrition, perpetuating the cycle of undernutrition, poverty and inequities.

Source: Adapted from UNICEF, 1990.

Fig. 20.1 Causal framework and consequences of maternal and child undernutrition (UNICEF (2013). *Improving child nutrition: the achievable imperative for global progress.* https://www.unicef.org/gambia/Improving_Child_Nutrition_-_the_achievable_imperative_for_global_progress.pdf).

Millennium Development Goals

The World Food Summit in 1996 set eight millennium goals for 2015 to help reduce hunger (see Box 20.1).

Reviews of global and regional progress made towards the Millennium Development Goals (MDGs) suggest that significant progress was achieved across all goals and contributed to improved living conditions for millions of people around the world. However, uneven progress and shortfalls in many areas still require attention. For further information, see full report.[5]

Box 20.1 The Millennium Development Goals (1990–2015)

- GOAL 1: halve between 1990 and 2015, the proportion of people whose income is < $1 a day and halve between 1990 and 2015, the proportion of people who suffer from hunger.
- GOAL 2: ensure that by 2015, children everywhere, boys and girls alike, will be able to complete a full course of primary schooling.
- GOAL 3: eliminate gender disparity in primary and secondary education by 2005 and in all levels of education before 2015.
- GOAL 4: reduce the under-5 mortality rate by two-thirds between 1990 and 2015.
- GOAL 5: reduce the maternal mortality ratio by three-quarters between 1990 and 2015.
- GOAL 6: halt and begin to reverse the spread of HIV/AIDS by 2015; halt and begin to reverse the incidence of malaria and other major diseases by 2015.
- GOAL 7: integrate the principles of sustainable development into country policies and programmes; halve the proportion of people without sustainable access to safe drinking water by 2015; achieve a significant improvement in the lives of at least 100 million slum dwellers by 2020.
- GOAL 8: develop a global partnership for development.

Further information: ℬ http://mdgs.un.org/unsd/mdg/default.aspx and ℬ http://www.un.org/millenniumgoals.

---

5 The Millennium Development Goals Report (2015). Available at: ℬ http://www.un.org/millenniumgoals/2015_MDG_Report/pdf/MDG%202015%20rev%20(July%201).pdf).

World Health Assembly targets

In 2012, the World Health Assembly set six global nutrition targets on maternal, infant, and young child nutrition (MIYCN) to improve nutritional status.

The following targets were identified to be achieved by 2025:
- 40% reduction in the number of children under 5 who are stunted;
- 50% reduction of anaemia in women of reproductive age;
- 30% reduction in low birth weight;
- no increase in childhood overweight;
- increase the rate of exclusive breastfeeding in the first 6 months up to at least 50%;
- reduce and maintain childhood wasting to less than 5%.

In 2013, three diet-related non-communicable disease (NCD) targets to be achieved by 2025 were set by the World Health Assembly (see below):
- 30% relative reduction in mean population intake of salt;
- 25% relative reduction in the prevalence of raised blood pressure or contain the prevalence of raised blood pressure, according to national circumstances;
- halt the rise in diabetes and obesity.

Sustainable Development Goals

In 2015, as part of a new sustainable development agenda, countries adopted the Sustainable Development Goals (SDGs), also called Global Goals, to end poverty, protect the planet, and ensure prosperity for all by 2030. These goals build on the success of the MDGs. A total of 17 goals were set, of which 12 are particularly relevant for nutrition (see Box 20.2). The MIYCN and diet-related NCD targets overlap with SDG 2 and 3, more specifically goals 2.2 and 3.4.

Reviews of progress made to date towards the 17 SDGs show that, in many areas, the rate of progress needed to achieve the targets set by 2030 is too slow. Further information is presented in the SDG Report 2017. Further information on the progress made towards the World Health Assembly targets is presented in the Global Nutrition report 2017.[6]

6 Global Nutrition Report (2017). Available at: ℜ http://www.globalnutritionreport.org/

Box 20.2 Sustainable Development Goals

- **GOAL 1:** end poverty in all its forms everywhere.
- **GOAL 2:** end hunger, achieve food security and improved nutrition, and promote sustainable agriculture.
- **GOAL 3:** ensure healthy lives and promote wellbeing for all at all ages.
- **GOAL 4:** ensure inclusive and equitable quality education and promote life-long opportunities for all.
- **GOAL 5:** achieve gender equality and empower all women and girls.
- **GOAL 6:** ensure availability and sustainable management of water and sanitation for all.
- **GOAL 7:** ensure access to affordable, reliable, sustainable, and modern energy for all.
- **GOAL 8:** promote sustained, inclusive, and sustainable economic growth, full and productive employment, and decent work for all.
- **GOAL 9:** build resilient infrastructure, promote inclusive and sustainable industrialization, and foster innovation.
- **GOAL 10:** reduce inequality within and among countries.
- **GOAL 11:** make cities and human settlements inclusive, safe, resilient, and sustainable.
- **GOAL 12:** ensure sustainable consumption and production patterns.
- **GOAL 13:** take urgent action to combat climate change and its impact.
- **GOAL 14:** conserve and sustainably use the oceans, seas, and marine resources for sustainable development.
- **GOAL 15:** protect, restore, and promote sustainable use of terrestrial ecosystems, sustainably manage forests, combat desertification, and halt and reverse land degradation and halt biodiversity loss.
- **GOAL 16:** promote peaceful and inclusive societies for sustainable development, provide access to justice for all, and build effective, accountable, and inclusive institutions at all levels.
- **GOAL 17:** strengthen the means of implementation and revitalize the global partnership for sustainable development.

Further information

⌖http://www.un.org/sustainabledevelopment/sustainable-development-goals/

Iron deficiency anaemia globally

- Most common nutritional deficiency worldwide, affecting over 30% of global population, especially the under-5s and women.[7]
- Estimated 2016 anaemia prevalence in women of reproductive aged 15-49 years: 32% for non-pregnant women; 40% for pregnant women.
- Estimated 2011 anaemia prevalence in children (6-59 months): 42.6%.
- Highest prevalence for all women of reproductive age (15-49 years) is in SE Asia > Sub-Saharan Africa > Eastern Mediterranean region.
- Low iron intakes → ↓ physical activity → ↓ productivity.
- Affects low, middle, and high income countries, especially the poor and least educated, children, and pregnant/lactating women.

Main causes of iron deficiency

- Poor diet: food insecurity; reliance on plant-based staple foods.
- Poor iron stores: habitually poor diet and high demands.
- Pregnancy: blood loss after delivery and pregnancies close together.
- Malabsorption: intestinal infections (diarrhoea).

Public health consequences of iron deficiency

- *Infant deficiencies:* poor physical growth, cognitive, and motor development:
  - *severe health implications:* ↑ child deaths;
  - *educational implications:* ↓ school achievement;
  - *national productivity:* ↓ physical and mental ability of adolescents and adults ∴ ↓ productivity;
- *Maternal deficiencies:* increased risk of prematurity and low birth weight and increased risk of maternal and perinatal mortality. Additionally, babies born with low reserves; breastmilk may be low in iron, if diet is low in iron.
- *Adult deficiencies:* ↓ immune status and ↑ morbidity from infections.

Preventing iron deficiency anaemia

The WHO suggests that iron deficiency anaemia is best dealt with by tackling all risk factors simultaneously by:

- *improving iron intakes*, e.g. fortification/supplementation/education;
- *infection control*, e.g. combat hookworm and malaria;
- *general dietary improvements* in nutritional quality and dietary diversity. See ➜ Chapter 6, 'Iron', p. 148 for further information.

---

7 WHO (2017). Available at: ℘ http://www.who.int/nutrition/topics/ida/en/.

Iodine deficiency disorders globally

The WHO[8] estimates that iodine deficiency remains a public health problem globally, with 54 countries still affected, but the prevalence has fallen (see Box 20.3). Two billion people have insufficient iodine intake globally, with Europe and the Eastern Mediterranean most affected. The proportion of school-aged children affected is 36.5%.

Iodine deficiency disorders are the most important cause of preventable mental retardation worldwide, and their elimination could contribute to at least four of the SDGs (see Box 20.2):

- end poverty in all its forms everywhere;
- end hunger, achieve food security and improved nutrition, and promote sustainable agriculture;
- ensure healthy lives and promote wellbeing for all at all ages;
- ensure inclusive and equitable quality education and promote life-long opportunities for all.

Iodization of salt is the most effective and least expensive strategy to control iodine deficiency, which also contributes to economic and social development. Worldwide, the number of households having access to iodized salt is estimated at 66%, therefore reducing iodine deficiency.

International action is organized by a coalition of international organizations, including International Council for Control of Iodine Deficiency (ICCID), WHO, Micronutrient Initiative, and UNICEF, national iodine-deficiency disorders control committees, and the salt industry.

8 Available at: ℘ http://www.who.int/vmnis/database/iodine/iodine_data_status_summary/en/.

Box 20.3 Public health implications of iodine deficiency

Children
- Cretinism, goitre
- Growth impairments
- Brain growth, mental impairment.

Adults
- Goitre
- Mental impairment (apathy, loss of initiative, decision-making)

Pregnancy
- Still birth
- Spontaneous abortion
- Congenital abnormalities such as cretinism

Communities
- Loss of economic development
- Lower productivity
- Social problems
See ➲ Chapter 6, 'Iodine', p. 160 for further information.

Vitamin A deficiency globally

- Vitamin A deficiency (VAD), defined as serum (plasma) retinol concentration <0.70 μmol/L (<20 μg/dL), is the most common manifestation of poor nutrition globally besides undernutrition.
- Global prevalence of VAD: 33.3% in preschool-age children (190 million);[9] 15.3% in pregnant women (19.1 million).
- Global prevalence of night blindness: 0.9% in preschool-age children (5.2 million); 7.8% in pregnant women (9.8 million) Most affected areas: Africa, SE Asia, Eastern Mediterranean.
- VAD → xerophthalmia, which can → blindness: 250,000–500,000 children go blind each year as a result of deficiency.
- VAD results in ↑ susceptibility to infection, such as diarrhoea and respiratory infections, and ↑ deaths.

See ❸ Chapter 6, 'Vitamin A', p. 102 for further information.

Risk factors for deficiency

- *Poor growth:* VAD associated with stunting.
- *Presence of other nutrient deficiency:*
  - undernutrition;
  - zinc, selenium, iodine deficiencies.
- *Low socio-economic status:*
  - poverty is the main risk factor for VAD;
  - clinical VAD will only be seen in the most impoverished nations.
- *Young age:*
  - occurs at all ages, but rare in children under 2;
  - 2–4-year-olds at greatest risk.
- *Poor diet:*
  - poorer countries have low intakes of animal produce (meat, eggs);
  - reliance on carotenoids, but carotenoid bioavailability only 3–10% vs. 80% for retinol;
  - where rice is staple food (S and SF Asia), VAD will be more likely.

Prevention of VAD

Food-based approaches

- Aim to educate, provide opportunity to take more vitamin A in diet.
- Diet diversification.
- Fortification.

Supplementation

- Aim to provide a high dose of vitamin A, two to three times per year.
- For example, schools to run vitamin A days, national campaigns.
- Target women at end of pregnancy—they will pass on vitamin A in breastmilk.

9 World Health Organization. (2009). Global prevalence of vitamin A deficiency in populations at risk 1995-2005: WHO global database on vitamin A deficiency. Available at: ℛ http://apps.who.int/iris/bitstream/10665/44110/1/9789241598019_eng.pdf.

Immunization/supplementation

♠Vitamin A supplementation has been the cause of controversy.[10] The World Public Health Nutrition Association has questioned the motives and validity of the current practice of providing regular supplements of massive medicinal doses of vitamin A to children aged 6-59 months. They suggest that food-based approaches are more sustainable, favouring vitamin A-rich plant oils, e.g. palm oil, promoting breastfeeding, and use of plant sources of carotenoids. Others argue that this needs to be balanced with vitamin A supplementation, which is one of the most cost-effective interventions that exists for preventing mortality, illness, and blindness in children under 5, as outlined in the *Lancet* 2008 series and the Copenhagen Consensus 2008, so arguably it is more a matter of assessing needs better.

10 Latham, M. (2010). The great Vitamin A fiasco. *World Nutr.* **1**, 12–45. Available at: ℛ www. wphna.org.

Nutrition transition

Nutrition transition[11] is defined as a shift from a traditional diet using local foods to eating more:
- processed foods;
- food of animal origin: dairy, meat, eggs;
- food energy, especially from fat, sugar;
- 'fast foods' and soft drinks, which become easily available and affordable;
- reduced intake of fruit and vegetables, cereals, and fibre-rich foods.

Nutrition transition is stimulated by a number of factors:
- ↓ in relative price of certain foods (oil/sugar);
- ↑ urbanization, which modifies lifestyle, food patterns, and energy expenditure. 63%, 39%, and 30% of the population in upper-middle, lower-middle and low income countries live in urban areas, respectively.
- culture—obesity and overweight as signs of affluence;
- globalization of markets ∴ making energy dense nutrient-poor processed foods more available and accessible;
- advertising and marketing ∴ making energy dense nutrient-poor processed foods more desirable;
- low birth weight infants leads to programming of ill-health → ↑ likelihood of obesity/nutrition-related NCDs in later life.

Health consequences of the transition
- Large ↑ in nutrition-related noncommunicable diseases (NR-NCD) in adults (and now in children). → Coronary heart disease, strokes, type II diabetes, cancers, obesity.
- 80% of NCD deaths occur in low and middle income countries.
- Over three-quarters of deaths from diabetes are in low and middle income countries.
- Over half of the new cases in the world are found in India and China.
- The age-specific burden is relatively much higher at a younger age in poorer countries.
- Increasing prevalence of overweight and obesity in low income/food insecure households—a seemingly paradoxical association. One explanation is the dependency on low cost foods that are flour/tuber-based and also high in added sugar, fats/oils.
- Limited variety of food consumed relying on a few 'stomach-filling' high energy foods.
- Evidence of overweight mother/underweight or stunted child in the same household among the poor—a challenging situation for public health.

Preventing obesity
See ➲ Chapter 18, 'Obesity prevention', p. 398.

11 Popkin, B.M. (2001). The nutrition transition and obesity in the developing world. *J Nutr* **131**(3), 871S–3S.

Further reading

Delpeuch, F., Maire, B., Monnier, E., Holdsworth, M. (2009). *Globesity—a planet out of control*. Earthscan Books, London. Available at: ℘ http://www.earthscan.co.uk/?tabid=56997.

GBD 2015 Risk Factors Collaborators (2016). Global, regional, and national comparative risk assessment of 79 behavioural, environmental and occupational, and metabolic risks or clusters of risks, 1990–2015: a systematic analysis for the Global Burden of Disease Study 2015. *Lancet* **388**(10053), 1659–724.

Global Nutrition report (2018). Available at: ℘ http://www.globalnutritionreport.org/.

Maire, B., Delpeuch, F. (2005). *Nutrition indicators for development*. FAO. Available at: ℘ http://www.fao.org/docrep/008/y5773e/y5773e00.HTM.

World Health Organization (2013). Global action plan for the prevention and control of NCDs 2013–2020. Available at: ℘ http://www.who.int/nmh/publications/ncd-action-plan/en/.

Nutrition in emergencies

'Nutrition in Emergencies' (NIE) has progressed and expanded greatly over the past 20 years with the renewed political interest in tackling hunger and famine. Humanitarian funding demands that activities work to internationally accepted professional standards.[12] Detailed assessment methods, programme design, training manuals,[13] and monitoring and evaluation systems are all widely documented and available at no cost.

Tools exist to fully address undernutrition and the challenge is to increase the knowledge of personnel in emergency prone countries. The 'emergency' tends to relate to context, e.g. war/famine, but with a case fatality rate of 20–30%, undernutrition can be viewed as an emergency.

The undernutrition crisis

Regrettably, climate change, population growth, and rising oil prices will exacerbate the crisis. It is important within emergency contexts to protect nutritional status in all people if excess morbidity and mortality are to be avoided. South Asia is the continent with the highest numbers[14] of the acutely malnourished. Sub-Saharan Africa has frequent and high profile 'famines', although the mortality rates tend to be lower than that of South Asia. Reasons behind this include:
- even poorer status of women in South Asia;
- lack of sanitation;
- urbanization;
- higher numbers of natural disasters, which can worsen an already poor situation.

Treating undernutrition in emergencies

The case fatality rate for acute malnutrition in a non-emergency setting is 20–30%. In emergencies addressed by the humanitarian community, this is typically reduced to <10%. A significant reduction in mortality can be attained by understanding the factors that lead to death; these principles are incorporated into clinical management protocols for treatment of undernutrition by host governments, UN agencies, and non-governmental agencies (NGAs):
- *Hypothermia:* thermogenesis is impaired because of lack of energy. It can be addressed with kangaroo care, provision of blankets at night.
- *Hypoglycaemia:* gluconeogenesis impaired because of lack of energy intake. It can be addressed by feeding through the night.
- *Dehydration:* can be addressed by careful rehydration with appropriate rehydration solution.
- *Infections:* usually present, but undetected in the undernourished because of impaired responses. Addressed by routine administration of broad spectrum antibiotics, as per host government guidelines.

12 Sphere (2004). *Humanitarian charter and minimum standards in disaster relief.*

13 UN (2008). *Harmonised training package for nutrition in emergencies.* Available at: ℅ https://www.unicef.org/nutrition/training/.

14 Black, R.E., *et al.* (2013). Maternal and child undernutrition and overweight in low-income and middle-income countries. *Lancet* **382**(9890), 427–51.

Common types of malnutrition seen in humanitarian emergencies

The focus of nutrition in emergencies is on acute undernutrition in <5-year-olds and pregnant/lactating women. However, chronic undernutrition is also very likely to be prevalent in emergency contexts. The negative impacts of undernutrition are largely reversible in <2-year-olds, i.e. 9–24 months.

Global acute malnutrition (GAM) is the proxy indicator of the prevalence of undernutrition (i.e. wasting) in a population.

GAM = moderate acute malnutrition (MAM)+SAM.

To reduce GAM, both preventative and curative methods are required. Undernutrition is also defined using the following measures:

- low birth weight (LBW) in newborns;
- low mid-upper arm circumference (MUAC)[15] in children aged 6-60 months (typically <12.5 cm and <11.5 cm for moderate and severe acute malnutrition, respectively). MUAC is commonly used in community settings and its use is increasing in health facilities. Measuring MUAC is relatively cheaper and simpler than measuring weight and length/height;
- micronutrient deficiencies;
- there is no consensus on the cut-off points for MUAC in adults, but results of a meta-analysis[16] propose that a MUAC ≤24.0 cm can be used to indicate low BMI.

The main nutritional problems commonly addressed in emergencies are:
- *Acute undernutrition in pregnant and lactating women.*
- *Micronutrient deficiencies*: vitamin A and zinc should be routinely addressed. Outbreaks of scurvy (vitamin C), beri-beri (thiamine) and pellagra (nicotinic acid) have been documented in the past 20 years (see → Chapter 6, p. 100, for further information) .
- *Acute undernutrition in young children, kwashiorkor and marasmus*:
  - *marasmus* (Fig. 20.2) is the name given to uncomplicated starvation.
  - *kwashiorkor* is the name given when there is the presence of bilateral oedema. The causation of kwashiorkor remains unknown, but it is NOT a result of protein deficiency, as was previously believed, and indeed a low protein diet is needed to treat these syndromes.

▶ Mild cases of marasmus and kwashiorkor are difficult to detect visually and need to be carefully assessed, by taking weight and height/length, MUAC, and/or checking for bilateral oedema (Box 20.4).

15 Available at: ℜ https://www.unicef.org/supply/files/Mid_Upper_Arm_Circumference_Measuring_Tapes(1).pdf.

16 Available at: ℜ https://www.fantaproject.org/sites/default/files/resources/Global-MUAC-Cutoffs-nonPregnant-Adults-Jun2017.pdf.

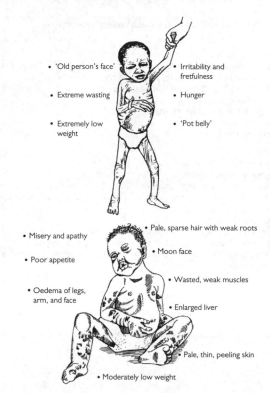

- 'Old person's face'
- Extreme wasting
- Extremely low weight
- Irritability and fretfulness
- Hunger
- 'Pot belly'

- Misery and apathy
- Poor appetite
- Oedema of legs, arm, and face
- Pale, sparse hair with weak roots
- Moon face
- Wasted, weak muscles
- Enlarged liver
- Pale, thin, peeling skin
- Moderately low weight

Fig. 20.2 Clinical features of marasmus (top) and kwashiorkor (bottom).

Reproduced from *Oxford Handbook of Tropical Medicine*, 2nd edn, Eddison, M., Davidson, R, Wilkinson, R, Pierini, S. p. 595 (Oxford: 2005). With permission from Oxford University Press.

Box 20.4 Marasmus and kwashiorkor symptoms

Marasmus
- Extremely emaciated
- Fat and muscle tissue greatly reduced
- Prominence of the scapulae, spine, and ribs
- Thin, flaccid skin, 'old man's' appearance
- Normal hair
- Frequent infection with minimal signs
- Electrolyte imbalance
- Alert and irritable

Kwashiorkor
- Bilateral pitting oedema
- Higher mortality
- Reduced fat and muscle tissue, which may be masked by oedema
- Skin lesions: hyper-pigmentation, skin cracked and peeling off, prone to ulceration and infection
- Pale appearance
- Hair colour becomes paler/redder, brittle, thin
- Frequent infections, e.g. upper respiratory tract, otitis media
- Generally apathetic lethargic and miserable when left alone. Irritable when handled

Anthropometric surveys to assess for acute undernutrition

The objective of an anthropometric survey is to quantify the prevalence of global acute malnutrition (GAM) within a population to determine whether an emergency response is needed. GAM is used as a proxy indicator of the health of the whole population.

Cross-sectional anthropometric surveys are implemented using either simple random sampling, e.g. in a refugee camp situation, or stratified cluster sampling, e.g. for a district level survey.

The WHO Child Growth Standards (2006) have been widely adopted and replace the National Center for Health Statistics growth standards (see ➲ Chapter 13, 'Infant growth and development', p. 258; see Table 20.1 for the WHO classification rates). Weight and height/length are collected in children aged 0–59 months. MUAC data are collected on children 6–59 months. Presence of bilateral oedema is assessed.

Additional information can also be gathered, e.g. measles vaccination, retrospective mortality, and whether the child is registered for a therapeutic or supplementary feeding programme.

Interpretation of anthropometric data

Prevalence of undernutrition must be interpreted in relation to the seasonal patterns of undernutrition.

For example, 15% wasting during the hungry season in a stable, rural population is not as alarming as a prevalence of 15% wasting post-harvest when conditions are at their best or if the mortality rate is increasing.

For mortality, the following thresholds are used:
- <5 years mortality rate of 2/10,000/day = serious situation.
- <5 years mortality rate of 4/10,000/day = an emergency out of control.

Conceptual framework for undernutrition in emergencies

Emergency contexts can affect nutritional status in many ways → to high rates of undernutrition and preventable mortality. These may be caused by epidemics, poor food security, or a poor public health environment. Influences such as food price fluctuations, gender equality, climate change, and population growth mean that nutritional emergencies are likely to be commonplace for some time despite the renewed international interest in tackling these. See ➲ this Chapter, 'Causes of global undernutrition', p. 442.

Food security

See Chapter 19, 'Food security', p. 429.

Table 20.1 WHO classification of rates of global acute malnutrition (GAM), 2003

Severity	Prevalence of GAM (i.e. wasting)
Acceptable	<5%
Poor	5–9.9%
Serious	10–14.9%
Critical	≥15%

Tackling undernutrition in low income countries

In recent years, there has been a focus on building the evidence for interventions aimed at addressing undernutrition. In 2013, the *Lancet* 'Maternal and Child Nutrition series'[14] produced a framework that highlighted the dietary, behavioural, and health determinants of optimal nutrition and growth, and strategies to address both immediate and underlying determinants of poor nutrition (see Figure 20.3).

Nutrition-specific and nutrition-sensitive interventions

Nutrition-specific interventions are those that address the *immediate causes* of poor nutrition, including:

• adolescent health and preconception nutrition; maternal dietary supplementation; breastfeeding and complementary feeding; dietary supplementation for children; treatment of severe acute malnutrition; disease prevention and management; and nutrition interventions in emergencies.

Nutrition sensitive interventions address *underlying causes* of poor nutrition, including:

• agriculture and food security; education; early child development; social safety nets; women's empowerment; water and sanitation.

In the 2013 *Lancet* series on 'Maternal and Child Nutrition', it was stated that '3.1 million deaths in children younger than 5 years were due to undernutrition and that nearly 15% of these deaths could be reduced if 10 core nutrition-specific interventions (see Box 20.5) identified were scaled up'. Furthermore, the series also concluded that nutrition-sensitive approaches and programmes are essential to support the scaling-up of nutrition-specific interventions.[17]

Community based management of acute malnutrition (CMAM)

CMAM is a type of therapeutic feeding programme[18] that treats the majority of children in their own homes. This avoids risks associated with infectious diseases in crowded environments. Children with no appetite/complications must be admitted to an inpatient stabilization centre.

Advances in food packaging and food technology → the production of ready to use therapeutic food (RUTFs). RUTF provides all the required nutrition for the child in clean packaging. Children treated at home need

17 Ruel, M.T., Alderman, H., Maternal and Child Nutrition Study Group. (2013). Nutrition-sensitive interventions and programmes: how can they help to accelerate progress in improving maternal and child nutrition? *Lancet* **382**, 536–51.

18 Valid International (2006). *Community based therapeutic care—A field manual*. Available at: ✆ http://www.validinternational.org/bahwere-et-al-community-based-therapeutic-care-ctc-a-field-manual/.

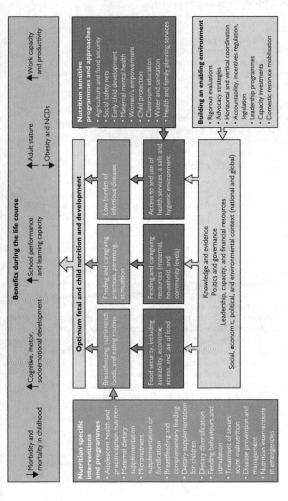

Fig. 20.3 Framework of actions to achieve optimal fetal and child nutrition and development.

Box 20.5 10 core nutrition-specific interventions to address undernutrition-based interventions in low and middle income countries

The following activities have proven to be effective and efficacious to address undernutrition:
1. Folic acid supplementation.
2. Maternal multiple micronutrient supplementation.
3. Maternal calcium supplementation.
4. Addressing maternal wasting and food insecurity with balanced energy and protein supplementation.
5. Exclusive breastfeeding.
6. Complementary feeding.
7. Vitamin A supplementation (6-59 months).
8. Preventive zinc supplementation.
9. Management of SAM.
10. Management of MAM.

See ➲ p. 464 for CMAM.

regular and frequent follow-up by trained personnel, and CMAM programmes need support from the local community to be effective.

Food aid

Over half of all humanitarian spending goes on the distribution of food aid. Food aid is a bilateral gift from one country to another and is highly vulnerable to political considerations. It is only rarely and in high profile emergencies that food aid requirements are adequately met by the international community. Food aid should be a preventative measure brought in before the onset of a nutritional emergency.

It can be very useful in the early stages of an acute emergency. However, in the longer term its use can become controversial, as the provision of large quantities of free food in the marketplace can reduce prices and become a strong disincentive to local marketing and agricultural production.

An emergency food aid basket usually provides a cereal grain, pulses, vitamin A fortified vegetable oil, and iodized salt. A full ration provides 2100 kcal/day per person with 10–12% of energy coming from protein.

It can be used in a number of ways[19] in emergencies:
- *General food distribution (GFD)* refers to the free distribution of a combination of food commodities to the affected population as a whole. If the population is cut off from its food supply, or suffers abnormally high rates of malnutrition, food rations should meet all nutritional needs.
- *Food for work (FFW)* activities largely involve providing food aid to unskilled labourers in exchange for work.

19 Jaspars, S. (2000). *Solidarity and soup kitchens. A review of principles and practice for food distribution in conflict.* Overseas Development Institute, London. Available at: ⏣ www.odi.org.uk/resources/download/247.pdf.

- *School feeding* is the provision of foods as a meal or snack at
- *Blanket supplementary feeding* for all under-5s is used to prote security.

Further reading

Bhutta, Z.A., Das, J.K., Rizvi, A., Gaffey, M.F., Walker, N., Horton, S., Webb, P., Lartey, A., Bla (2013). Evidence-based interventions for improvement of maternal and child nutrition: wh. be done and at what cost? *Lancet* **382**(9890), 452–77.

DFID (2010). *The neglected crisis of undernutrition*. UKaid, London. Available at: ℘ http. webarchive.nationalarchives.gov.uk/+/ ℘ https://www.gov.uk/government/publications the-neglected-crisis-of-undernutrition-evidence-for-action-2009

Navarro-Colorado, C., Mason, F., Shoham, J. (2008). *Measuring the effectiveness of supplementary feeding programmes in emergencies*. ODI. HPN Network, Paper 63.

UN (2011). *Harmonized training package for nutrition in emergencies*. ℘ http://www.ennonline.net/ ourwork/capacitydevelopment/htpversion2.

WHO (1999). *The treatment of severe malnutrition, a guide for senior health professionals in developing countries*. WHO, Geneva. ℘ http://apps.who.int/iris/bitstream/10665/41999/1/a57361.pdf.

Useful websites/international nutrition organizations

IFPRI ℘ http://www.ifpri.org/
GAIN ℘ https://www.gainhealth.org/
UNICEF ℘ https://www.unicef.org/
FAO ℘ http://www.fao.org/home/en/
WHO ℘ http://www.who.int/en/
Action Against Hunger ℘ https://www.actionagainsthunger.org.uk/
World Cancer Research Fund ℘ https://www.wcrf-uk.org/

Chapter 21

Obesity

Overview 470
Prevalence 472
Causes and consequences 474
Weight management: assessment 476
Weight management: overview 477
Weight management: dietary approaches 478
Weight management: physical activity 482
Weight management: behavioural approaches 483
Pharmacotherapy 484
Bariatric surgery 486
Structure of treatment 488
Conditions associated with obesity 490

Overview

Obesity is a major cause of morbidity and mortality worldwide and is common in adults and children. It arises as a result of a prolonged energy imbalance within an obesogenic environment, especially in genetically susceptible individuals. Lifestyle weight management is the cornerstone of treatment, including diet, physical activity, and behaviour change. Multicomponent interventions have been demonstrated to result in modest weight loss, which can be increased further by the addition of adjunct pharmacotherapy. Bariatric surgery has the greatest impact on weight loss and co-morbidities but is associated with the greatest risk of complications. Whatever treatment is used, lifelong vigilance to prevent weight regain is required. Prevention of excess weight gain is key, using multi-sectoral public health approaches.

Definition

Obesity is a disease characterized by excessive body fat accumulation with multiple organ-specific consequences and is most commonly diagnosed in adults using body mass index (BMI). Individuals are classified according to their risk of metabolic complications associated with excess weight (Table 21.1).

Although BMI is commonly used and useful at a population level, it is an indirect measure of body fatness that cannot distinguish between different tissue types, nor does it describe the health risks associated with fat distribution (see ➲ Chapter 4, 'Body mass index'). BMI alone should be used with caution; ideally measures of fat distribution such as waist circumference (WC) should also be used, although at BMI >35 kg/m², WC does not improve prediction of co-morbidities.

WC is a single simple measurement and is a good indicator of intra-abdominal fat deposition, which is associated with adverse health consequences. Using WC (measured at the midpoint between the lower border of the ribcage and the iliac crest), the following cut-off points have been described (Table 21.2).

BMI and WC cut-offs for different populations

Different populations vary in their risk of metabolic abnormalities and population-specific WC cut-off points have been defined (Table 21.3).

Individuals of south Asian origin (Bangladeshi, Indian, and Pakistani origin) have greater prevalence of metabolic abnormalities at lower BMI than would be expected and it has been proposed that for these populations, lower cut-off points for public health action should be used.

Although there is a lack of UK-based evidence for ethnicity-specific cut-off points, because of increased risks at lower BMI (<25 kg/m²) experienced by members of black, Asian, and other ethnic groups, it is recommended that the lower cut-off points of 23.0 kg/m² for increased risk and 27.5 kg/m² for high risk are used to indicate need for action to prevent type 2 diabetes.

Other measures, such as waist-to-height ratio, are useful predictors of metabolic risk[1] but less well understood by most healthcare professionals. More complex measures of body composition, such as bioimpedance, are not recommended as alternatives to BMI in clinical practice.

1 Ashwell, M., Gibson, S. (2016). Waist to height ratio as an indicator of 'early health risk': simpler and more predictive than using a 'matrix' based on BMI and waist and circumference *BMJ Open* 6(3), e010159. doi: 10.1136/bmjopen-2015-010159.

Table 21.1 Classification of weight using body mass index*

BMI range, kg/m²	Classification	Risk of co-morbidities
<18.5	Underweight	Low (but may be other health problems)
18.5-24.9	Healthy weight	Average
25.0-29.9	Overweight	Increased
30.0-34.9	Obesity I	Moderate
35.0-39.9	Obesity II	Severe
≥40.0	Obesity III	Very severe

*Reproduced with permission from World Health Organization (WHO). *Obesity: preventing and managing the global epidemic. WHO Technical Report Series 894*. Geneva, Switzerland: World Health Organization. Copyright © 2000 WHO ℗ http://www.who.int/nutrition/publications/obesity/WHO_TRS_894/en/.

Table 21.2 Cut-off points for risk of metabolic complications in Caucasian adults with obesity according to waist circumference*

Risk of metabolic complications	Waist circumference, cm	
	Men	Women
Increased	≥94	≥80
Substantially increased	≥102	≥88

*Source: data from Ashwell, M., Gibson, S. (2016). Waist to height ratio as an indicator of 'early health risk': simpler and more predictive than using a 'matrix' based on BMI and waist and circumference *BMJ Open* 14, 6(3):e010159. doi: 10.1136/bmjopen-2015-010159.

Table 21.3 Waist circumference cut-off points according to ethnicity*

Population	Gender	WC in cm (inches)
European	Men	≥94 (37)
	Women	≥80 (31.5)
South Asian, Chinese and Japanese	Men	≥90 (35)
	Women	≥80 (31.5)
Ethnic south and central Americans	Use South Asian recommendations in lieu of more specific data	
Sub-Saharan Africans	Use European recommendations in lieu of more specific data	

*Reproduced with permission from Alberti, K.G.M.M., et al. International Diabetes Federation: a consensus on type 2 diabetes prevention. *Diabetic Med.* 24, 451-63.

...ce

...onal

...a global public health problem affecting both adults and children
...d middle income as well as high income countries. In 2016, 39% of
...globally were overweight and of those 13% were classed as obese.[2]
...represents more than 1.9 billion adults being at least overweight, of
...om more than 600 million were obese (266 million men and 375 million
...omen).[3] A recent study reported that overweight and obesity has doubled
...n more than 70 countries since 1980 and increased steadily in almost all
other countries.[4]

UK

Prevalence of excess weight in England increased by 72% between 1989
and 2013, and prevalence of obesity among adults rose from 15% to 27%
between 1993 and 2015.[5] Within the UK, 65% of adults were classed as
overweight or obese in 2017.

By 2050 obesity is predicted to affect 60% of adult men, 50% of adult
women, and 25% of children. Prevalence in the UK is comparatively
high and ranked 8th for obesity prevalence in men (25.7%) and 11th for
women (26.6%) out of 23 Organisation for Economic Co-operation and
Development (OECD) countries in 2016.[6]

Who is at risk?

Major demographic risk factors for obesity include age, gender, ethnicity,
and socioeconomic status. Prevalence of obesity is generally higher in older
than younger adults, except for oldest adults. The relationship between ethnicity and obesity prevalence is complex and varies with gender and method
of assessing obesity. Prevalence of overweight and obesity is higher in men
than women (67% and 62%, respectively, in England in 2019);[7] however, the
prevalence of obesity was similar in both genders. An inverse relationship
between socio-economic status and excess weight is seen in women but
not men.

2 WHO (2018) Obesity and overweight. Key facts. Available at: https://www.who.int/en/news-
room/fact-sheets/detail/obesity-and-overweight.

3 NCD Risk Factor Collaboration (NCDRisC) (2016). Trends in adult body-mass index in 200 countries from 1975 to 2014: a pooled analysis of 1698 population-based measurement studies with
19.2 million participants. Lancet 387, 1377–96.

4 GBD 2015 Obesity Collaborators (2017). Health effects of overweight and obesity in 195 countries over 25 years. N. Engl. J. Med. 377, 13–27. Available at: ℗ http://www.nejm.org/doi/full/
10.1056/NEJMoa1614362.

5 Ng, M., et al. (2014). Global, regional and national prevalence of overweight and obesity in children
and adults during 1980-2013: a systematic analysis for the Global Burden of Disease Study 2013.
Lancet 384, 766–81.

6 OECD (2018). Health statistics 2018, frequently requested data. Available at: ℗ http://www.
oecd.org/health/health-data.htm.

7 NHS Digital (2019) Statistics on obesity, diet and physical activity. Available from https://digital.
nhs.uk/data-and-information/publications/statistical/statistics-on-obesity-physical-activity-and-diet.

Causes and consequences

Obesity arises in genetically susceptible individuals exposed to obesogenic environments. As such it can be viewed as a normal response to an abnormal environment. The genetic heritability of BMI is estimated to range from 40% to 70%,[8] and there are numerous potential mechanisms through which genes may mediate effects on body weight, e.g. on appetite, food and activity preferences.

However, the rapid increase in prevalence globally indicates that social and environmental factors are also important. Factors favouring weight gain include increased consumption of energy dense, nutrient-poor foods often in large portion sizes, reduced physical activity and increased time spent in sedentary activities, inadequate and/or disturbed sleep, and stress. The roles of prenatal influences, epigenetics and the gut microbiome have also received attention. Food prices and time cost of fast foods, marketing and advertising, fast food consumption, and related behaviours may also contribute. That obesity is caused by numerous physical, biological/physiological, environmental, societal (cultural and economic), and psychological factors which interact in a complex matrix appears to be beyond doubt,[9] and action across all sectors is required to address this. See ➲ Chapter 18, 'Obesity prevention', p. 398.

Co-morbidities and costs of obesity

High BMI is the third highest contributor to disease burden expressed as a percentage of UK disability-adjusted life-years, after smoking and high blood pressure. BMI has been shown to strongly predict overall mortality; life expectancy both above and below the optimal 22.5kg/m^2 is comparatively reduced. Reductions of 2-4 years for BMI category 30-35 kg/m^2, and 8-10 years for BMI category 40-50kg/m^2 are estimated.

Co-morbidities include:

Metabolic: type 2 diabetes, cardiovascular disease, hypertension, hyperlipidaemia, some types of cancer, increased risk of liver and kidney disease, dementia, and reduced fertility as well as adverse outcomes of pregnancy, gallstones, stroke, and polycystic ovary syndrome.

Physical: osteoarthritis, sleep apnoea, back pain, poor mobility, and increased risk of accidents.

Psychosocial: low self-esteem, poor body image, and depression. Obesity is a highly stigmatized condition, perhaps the only remaining socially acceptable stigma. Stigma and bias can result in worse treatment outcomes, poor adherence to treatment plans, and reluctance to seek help.

Financial impact of obesity includes direct and indirect costs such as lost productivity, welfare payments, and increased morbidity and mortality. Additional hidden costs of obesity include increased fuel required for greater food production and transport of heavier people, increasing greenhouse emissions and carbon footprint.

8 Herrera, B.M., et al.(2011). Genetics and epigenetics of obesity *Maturitas* **69**, 41–9.

9 Foresight (2007). Obesity Systems Map. Available at: ℜ https://www.gov.uk/government/uploads/system/uploads/attachment_data/file/296290/obesity-map-full-hi-res.pdf.

...o develop a tailored individualized care plan is fun-
...ctice. Suggested areas for assessment are shown in
...should not be the sole focus of either assessment or
...e healthy changes to behaviours, improving diet and ac-
...increase the likelihood that changes will be sustained.

...e 21.4 Assessment topics in weight management*

A. Anthropometrics
- *Height;*
- *Weight;*
- *Body mass index;*
- *Waist circumference.*

B. Medical
- *Potential causes,* e.g. endocrine, neurological, medications, genetic influences (age of onset, family history);
- *Co-morbidities:* current and future risk;
- *Severity of obesity and extent of physical disability.*

C. Psychological
- *Identify psychological factors,* e.g. depression, addictive behaviours;
- *Eating disorders:* binge eating, bulimia nervosa, disordered eating;
- *Risk of potential barriers to treatment,* e.g. psychiatric history.

D. Nutritional
- *Weight history:* extremes of adult weight, patterns of weight gain and loss, age of onset, triggers to weight gain, triggers to disordered or excessive eating;
- *Dieting history:* number and types of diet, weight loss medications, success of previous attempts to manage weight, alternative or complementary approaches to weight management;
- *Current eating patterns:* meal patterns (meals skipped, snack consumption, largest meal eaten);
- *Nutritional intake:* nutrient density, nutritional supplements;
- *Environmental factors:* meals eaten away from home, fast food consumption, restaurant meals, ethnic foods, lifestyle factors (time, financial);
- *Exercise history:* current exercise, activities of daily living, exercise history, barriers to exercise;
- *Readiness to change:* reasons to lose weight, weight loss goals, support systems, likely difficulties, readiness for making changes.

*Source: data from American Dietetic Association (2009). Position of the American Dietetic Association: Weight Management. *J. Am. Diet. Assoc.* **109**:330-46.

Weight management: overview

First line treatment is lifestyle intervention to change eating and ac
haviours and achieve negative energy balance and weight loss. Mod.
of the Eatwell Guide may be used[10] (see ➔ Chapter 2), although th
be too unstructured an approach for those who struggle with portion

The aim of treatment is usually loss of 5-10% of initial body we,
although this should relate to initial body weight, so those with a Br
<40 kg/m^2 may aim for 5% and those with BMI of >40 kg/m^2 aim for
>10%. Weight loss at this level is achievable, sustainable, and incurs signifi-
cant clinical benefit. The majority of weight loss occurs in the first 6 months,
with weight regain thereafter in most individuals. Multicomponent interventions (i.e. those tackling diet, physical activity, and behaviour change) are
recommended.

10 Public Health England. (2018). Eatwell Guide. Available at: ℘ https://www.gov.uk/government/
publications/the-eatwell-guide.

management: dietary approaches

macronutrient composition of a weight loss diet is hotly con-
and a variety of approaches have been shown to result in modest
losses in the short term. Studies lasting longer than a year typically
ot show significant weight differences between different dietary groups,
er in terms of weight lost or weight loss that is maintained. Adherence
weight management interventions in the long term is critical to success.
odest weight losses at the individual level have the potential for a large
impact on public health. This suggests that so long as a hypocaloric weight
loss diet is otherwise nutritionally complete, individual preferences can dictate the type of diet followed, and may help improve adherence to the
programme.

There is evidence to support a range of dietary approaches resulting in
moderate weight loss of approximately 5-8.5 kg (5-9%) in the first 6 months.
These include an energy-restricted diet (generally 500-600 kcal below requirements), a low fat diet (<30% energy from fat), and meal replacements.
This modest effect may reduce adherence to diets and expectations both
of patients and commissioners must be addressed to reduce this possibility.

Low carbohydrate

Low carbohydrate diets appear to result in modestly greater weight loss
compared with low fat diets. Systematic reviews[11,12] found that low carbohydrate diets (≤120 g/day and ≤60 g/day, respectively) resulted in significantly greater weight loss and improved lipid profiles compared with low fat
diets (≤30% energy from fat) and low energy diets (600 kcal deficit diet).

However, the long-term safety of low carbohydrate diets is unclear.
Studies using low carbohydrate diets are heterogeneous, using different inclusion criteria, different levels of carbohydrate restriction, different study
durations and follow-up, all of which may affect assessment of their clinical
value. Additionally, many studies do not include intention-to-treat analysis,
thus possibly overestimating their benefits.

Low GI/GL

Studies of low glycaemic index (GI) and glycaemic load (GL) tend to be
small and heterogeneous. A systematic review[13] concluded that low GI
diets resulted in significantly greater weight loss and improved risk factors
when compared with other diets. Even *ad libitum* low GI diets were at least
as good as conventional energy restricted diets. However, only six small
studies were included, duration of studies was short, ranging from 5 weeks
to 6 months, and only two studies included obese adults. They are generally not recommended as a sole dietary management approach because of

11 Sackner-Bernstein, J., *et al.* (2015). Dietary intervention for overweight and obese adults: comparison of low-carbohydrate and low-fat diets. A meta-analysis. *PLoS One* **10**, e0139817.

12 Noto H., *et al.* (2012). Low-carbohydrate diets and all-cause mortality: a systematic review and
meta-analysis of observational studies. *PLoS One* **8**, e55030.

13 Thomas D., *et al.* (2007). Low glycaemic index or low glycaemic load diets for overweight and
obesity (review). *Cochrane Database Syst. Rev.* **3**, CD005105.

a lack of well-controlled long-term studies. However, in those with insulin sensitivity or resistance, hypocaloric low GI/GL diets may be preferred and if they suit personal preference and are of adequate nutritional quality they may be a useful strategy for some individuals.

Intermittent fasting

Intermittent fasting or intermittent energy restriction (IER)[14,15] can take a number of forms, but is defined as periods of energy restriction interspersed with normal energy intake. Studies have shown that IER approaches result in similar weight loss to interventions using continuous energy restriction, but a variety of different approaches to IER are used and many studies are short term. Weight loss outcomes in IER compared with continuous restriction for a minimum of 6 months do not differ significantly. Longer-term effects of IER, particularly if non-restricted days are used to either fast or feast are unclear. Therapeutic fasting practised too often or for too long may have negative effects. The approach has potential value for overweight or obese individuals who find continuous restriction difficult, because an intermittent approach means that usual intake can be consumed on non-restricted days, and IER was not shown to result in adaptive responses to restricted energy intake. There is some evidence that IER improves some aspects of mental health in overweight or obese individuals, but more research is needed using sufficiently powered studies to identify optimal IER patterns, whether there are differences in body composition between continuous restriction and IER and whether there are differential effects in men compared to women using this approach. In addition, potential longer-term effects, both positive and negative, need to be identified.

Meal replacements

These portion-controlled products supplemented with vitamins and minerals are designed to replace one to two meals per day, with one remaining meal using conventional foods, and an overall aim of achieving intakes of 1200-1600 kcal/day. They have been shown to be beneficial in short- and long-term use, in primary care and unsupervised 'off-the-shelf' use. A role in weight maintenance has also been demonstrated. For example, in the Look AHEAD trial,[16] weight loss of 4.7% at 8 years in the intervention arm was seen. Meal replacements were one of the dietary strategies used in both the weight loss and maintenance phases of this trial involving 5145 ethnically diverse adults with type 2 diabetes. For those who have difficulty with portion control or food selection, they may be a useful strategy for both weight loss and weight maintenance.[17] Because they are neither

14 Harvie, M., *et al.* (2017). Potential benefits and harms of intermittent energy restriction and intermittent fasting amongst obese, overweight and normal weight subjects – a narrative review of human and animal evidence. *Behav. Sci.* **7**, pii.E4. DOI: 10.3390/bs7010004.

15 Horne, B.D., *et al.* (2015). Health effects of intermittent fasting: hormesis or harm? A systematic review. *Am. J. Clin. Nutr.* **102**, 464–72.

16 LookAHEAD Research Group. (2014). Eight-year weight losses with an intensive lifestyle intervention: the Look AHEAD study. *Obesity* **22**, 5–13.

17 American Dietetic Association (2009). Position of the American Dietetic Association: Weight Management. *J. Am. Diet. Assoc.* **109**, 330–46.

extreme dietary approaches nor total diet replacements, they can be used indefinitely.

Very low energy diets

Very low energy diets (VLED) or very low calorie diets (VLCD) are complete dietary replacements, providing 450-800 kcal/day, and are nutritionally complete apart from energy. They can be used for a maximum of 12 weeks continuously or intermittently as part of a comprehensive strategy with ongoing clinical support and should not be routinely used to manage obesity. The use of VLED has been shown to result in rapid substantial weight loss followed by rapid weight regain. They may be useful in situations where rapid weight loss is needed under clinical supervision and with a planned reintroduction of conventional foods.

Over >6 months, there appears to be little difference in the weight loss achieved by following diets differing in macronutrient composition. Adherence to the diet is what counts and what predicts weight loss, and this seems to be more important than the exact macronutrient breakdown. Part of a tailored approach may be modifying diets in terms of their macronutrient composition depending on the preferences and health status of the individual; with the proviso that the nutritional quality of the diet is a critical consideration.

Potential concerns associated with VLED include malnutrition and keto-acidosis but these were not identified as adverse effects by a recent systematic review.[18]

18 Parretti, H.M., et al. (2016). Clinical effectiveness of very-low-energy diets in the management of weight loss: a systematic review and meta-analyis of randomised controlled trials *Obes. Rev.* **17**, 225–34.

...t management: physical activity

...activity alone is less effective in bringing about weight loss than ...nd physical activity combined.[19] Regardless of its impact on weight, ...cal activity should always be recommended because of its beneficial ...cts on health and wellbeing. It is also thought to be a critical factor in ...eight maintenance. Those who successfully lost 10% body weight and kept ...off at 24 months follow-up spent more time being physically active than those who did not. Successful weight loss maintainers report daily physical activity, both planned and activities of daily living, and this may be the key to their success.

19 Johns, D.L., *et al.* (2014) Diet or exercise interventions vs combined behavioural weight management programs: a systematic review and meta-analysis of direct comparisons. *J. Acad. Nutr. Diet.* **114**, 1557–68.

Weight management: behavioural approaches

Multicomponent interventions including diet, physical activity, and behaviour change are more effective than either diet or activity alone.

Current UK guidance[20] suggests that the following strategies should be included in behavioural interventions for adults, as appropriate:

- self-monitoring of behaviour and progress;
- stimulus control;
- goal setting;
- slowing rate of eating;
- ensuring social support;
- problem solving;
- assertiveness;
- cognitive restructuring (modifying thoughts);
- reinforcement of changes;
- relapse prevention;
- strategies for dealing with weight regain.

20 National Institute for Health and Care Excellence (NICE). (2014). *Obesity: identification, assessment and management. Clinical guideline 189*. Available at: ℜ https://www.nice.org.uk/guidance/cg189/chapter/1-Recommendations#identification-and-classification-of-overweight-and-obesity.

Pharmacotherapy

Currently only one medication, orlistat (brand names include Xenical and Alli) is licensed for use in the UK. Orlistat is a pancreatic lipase inhibitor which reduces absorption of dietary fat by approximately 30% when given with a diet comprising approximately 30% fat. Used in combination with lifestyle change, weight loss of 2.9 kg greater than placebo was observed. Orlistat is not well absorbed so systemic side effects are minimal; the largest problems relate to unabsorbed dietary fat until patients learn to reduce their dietary fat intakes. There may be some reduced absorption of fat-soluble vitamins and reduced absorption of the drug aciclovir. Severe adverse effects are very rare but may include acute kidney injury so orlistat should be used with caution in renal impairment.

Current guidance in the UK:[20]

- Prescribe for adults with a BMI of ≥28 kg/m^2 plus co-morbidity or BMI ≥30 kg/m^2 as part of a plan to manage obesity.
- Continued prescribing should only occur in those who have lost at least 5% of their initial body weight, although lower targets may be set for those with type 2 diabetes, in whom weight loss tends to be lower.
- Supplements are generally not considered necessary unless orlistat is used in vulnerable groups, e.g. young people.

Sibutramine, an appetite suppressant, was withdrawn from licence for treating obesity in the UK in 2010 and in several other countries including the European Union, India, and USA because of associated cardiovascular risks. Other appetite suppressants, including dexfenfluramine and rimonabant, have had approval withdrawn because of health risks exceeding possible benefits. However, unlicensed drugs are available to purchase online so health professionals need to be aware of the risks associated.

Drugs that aim to promote satiety via gastrointestinal effects, e.g. methylcellulose and sterculia, are not recommended because of lack of evidence that they are effective.

Ongoing obesity pharmacology development indicates that new drugs may become available in the near future.[21]

21 Coulter, A.A., et al. (2018). Centrally acting agents for obesity: Past, present and future. *Drugs* **78**(11), 1113-32.

…surgery

…y is the most effective intervention for achieving weight loss …ts,[22] but has more complications than non-surgical methods. …f bariatric surgery are associated with significantly greater re- …f diabetes compared with controls at 10 years and 15 years post- …, and significant improvements to weight-related complications. …rent UK guidance[20] recommends bariatric surgery:

- …first line treatment in those with BMI ≥50 kg/m^2 in whom other …nterventions have failed;
- as a treatment option in those with BMI ≥40 kg/m^2 or between 35 and 40 kg/m^2 and significant disease that would benefit from weight loss;
- all appropriate non-surgical measures have been tried but adequate weight loss has not occurred or been maintained;
- patients receiving intensive management in a tier 3 service;
- patients generally fit for anaesthesia and surgery;
- committed to need for long-term follow-up;
- expedited referral to bariatric surgery should be offered to those with BMI ≥35 kg/m^2 diagnosed with type 2 diabetes in the last 10 years, so long as they will receive assessment in tier 3 or equivalent service.

A **gastric band** is an inflatable band placed around the upper portion of the stomach resulting in a reduced stomach capacity above the band. The degree of tightness of the band can be altered using sterile saline injected through a port under the skin, thus potentially inducing satiety (% https://asmbs.org/patients/bariatric-surgery-procedures#band).

Roux-en-Y gastric bypass is the most common form of bypass; a small stomach pouch (approximately 30 mL) is made by dividing the top from the rest of the stomach. This is connected to the small bowel (this is the Roux limb). The Roux limb is connected by a Y join to the lower part of the small intestine so the stomach acid and enzymes from the bypassed stomach and first part of the small intestine can mix with the food and the remaining stomach is left undisturbed. Re-routing the stomach alters gut hormones promoting satiety and suppressing hunger, and the small stomach pouch results in satiety after small meals. In addition, there may be some malabsorption (% https://asmbs.org/patients/bariatric-surgery-procedures#bypass).

Sleeve gastrectomy: approximately 80% of the stomach is removed, restricting the volume of food that can be consumed. Hormonal changes also impact on satiety, hunger, and control of blood sugar (% https://asmbs.org/patients/bariatric-surgery-procedures#sleeve).

Long-term follow-up of morbidities, medication, and nutritional status are required (Table 21.5); the nature and frequency of monitoring and type of supplementation required will depend on the procedure the patient has undergone.

22 Picot, J., et al. (2009). The clinical effectiveness and cost-effectiveness of bariatric (weight loss) surgery for obesity: a systematic review and economic evaluation. *Health Technol. Assess.* **13**(41), 1-190, 215-357, iii-iv..

Table 21.5 Recommendations for annual blood test monitoring and supplements according to bariatric procedure**

Procedure	Supplement recommendation	Annual blood test monitoring recommendations
Gastric band	Comprehensive multivitamin and mineral supplement recommended	
Gastric bypass	Over the counter (OTC) daily multivitamin and mineral supplement Vitamin B$_{12}$ injections every 3 months Calcium and vitamin D (additional vitamin D may be required) Iron (start with 200 mg daily and monitor dosage especially in premenopausal women)	Liver function tests Full blood count Ferritin Folate Vitamin B$_{12}$* Calcium and vitamin D Parathyroid hormone Zinc and copper Vitamin A (if long-limb bypass, night blindness, or symptoms of steatorrhoea present) Selenium (only measure if concern about possible deficiency)
Sleeve gastrectomy	OTC daily multivitamin and mineral supplement. Vitamin B$_{12}$ injections every 3 months Calcium and vitamin D (additional vitamin D may be required). Iron (start with 200 mg daily and monitor dosage especially in premenopausal women)	Liver function tests Full blood count Ferritin Folate Vitamin B$_{12}$* Calcium and vitamin D Parathyroid hormone Zinc, copper, and selenium (measure if concerns about possible deficiency)

*Annual checks may be unnecessary if patient is receiving 3-monthly injections of vitamin B$_{12}$.

**Source: data from O'Kane, M., et al. (2014). *BOMSS Guidelines on perioperative and postoperative biochemical monitoring and micronutrient replacement for patients undergoing bariatric surgery.* ℬ http://www.bomss.org.uk/wp-content/uploads/2014/09/BOMSS-guidelines-Final-version1Oct14.pdf.

Structure of treatment

Many weight loss interventions are delivered within group settings and group treatment may be more effective than individual treatment, providing social support and cost-effective delivery. Commercial weight-management services are delivered within groups and have been shown to be cost-effective.[23] However, if these services are offered to patients it is important that only programmes which follow best practice guidance are offered and that healthcare professionals continue to monitor patients.

Weight loss maintenance

A variety of lifestyle approaches induce weight loss, but typically when interventions stop, weight regain occurs. Keeping lost weight off is a life-long challenge and different behaviours are needed to keep weight off from those to lose weight. Those who successfully keep weight off use a variety of strategies including diet, physical activity (activities of daily living and structured), and a high degree of self-monitoring. Physical activity has been identified as a critical influence protecting against weight regain.

Prevention and public health approaches

The first aim of public health should be preventing gradual weight gain in adults. Simplistic messages about making small changes (such as eating less and moving more) ignore the complex nature of energy balance. Public health approaches should target the food, physical activity, and socio-economic environments, have a direct influence on behaviours, and support clinical interventions and health services. A healthy environment in which healthy choices are the easy choices is advocated with action taken across the lifecourse.

See ➔ Chapter 18, 'Obesity prevention', p. 398.

23 Jolly, K., et al. (2011). Comparison of range of commercial or primary care led weight reduction programmes with minimal intervention control for weight loss in obesity: Lighten Up randomised controlled trial. *BMJ* **343**, d6500.

Conditions associated with obesity

A number of conditions are associated with obesity.

Down syndrome

Obesity is not inevitable for those with Down syndrome but it may be more common. As with other individuals, preventing excess weight gain using diet and physical activity is better than managing excess weight gain. Those with Down syndrome do not need different lifestyle approaches compared with others, and similarly to others information needs to be tailored and accessible. Sustainable changes to diet and activity to encourage healthier lifestyles should be encouraged, within a supportive family environment.

Polycystic ovary syndrome (PCOS)

This condition affects about 5-10% of women and is characterized by weight gain, hirsuitism (on the face or body), irregular menstrual cycles, anovulation, reduced fertility, hormonal abnormalities, and skin changes. Women with PCOS have an increased risk of developing type 2 diabetes and heart disease. Losing weight can significantly improve PCOS and reduce risks of co-morbidities. Aiming for 5-10% weight loss is achievable, sustainable, and associated with clinical benefits. Modification of diet and lifestyle is first-line treatment.

Prader-Willi syndrome

This rare genetic condition is characterized by reduced growth and muscle tone, a constant feeling of hunger and drive to eat, learning difficulties and immature sexual development. Because there is no cure, management of symptoms is key. Maintaining a healthy weight is key but is difficult to achieve, as eating behaviours can be obsessive. A care plan will be developed with healthcare professionals, ideally a paediatric dietitian, and this will be monitored and assessed over time. The family should be involved in the development of the care plan.

Further information

📖 https://www.downs-syndrome.org.uk/
📖 http://www.pcos-uk.org.uk/about-pcos.html
📖 https://www.pwsa.co.uk/

Obesity: further information

Butland, B., Jebb, S., et al. (2007). Tackling Obesities: Future Choices—Project Report. 2nd edn. Government Office for Science: Department of Innovation, Universities and Skills. Available at: 📖 https://www.gov.uk/government/uploads/system/uploads/attachment_data/file/287937/07-1184x-tackling-obesities-future-choices-report.pdf.

Mackenbach, J.D., Rutter, H., Compernolle, S., et al. (2014). Obesogenic environments: a systematic review of the association between the physical environment and adult weight status: the SPOTLIGHT project. BMC Public Health **14**, 233.

National Institute for Health and Care Excellence (NICE) (2006). Obesity: guidance on the prevention, identification, assessment and management of overweight and obesity in adults and children. [CG43]. Available at: 📖 https://www.nice.org.uk/guidance/cg189/evidence/obesity-update-appendix-p-6960327450.

National Institute for Health and Care Excellence (NICE) (2013). BMI: preventing ill health and premature death in black, Asian and other minority ethnic groups. PH46. Available at: 📖 www.nice.org.uk/guidance/ph46.

National Institute for Health and Care Excellence (NICE) (2014). *Weight management: lifestyle services for overweight or obese adults*. PH53. Available at: ℘ https://www.nice.org.uk/guidance/ph53.

National Institute for Health and Care Excellence (NICE) (2016). *Obesity: clinical assessment and management*. [QS127]. Available at: ℘ https://www.nice.org.uk/guidance/qs127.

Phelan, S.M., Burgess D.J., Yeazel, M.W., *et al.* (2015). Impact of weight bias and stigma on quality of care and outcomes for patients with obesity. *Obesity Rev.* **16**, 319–26.

Public Health England (2015) Sugar reduction: from evidence into action. Available at: ℘ https://www.gov.uk/government/publications/sugar-reduction-from-evidence-into-action.

Chapter 22

Diabetes

Classification and prevalence 494
Contributing causes and clinical consequences 496
Targets 498
Key priorities for management 500
Goals and principles of dietary management 502
Management of type 1 diabetes 506
Management of type 2 diabetes 510
Hypoglycaemia 512
Structured education in diabetes 514
Weight management 515
Diabetes in pregnancy, children, and young people 516
Diabetes in the elderly 518

Classification and prevalence

Classification

Diabetes is a metabolic disorder characterized by chronic hyperglycaemia with disturbances of carbohydrate, fat, and protein metabolism resulting from defects in insulin secretion, insulin action, or both.

- Type 1 diabetes can occur at any age, but usually develops in children or adults aged <40 years. It is an autoimmune disease that destroys the β-cells of the pancreas resulting in absolute insulin deficiency. Type 1 diabetes is treated by insulin replacement and dietary management.
- Type 2 diabetes is usually diagnosed in older adults but is increasingly seen in younger adults and some children. It is characterized by impaired insulin resistance and insulin secretion (Box 22.1) and is strongly associated with overweight and obesity. Treatment includes lifestyle modification, oral hypoglycaemic agents, and injectable therapies including insulin.
- Type 3c diabetes is related to pancreatic exocrine insufficiency. Although it is often misdiagnosed as type 2, management is similar to type 1 diabetes (see ➌ Chapter 27 'Chronic pancreatitis', p. 682).
- Gestational diabetes is hyperglycaemia diagnosed during pregnancy. It is treated with lifestyle modification, including diet, physical activity, and weight management, metformin and insulin.

Prevalence

Globally, it is estimated that 415 million people had diabetes in 2015 and that this will rise to 642 million by 2040. Countries with the highest numbers of people with diabetes include China, India, the USA, Brazil, and the Russian Federation.[1] In the UK, 3.5 million people (6.2% of the population) have been diagnosed with the condition and the majority of these (90%) have type 2 diabetes. It is estimated that a further 1.1 million individuals in the UK may have undiagnosed type 2 diabetes.[2]

Box 22.1 Insulin resistance

There is considerable individual variation in the cellular response to insulin. A lower than normal response is described as insulin resistance. Insulin resistance leads to ↓ glucose uptake by the skeletal muscles and/or liver, ↓ lipolysis in adipose tissue, and altered amino acid metabolism, either alone or in combination. As a consequence of insulin resistance, blood glucose concentrations ↑ and this leads to further stimulation of the pancreas resulting in hyperinsulinaemia and, eventually, leading to pancreatic β-cell failure and impaired insulin secretion. Insulin resistance is strongly associated with obesity.

---

1 International Diabetes Federation (2016). *Diabetes Atlas 7th Edition*. IDF.

2 Diabetes UK (2016). *Facts and Stats 2016*. Diabetes UK, London.

Risk factors

Risk factors for type 1 diabetes are broadly unknown, although there is evidence of some heritability, with the risk among first-degree relatives about 15 times higher than among the general population. Type 2 diabetes is associated with both modifiable and non-modifiable risk factors. Non-modifiable risk factors include age, family history and ethnicity, with people from South Asian or Black communities at two to four times the risk of White people. Modifiable factors for type 2 diabetes include obesity, unhealthy diet, and lack of physical activity.

Studies have shown that the incidence of type 2 diabetes can be reduced by ~50% by lifestyle modification including weight management, a healthy (low fat, high fibre) diet and increased physical activity levels.[3]

Diagnosis

Table 22.1 Values for the diagnosis of diabetes mellitus and other categories of hyperglycaemia[***]

	Fasting venous plasma glucose concentration		2-hour venous plasma glucose concentration after 75 g glucose load		HbA1c	
	mmol/L	mg/dL	mmol/L	mg/dL	mmol/mol	%
Diabetes	≥7.0	≥126	≥11.1	≥200	≥48	≥6.5*
Impaired glucose tolerance**	<7.0	<126	≥7.8–<11.1	≥140–<200	-	-
Impaired fasting glucose	6.1–6.9	110–125	<7.8	<142	-	-

* In the absence of symptoms, diagnosis should not be made on the basis of a single HbA1c test. An additional test (HbA1c or plasma glucose) is required to confirm the diagnosis.

** Impaired glucose tolerance is diagnosed in the presence of both abnormal fasting glucose and 2-hour glucose concentrations.

***Source: data from World Health Organization. (2006). *Definition and diagnosis of diabetes mellitus and intermediate hyperglycaemia*. WHO, Geneva; World Health Organization. (2011). *Use of glycated haemoglobin (HbA1c) in the diagnosis of diabetes mellitus*. WHO, Geneva.

3 World Health Organization (2006). *Definition and diagnosis of diabetes mellitus and intermediate hyperglycaemia*. WHO, Geneva.

Contributing causes and clinical consequences

Contributing causes

Type 1 diabetes

Insulin secretion by the pancreatic β-cells is ↓ following damage mediated by an autoimmune T-cell reaction. Genetic factors and environmental factors, such as viral infections, may be implicated.

Type 2 diabetes

Type 2 diabetes is closely associated with obesity and genetic factors. Approximately 15–30% of first-degree relatives of people with type 2 diabetes develop impaired glucose tolerance or diabetes. However, the substantial contribution made by obesity is particularly important as this is a potentially modifiable risk factor. Excess body fat, stored as lipid in adipocytes, is associated with ↑ concentration of circulating hormones, cytokines, and metabolic fuels (e.g. free fatty acids), which modulate the effect of insulin. Large adipocytes, especially in abdominal fat, are resistant to the lipolytic effects of insulin, which leads to further release of free fatty acids and ↑ in circulating concentrations. These changes inhibit the insulin signalling cascade, resulting in impaired glucose metabolism in skeletal muscle and stimulated hepatic gluconeogenesis with consequent hyperglycaemia.

Clinical consequences

Diabetes is associated with ↑ risk of morbidity, disability, and premature mortality. Long-term complications include macrovascular disease, leading to cardiovascular disease (CVD) and ↑ risk of stroke, and microvascular disease leading to retinopathy, nephropathy, and neuropathy. People with diabetes also have ↑ risk of suffering from infections, cataracts, depression, and sexual dysfunction. Studies have demonstrated that effective blood glucose control and management of CVD risk factors can ↓ the risk of these complications (see Box 22.2).

Box 22.2 Benefits of effective glycaemic control in diabetes

*Type 1 diabetes**

- Risk of new eye disease reduced by 76%
- Risk of nerve damage reduced by 60%
- Risk of death, non-fatal heart attack or stroke reduced by 57%
- Worsening of existing eye disease reduced by 54%
- Risk of kidney disease reduced by 50%
- Risk of cardiovascular events reduced by 42%

*Type 2 diabetes***

- Risk of microvascular disease reduced by 25%
- Risk of myocardial infarction reduced by 15%
- All-cause mortality reduced by 12%
- Any diabetes-related endpoint reduced by 12%

*Source: data from US Dept of Health and Human Services (2008). *DCCT and EDIC*. NIH Publication No 08-3874.

Source: data from Holman R *et al*. (2008). 10-year follow-up of intensive glucose control in type 2 diabetes. *N. Eng. J. Med.* **359:1577-89.

Targets

Glycaemic control

Glycated haemoglobin

In the UK, glycated haemoglobin (HbA1c) targets are <48 mmol/mol (6.5%) for adults and children with type 1 diabetes,[4,5] and for those with type 2, individualized targets of 48-59 mmol/mol (6.5-7.5%) are recommended.[6] Pregnant women with diabetes or gestational diabetes are advised to optimize glycaemic control, although HbA1c is not a reliable test during pregnancy.[7]

Self-blood glucose monitoring

Self-blood glucose monitoring (SBGM) is recommended at least four times daily in those with type 1 diabetes and more monitoring may be required when exercising, driving, in sickness, during pregnancy, and in those experiencing hypoglycaemia. Targets in the UK are:

- Children and adolescents with type 1 diabetes:[4]
  - on waking (fasting plasma glucose): 4-7 mmol/L;
  - before meals: 4-7 mmol/L;
  - after meals: 5-10 mmol/L.
- Adults with type 1 diabetes:[5]
  - on waking (fasting plasma glucose): 5-7 mmol/L;
  - before meals: 4-7 mmol/L;
  - ≥90 minutes postprandial: 5-9 mmol/L.
- During pregnancy:[7]
  - fasting: <5.3 mmol/L;
  - 1 hour post meal <7.8 mmol/L;
  - 2 hours post meal <6.4 mmol/L.

In the UK, it is no longer recommended that routine SBGM is offered to people with type 2 diabetes unless they are treated with insulin, have evidence of hypoglycaemia or are driving or operating machinery and take oral medication that increases the risk of hypoglycaemia. Women with type 2 diabetes planning pregnancy or who are pregnant should also have access to SBGM.

4 National Institute for Health and Care Excellence. (2015). *Diabetes (type 1 and type 2) in children and young people: diagnosis and management.* NG18. Available at: ℘ https://www.nice.org.uk/guidance/ng18.

5 National Institute for Health and Care Excellence. (2015). *Type 1 diabetes in adults: diagnosis and management.* NG17. Available at: ℘ https://www.nice.org.uk/guidance/ng17.

6 National Institute for Health and Care Excellence. (2015). *Type 2 diabetes in adults: management.* NG28. Available at: ℘ https://www.nice.org.uk/guidance/ng28.

7 National Institute for Health and Care Excellence. (2015). *Diabetes in pregnancy: management from preconception to the postnatal period.* NG3. Available at: ℘ https://www.nice.org.uk/guidance/ng3.

Co-morbidities

Adults with type 1 diabetes[5]

- Blood pressure <135/80 mm/Hg (or <130/80 mm/Hg for those w
  abnormal albumin excretion or ≥2 features of metabolic syndrome).
- No specific targets for lipid concentrations. Therapy should be offered
  to those aged ≥40 years, with established nephropathy or with ≥10%
  risk of CVD assessed by QRISK2 tool.

Adults with type 2 diabetes[6]

- Blood pressure <140/80 mm/Hg (or <130/80 mm/Hg in those with
  evidence of complications).
- No specific targets for lipid concentrations (aim should be lowest
  possible). Therapy should be offered to those with ≥10% risk of CVD
  assessed by QRISK2 tool (predictive algorithm).

Diabetes UK recommend the following lipid concentrations for people with
diabetes:[8]

- Total cholesterol <4.0 mmol/L
- LDL cholesterol <2.0 mmol/L
- HDL cholesterol ≥1.0 mmol/L in men and ≥1.2 mmol/L in women
- Triglycerides <1.7 mmol/L

8 Diabetes UK (2017). Testing. Available at: ℬ https://www.diabetes.org.uk/Guide-to-diabetes/
Monitoring/Testing/.

priorities for management

e 1 diabetes

ucation is a central part of management of type 1 diabetes for adults,
ildren, and young people, and dietary aspects play an important role.
Recommendations for dietary interventions include:

- offering nutritional information from diagnosis onwards;
- providing information that is sensitive and tailored to personal needs and culture, and that is delivered by professionals with specific and approved training;
- providing structured education, either as group sessions or to individuals;
- enabling people to make optimal choices about foods they consume;
- facilitating insulin dose changes according to carbohydrate intake;
- discuss timing and composition of snacks and issues associated with fasting and feasting;
- providing information about a cardioprotective diet;
- including information about excess weight, underweight, eating disorders, raised blood pressure, renal failure;
- reviewing education needs annually;
- providing ongoing education with access to information and opportunities for discussion at clinic visits.

Table 22.2 Key priorities for implementation in adults, children, and young people with type 1 diabetes

Adults*	Children and young people**
• Patient-centred care	• Patient-centred care
• Structured education	• Structured education
• Blood glucose management	• Insulin therapy
• Insulin therapy	• Dietary management
• Awareness and management of hypoglycaemia	• Glycaemic targets
• Care in hospital	• Hyperglycaemia and diabetic ketoacidosis
	• Psychological and social issues
	• Diabetic kidney disease

* National Institute for Health and Care Excellence (2015). *Type 1 diabetes in adults: diagnosis and management.* NG17. ♫ https://www.nice.org.uk/guidance/ng17

** National Institute for Health and Care Excellence (2015). *Diabetes (type 1 and type 2) in children and young people: diagnosis and management.* NG18. ♫ https://www.nice.org.uk/guidance/ng18; Smart, C.E., Annan, F., Bruno, L.P., et al. (2014). ISPAD Clinical Practice Consensus Guidelines 2014. *Pediatr. Diabetes* **15**, 135-53.

Type 2 diabetes

Recommendations for key priorities for implementation in adults include:[6]

- patient-centred care;
- structured education;
- dietary advice;
- blood pressure management;
- blood glucose management;
- drug treatment.

Structured education should be offered to all adults with type 2 diabetes incorporating dietary interventions that are recommended to:

- provide individualized dietary advice that is sensitive to the person's needs, culture, and beliefs, and which is delivered by a healthcare professional with specific expertise and competence in nutrition;
- emphasize healthy balanced eating including carbohydrate management;
- encourage weight loss in those who are overweight;
- limit amounts of sucrose-containing foods to <5% of total energy intake;
- discourage the use of so-called 'diabetic' foods.

Goals and principles of dietary management

Goals of dietary management

- Support self-management and maintain health through the use of appropriate and healthy food choices.
- Achieve individual targets for glycaemia, blood pressure, lipids, and body weight to delay or prevent complications of diabetes.
- Promote quality of life.
- Provide flexibility and meet the needs of all individuals, including those with co-morbidities such as coeliac disease and cystic fibrosis.

Dietary advice should be seen as part of the holistic context of care, which includes supporting patients to manage their diabetes and make their own decisions; it should also complement other treatment including pharmacological, physical activity, and behavioural and smoking cessation programs. If it is to be effective, dietary advice must take account of the individual's personal preferences, cultural background, and lifestyle.

Principles of dietary management

People with diabetes should not need to follow a 'special diet' or comply with narrow restrictions and measured portions of food that were considered central to dietary advice in previous years. However, diet and nutrition are key factors in diabetes control and they contribute to quality of life, general health, and improved long-term health outcomes. The optimum healthy choice of food for people with diabetes is similar to that recommended to the general population, although carbohydrate management is an additional key strategy for those with diabetes. Recommendations for healthful diets are now made in terms of foods, rather than nutrients, as it is widely recognized that there is little evidence for the optimum macronutrient content of the diet in people with diabetes (see Box 22.3).

All people with newly diagnosed diabetes should have access to dietary advice provided by a healthcare professional with appropriate skills and training, preferably a dietitian. Dietary education should be delivered as part of a structured education programme, whether in groups or individually. Further dietetic intervention should then be offered when required, e.g. at annual review or when deemed appropriate by another healthcare professional or the person with diabetes.

Ways to eat well with diabetes[9]

1. Eating regular meals including breakfast.
2. Keeping an eye on portion sizes to manage body weight.
3. Including some carbohydrate. Healthier sources include wholegrains, fruit, vegetables, legumes, and some dairy foods, e.g. milk, yogurt.
4. Reducing the amount of saturated or animal fat found in butter, red and processed meat products, palm oil, coconut oil, ghee, cakes, and pastries.

9 Diabetes UK (2017) *Ten ways to eat well with diabetes.* https://www.diabetes.org.uk/guide-to-diabetes/enjoy-food/eating-with-diabetes/10-ways-to-eat-well-with-diabetes

5. Including at least five portions of fruit and vegetables daily.
6. Reducing salt by adding less in cooking and at the table and eating fewer processed foods. Approximately 75% of salt eaten is found in processed foods.
7. Substituting fish for meat and aiming to eat two portions of oily fish each week.
8. Using more legumes such as beans, lentils and pulses.
9. Reducing sugar intake by keeping sugary foods and drinks to an occasional treat.

Box 22.3 Key recommendations for a healthy eating pattern[10]

A healthy eating pattern includes:
- A variety of different vegetables
- Fruit, especially whole fruit
- Wholegrains
- Low fat dairy products
- Seafood, lean meat, poultry, and eggs
- Nuts, seeds, and legumes (beans and peas)
- Vegetable oils

A healthy eating pattern limits:
- Red and processed meats
- Refined carbohydrate foods
- Sugar, especially sugar-sweetened beverages

Carbohydrate management

Adopting a healthy eating pattern is recommended for long-term health, but for people with diabetes, carbohydrate management is also a key strategy for glycaemic control. Both the quantity and the quality of carbohydrate influence blood glucose concentrations, but the total amount of carbohydrate eaten is the main predictor of postprandial glycaemic response. Adults, children, and young people with type 1 diabetes are advised to adopt carbohydrate counting and insulin dose adjustment to manage postprandial glucose excursions, and it is recommended that this is delivered as part of structured education. For those with type 2 diabetes, general carbohydrate monitoring and management is recommended. In terms of the quality of carbohydrate, people with diabetes are advised to adopt the healthy eating patterns described above and include unrefined, unprocessed, wholegrain carbohydrates (wholegrains, vegetables, fruit, legumes, and pulses) and restrict refined (white bread, white rice, pasta) and sugary carbohydrates. Recent recommendations for free sugars (those added during processing, preparation and cooking) for the general population have advised that they

10 Mozaffarian, D. (2016). Dietary and policy priorities for cardiovascular disease, diabetes, and obesity: A comprehensive review. *Circulation* 133, 187–225.

should be limited to <5% total energy intake, and this applies equally to people with diabetes.[11]

Glycaemic index

Glycaemic index (GI) is a term designed to give an indication of the blood glucose response to different types of carbohydrate (see ➔ Chapter 5 'Glycaemic index'). Low GI foods reduce the degree of post-prandial hyperglycaemia and associated insulin secretion and should be of benefit to people with diabetes. There has been controversy over the use of GI and its role in diabetes, and although it is still recommended in some parts of the world, e.g. Australia, it is no longer generally considered an effective strategy. In the UK it is positively discouraged by NICE for adults with type 1 diabetes and for those with type 2 it is regarded as a useful adjunct but should not be relied on as a primary strategy for glycaemic control.

11 World Health Organization. (2015). *Sugars intake for adults and children*. WHO, Geneva. Available at: ⌕http://www.who.int/nutrition/publications/guidelines/sugars_intake/en/.

Management of type 1 diabetes

Insulin therapy

Insulin therapy delivered by multiple daily doses of injected insulin (MDI) or by continuous subcutaneous insulin infusion (CSSI or pump therapy) is the treatment for type 1 diabetes. It is recommended that the choice of insulin regimen should take into account the person's lifestyle, culture, and habits, although as carbohydrate counting and insulin adjustment are recommended for all with type 1 diabetes, most people are encouraged to start with MDI. There are many different types of insulin available and their characteristics are summarized in Table 22.3. Insulin is derived from three sources; animal insulin (porcine and bovine), which is now rarely prescribed; human insulin produced by recombinant DNA technology; and analogue insulin produced by modifying human insulin. Analogue insulins are widely recommended as they more closely match the profile of endogenous insulin.

Insulin regimens

MDI commonly consists of one or two daily injections of slow-acting background or basal insulin and three or more injections of rapid-acting prandial or bolus insulin taken with meals and snacks. Less commonly, two injections of mixed insulin are used, usually taken before breakfast and before the evening meal. Rapid-acting analogue insulin is used in pump therapy. Insulin therapy is associated with a risk of hypoglycaemia and education about and management of hypoglycaemia should be addressed, preferably within structured education programmes.

Insulin dosing

Children and adults with type 1 diabetes are encouraged to match prandial insulin to carbohydrate on a meal-by-meal basis. Carbohydrate counting should be facilitated as part of a structured education course, and this can be supported by the use of apps and reference books. There is variation in individual carbohydrate:insulin ratios, although many adults take one unit of insulin for every 10-15 g carbohydrate eaten. Ratios vary more in children and are often subject to great change during adolescence. In addition, a correction factor can be applied if blood glucose concentrations are out of target before a meal. Considerations for adjusting insulin dose are shown in Box 22.4.

CSSI (pump) therapy

Pumps use fast-acting analogue insulin administered as a basal rate providing background insulin, together with a bolus of insulin delivered with food. Many of the newer pumps are able to calculate the required dose of insulin based upon pre-programmed insulin: carbohydrate ratio and preprandial blood glucose level. Pumps offer flexibility in dosing by:

• delivering insulin in 0.1 unit increments;
• offering different bolus dosing including:
  • standard bolus where the total amount of insulin is delivered in a single dose. This may not match foods eaten over a long period of time, or those that are digested slowly, e.g. pizza;

Table 22.3 Examples of commonly used insulin

Type	Examples	Onset (mins)	Peak (hours)	Duration (hours)
Prandial/bolus:				
Human	Actrapid® (Novo Nordisk)	30	1-3	6-8
	Humulin S® (Lilly)			
Analogue	NovoRapid® (aspart, Novo Nordisk)	5	1-1.5	3-5
	Humalog® (lispro, Lilly)			
	Apidra® (glulisine, Sanofi)			
Basal/background:				
Human	Insulatard® (Novo Nordisk)	90-120	5-8	12-24
	Humulin I® (Lilly)			
	Insuman Basal® (Sanofi)			
Analogue	Levemir® (detemir, Novo Nordisk)	Flat	Flat	18-24
	Lantus® (glargine, Sanofi)			
	Abasaglar® (glargine, Lilly)			
	Degludec® (tresiba, Novo Nordisk)	Flat	Flat	42
Mixed insulin:				
Human	Humulin M3® (Lilly)	30	2-8	12-24
	Insuman Comb 15/25/30® (Sanofi)			
Analogue	NovoMix 30® (Novo Nordisk)	12-20	1-4	18-20
	Humalog Mix 25/30® (Lilly)			

Box 22.4 **Practical considerations for insulin dose adjustment**[12,13]

Meal-time dosing

Amount

- Calculate amount of carbohydrate in each meal and administer insulin according to individual ratio.
- Reduce or increase amount of insulin according to preprandial blood glucose concentrations and individual correction factor.
- To improve glycaemic control, account should be taken of previous bolus doses of insulin (often called active insulin or insulin on-board). Bolus calculators in pumps and smart blood glucose meters are useful to calculate total bolus insulin dose.

Timing

- Human insulin should be injected 30 minutes before eating; this limits the flexibility of carbohydrate counting.
- Analogue insulin is most effective when administered immediately before eating, even when preprandial blood glucose concentrations are lower than target, but can be administered after eating when:
  - toddlers and small children have erratic appetite and eating habits;
  - eating out, where there is uncertainty about the amount of carbohydrate in the meal;
  - a very high fat or low GI meal is eaten.

Dosing for snacks

- Between-meal snacks are generally considered unnecessary to prevent hypoglycaemia in people using analogue insulin, snacking depends on personal preference.
- A snack before bed is generally considered unnecessary in those using long-acting analogue insulin.
- In the absence of hypoglycaemia, snacks providing >15 g carbohydrate usually require an insulin bolus.

Insulin adjustment for exercise

- To avoid the risk of hypoglycaemia during and after exercise, the following strategies can be employed:
  - reduce pre-exercise dose of prandial insulin.
  - take additional carbohydrate (without insulin) during exercise.
- Reduce basal insulin following exercise.

12 Annan, F. (2016). What matters for calculating insulin bolus dose? *Diabetes Technol. Ther.* **18**, 203–5

13 Gallen, I.W., *et al.* (2011). Fuelling the athlete with type 1 diabetes. *Diabetes Obes. Metab.* **13**, 130–6.

- extended or square wave bolus, where the insulin is delivered evenly over a defined period of time (30 minutes to several hours). This is useful when eating continually over a period of time, although the total amount of carbohydrate must be calculated before setting the bolus;
- dual or multi-wave bolus which is useful for meals with large amounts of carbohydrate or high fat foods and where 50% of the calculated dose is given with food and the remainder using an extended bolus.

Management of type 2 diabetes

Hypoglycaemic agents

Algorithms for treating type 2 diabetes using oral hypoglycaemic agents have been published, but all stages of therapy are underpinned by lifestyle modification, including weight management, dietary change, and physical activity.[14] Table 22.4 summarizes the action of commonly used hypoglycaemic agents. Type 2 diabetes is seen as a progressive condition and most people require a combination of oral and injectable therapies to achieve therapeutic targets. In response to the need for combination therapy, some combined formula medications are now available, including metformin in combination with pioglitazone, metformin with dipeptidyl peptidase-4 (DPP-4) inhibitors and metformin in combination with sodium-glucose linked transporter SGLT-2 inhibitors. In addition, mixed injection therapy has been developed combining fixed doses of insulin and glucagon-like peptide GLP-1 receptor agonists.

14 Inzucchi, S.E., et al. (2015). Management of hyperglycaemia in type 2 diabetes, 2015: a patient-centred approach. Update to a position statement of the American Diabetes Association and the European Association for the Study of Diabetes. *Diabetologia* **58**, 429–42.

Table 22.4 Hypoglycaemic agents

Type of agent	Examples	Mode of action
Oral agents		
Biguanide	Metformin	Increases insulin sensitivity and suppresses gluconeogenesis
Sulfonylurea	Gliclazide, glipizide, glibenclamide	Stimulates insulin secretion
Prandial glucose regulator	Nateglinide, repaglinide	Stimulates insulin secretion
α-glucosidase inhibitor	Acarbose	Slows down digestion and absorption of carbohydrate
Thiazolidinedione	Pioglitazone	Increases insulin sensitivity and suppresses gluconeogenesis
SGLT-2 inhibitor	Canagliflozin, dapagliflozin, empagliflozin	Promotes excretion of glucose in the urine by preventing reabsorption in the kidney
Dipeptidyl peptidase-4 DDP-4 inhibitor	Alogliptin, linagliptin, saxagliptin, sitagliptin, vildagliptin	Increases insulin secretion in a glucose-dependent manner and suppresses gluconeogenesis
Injectable agents		
Incretin mimetics (GLP-1 receptor agonists)	Exenatide, liraglutide, dulaglutide, albiglutide	
Insulin (Table 22.3)		

Hypoglycaemia

Hypoglycaemia in people with diabetes is defined as a blood glucose concentration <4 mmol/L.

Causes
- Excess insulin or oral insulin secretagogues (sulfonylurea or prandial glucose regulator)
- Insufficient carbohydrate intake
- Missed or delayed meal or snack
- Increased physical activity
- Alcohol

Symptoms
Early symptoms are associated with release of counter-regulatory hormones in response to low blood glucose concentrations and include:
- Hunger
- Sweating
- Tingling lips
- Dizziness or light-headedness
- Tiredness or fatigue
- Blurred vision
- Trembling or shakiness
- Pallor

More advanced symptoms are associated with lack of glucose in the brain and include:
- Irritability
- Difficulty concentrating
- Confusion
- Disorderly or irrational behaviour
- May lead to coma or (rarely) death

Treatment
Hypoglycaemia should be treated immediately in the conscious patient by:
1. Oral administration of 15-20 g fast-acting glucose;
2. Re-testing blood glucose concentrations after 15 minutes to check they are rising;
3. If no change, or concentrations still decreasing, repeat treatment;
4. An extra 15-20 g carbohydrate from any source may be necessary if next meal is not due;
5. Insulin may need to be reduced at next meal.

Hypoglycaemia should not be treated orally in the unconscious patient, either a glucagon injection should be administered or an ambulance called.

Box 22.5 Sources of 15 g fast-acting carbohydrate for hypoglycaemia treatment
- Five small or four large glucose tablets
- Five jelly babies, fruit pastilles, or wine gums
- 10 jelly beans
- 150 mL (mini can) cola
- 170 mL Lucozade*

* Formula revised April 2017.

Structured education in diabetes

Structured education provides training and learning opportunities for people with diabetes and their family, and has an evidence-based curriculum which suits the needs of individuals.[15] Specific aims and learning objectives support people to develop attitudes, beliefs, knowledge, and skills to enable them to self-manage diabetes. The programmes are delivered by trained educators, and are quality assured and regularly audited.

Structured diabetes education and self-management (DESM) is effective for people with both type 1 and type 2 diabetes. In type 1 diabetes, DESM has been reported to improve glycaemic control, quality of life, and diabetes distress, and reduce the risk of severe hypoglycaemia and diabetic keto-acidosis.[16] For those with type 2 diabetes, DESM resulted in improved biomedical, lifestyle, and psychosocial outcomes when compared to standard care.[17] DESM is cost-effective for both type 1 and type 2 diabetes.[18,19]

In the UK, DESM is recommended at diagnosis by NICE,[5,6] and the importance of ongoing education is emphasized. There are guidelines available for the key components of DESM in the UK,[20] and accreditation of programmes is recommended.[21] Accredited courses include DAFNE, DESMOND, and the X-PERT programme, although there are many smaller, local programmes.

Further information is available at: ℅ http://www.diabetes-education.net.

15 National Institute for Health and Care Excellence. (2016). Quality statement 3: Structured education programmes for adults with type 1 diabetes. Available at: ℅https://www.nice.org.uk/guidance/qs6/chapter/Quality-statement-3-Structured-education-programmes-for-adults-with-type-1-diabetes.

16 Speight J., et al. (2010). Long-term biomedical and psychosocial outcomes following DAFNE structured education to promote intensive insulin therapy in adults with sub-optimally controlled type 1 diabetes. Diabetes Res. Clin. Prac. **89**, 22–9.

17 Steinsbekk, A., et al. (2012). Group based diabetes self-management education compared to routine treatment for people with type 2 diabetes mellitus. A systematic review with meta-analysis. BMC Health Serv. Res. **12**, 213.

18 Kruger, J., et al. (2013). The cost-effectiveness of the Dose Adjustment for Normal Eating (DAFNE) structured education programme: an update using the Sheffield Type 1 Diabetes Policy Model. Diabet. Med. **30**, 1236–44.

19 Lian, J.X., et al. (2017). Systematic review on the cost-effectiveness of self-management education programme for type 2 diabetes mellitus. Diabetes Res. Clin. Pract. **127**, 21–34.

20 Department of Health and Diabetes UK. (2005). Structured Patient Education in Diabetes. Diabetes UK and DOH, London.

21 Quality Institute for Self-Management Education and Training. (2017). Certification. Available at: ℅ http://www.qismet.org.uk/certification/.

Weight management

There is little published evidence of the prevalence of overweight in people with type 1 diabetes or for the efficacy of weight loss. Approximately 86% of people with type 2 diabetes are overweight or obese and there is strong evidence for the benefits of weight loss, including improvements in glycaemic control, quality of life, mobility, sleep apnoea, depression, sexual function, reductions in cardiovascular risk, and even a suggestion that dietary restriction and weight loss can induce remission of diabetes.[22]

Multicomponent strategies, incorporating diet, physical activity, and behavioural approaches are recommended, although there is little evidence for the most effective diet for weight loss.[23] Evidence suggests that a range of dietary strategies, including low fat, low carbohydrate, high protein, and high monounsaturated fat diets, are effective and that the degree of adherence predicts outcomes rather than a specific diet. Both NICE and Diabetes UK state that any dietary, pharmaceutical, or surgical strategy that is currently recommended for people without diabetes is appropriate for those with diabetes (see ➔ Chapter 21 'Obesity', p. 477).

Realistic weight loss targets of 5-10% initial weight are advocated, as 2-5% weight loss lowers HbA1c by 2-3 mmol/mol (0.2-0.3%) and 5-10% weight loss is associated with reductions of 7-11 mol/mol (0.6-1.0%).[24]

22 Wilding, J. (2014). The importance of weight management in type 2 diabetes mellitus. *Int. J. Clin. Pract.* **68**, 682–91.

23 Diabetes UK. (2011). *Evidence-based nutrition guidelines for the prevention and management of diabetes.* Available at: ✍ https://www.diabetes.org.uk/Documents/Reports/nutritional-guidelines-2013-amendment-0413.pdf.

24 Franz, M.J., et al. (2015). Lifestyle weight-loss intervention outcomes in overweight and obese adults with type 2 diabetes: a systematic review and meta-analysis of randomized clinical trials. *J. Acad. Nutr. Diet.* **115**, 1447–63.

Diabetes in pregnancy, children, and young people

Diabetes in pregnancy

In the UK, it is estimated that approximately 5% of all pregnancies occur in women with diabetes, with gestational diabetes (GDM) accounting for 87.5% of these pregnancies, women with type 1 diabetes for 7.5% and women with type 2 diabetes for 5%.[7] Gestational diabetes has increased by 30% over the past decade and the International Diabetes Federation estimated that global prevalence of hyperglycaemia in pregnancy was 16.9% in 2013.[25] Increases in GDM are related to changes in diagnostic thresholds, screening criteria, and an increasing prevalence of overweight and obesity. GDM is more common in women whose family origins are South Asian, Chinese, Afro-Caribbean, or Middle Eastern.

Preconception care for women with diagnosed diabetes

Preconception care, including the following components is associated with improved pregnancy outcomes:
- Optimize glycaemic control, aim for HbA1c 48 mmol/mol (6.5%).
- Weight management for women with BMI >27 kg/m^2 to achieve acceptable weight before pregnancy.
- Folic acid supplementation (5 mg/day) before pregnancy until 12 weeks gestation.

Care during pregnancy

Women with diagnosed diabetes

Dietary advice from a dietitian is recommended to achieve adequate nutritional intake, optimal glycaemic control and appropriate weight gain.

Women with GDM

GDM is associated with adverse maternal and fetal outcomes, and lifestyle interventions are first-line therapy. Recommendations include:[7]
- referral to a dietitian;
- individualized diet and exercise advice;
- advice about a healthy diet including:
  - replacing high GI with low GI carbohydrates;
  - maintaining high intake of fruit and vegetables;
  - including lower fat protein foods;
  - substituting unsaturated (either polyunsaturated or monounsaturated) for saturated fat;
- regular exercise, including walking for 30 minutes after a meal to lower postprandial glucose concentrations.

25 Guariguata, L., et al. (2014). Global estimates of the prevalence of hyperglycaemia in pregnancy. *Diab. Res. Clin. Prac.* **103**, 176–85.

Postnatal care

Breastfeeding should be encouraged in all women. Women with type 1 diabetes are at increased risk of hypoglycaemia during breastfeeding and may need snacks before or during feeds. Women with GDM who are able to breastfeed immediately after delivery may reduce the risk of neonatal hypoglycaemia. Breastfeeding should be continued for at least 3 months to reduce the risk of childhood obesity (see ➔ Chapter 13, 'Breast versus bottle feeding', p. 262). Women with previous GDM have an increased lifetime risk of development of type 2 diabetes and their children are at higher risk of developing childhood obesity, therefore postpartum advice on lifestyle modification and regular monitoring is recommended.

Diabetes in children and young people

Management of diabetes in children and young people aims to optimize glycaemic control, reduce the risk of diabetes complications, and there is additional emphasis on providing sufficient energy and nutrients for optimal growth. Recommendations for those with type 1 diabetes include:[26]

- multi-disciplinary team approach, including a specialist paediatric dietitian;
- adaptable, flexible dietary advice that is reviewed regularly;
- energy intakes allowing for optimal growth while maintaining target blood glucose levels and minimizing the risk of overweight and obesity;
- no specific carbohydrate restriction but emphasis on unprocessed, unrefined, or wholegrain carbohydrate and limited amounts of free sugars, especially sugar-sweetened beverages;
- balanced diet as recommended for the general population providing adequate protein, fat, vitamins, and minerals;
- promoting physical activity with care planning to avoid hypoglycaemia.

Type 2 diabetes is increasing in children, although it is rarely diagnosed before puberty. The true prevalence is unknown, in the UK in 2016 it was estimated that ~1,200 young people were living with type 2 diabetes.[27] Type 2 diabetes in children is strongly associated with obesity and is more common in non-white ethnic groups and in females. It is recommended that lifestyle change is initiated at diagnosis aiming for weight loss with a combination of diet and physical activity.[28]

26 Smart, C.E., et al. (2014). ISPAD Clinical Practice Consensus Guidelines 2014. *Pediatr. Diabetes* 15, 135–53.

27 Royal College of Paediatrics and Child Health. (2016). *National Paediatric Diabetes Report* Available at: ℜ http://www.rcpch.ac.uk/improving-child-health/quality-improvement-and-clinical-audit/national-paediatric-diabetes-audit-n-0.

28 Zeitler, P., et al. (2014). ISPAD Clinical Practice Consensus Guidelines 2014. Type 2 diabetes in the child and adolescent. *Pediatr. Diabetes* 15(Suppl 20), 26–46.

Diabetes in the elderly

Age is a recognized risk factor for type 2 diabetes, and prevalence rates are higher in those aged >65 years. General growth and ageing of the population has led to estimates that the number of people with type 2 diabetes will increase by 20% in high income countries. Physiological changes associated with ageing such as abdominal obesity, high BMI, reduced physical activity, and poor nutrition are all associated with increased risk, and additional psychosocial factors such as depression, illness, stress, and lower social support also contribute. Nutritional status may be compromised as people age, and undernutrition is a key feature. There are challenges meeting the increased requirements for protein and some vitamins and minerals as appetite and food intake generally decrease. Individualized advice is recommended to maintain adequate dietary intake and appropriate levels of physical activity.

Further information

Goff, L., Dyson, P. (Ed) (2016). *Advanced Nutrition and Dietetics in Diabetes*. Wiley Blackwell, Chichester.

Nutrition guidelines

Diabetes UK evidence-based nutrition guidelines for the prevention and management of diabetes. Available at: ℑ https://www.diabetes.org.uk/nutrition-guidelines.

Evert, A.B., Boucher, J.L., Cypress, M., et al. (2013). Nutrition therapy recommendations for the management of adults with diabetes. *Diabetes Care*. 36, 3821–42.

Structured education

The UK Diabetes Education Network: ℑ www.diabetes-education.net.

Dose Adjustment for Normal Eating (DAFNE): ℑ www.dafne.uk.com.

Diabetes Education and Self-Management for Ongoing and Newly Diagnosed Diabetes (DESMOND): ℑ www.desmond-project.org.uk.

The X-PERT programme: ℑ www.xperthealth.org.uk.

Other information

Glycaemic index: ℑ www.glycemicindex.com.

Carbohydrate counting: ℑ www.carbsandcals.com.

Cardiovascular disease

Classification, prevalence, and contributing causes *520*
Cardioprotective diet *524*
Familial hypercholesterolaemia *528*
Heart failure *530*
Stroke, including dysphagia *532*
Hypertension *538*
Peripheral arterial disease *540*

Classification, prevalence, and contributing causes

Classification
Cardiovascular disease (CVD) includes the following.
- *Coronary heart disease:* narrowing of the lumen of arteries supplying blood to the heart muscle as a result of atheromatous plaque on the arterial walls. This limits the blood supply to the heart muscle causing pain (angina) and breathlessness on exertion. Damaged plaque leads to a clotting response, which may result in a thrombus detaching from the artery wall and occluding the lumen with subsequent heart muscle death (myocardial infarction).
- *Cerebral infarction:* thrombus occlusion of an artery supplying blood to the brain leading to irreversible damage to brain tissue (stroke or transient ischaemic attack). The thrombus may arise from atheromatous plaque from within the brain or another blood vessel and the risk of occlusion is ↑ in narrowed arteries.
- *Peripheral arterial disease:* atheromatous plaque leads to narrowing of peripheral blood vessels, most commonly in the legs. This results in poor blood supply and pain on exertion (claudication).

Prevalence
Globally, CVD is the greatest cause of death, 17.7 million (31%) per year, and >75% of these deaths occur in low and middle income countries. The prevalence is increasing in countries adopting an unhealthy lifestyle (see Box 23.1 for risk factors), and with rates rising rapidly in developing countries in parallel with obesity, urbanization, and longevity (Fig. 23.1). The greatest ↑ in premature CVD deaths in the last 20 years have been reported from East, South, and South-East Asia, and parts of central America. In contrast, a substantial ↓ in premature CVD deaths has been reported from Eastern Europe following rapid ↑ during the previous decade; in spite of this, CVD mortality remains high.[1]

In the UK, CVD is the cause of death of 0.16 million (26%) patients per year. The CVD mortality rate has fallen in the UK since peak levels in the early 1970s, because of improvements in prevention, diagnosis, and treatment and ↓ prevalence of smoking, although CVD remains the second most common cause of death (Table 23.1).

CVD prevalence is higher in men than women before the menopause and increases with age. It is higher in central Scotland, the north of England, and south Wales compared to the south of England, and is higher than average in lower socio-economic groups and South Asians.

1 Roth, G.A., *et al.* (2015). Global and regional patterns in cardiovascular mortality from 1990 to 2013. *Circulation* **132**, 1667–78.

Box 23.1 Risk factors for CVD[2]

Non-modifiable risk factors include

- Increasing age
- Male gender
- Females (post-menopause)
- Family history
- Ethnic background (people of South Asian origin are at higher risk than those of European origin)

Modifiable risk factors include

- Smoking
- ↓ Serum HDL cholesterol
- ↑ Serum total cholesterol
- ↑ Serum LDL cholesterol
- Sedentary lifestyle/physical inactivity
- Unhealthy diet
- Alcohol intake above recommended levels
- Overweight and obesity

Co-morbidities* that increase CVD risk include:

- High blood pressure
- Diabetes and pre-diabetes
- Dyslipidaemia (familial and non-familial)
- Atrial fibrillation
- Systemic inflammatory disorders, e.g. rheumatoid arthritis
- Obesity, especially if associated with sleep apnoea
- Influenza
- Serious mental health problems
- Periodontal disease

Other factors to consider when assessing risk

- ↓ Socio-economic status
- Ratio of blood apolipoprotein B100 to apolipoprotein A1†
- C-reactive protein†
- Fibrinogen†
- Lipoprotein (a)†

*Some risk factors, such as these co-morbidities, do not fit neatly into the categories of modifiable or non-modifiable.

†Not routinely used to assess risk of CVD in the UK.

2 National Institute of Care and Health Excellence (NICE). (2014). *CVD risk assessment and management*. Available at: ℞ https://cks.nice.org.uk/cvd-risk-assessment-and-management#!backgroundsub:2.

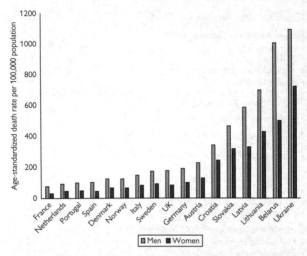

Fig. 23.1 Age-standardized death rates per 100,000 population from ischaemic heart disease in men and women of all ages in selected European countries (most recent data). Data from European Heart Network. (2017). *European cardiovascular disease statistics.* ✍ http://www.ehnheart.org/cvd-statistics.html.

Table 23.1 Deaths and morbidity from circulatory system disease and coronary heart disease in the UK*

	Number (%)	
	Male	Female
Circulatory system deaths, all	80,105 (27%)	78,050 (25%)
Coronary heart disease	41,959 (14%)	27,826 (9%)
Inpatient episodes, coronary heart disease	318,163	162,421

*British Heart Foundation. (2017). ✍ https://www.bhf.org.uk/research/heart-statistics.

Cardioprotective diet

Dietary advice[3] for cardiovascular risk is associated with health benefits in healthy adults. Two evidence-based aspects are important: (a) the content, i.e. optimum nutrient/food intake; and (b) the delivery, i.e. a behaviour change approach.

Nutrient/food intake

Public health guidelines[4] on cardiovascular prevention focus on addressing lifestyle including diet and accessibility to healthy food with two main nutrient targets:

- reducing salt intake to <6 g/day (target is <3 g by 2025);
- reducing saturated fat intake to <11% of food energy intake.

These targets are included in nutritional recommendations for the general population and with UK food-based guidelines, the Eatwell Guide (see ➔ Chapter 2 'Food-based dietary guidelines', p. 27).

Clinical guidelines[5] for people at high risk of, or with, CVD advise:

- total fat intake to ≤30% of total energy intake;
- saturated fat intake to ≤7% of total energy intake;
- dietary cholesterol <300 mg/day.

Table 23.2 describes foods that contribute to a cardioprotective diet. These are compatible with the concept of a Mediterranean diet, which is described as cardioprotective and associated with multiple health benefits[6] (Box 23.2).

Which type of fat is best?

Although there is strong evidence to support ↓ saturated fat intake, evidence[7] is less clear about what should replace this, i.e. polyunsaturated (PUFA) or monounsaturated (MUFA) fat or carbohydrate (see ➔ Chapter 6 'Fats'). However, cardioprotective diets should not focus on a single nutrient, i.e. just fat, but include a wide range of foods that people enjoy and which help to maintain ideal body weight (see ➔ Table 4.8 International BMI classification).

Oily fish and omega-3

After myocardial infarction, people are no longer advised to eat two to four portions of oily fish per week or to take omega-3 supplements

3 Rees, K., et al. (2013). Dietary advice for reducing cardiovascular risk. *Cochrane Database Syst. Rev.* CD002128.pub5.

4 National Institute of Health and Care Excellence (NICE). (2010). *Cardiovascular disease prevention.* Public health guideline PH25. Available at: ℵ https://www.nice.org.uk/guidance/ph25.

5 National Institute of Health and Care Excellence (NICE) (2016). *Cardiovascular disease: risk assessment and reduction, including lipid modification.* Clinical guideline CG181. Available at: ℵ https://www.nice.org.uk/guidance/cg181.

6 Dinu, M., et al. (2017). Mediterranean diet and multiple health outcomes: an umbrella review of meta-analyses of observational studies and randomised trials. *Eur. J. Clin. Nutr.* **72**(1), 30-43.

7 Hooper, L., et al. (2015). Reductions in saturated fat intake for cardiovascular disease. *Cochrane Database Syst. Rev.* CD011737.

as there is no strong evidence of either cardioprotective benefit or harm.[8,9]

Eggs

Blood cholesterol levels respond more to dietary intake of saturated fat than to dietary cholesterol. An average hen's egg contains approximately 190 mg of cholesterol and previous advice has been to limit intake to less than two eggs per week. A recent meta-analysis[10] has reported no ↑ CVD risk associated with consuming one egg daily compared with less than two per week. Eggs are nutritious, and consuming one daily is compatible with a cardioprotective diet.

Delivery of cardioprotective advice

The delivery of advice should not simply provide information but should follow a set of principles[11] that will help people change their behaviour and adopt a healthier lifestyle. This might include assessing readiness to change, motivational interviewing, goal-setting, empowering, and, importantly, should listen to the individual and consider their specific needs (see ➔ Chapter 17 'Nutrition interventions with patients and individuals', (see p. 365).

Considering that the prevalence of CVD is higher in lower socio-economic groups and in certain ethnic groups and geographical regions, the advice given must be tailored to the target individual or group's needs so that it is practical and culturally appropriate. Individuals who have either suffered recently from myocardial infarction or other CVD event or have a close family member who has, are often more amenable to acting on dietary advice.

Registered dietitians are well-trained to deliver cardioprotective dietary interventions but where access is limited, their workload should be prioritized to:

- optimize the advice provided by other health professionals, e.g. cardiac rehabilitation nurses, practice nurses, etc.;
- support individuals who are struggling with dietary advice or who have other medical conditions, e.g. diabetes;
- provide high quality written information to all people with CVD.

8 National Institute of Health and Care Excellence (NICE). (2013). *Myocardial infarction: cardiac rehabilitation and prevention of further cardiovascular disease.* Clinical guideline CG172. Available at: ℜ https://www.nice.org.uk/guidance/cg172.

9 Abdelhamid, A.S., *et al.* (2018). Omega-3 fatty acids for the primary and secondary prevention of cardiovascular disease. *Cochrane Database Syst. Rev.* 7, CD003177. DOI: 10.1002/14651858. CD003177.pub3.

10 Alexander, D.D., *et al.* (2016). Meta-analysis of egg consumption and risk of coronary heart disease and stroke. *J. Am. Coll. Nutr.* 35, 704–16.

11 National Institute of Health and Care Excellence (NICE) (2014). *Behaviour change: individual approaches.* Public health guideline PH49. Available at: ℜ https://www.nice.org.uk/guidance/ph49.

Table 23.2 Cardioprotective diet for those at risk from or with CVD[12]

Foods/nutrients*	Details
Fruit and vegetables	Five or more portions per day
Fish	Two portions per week, including one of oily fish
Nuts, seeds, and legumes	Four or more portions per week; choose unsalted nuts
Fat	Limit amount of all fat eaten, e.g. select lean meat and lower fat dairy products, use ↓ oil and fat in cooking, ↓ full fat spreads, eat ↓ fried food and high fat foods such as cakes, biscuits, pastries, and savoury snacks
Oils and spreads	Choose plant-based oils/spreads that are ↑ in mono- or polyunsaturates and ↓ in saturates, e.g. olive, rapeseed, or sunflower oil
Plant stanols and sterols	Not recommended
Salt	Reduce intake by using ↓ at table and in cooking and by eating ↓ processed foods
Starchy food	Choose wholegrain varieties of starchy foods, e.g. wholemeal or granary bread, oats, high fibre breakfast cereals
Sugar	Limit intake of sugar and foods containing refined sugars including fructose
Alcohol	Keep to lower risk alcohol guidelines, i.e. ≤14 units per week for men and women
Energy intake	Limit energy intake if overweight or obese

*These focus on key aspects of a cardioprotective diet and are not a comprehensive list of all foods.

Box 23.2 A Mediterranean diet is not a single entity, but includes:
- More oily fish and less meat
- Fresh fruit and vegetables
- Olive oil rather than saturated animal fats
- Wholegrains
- Legumes (pulses), nuts, and seeds
- Red wine in moderate amounts

12 British Dietetic Association. (2017). *Heart health*. Available at: ℘ https://www.bda.uk.com/foodfacts/hearthealth.pdf.

Other lifestyle interventions

Dietary advice should be given in conjunction with guidance/support about other aspects of life including:[5]

- promotion of physical activity:
  - ≥150 minutes of moderate intensity aerobic activity weekly *or* 75 minutes of vigorous intensity aerobic activity *or* a mix of moderate and vigorous aerobic activity
  - muscle-strengthening activities on ≥2 days/week
  - if unable to perform moderate intensity physical activity because of co-morbidity, medical conditions, or personal circumstances, to exercise at their maximum safe capacity;
- smoking cessation;
- stress management.

Familial hypercholesterolaemia

Diagnosis

A diagnosis of familial hypercholesterolaemia (FH) should be suspected in adults with a total cholesterol level >7.5 mmol/L and/or a personal or family history of premature coronary heart disease, i.e. an event before aged 60 years in index individual or first-degree relative.[13] A diagnosis of FH should be made using the Simon Broome criteria which include a combination of family history, clinical signs (specifically tendon xanthomata), cholesterol concentration (see Table 23.3), and DNA testing (see appendix ➔ of the NICE guideline[14]).

Management

Lifestyle advice should be a component of management offered by the multi-disciplinary team, but is not an alternative to the lipid-modifying drug therapy described below. In addition to discouraging smoking, patients with FH should be offered the following:

- Individualized dietary advice provided by an appropriate healthcare professional with nutrition expertise, e.g. registered dietitian.
- A ↓ fat diet compatible with the 'Eatwell Guide' (see ➔ Chapter 2, p. 27), which includes ≤30% energy from fat and ≤10% energy from saturated fat.
- Monounsaturated and polyunsaturated fats should be used to replace saturated fat.
- Dietary cholesterol intake should be limited to ≤300 mg/day.
- Eat at least five portions of fruit and vegetables each day.
- Eat at least two portions of fish per week, including at least one oily fish. For women who are pregnant or trying to conceive, see ➔ Chapter 12 'Eating fish in pregnancy', p. 242.
- Advise people who wish to take food products containing stanols and sterols that they need to be taken consistently to be effective.
- Do not routinely advise people to take omega 3 supplements.
- Alcohol intake should be limited to lower risk levels, i.e. ≤14 units per week, and binge drinking of alcohol avoided.
- Weight management advice should be offered to those who are overweight or obese (see ➔ Chapter 21, 'Weight management', p. 477).
- For people with FH who have already had a myocardial infarction, dietary advice should be in line with a cardioprotective diet, see ➔ this chapter, Table 23.2.
- Advise >30 minutes of physical activity/day. This should be of moderate intensity on at least 5 days per week. If not able to undertake moderate intensity activity because of co-morbidities or other reasons, a person should be encouraged to exercise at their maximum safe capacity. Accumulated bouts of activity of ≥10 minutes are as effective as longer sessions.

13 National Institute for Health and Care Excellence (NICE) (2008). *Identification and management of familial hypercholesterolaemia*. Clinical guideline 71. https://www.nice.org.uk/guidance/cg71

14 National Institute for Health and Care Excellence (NICE) (2017). *Familial hypercholesterolaemia: Identification and management*. Available at: ℛ https://www.nice.org.uk/guidance/cg71.

Table 23.3 Cholesterol levels used in diagnosing in FH in index cases*,†,‡

	Total cholesterol (mmol/L)	LDL cholesterol (mmol/L)
Child/young person	>6.7	>4.0
Adult	>7.5	>4.9

*Cholesterol levels pre-treatment or highest on treatment.

†These levels should not be used alone but in conjunction with Simon Broome criteria.

‡These levels should not be used in relatives of the index case as this may result in underdiagnosis.

Lipid-modifying drug therapy[13]

Statins should be prescribed as initial treatment in adults and in children and young people with FH. Other medication is an option if statins are contraindicated or not tolerated. Treatment with bile acid sequestrants can be considered if other medication is contraindicated or not tolerated but should be advised by a specialist in FH. If bile acid sequestrants are prescribed for long-term treatment, supplementation with fat-soluble vitamins (A, D, and K) and folate should be considered.

Heart failure

Heart failure results when damage to the heart leads to reduced efficiency in pumping blood around the body with consequent symptoms of breathlessness, fatigue, and fluid retention. Medical treatment, including the prescription of ACE (angiotensin-converting enzyme) inhibitors and diuretics, may be supported by dietary management.

- *Restricting dietary sodium:* current guidelines[15] recommend a salt intake of <6 g/day. Limiting sodium intake will theoretically help maximize effects of diuretics and thus moderate the heart's workload by reducing circulating volume. However, low sodium diets may not be effective[16] and can be unpalatable so a compromise between avoiding excessive salt and maintaining an adequate nutritional intake is needed. A less restrictive 'no added salt' diet provides <6 g salt and excludes salt added at the table (use just a pinch in cooking), stock cubes, meat/vegetable extracts, cured meat, tinned fish/meat, tinned/packet soup, salted nuts/crisps, soy sauce, monosodium glutamate (see ➔ Chapter 28, 'Low sodium diets', p. 696).
- *Fluid restriction:* patients with severe heart failure should be advised to restrict their fluid intake to 1.5–2.0 L/day. Patients with mild or moderate heart failure are unlikely to benefit from fluid restriction.
- *Obesity:* patients with excess body weight (body mass index [BMI] >30 kg/m²) should be advised to reduce slowly to reduce progression of heart failure, ↓ symptoms, and improve wellbeing. In moderate to severe heart failure, routine weight loss advice is inappropriate because unintentional weight loss and anorexia is common.
- *Nutritional adequacy:* in more advanced cases, appetite can be very poor and food intake limited by symptoms. Patients should be regularly screened for undernutrition (see ➔ Chapter 25, 'Nutrition screening', p. 558). Changes in body weight may indicate fluid retention so a holistic assessment taking into account food intake is required. Ensuring a nutritionally adequate intake by encouraging small, frequent, nutrient dense meals may help maintain body weight. This may conflict with the principles of the cardioprotective diet so advice must take into account the likely prognosis.
- *Alcohol:* consuming alcohol is associated with a negative effect on cardiac muscle contraction, ↑ blood pressure, and risk of arrhythmias. Patients should be advised to limit their intake of alcohol to 10–20 g alcohol (approximately 1–2 units, see ➔ Chapter 9, 'Alcohol', p. 206). If patients have alcohol-related cardiomyopathy, they should be advised to abstain from alcohol completely.

15 Ponikowski P *et al.* (2016). ESC guidelines for the diagnosis and treatment of acute and chronic heart failure. *Eur. Heart J.* **37**:2129–200.

16 Rifai L *et al.* (2016). A review of the DASH diet as an optimal dietary plan for symptomatic heart failure. *Prog. Cardiovas. Dis.* **57**:548–54.

Stroke, including dysphagia

Stroke or cerebrovascular accident (CVA) is the cause of approximately 40,000 (7%) of deaths in the UK, the second most common cause of dementia, and the most important single cause of severe disability in people living in their own homes. Approximately 200,000 episodes of inpatient care result from stroke each year in the UK and the incidence increases with ↑ age. Approximately 85% of strokes are caused by cerebral infarction, 10% by primary haemorrhage, and 5% subarachnoid haemorrhage. Nutrition has two key roles to play:

• Prevention
  • 1°: a healthy, well-balanced diet including components of a Mediterranean diet can help reduce risk in a healthy population;
  • 2°: diet can also reduce CVD risk factors in individuals who have had a stroke.
• Treatment
  • an appropriate, modified diet may be required to help maintain adequate nutritional intake and hydration following stroke.

Nutrition and diet in 1° stroke prevention

Public health guidance[4] to reduce stroke risk addresses lifestyle changes including diet and accessibility to healthy food. It includes two main nutrient targets (see ➲ this chapter, 'Cardioprotective diet', Table 23.2 and Chapter 2 'Food-based dietary guidelines', p. 26):

• Reducing salt intake to <6 g/day (target is <3 g by 2025);
• Reducing saturated fat intake to <11% of food energy intake.

Dietary advice

• There is evidence that some components of a Mediterranean diet can help reduce stroke risk in a healthy population (Table 23.4).
• Reduce weight in obesity. Excess body weight is associated with increased stroke risk. A reduction of 3-9% in body weight is associated with a 3 mmHg reduction in systolic and diastolic BP. Ideally, this should be accompanied by an increase in regular, low intensity activity such as walking. Note that the relationship between BMI and mortality from stroke is not linear.
• Avoid binge drinking of alcohol, i.e. ≥6 units of alcohol/day. A J-shaped curve of relative risk of stroke against alcohol intake suggests that there may be benefits from consuming up to 1–2 units of alcohol/day but definite risk of harm from heavy drinking[17] (see ➲ Chapter 9, 'Alcohol').
• Reduce excessive salt intake. Cutting salt intake from 9 to 6 g/day is estimated to reduce systolic BP by 3 mmHg. This could be achieved by avoiding adding salt to food at the table, using just a pinch of salt in cooking, and limiting processed foods including stock cubes, meat and vegetable extracts, cured meat, tinned fish and meat, tinned and packet soup, salted nuts, crisps, soy sauce, and monosodium glutamate.

---

17 Mostofsky, E., et al. (2016). Alcohol and immediate risk of cardiovascular events: a systematic review and dose-response meta-analysis. *Circulation*. **133**, 979–87.

- Increase fruit and vegetable intake. A minimum of five portions per day, including green leafy vegetables, will help increase potassium and folate intake and provide the antioxidants, vitamin C, carotenoids, and flavonoids. There is no evidence that supplements with B vitamins including folate are beneficial.
- There is good evidence to show that supplementation with the following micronutrients does not reduce risk of stroke in healthy populations:[18] antioxidant vitamins (β-carotene, vitamin C, vitamin E), folic acid and vitamin B_{12}.
- There is little evidence that supplementation with Ω-3 polyunsaturated fatty acids reduces risk of stroke in healthy populations.[19]
- In people with diabetes, ensure good blood sugar control.

Stroke risk increases with age. In some older people, a reduced food intake resulting from bereavement, difficulty in shopping, cooking, eating, or lack of appetite, often leads to a reduced intake of fruit and vegetables and ↑ consumption of nutrient-poor, processed foods. Social and practical support may be required to counter this with an adequate, well-balanced diet.

Table 23.4 Components of the Mediterranean diet and their effect on stroke risk[20]

Reduced risk	Increased risk	No effect on risk
Fruit and vegetables	Red and processed meat	Nuts
Fish	Alcohol	Legumes
Olive oil		
White meat		

Nutrition and diet in 2° stroke prevention

Individualized advice following stroke can reduce CVD risk factors but there is limited evidence about their impact on recurrence or mortality[21] (Box 23.3).

Nutritional support following stroke

Anyone with a suspected stroke should be admitted to a specialist stroke unit as soon as possible for urgent assessment, brain imaging, and possibly thrombolysis/thrombectomy. Following acute stroke, many people are unable to swallow safely and therefore need support with hydration and nutrition.

18 Hankey, G.J. (2012). Vitamin supplementation and stroke prevention. *Stroke* 43, 2814–8.

19 Siscovick, D.S., et al. (2017). Omega-3 Polyunsaturated fatty acid (fish oil) supplementation and the prevention of clinical cardiovascular disease: A science advisory from the American Heart Association. *Circulation* 135, e867–84.

20 Lakkur, S., et al. (2015). Diet and stroke: recent evidence supporting a Mediterranean style diet and food in the primary prevention of stroke. *Stroke* 46, 2007–11.

21 Hookway C et al. (2015) Royal College of Physicians Intercollegiate Stroke Working Party evidence-based guidelines for the secondary prevention of stroke through nutritional or dietary modification. *J. Hum. Nutr. Diet.* 28:107–25.

Box 23.3 Nutritional recommendations for 2° prevention following stroke or transient ischaemic attack[22]

- Eat at least five portions of fruit and vegetables per day from a variety of sources;
- Eat at least two portions of oily fish per week (salmon, trout, herring, pilchards, sardines, fresh, tuna);
- Reduce and replace saturated fat with polyunsaturated diet by using low-fat dairy products, replacing butter, ghee, and lard with products based on vegetable and plant oils, limiting red meat, especially fatty cuts and processed meat;
- Reduce salt intake by not adding salt at the table, using little or no salt in cooking, avoiding high salt foods, e.g. processed meat such as ham and salami, cheese, stock cubes, pre-prepared soups and savoury snacks such as crisps and salted nuts;
- If overweight or obese, offer support to reduce weight through adopting a healthy diet, limiting alcohol to ≤2 units per day and regular exercise;
- If drinking alcohol, limit intake to 14 units per week spread over at least 3 days;
- Avoid taking the following micronutrient supplements unless advised for other medical conditions: B vitamins, folate, antioxidants (vitamins A, C, E, and selenium), calcium with or without vitamin D.

Assessment of swallowing function[23]
- On admission following acute stroke and before being given any oral food, fluid, or medication, swallowing function should be screened by an appropriately trained healthcare professional.
- If screening identifies a problem with swallowing, a specialist assessment of swallowing should be undertaken preferably <24 hours and no more than 72 hours after admission.
- If specialist assessment identifies suspected aspiration or need for tube feeding or dietary modification for 3 days, the patient should be referred for dietary advice.
- People who are unable to take adequate nutrition and fluids orally should receive a nasogastric (NG) tube <24 hours after admission. If they are unable to tolerate an NG tube, a nasal bridle or gastrostomy should be considered. A detailed nutritional assessment, individualized advice, and monitoring should be undertaken by an appropriately trained healthcare professional.

Screening of nutritional and hydration status[22]
- On admission to hospital, stroke patients should undergo screening for malnutrition and risk of malnutrition (see ➲ Chapter 25, 'Nutrition screening', p. 558).

22 Royal College of Physicians. (2016). *National clinical guideline for stroke*, 5th edn. Available at: 🔗 https://www.rcplondon.ac.uk/guidelines-policy/stroke-guidelines.

23 National Institute for Health and Care Excellence (NICE) (2017) *Stroke and transient ischaemic attack in over 16s: diagnosis and initial management.* Clinical guideline CG68 https://www.nice.org.uk/guidance/cg68

- Screening should be undertaken by an appropriately trained healthcare professional and be repeated weekly during admission.
- Screening should consider BMI, unintentional weight loss, duration of unintentional reduced nutrient intake, and likelihood of future impaired intake.
- The impact of dysphagia, poor oral health, and reduced ability to self-feed should be considered during screening.
- People who are adequately nourished on admission should not be routinely offered nutritional supplementation.
- People who are malnourished or at risk of malnutrition should be provided with nutritional support, which might include oral nutritional supplements, specialist dietary advice, and/or tube feeding.
- Hydration status should be assessed on admission, regularly reviewed, and managed to ensure normal hydration.

Tube feeding

Following assessment that adequate nutritional intake cannot be achieved orally, NG feeding should commence. People should be considered for gastrostomy feeding if they need but are unable to tolerate NG feeding, are unable to swallow adequate food and fluid orally by 4 weeks after onset of the stroke, or are at high risk of malnutrition.[22] Inserting a gastrostomy is an invasive procedure and ethical consideration must be given to the associated risks and ongoing management as well as potential benefits (see ➡ Chapter 25, 'Enteral feeding', p. 574).

Dysphagia

Dysphagia (discomfort, difficulty, or pain when swallowing) is common following stroke. Swallowing has four stages:
- *Preparation:* transfer of food into the mouth, sealed with lips.
- *Oral:* chewing, mixing with saliva, bolus formation, and transfer toward pharynx.
- *Pharyngeal:* complex stage where bolus is involuntarily transferred towards oesophagus with simultaneous closure of larynx and pause in respiration.
- *Oesophageal:* transfer to stomach by peristalsis and gravity.

❗ Impaired swallowing leads to high risk from aspirating food or liquid into the respiratory tract.

Modification of texture of food and fluid

If swallowing is impaired, modifying the texture of food or viscosity of fluid may facilitate safe oral intake. A speech and language therapist should assess what each patient is capable of swallowing safely. Standardized descriptions of food and fluid are used to safely translate the assessment findings into appropriately modified food and drink. The International Dysphagia Diet Standardization Initiative (IDDSI) provides a framework of terminology and definitions, including an objective measurement of liquid thickness (Fig. 23.2).

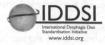

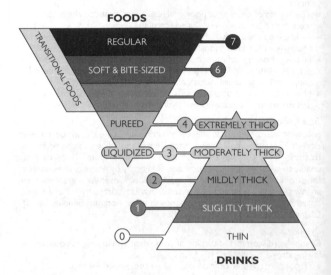

Fig. 23.2 Framework for terminology and definitions of food and fluids for individuals with dysphagia. Reproduced from the International Dysphagia Diet Standardization Initiative. (2016). ℘ http://iddsi.org/framework/. Copyright © 2016 The International Dysphagia Diet Standardization Initiative. The IDDSI Framework and Descriptors are licensed under the CreativeCommons Attribution Sharealike 4.0 Licence ℘ https://creativecommons.org/licenses/by-sa/4.0/legalcode

Additional information including descriptions and video are available to explain how to:
- test foods (e.g. does the consistency flow through the prongs of a fork): ℘ http://iddsi.org/framework/food-testing-methods/;
- test drinks (e.g. 10 mL syringe test): ℘ http://iddsi.org/framework/drink-testing-methods/.

Post-acute and longer term care
The patient's nutritional status and ability to swallow should be regularly monitored and adjustments made to their nutritional management accordingly. Dysphagia frequently resolves in the first 6 months following a stroke, although it may persist. Switching to overnight tube feeding to encourage oral intake during the day may facilitate a return to a normal eating pattern.

Patients may continue to need assistance with meals and, importantly, time to maximize their ability to eat an adequate diet. Neurological damage after stroke varies with the following losses of function that may impact on eating:

- altered levels of consciousness in 30–40% of patients;
- difficulty in swallowing in 30%;
- motor weakness in 50–80%;
- slurred speech in 30%;
- dysphagia/aphasia in 30%;
- visual field defects in 7%.

As a result, inadequate intake and resulting undernutrition is a common problem, especially in altered states of consciousness, and becomes significantly worse as hospital stay continues; it is associated with ↑ morbidity and reduced survival.

Nutritional support should continue for people discharged from specialist hospital care. For those receiving palliative care, burdensome restrictions on oral food and fluid intake should be lifted if they exacerbate suffering.[22]

Nutritional requirements

Energy and protein requirements may be ↑ as a result of hypermetabolism, which persists for 4–8 weeks, and in frail elderly people who have pre-existing undernutrition (see ➔ Chapter 25, 'Estimating requirements in disease states', p. 596).

Free radicals may play a role in brain damage after infarction/reperfusion. This suggests that an adequate antioxidant intake may be important although dietary intake may be compromised in dysphagia. It is important to remember that modified textured food, e.g. puréed items, may contain less energy and ↓ quantities of macronutrients than un-puréed food be cause of the dilution effect of adding fluid to facilitate blending. In addition, the blending process breaks down plant cell walls and exposes antioxidants and other micronutrients to potential oxidation thus reducing bioavailability. However, at present there is no evidence[18] to support antioxidant supplementation post-stroke and this cannot be recommended. However, attention should be given to the adequacy of all nutrient intake from food.

Further information

British Heart Foundation. Available at: ℛ https://www.bhf.org.uk/heart-health/preventing-heart-disease/healthy-eating.

National Institute for Health and Care Excellence (NICE). (2017). *Stroke and transient ischaemic attack in over 16s: diagnosis and initial management*. Clinical guideline 68. Available at: ℛ https://www.nice.org.uk/guidance/cg68.

Royal College of Physicians. (2016). National clinical guideline for stroke, 5th edn. Available at: ℛ https://www.rcplondon.ac.uk/guidelines-policy/stroke-guidelines.

Stroke Association. Available at: ℛ http://www.stroke.org.uk.

Hypertension

Hypertension (HT) is defined as persistent systolic blood pressure (SBP) above 140 mmHg, diastolic blood pressure (DBP) above 90 mmHg, or when levels below this are maintained by antihypertensive medication.

Average blood pressure has fallen over the last decade in the UK but it remains a significant health problem with approximately 9.5 million people on the HT register. Prevalence increases with age and is higher in Black and South Asian communities. In the UK, hypertensive disease is the cause of death in approximately 7,000 people annually.

HT is a major risk factor for cardiovascular disease (especially stroke, angina, myocardial infarction, heart failure, and left ventricular failure), renal disease, and retinopathy.

Factors contributing to HT include:
- obesity, especially if central adiposity;
- insulin resistance;
- diabetes mellitus;
- low levels of physical activity;
- psychosocial stress;
- high salt intake;
- high alcohol intake, especially if regular heavy or binge drinking;
- increasing age.

Management

Lifestyle advice should be offered as the first line of treatment.[24] This should include the promotion of a healthy diet (see ➔ this chapter, 'Cardioprotective diet', Table 23.2 and Box 23.4), regular exercise, and smoking cessation. Those with diabetes, hyperlipidaemia, or previous coronary heart disease should receive additional advice.

Box 23.4 Dietary Approaches to Stop Hypertension

The principles described above are incorporated into the Dietary Approaches to Stop Hypertension (DASH) diet (↓ salt, ↓ fat, ↑ fruit and vegetables), which has been developed and evaluated in the USA. Adherence is associated with improved health outcomes including ↓ hypertension.

⅍ http://dashdiet.org

Dietary advice
- Reduction of excess body weight diet (see ➔ Chapter 21, 'Obesity'). Losing 3–9% body weight if overweight or obese is associated with 3 mmHg reduction in SBP and DBP.
- Limit alcohol intake to within lower risk levels, i.e. ≤14 units per week for men and women spread out over ≥3 days. Structured intervention to reduce excess intake is associated with a mean reduction of

---

24 National Institute of Health and Care Excellence (NICE). (2016). *Hypertension in adults: diagnosis and management.* Clinical Guideline 127. Available at: ⅍ https://www.nice.org.uk/guidance/cg127.

3-4 mmHg SBP and DBP, with a third of patients achieving >10 mmHg reduction in SBP.
- Limit salt intake to <6 g/day (2.4 g or 100 mmol Na$^+$). This reduction does not mean consuming 6 g of 'added salt' (i.e. heaped teaspoonful!). Most people consume a substantial proportion of salt from manufactured food products and this should be included within the 6 g limit. This could be achieved by not adding any salt to food at the table, using just a pinch of salt in cooking, and limiting processed foods including stock cubes, meat and vegetable extracts, cured meat, tinned fish and meat, tinned and packet soup, salted nuts and crisps, soy sauce, and monosodium glutamate. Some people use potassium-containing salt substitutes but others find them metallic-tasting and unpleasant. Experimenting with herbs, spices, lemon juice, and garlic etc can help promote flavour and enjoyment in eating. There are additional health benefits from lower salt intakes <3 g/day and this is a national target for average intake for adults in the UK by 2025. Re-formulation of manufactured food products has helped to reduce average salt intake by approximately 1 g between 2004 and 2014 and this is thought to have contributed to the fall in average blood pressure.[25] Further reductions require continuation of this initiative as well as advising people to continue limiting salt intake.
- Discourage excessive consumption of coffee and other caffeine-rich products. No specific limit is advised.
- Calcium, potassium, and magnesium supplements are not recommended.

Further information

Blood Pressure Association. Available at: http://www.hpassoc.org.uk.
British Hypertension Society. Available at: http://www.bhsoc.org/.
Consensus Action on Salt and Health. Available at: http://www.actiononsalt.org.uk/salthealth/.
National Institute of Health and Care Excellence (NICE). (2016). *Hypertension in adults: diagnosis and management*. Clinical Guideline 127. Available at: https://www.nice.org.uk/guidance/cg127.

25 He, F.J., et al (2014). Salt reduction in England from 2003 to 2011: its relationship to blood pressure, stroke and ischaemic heart disease mortality. *BMJ Open* 4, e004549.

Peripheral arterial disease

Peripheral arterial disease (PAD) is caused by atheromatous plaque and chronic inflammation leading to narrowing of peripheral blood vessels, most commonly in the legs. This results in poor blood supply and pain on exertion (claudication) and may lead to ulceration, limb loss, and ↑ risk of death from myocardial infarction and stroke. Poor quality of life and depression are associated.

- *Prevalence:* although reported as poorly diagnosed, it is estimated that approximately 350,000 people in England are affected.
- *Risk factors:* include ↑ age, smoking, diabetes mellitus, hyperlipidaemia, and hypertension.

Nutrition

- *Prevention:* epidemiology[26] indicates that ↑ intake of dietary antioxidants (vitamins A, C, and E), vitamin B$_6$, folate, fibre, and omega-3 fatty acids have a protective effect independent of other cardiovascular risk factors. However, there is insufficient evidence to support recommending supplements.[27]
- *Cardioprotective diet:* people with PAD should be offered diet and lifestyle advice to reduce risk of CVD[28] (see ⮕ this chapter, 'Cardioprotective diet').
- *Folate:* patients with PAD have significantly ↑ total plasma homocysteine levels compared with controls. This is associated with low folate intake but, at present, there is insufficient evidence to recommend folate supplements.[29]
- *Vitamin D:* low serum vitamin D levels are associated with ↑ prevalence of PAD.[30] To date, no intervention studies have examined the effects of vitamin D supplementation.

26 Lane, J.S., *et al.* (2008). Nutrition impacts the prevalence of peripheral arterial disease in the United States. *J. Vasc. Surg.* **48**, 897–904.

27 Nosovo, E.V., *et al.* (2015). Advancing beyond the "heart-healthy diet" for peripheral arterial disease. *J. Vasc. Surg.* **61**, 265–74.

28 National Institute of Health and Care Excellence (NICE). (2012). *Peripheral arterial disease; diagnosis and management.* Clinical Guideline 147. Available at: ⮕ https://www.nice.org.uk/guidance/cg147.

29 Andras, A., *et al.* (2013). Homocysteine lowering interventions for peripheral arterial disease and bypass grafts. *Cochrane Database Syst. Rev.* **19**, CD003285.

30 Nsengiyumva, V., *et al.* (2015). The association of circulating 25-hydroxyvitamin D concentration with peripheral arterial disease: a meta-analysis of observational studies. *Atherosclerosis* **242**, 645–51.

Cancer

Aetiology and dietary recommendations 542
Cancer cachexia 544
Cancer treatment 546
Managing nutritional status in cancer 548
Living with and beyond cancer 550
Frequently asked questions 551
Neutropenia and food hygiene 552
Late effects 553
Palliative care in cancer 554

Aetiology and dietary recommendations

The incidence of cancer is increasing and, at present, a third of the UK population will be diagnosed with cancer at some point in their lifetime. The aetiology of cancer is complex, with 5% being caused by genetic factors and the remainder the result of a wide range of environmental factors. Diet can be part of this complex picture. The effects of diet probably start during childhood and then continue into adult life. This may be directly caused by the foods eaten, but also through influence of the food on body weight and growth. Other environmental factors include:

- tobacco;
- infection;
- industrial pollutants, e.g. asbestos;
- ionizing radiation;
- sunlight.

Estimates of cancer preventability by appropriate diet, nutrition, physical activity, and body fatness have been undertaken by the World Cancer Research Fund for four countries and described as the Population Attributable Fraction (PAF). PAF is the proportional reduction in population disease or mortality that would occur if exposure to a risk factor were reduced to an alternative ideal exposure scenario (e.g. no alcohol use). Detailed statistics are available online: ♫http://www.wcrf.org/int/cancer-facts-figures/preventability-estimates/cancer-preventability-estimates-diet-nutrition.

The World Cancer Research Fund has recommended the following basic principles to a healthy eating diet that may support cancer prevention:

- Maintain your weight within the normal body mass index (BMI) range.
- Be physically active for at least 150 minutes every week and sit less.
- Reduce your intake of high calorie foods and avoid sugary drinks.
- Eat at least five portions of fruit/vegetables every day.
- Eat a portion of pulses or wholegrain foods with every meal.
- Reduce your intake of red meat to no more than 350–500 g (12–18 oz) a week and eat minimal amounts of processed meats.
- Limit or avoid alcohol. If consumed, limit your alcohol intake to 2 units a day for men and 1 unit a day for women.
- Breastfeed your baby.
- Do not use dietary supplements for the prevention of cancer.

They recommend that a typical meal should ideally consist of three-quarters of the plate as wholegrain cereals, pulses, vegetables, and fruit, with the remaining one-quarter containing a source of protein such as fish, chicken, egg, or lean meat (Fig. 24.1).

Healthy plate guide:

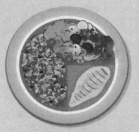

3/4
(or more)
wholegrains,
vegetables,
fruit and
pulses

1/4
(or less) meat,
fish and other
protein foods

Meal examples:

▶ Mixed salad and wholemeal pasta, with grilled salmon fillet
▶ Steamed green vegetables, carrots and new potatoes, with baked chicken breast
▶ Vegetable and brown rice stir-fry, with tofu

Fig. 24.1 Healthy plate guide. Reproduced from 'Eat well for life', with permission from the World Cancer Research Fund. © World Cancer Research 2019. ℘ https:// www.wcrf-uk.org/sites/default/files/eat-well-for-life-booklet.pdf. More information and recipe ideas are available at: ℘ www.wcrf-uk.org.

Cancer cachexia

Cancer cachexia is a multi-factorial syndrome which is defined by an on-going loss of skeletal muscle mass, with or without loss of fat mass, that cannot be fully reversed by conventional nutritional support. It leads to progressive functional impairment and can influence tolerance to cancer treatment (see ➔ Chapter 25 'Undernutrition').

The diagnostic criteria are:

- weight loss >5%; or
- weight loss >2% in individuals showing depletion according to current bodyweight and height (BMI < 20 kg/m^2) or skeletal muscle mass (sarcopenia).

The cachexia syndrome can develop progressively through various stages from pre-cachexia, cachexia, to refractory cachexia. The severity can be classified depending on the degree of depletion of energy stores and body protein in combination with the amount of weight loss.[1]

It is more common in some tumour types such as lung and gastrointestinal cancer and less common in other types of cancer, for example, breast and prostate cancer. Progression of disease increases the risk of cachexia, and refractory cachexia occurs in advanced cancer.

The metabolic features of cancer cachexia are:

- Protein metabolism: systemic inflammation is associated with altered protein turnover, a loss of fat and muscle mass, and an increase in the production of acute phase proteins.
- Carbohydrate metabolism: systemic inflammation is frequently associated with insulin resistance and impaired glucose tolerance.
- Lipid metabolism: the capacity for lipid oxidation is maintained or even increased in cancer patients, and especially so in the presence of weight loss.[2]

Nutrition screening should be used to identify malnutrition and cachexia as early as possible to facilitate a full nutritional assessment and implementation of a nutrition care plan. Nutrition screening tools which include symptoms that affect food intake are more sensitive to identifying those with cancer who are at risk of undernutrition.[3] A full nutrition assessment should be undertaken by a healthcare professional experienced in nutrition and cancer (see ➔ Chapter 4 'Nutrition assessment'). The Patient Generated Subjective Global Assessment (PG-SGA) is a useful tool providing a

1 Fearon, K., *et al.* (2011). Definition and classification of cancer cachexia: an international consensus. *Lancet Oncol.* **12**, 489–95.

2 Arends, J., *et al.* (2017). ESPEN guidelines on nutrition in cancer patients. *Clin. Nutr.* **36**, 11–48.

3 Shaw, C., *et al.* (2015). Comparison of a novel, simple nutrition screening tool for adult oncology inpatients and the Malnutrition Screening Tool (MST) against the Patient-Generated Subjective Global Assessment (PG-SGA). *Support Care Cancer* **23**, 47–54.

framework for a full assessment. It includes assessment of weight change, symptoms affecting food intake, current food intake, physical function, impact of disease, and a physical examination to assess muscle and fat stores. It has been validated in oncology and been shown to be a prognostic indicator.[4]

4 Ottery, F.D. (1996). Definition of standardized nutritional assessment and interventional pathways in oncology. *Nutrition* **12**(Suppl. 1), S15–9.

Cancer treatment

The diagnosis of cancer requires a multi-professional discussion and plan for the appropriate treatment. Multi-modality treatment is often planned with treatments running concurrently or consecutively and can include any of the following.

- *Chemotherapy*—the use of drugs, either systemically or orally, given with the intention of killing cancer cells. Their actions affect both normal and cancer cells, producing toxicity in normal tissues and organs such as stomatitis, diarrhoea, and bone marrow depression. May be administered intermittently, allowing the body to recover between administration, or continuously. Often produce symptoms that affect food intake including anorexia, nausea, sore mouth, and taste changes. High dose chemotherapy may be given in haematological cancers with the intention of destroying the cancer contained in the immune system. Such procedures require support in the form of a bone marrow transplant or stem cell rescue to restore the function of the immune system.

- *Radiotherapy*—the use of ionizing radiation given with the intention of killing cancer cells. Radiotherapy is directed at the tumour cells. It kills both normal and cancer cells and is given at doses that allow the normal cells to recover and regenerate. Side effects of the treatment are primarily confined to the area treated, for example, a sore mouth or throat when the head or neck is treated or diarrhoea when organs in the pelvis are treated. It may be used in combination with chemotherapy which sensitizes the tissues.

- *Surgery*—may be used before or after other treatments. Usually involves excision of the tumour with adjacent lymph nodes to which the cancer may have spread. May also be used for palliation, for example, to bypass an intestinal obstruction. The effect on nutritional status will vary depending on the extent of the surgery and whether it impacts on intestinal function.

- *Hormone treatment*—cancers that are dependent on hormones to promote growth may be treated with drugs to alter the availability of hormones in the body. These then block or reduce the growth of tissues that rely on hormones. They may influence nutrition via their effects on promoting weight gain and reducing bone density.

- *Novel therapies*—these include experimental and new treatments that may be used in combination with conventional therapies or on their own. They include drugs such as growth factor inhibitors and immunotherapy.

Aims of cancer treatment

Nutritional management can plan an important role during each of the three aims of cancer treatment:

- cure—to obtain a complete response;
- control—to extend life and quality of life if cure is not possible;
- palliation—to provide comfort where cure and control are not possible, to relieve symptoms and maximize quality of life.

Nutritional status during cancer treatment

Weight loss and poor nutritional status can have a negative impact on the ability to withstand cancer treatment. Changes in nutritional status can occur at any time before or after a diagnosis of cancer so it is important that people are screened and assessed on a regular basis. Nutritional interventions and support should be aimed at providing adequate nutritional intake, to maintain muscle mass in conjunction with physical activity and to improve quality of life. The aim is to prevent further deterioration in nutritional status or improve nutritional parameters, reducing the risk of breaks from treatment related to toxicity and to enable planned cancer treatment to be undertaken.

Nutritional requirements

Altered energy expenditure may occur in some people with cancer; however, this is often balanced by a reduction in physical activity. The provision of any form of nutritional status requires an estimation of energy, protein, fluid, and micronutrient requirements with appropriate monitoring. Nutritional requirements can be estimated by the following:

- 25–30 kcal/kg body weight
- 1.0–1.5 g protein/kg body weight.[2]

When planning artificial nutrition support it is advisable to assess each individual using the Henry equations (see ➔ Chapter 25 'Estimating requirements in disease states') with the appropriate estimated stress and activity factors.

The optimal ratio of carbohydrate to fat intake has not yet been established. In patients with insulin resistance, uptake and oxidation of glucose by muscle cells is impaired while the use of fat is normal or increased.[3] It may be prudent when planning higher energy diets to promote weight gain to increase the ratio of fat to carbohydrate to meet energy requirements.

Micronutrient requirements are assumed to be similar to those of healthy individuals. It is unclear how high doses of vitamins, particularly antioxidants, influence toxicity of treatment, particularly chemotherapy and radiotherapy and overall survival.[5]

5 Harvie, M. (2014). Nutritional supplements and cancer: potential benefits and proven harms. *Am. Soc. Clin. Oncol. Educ. Book* e478–86.

Managing nutritional status in cancer

The risk of malnutrition in cancer should be identified early to allow interventions to be planned, preventing a further deterioration in nutritional status. Nutritional therapy in cancer patients who are malnourished or at risk of malnutrition has been shown to improve body weight and energy intake but not survival.[2]

Dietary counselling, by healthcare professionals with the relevant knowledge and experience in cancer, should provide advice and support focused on eating and drinking, whenever this is possible. Although the research evidence does not suggest routine use of artificial nutritional support, it may be required in some circumstances when oral intake is insufficient because of the tumour itself or because of the side effects of planned treatment. If the gastrointestinal tract is functioning and can be accessed, then this should be the route of choice. Timing of the placement of an enteral feeding tube is important to ensure that this is done when the person is able to withstand the procedure and not when they are at increased risk of infection. Parenteral nutrition should be reserved for those with a non-functioning gastrointestinal tract, for example, in bowel obstruction or with a high output fistula (see ➲ Chapter 26 'Fistulae').

Managing symptoms

Symptoms affecting food intake are common in people with cancer and increase the risk of weight loss and malnutrition.[6] The most frequent symptoms include no appetite, early satiety, taste changes, nausea, dry mouth, constipation, dry mouth, vomiting, and difficulties with swallowing. Medical management is essential for patient comfort and to reduce the impact on the oral intake of food and fluids. Dietary interventions can also help manage symptoms (Table 24.1).

Table 24.1 Dietary interventions to help manage symptoms[7]

Symptom	Dietary advice and suggestions
Weight loss	Food fortification—use of higher fat alternatives and addition of energy dense foods to meals and snacks
	Changes to meal patterns to promote small frequent meals and snacks
	High energy snacks, e.g. nuts, seeds, cheese, chocolate, fruit and nut bars
	Use of high energy drinks, e.g. milky drinks including coffee and hot chocolate, milkshakes, smoothies
	Use of commercial oral nutritional supplement drinks
	Use of commercial energy supplements to add to food, drinks, or to be taken separately

(Continued)

6 Khalid, U., *et al.* (2007). Symptoms and weight loss in patients with gastrointestinal and lung cancer at presentation. *Support Care Cancer* **15**, 39–46.

7 Shaw, C. (2015). *The Royal Marsden Cancer Cookbook*. Kyle Books, London.

Table 24.1 (Contd.)

Poor appetite	Serving small portions
	Meal pattern of little and often throughout the day
	Food fortification
	Relying on foods that are palatable
Nausea	Use of anti-emetics prior to eating
	Avoiding the smell of food
	Cold foods may be preferable as they have less odour
	Choose carbohydrate-based foods such as crackers, toast, plain biscuits, or cookies
	Sip glucose-containing drinks
	Try drinks and foods that contain ginger, for example, ginger tea or ginger ale
Sore mouth	Appropriate mouthcare as advised by medical team
	Plenty of fluids and use a straw if lips are sore
	Avoid the use of salty, spicy, and sharp foods
	Reduce seasoning, especially salt, in food
	Foods that are soft, bland, and easy to eat
	Cook cereals until they are soft and mash vegetables
	Use of high energy drinks, e.g. milky drinks including coffee and hot chocolate, milkshakes, smoothies
	Use of commercial oral nutritional supplement drinks avoiding sharp fruit flavours
Taste changes	Often taste for tea and coffee is affected, if so, try fruit and herb teas, for example, berry, mint or camomile
	If unable to detect flavours then increase seasoning, use herbs, salt, or citrus fruits such as lime and lemon
	Try hot or warm foods
	If foods such as meat taste metallic, then try different sources of protein including eggs, yogurt, and cheese
Dysphagia	Foods that are soft and easy to eat
	May require puree foods with advice about food fortification
	Use of high energy drinks, e.g. milky drinks including coffee and hot chocolate, milkshakes, smoothies
	Use of commercial oral nutritional supplement drinks
Early satiety	Consider anti-emetics that promote gastric emptying
	Small frequent meals and snacks
	Avoid large volumes fluid consumed before or during mealtimes

Living with and beyond cancer

A diagnosis of cancer often leads people to research whether any particular foods or diet may influence the growth of their disease. This subject is highly complex and can be controversial. Dietary recommendations produced by the World Cancer Research Fund, following a systematic review of the available research evidence, are recommended for people who do not have any specific difficulties with eating and drinking. These principles are generally the same as those outlined in earlier in this chapter, 'Aetiology and dietary recommendations'. However, for some diagnostic groups there may be specific considerations, e.g. indication of links between better survival and consuming foods containing soy in people with breast cancer.[8]

There is emerging evidence of the benefit of maintaining a body weight in the normal range, eating a healthy balanced diet, and being physically active after diagnosis. The evidence is strongest in colo-rectal, breast, and prostate cancers, with the impact being on either cancer-related mortality or overall health in the prevention of other chronic diseases such as cardiovascular disease and diabetes.[9]

8 World Cancer Research Fund. (2014). *Diet, nutrition, physical activity and breast cancer survivors.* Available at: ℗ http://www.wcrf.org/sites/default/files/Breast-Cancer-Survivors-2014-Report. pdf.

9 Moug, S.J., *et al.*(2017). Lifestyle interventions are feasible in patients with colorectal cancer with potential short-term health benefits: a systematic review. *Int. J. Colorectal Dis.* 32, 765–75.

Frequently asked questions

Sugar People do not need to avoid sugar to prevent or cure cancer. Cancer cells, like all other cells in the body, use glucose for energy. Some people have suggested that reducing sugar intake can minimize cancer cell growth. However, restricting the amount of sugar has not been proven to slow down or control the growth of cancer cells and, therefore, it does not need to be avoided. Reducing sugar in the diet can be a useful way to help someone lose weight.

Vitamin and mineral supplementation If an individual follows the principles of healthy eating, then the diet is likely to provide all the vitamins and minerals required. However, there may be times when eating is more difficult and an individual is unable to eat sufficiently to meet their requirements. In this situation, a one-a-day multivitamin and mineral supplement would be recommended to meet the needs of the individual.

At present, there is no evidence that taking extra vitamins as supplements will reduce the chance of cancer coming back. Very high doses, i.e. well above the reference nutrient intake, may be harmful and have unpleasant side effects or may interact with medication.[5]

Alternative and complementary diets People with cancer often obtain dietary information from the Internet, media, family, and friends. This may relate to individual foods, vitamins, minerals, supplement, or diets that claim to influence the growth of cancer. Such diets may vary widely in the foods they advise, but there are some common features including high consumption of vegetables, vegetable juices, and low sugar fruits and often avoid sugar or refined carbohydrates, grains, dairy, and meat. Some include a 'juice fast' or abstinence from nutrients for a period of time. Some are particularly prescriptive regarding the consumption of carbohydrate, limiting this with the aim of producing ketosis (ketogenic diet). The rationale behind the use of ketogenic diets is that normal tissues are able to use ketones but cancer cells are not and they continue to metabolize glucose.

A review of alternative cancer diets did not identify any clinical evidence to support their use.[10] Regimens suggested are often restrictive and put the person at risk of an unbalanced dietary intake and weight loss. Diets for which no clinical benefit has been shown, but which may entail risks should not be recommended. Patients seek such diets as they appear to provide hope and a cure. Advice and support for patients exploring such diets should take the psychological aspects into account.

10 Huebner J, *et al.* (2014). Counseling patients on cancer diets: a review of the literature and recommendations for clinical practice. *Anticancer Res.* **34**, 39–48.

Neutropenia and food hygiene

Neutropenia occurs when there is a low number of white blood cells called neutrophils. When neutrophils are low the immune system is weakened, making it harder to fight infection. This means a greater risk of food poisoning and illness. Neutropenia can be caused by a blood cancer or blood condition. It can also happen during or after treatment. Some of these treatments include: chemotherapy, a bone marrow or stem cell transplant, and medications that suppress the immune system (such as steroids, cyclosporine, and monoclonal antibodies). To help protect against food-borne organisms, it is important to follow good hygiene practices and avoid particular foods. The following advice should be given to all patients undergoing cancer treatment.

Food preparation

- Wash your hands thoroughly with soap and warm water before cooking, after touching the bin, going to the toilet, and before and after touching raw food.
- Wash all worktops and chopping boards before and after cooking.
- Use different chopping boards for raw and ready-to-eat foods.
- Keep raw food away from ready-to-eat foods such as bread, salad, and fruit.
- Store raw meat in a clean, sealed container on the bottom shelf of the fridge.
- Wash fruit and vegetables under cold running water before eating.
- When cooking, check food is piping hot throughout before eating.

Foods to avoid

It is recommended that these foods are avoided because they are associated with an increased risk of listeria, campylobacter, salmonella and toxoplasmosis:

- uncooked soft cheeses with white rinds, e.g. Brie, chevre (i.e. goats' cheese);
- uncooked blue cheeses, e.g. Gorgonzola, Roquefort, and Stilton;
- pâté—meat, fish, and vegetarian;
- raw and undercooked meat;
- raw shellfish;
- unpasteurized milk;
- raw and partially cooked eggs (follow local guidance).

People with prolonged, severe neutropenia such those undergoing a bone marrow transplant or peripheral stem cell transplant may require additional food restrictions. Guidance is published by the charity, Bloodwise: ℅ https://bloodwise.org.uk/sites/default/files/documents/Eating_Well_With_Neutropenia_2017_0.pdf

Late effects

There may be later consequences of cancer treatment that impact on dietary intake, nutritional status, and the risk of developing other diseases such as cardiovascular disease and diabetes (Table 24.2).

Table 24.2 Late effects of cancer diagnosis and treatment on nutrition

Cancer diagnosis	Late effects	Effect on nutrition
Head and neck cancer	Dysphagia, xerostomia, taste changes	Continued weight loss after treatment
Upper gastrointestinal cancer	Early satiety Stricture following surgery or radiotherapy Altered bowel habits Dumping syndrome	Continued weight loss after treatment Malabsorption Deficiency of vitamin B_{12} following gastrectomy and requirement for prophylactic vitamin B_{12} Anaemia
Gynae-oncology	Altered bowel habits following radiotherapy Risk of bowel obstruction because of disease, adhesions, or radiotherapy changes Surgery may result in formation of ileostomy or colostomy	Restricted dietary intake Early satiety, vomiting Malabsorption of food and fluids, e.g. with high output intestinal stoma Vitamin and mineral deficiencies
Haemato-oncology	Graft versus host disease Changes in bowel habits caused by radiotherapy Increased risk of metabolic syndrome	Weight loss Poor dietary intake Vitamin and mineral deficiencies
Urology, breast, brain, and central nervous system tumours	Increased risk of metabolic syndrome and increased adiposity Osteoporosis in hormone-related cancers such as prostate and breast	Obesity Poor vitamin D status
Childhood cancers	Recurrence of childhood cancer and risk of new cancer Altered gastrointestinal function	Poor growth Nutritional deficiencies

Palliative care in cancer

Palliative care is traditionally for those patients with advanced incurable disease. Nutrition has a role[2] and, as with all palliative care, should be considered in a holistic way considering all aspects of care and, importantly, the patient's wishes. All decisions should be validated and reviewed on an ongoing basis. It is vital that nutritional concerns are identified early. There is limited evidence of benefit from nutritional support in survival or comfort for patients with weight loss secondary to refractory cancer cachexia.[11] As with any patient identified with nutritional issues, holistic assessments should be made, establishing what is appropriate for that individual. This may include: food fortification advice, nutritional supplements, texture modification, or artificial nutritional support.

Artificial nutritional support should always be considered with care,[12] with the benefits and burdens being explored. Ethically and legally, artificial nutritional support is deemed a medical treatment and can be withdrawn if in the best interests of the individual; however, emotionally, nutrition can be seen as a 'source of life' and, as such, a lack of nutrition as causing starvation.[13] In particular, home parenteral nutrition (HPN) should only be considered:[11]

- if the patient has a WHO performance status of ≤2;
- when enteral nutrition is insufficient;
- when the expected survival because of tumour progression is >2-3 months;
- when HPN is expected to stabilize or improve performance status and quality of life; and
- the patient desires this mode of nutrition support.

See also ➲ Chapter 35, 'Palliative care'.

11 Bozzetti, F., *et al.* (2009). ESPEN guidelines on parenteral nutrition: non-surgical oncology. *Clin. Nutr.* **28**, 445–54.

12 Druml C et al. (2016). ESPEN guideline on ethical aspects of artificial nutrition and hydration. *Clin. Nutr.* **35**, 545–56.

13 Department of Health. (2013). *More care, less pathway. A review of the Liverpool care pathway.* Available at: ℘ https://www.gov.uk/government/publications/review-of-liverpool-care-pathway-for-dying-patients.

Chapter 25

Nutrition support

Nutrition screening 556
Malnutrition universal screening tool 558
Undernutrition 562
Treatment of undernutrition 568
Enteral feeding: introduction 572
Routes for enteral feeding 574
Enteral feeding regimens 580
Monitoring enteral feeding 582
Complications of enteral feeding 586
Enteral feeding and drugs 590
Blended enteral feeding 591
Parenteral nutrition 592
Estimating requirements in disease states 596
Refeeding syndrome 602
Metabolic response to injury 604
Critical care 606
Surgery 610
Spinal cord injury 612
Head injury 614
Burn injury 616
Clinically functional nutrients 620

Nutrition screening

This should be routinely undertaken to identify individuals who are at risk from under- or overnutrition and should be carried out by an appropriately trained and skilled person, but not necessarily a nutrition specialist. It differs from nutritional assessment, which is undertaken by a nutrition-trained healthcare professional, usually a registered dietitian, and which gives a more detailed nutritional profile of an individual. Screening for malnutrition is a multi-disciplinary responsibility.

Who and when to screen

All people in care settings[1] (Box 25.1)
- *All hospital inpatients*: on admission and repeated weekly or as per protocol.
- *All hospital outpatients*: on their first clinic visit and repeated when there is clinical concern.
- *All people in care homes*: on admission and repeated when there is clinical concern.
- *All people on GP lists*: on initial registration and repeated when there is clinical concern.

Hospital departments who see groups of patients who are low risk may opt out of screening following an explicit decision made in conjunction with nutrition experts.

How to screen

Many different nutrition screening tools are available. The tool selected for use must:
- have validity confirmed by peer reviewed publication;[1]
- be appropriate for the patient population;
- include the essential variables (see Box 25.2);
- have suitable cut-off points to maximize sensitivity and specificity (minimizing false positive and false negative results);
- provide outcomes that can be acted on when appropriate (link to care plans);
- reflect local needs and overcome resistance to implementation;
- be associated with a staff training programme;
- be user-friendly.

---

1 National Institute for Heath and Care Excellence (NICE) (2012). *Nutrition support in adults*. Quality Standard 24. Available at: https://www.nice.org.uk/guidance/qs24/chapter/Quality-statement-1-Screening-for-the-risk-of-malnutrition.

Box 25.1 Clinical concerns that should trigger early repeat screening
- Unintentional weight loss
- Fragile skin
- Poor wound healing
- Wasted muscles
- Apathy with ↓ intake
- Prolonged intercurrent illness
- Poor appetite
- Altered taste sensation
- Impaired swallowing
- Altered bowel habit
- Loose fitting clothes

Box 25.2 All screening must include evaluation of
- Body mass index (BMI), see ➲ Appendix 2
- Percentage unintentional weight loss
- Length of time that nutritional intake unintentionally reduced
- Likelihood of future impaired nutrient intake

See BMI ready reckoner for adults inside front cover.

🔗 http://www.nice.org.uk/guidance/CG32.

Malnutrition universal screening tool

The malnutrition universal screening tool[2] (MUST), developed by the multi-disciplinary British Association for Parenteral and Enteral Nutrition (BAPEN), is considered the most scientifically robust, practical, and versatile nutrition screening tool for adults (Boxes 25.3 and 25.4). It has been designed to detect undernutrition (malnutrition) and overnutrition (overweight/obesity).

Box 25.3 Use of Malnutrition Universal Screening Tool (MUST)

In all care settings including
- Hospital inpatients and outpatients
- Care homes
- GP surgeries and health centres
- Community

With different groups of adult patients, including but not exclusively
- Elderly
- Surgical
- Medical
- Orthopaedic
- Those requiring intensive care
- Mental health care
- Pregnancy and lactation (with adaptation)

By different healthcare professionals
- Nurses
- Doctors
- Dietitians
- Healthcare assistants
- Students

---

2 British Association for Parenteral and Enteral Nutrition (BAPEN) (2011). *Malnutrition Universal Screening Tool (MUST)*. Available at: ℬ http://www.bapen.org.uk/pdfs/must/must_full.pdf.

Box 25.4 The five MUST steps

1 Calculate BMI from weight and height (see ➜ Chapter 4, 'Anthropometry', p. 53). If height cannot be measured, see ➜ this Chapter 4 'Anthropometry' p. 56
   • BMI >20 = 0 (>30 = obese)
   • 18.5–20 = 1
   • <18.5 = 2
2 Note unplanned weight loss (%) in past 3–6 months.
   • <5% = 0
   • 5–10% = 1
   • >10% = 2
3 Consider the effect of acute disease.
   • If patient is acutely ill and there has been, or is likely to be, no nutritional intake for >5 days, score 2
4 Add scores from 1, 2, and 3 together to give overall risk of malnutrition. Total score
   • 0 indicates low risk
   • 1 indicates medium risk
   • ≥2 indicates high risk
5 Initiate appropriate nutritional management.
   Using local management guidelines (Table 25.1), prepare appropriate care plan.

   The 'Malnutrition Universal Screening Tool' ('MUST') is reproduced here with the kind permission of BAPEN (British Association for Parenteral and Enteral Nutrition). For further information on 'MUST' see ℛ www.bapen.org.uk.

Table 25.1 Malnutrition universal screening tool nutritional management guidelines*

Low risk (score 0)	*Routine clinical care*
	Repeat screening (hospital, weekly; care home, monthly; community, annually for special groups, e.g. those >75 years)
	See Box 25.1 for concerns that trigger early repeat screening
Medium risk (score 1)	*Observe*
	Document dietary intake for 3 days if subject in hospital or care home
	If improved or adequate intake, little clinical concern. Repeat screening (hospital, weekly; care home, at least monthly; community, at least every 2–3 months)
	If no improvement, clinical concern: follow local policy, set goals, improve and increase overall nutritional intake, monitor and review care plan regularly
High risk (score ≥2)	*Treat†*
	Refer to dietitian, nutritional support team, or implement local policy
	Set goals, improve and increase overall nutritional intake
	Monitor and review care plan (hospital, weekly; care home, monthly; community, monthly)
All risk categories	Treat underlying condition and provide help and advice on food choices, eating and drinking when necessary
	Record malnutrition risk category
	Record need for special diets and follow local policy
Obesity	Record presence of obesity. For those in hospital with underlying conditions, these are generally controlled before the treatment of obesity

*The 'Malnutrition Universal Screening Tool' ('MUST') is reproduced here with the kind permission of BAPEN (British Association for Parenteral and Enteral Nutrition). Further information on 'MUST' is available at: ℬ www.bapen.org.uk.

†Unless detrimental or no benefit is expected from nutritional support, e.g. imminent death.

If height cannot be measured

Where height cannot be measured, use recently documented or reported height if it appears realistic. If this is not possible, a surrogate measure can be used, e.g. ulna length, knee height, or demi-span. Ulna length is the easiest to obtain in bed-bound patients and can be measured as follows:

- The forearm is placed diagonally across the chest with fingers pointing towards the shoulder and palm inwards.
- The distance is measured between the central and most prominent part of the styloid process (bony knobble on outer wrist, little finger side) and centre tip of the olecranon process (elbow), see Figure 25.1.
- Estimated height ($_e$Ht) is calculated:
  - men <65 years: $_e$Ht (cm) = 79.2 + 3.60 × ulna length (cm);
  - men ≥65 years: $_e$Ht (cm) = 86.3 + 3.15 × ulna length (cm);
  - women <65 years: $_e$Ht (cm) = 95.6 + 2.77 × ulna length (cm);
  - women ≥65 years: $_e$Ht (cm) = 80.4 + 3.25 × ulna length (cm).
- Note that the calculated values may be inaccurate and particularly in Asian women, may produce an overestimate of height. Alternative equations are available for adults from non-White backgrounds.[3]

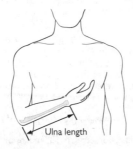

Ulna length

Fig. 25.1 Measurement of ulna length.

Self-screening for malnutrition

A self-screening tool has been developed for adults living in the community. It is well-accepted by users and the screening findings agree with those of healthcare professionals.[4]

Further information

MUST charts, toolkit, guidelines, and explanatory booklet can be downloaded from ◌ http://www.bapen.org.uk/screening-and-must/must.

3 Madden, A.M. et al. (2019) Improved prediction equations for estimating height in adults from ethnically diverse backgrounds. Clin. Nutr. doi: 10.1016/j.clnu.2019.06.007.

4 Cawood, A.L., et al. (2012) Malnutrition self-screening by using MUST in hospital outpatients: validity, reliability, and ease of use. Am. J. Clin. Nutr. 96, 1000–7.

Undernutrition

Undernutrition (often referred to as malnutrition) arises as a consequence of an inadequate intake of energy and macronutrients. It may also be associated with frank or subclinical micronutrient deficiencies in some people. The interplay between inadequate intake and disease is important and influences health outcomes. This is highlighted by two subgroups of undernutrition:

- *Sarcopenia* is defined as the loss of muscle mass and muscle strength. It is most often seen in older people but also in undernutrition and muscle disuse.[5]
- *Cachexia* is defined as a multi-factorial syndrome characterized by severe loss of weight, muscle, and fat, and increased protein catabolism caused by underlying diseases.

Using these definitions, all people with cachexia are undernourished but not all people who are undernourished are cachexic.

Classification

There is no single, universally accepted definition or classification of undernutrition, although a pattern of less than optimum body weight or loss of body weight is the main feature.

Body mass index (BMI)

Cut-off values between 18.5 and 20.0 kg/m² are most often used to identify risk of undernutrition in adults (Table 25.2). However, the use of BMI has its limitations. It cannot be used in children where height may be stunted as a result of poor nutrition, in the very elderly where a true height may be difficult to measure, or where unusual body morphology invalidates the ratio of weight to height.

$$BMI = weight\ (kg)/height^2(m^2)$$

See ➲ Chapter 1, 'Anthropometry', p. 53, and inside front cover.

Mid-upper arm circumference (MUAC)

Can be used if BMI cannot be calculated because of the absence of an accurate height measurement or because true weight is obscured by fluid retention (Table 25.3). (See ➲ Chapter 4, 'Anthropometry', p. 58).

Standard deviation score (Z-score)

Calculated from reference population data and used to determine risk of undernutrition in children (Table 25.4). No values for height are required and it is independent of age, making it useful in situations where these cannot be obtained.

$$Z\text{-}score = (patient's\ weight - median\ weight\ for\ population)/$$
$$SD\ value\ for\ population$$

See ➲ Chapter 4, 'Anthropometry', p. 54.

5 Muscaritoli, M., et al. (2010). Consensus definition of sarcopenia, cachexia and pre-cachexia: Joint document elaborated by Special Interest Groups (SIG) "cachexia-anorexia in chronic wasting diseases" and "nutrition in geriatrics". Clin. Nutr. **29**, 154–9.

Table 25.2 Categories of BMI for identifying undernutrition in adults

WHO classification of BMI, kg/m²	Interpretation
<18.50 (underweight)	Chronic undernutrition probable
18.50–24.99 (healthy/normal weight)	Chronic undernutrition possible if BMI <20
≥25.00 (overweight)	Chronic undernutrition unlikely (low risk)

Table 25.3 Classification of undernutrition in adults using MUAC*

MUAC, cm	Classification
Men	
≥22.5	Low risk of undernutrition
<22.5	Possible risk of undernutrition
Women	
≥17.7	Low risk of undernutrition
<17.7	Possible risk of undernutrition

*Source: data based on 5th percentiles from Bishop, C.W., et al. (1981). Norms for nutritional assessment of American adults by upper arm anthropometry. Am. J. Clin. Nutr. **34**, 2530–9.
Note: Although more recent data are available, the 1981 cut-offs are more useful for identifying undernutrition because of subsequent population increases in obesity prevalence.

Table 25.4 Classification of undernutrition in adults and children using Z-scores*

Z-score	Type and degree of undernutrition (ICD code)
–1 to +1	No undernutrition
–1 to –2	Mild undernutrition (E44.0)
–2 to –3	Moderate undernutrition (E44.1)
<–3	Severe undernutrition (E43)

*Adapted from Stratton, R.J., et al. (2003). *Disease-related malnutrition:* Reproduced with permission CABI publishing.

🔑 Malnourished patients are not always thin. They may be overweight or obese (sarcopenic obesity), but have suffered recent, unplanned weight loss.

🔑 Classifying undernutrition is concerned with establishing risk. None of the methods described above are fool proof but they do provide simple and reproducible means of undertaking this. The consequences of failing to identify and treat undernutrition are potentially serious and caution should be used when interpreting results. (For routine nutrition screening, see ➔ this chapter, 'Malnutrition universal screening tool'.)

Prevalence of malnutrition

The prevalence of undernutrition varies with the population, age group, presence and severity of disease, health, care setting, and the method used to identify undernutrition.

- 10-14% tenants in sheltered housing
- 14% of elderly people living at home;
- 30-42% of individuals living in care homes;
- 28% of patients admitted to hospital.

These figures show that undernutrition is not a rare event and so all healthcare staff working in all settings should be aware of this and ready to instigate and implement screening, prevention, and treatment policies. Identifying, treating, and preventing malnutrition are multi-disciplinary responsibilities.

Contributing causes

In most cases, the causes of undernutrition are multi-factorial and inter-linked (Fig. 25.2). An awareness of some specific contributory factors is a valuable first step in prevention. The following is just a brief summary.

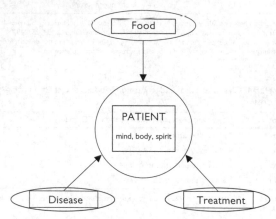

Fig. 25.2 To identify key causative factors of undernutrition, a holistic view of the patient, including their social context, is required.

Reduced nutritional intake
- Inadequate food availability (quantitative or qualitative):
  - patients nursed in isolation where meal trays may be left outside a single room or where they cannot be reached;
  - repeated deliberate starvation, e.g. nil by mouth for multiple tests or treatment;
  - slow motor co-ordination requiring feeding assistance;

- culturally inappropriate meals, e.g. providing non-halal or non-kosher food for Muslims or Jews (see ➜ Chapter 16).
- poor quality or unappetizing food.
- Anorexia (loss of appetite):
  - effects of disease, e.g. cancer, infection, inflammation;
  - nausea and vomiting;
  - psychological issues, e.g. depression, anxiety, loneliness;
  - effects of treatment, e.g. chemotherapy.
- Eating problems:
  - poor dentition;
  - changes in taste and smell, sometimes disease/treatment-related;
  - dry or painful mouth;
  - breathlessness;
  - disordered swallowing.

Reduced nutrient absorption
- Insufficient gastrointestinal (GI) secretions, including bile and all digestive enzymes, e.g. lack of pancreatic enzymes.
- Damage to absorptive GI surface, e.g. Crohn's disease.
- Gastrointestinal resection ± fistulae.
- Complication of drug therapy.

Increased requirements
- Disease-related hypermetabolism, e.g. liver cirrhosis, some cancers.
- Infection.
- Treatment-related, e.g. post-surgery.
- ↑ Losses, e.g. via GI tract, urine, skin, breath, or surgical drains.
- ↑ Activity, voluntary and involuntary, e.g. Parkinson's disease.

Consequences

The effects of undernutrition vary from subclinical with no obvious clinical impairment to death, and are dependent on the type, length, and degree of nutritional inadequacy and the age and nutritional and health status of the individual.

Survival in the total abstinence from any nutrient intake (water only) is:
- ~55–75 days in lean adults;
- ~32 days newborn infant;
- ~5 days pre-term infant.

In addition to a significant ↑ risk of mortality, undernutrition is associated with greater morbidity:
- Weight loss (predominantly fat and muscle).
- Impaired muscle function:
  - skeletal muscle—poor mobility, ↑ risk of falls;
  - respiratory—↑ risk of chest infection, ↓ reduced exercise capacity, delayed ventilator weaning;
  - cardiac—bradycardia, hypotension, ↓ cardiac output;
  - GI tract—↓ gut wall integrity increasing potential for micro-organism access.

- Reduced immune function:
  - ↓ phagocytosis, ↓ chemotaxis, ↓ intracellular bacterial destruction, ↓ T lymphocytes;
  - ↑ rates of infection;
  - poor response to vaccination.
- Impaired synthesis of new protein:
  - poor wound healing, ↑ risk of ulceration;
  - delayed recovery from surgery;
  - growth faltering or cessation in children;
  - ↓ fertility in women and men.
- Psychological impairment:
  - depression, anorexia, ↓ motivation;
  - ↓ quality of life;
  - intellectual impairment if malnourished in infancy.
- Increased economic cost:
  - ↑ complications;
  - ↑ length of stay in hospital and intensive care unit;
  - ↑ re-admission rates following discharge;
  - longer rehabilitation;
  - ↑ pharmaceutical cost;
  - ↑ visits to GP.

Treatment of undernutrition

Why bother treating undernourished patients? There is good evidence that nutritional support can increase energy and protein intake, which leads to increased body weight and attenuated weight loss, improved functional outcomes (muscle strength, walking distances, activity levels, mental health) and clinical outcomes (mortality, complications, length of hospital stay) in both hospital and community settings.

The following numbered sections correspond to the numbered stages in Figure 25.3:

1. Assessment

When undernutrition (malnutrition) is identified on screening, a full nutritional assessment should be undertaken to identify possible causes (see ➲ this Chapter 'Undernutrition') and provide a basis for treatment.

After assessment, the following steps can be taken. Although they are suggested in a sequential path, it may be appropriate to undertake a number simultaneously and utilize points that are relevant to the individual being treated.

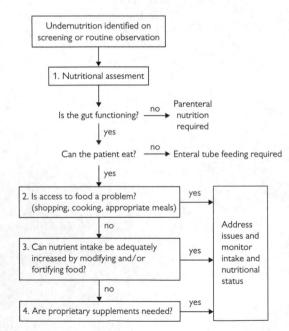

Fig. 25.3 Algorithm showing pathway of nutrition support for undernourished patients.

2. Food access

After assessment, it may become apparent that some relatively simple, non-technical measures are needed to help the undernourished individual access suitable food. Examples:

- arranging support through appropriate carers, e.g. shopping, cooking, company while eating;
- locating/repairing dentures;
- providing appropriate cutlery, dishes, utensils, etc. Seek expertise from occupational therapy;
- modifying texture of foods provided (see ➜ Chapter 23, 'Modification of texture of food and fluid');
- requesting suitable meals, e.g. vegetarian, halal, kosher (see Tables 16.1–16.3).

3. Food first: supplementation using food

The modification and/or supplementation of food and drink using ordinary food items can substantially increase energy and nutrient intake in many patients. This is a relatively straightforward step and should be tried before more complex interventions are initiated, i.e. 'food first'.[6] The patient's nutritional status must be monitored regularly. Examples:

- ensuring three or four meals each day;
- offering nutritious snacks between meals, e.g. small sandwiches, cheese and biscuits, yogurt;
- replacing all low fat items with higher fat alternatives (e.g. full cream milk);
- limiting drinks or foods that provide little energy or nutrients, e.g. low calorie drinks, salads, clear soups;
- increasing energy/protein density of meals and drinks by fortifying, e.g. adding butter, margarine, olive oil, grated cheese to mashed potato or savoury sauces, or adding sugar, honey, jam, milk powder, cream to desserts, milky drinks, etc.

❥ Care must be taken to ensure micronutrient intake is adequate when using fortifying food with energy or protein only;

- 'treats' like cake, biscuits, chocolate, crisps, etc., can provide valuable additional calories but should not replace meals providing protein and range of other nutrients;
- alcohol, as an aperitif or added to milky drinks, can stimulate the appetite and provide some extra energy.

Advantages include flexibility, palatability, the non-medicalization of eating, and lower cost. Success depends on the patient being able to consume enough food and a dedicated team of carers and/or health professionals.

Disadvantages include the requirement of a high level of motivation and effort ± culinary skills in patient, carers, and health professionals, the limited availability of appropriate ingredients in institutional food production, the difficulty in measuring ↑ intake, and potential need for additional micronutrient supplementation.

6 Available at: ℘ https://www.bapen.org.uk/nutrition-support/nutrition-by-mouth/food-first-project-leaflets.

Table 25.5 Examples of proprietary oral nutrition supplements available on prescription

Type	Brand name (manufacturer)
Milk-based drinks	Complan® Shake (Nutricia); Fresubin® Original (Fresenius Kabi); Resource® Energy (Nestlé Health Science)
Juice-based drinks	Ensure® Plus Juice (Abbott); Fortijuice® (Nutricia)
Savoury drinks	Ensure® Plus savoury (Abbott); Vitasavoury® (Vitaflo)
Desserts	Clinutren® Dessert (Nestlé); Forticreme® Complete (Nutricia

4. Supplementation using proprietary oral nutrition supplements

Many ready-to-use oral nutrition supplements (ONS), often called sip feeds, are available that can contribute to a nutritionally well-balanced intake. These may be used in conjunction with the 'food first' approach described above or used to make up a deficit if an individual cannot eat sufficient food. Some products are prescribable for patients who are under-nourished (Table 25.5; see also ➜ Chapter 38, 'Drug-nutrient interactions and prescription of nutritional products').

These products can also be bought without a prescription but are relatively expensive. Non-prescribable supplements, including some powdered products which need to be mixed with milk or water. These are a cheaper alternative and are available in some supermarkets, e.g. Meritene® (Nestlé), Nurishment® (Grace Foods).

Advantages of ONS include their known composition, most provide well-balanced intake of energy, macro- and micro-nutrients (but see caution at the end of this section), availability of ready-to-use form requiring little or no preparation, range of products and flavours, and no cost to patient if prescribed.

Disadvantages include the 'quick fix' of readily dispensed products without full evaluation of the patient's needs, flavour-fatigue after prolonged use, prescribing cost, medicalization of nutritional intake may further discourage eating, and ready-to-use products are bulky/heavy and require storage space for patients at home.

🌑 Care must be taken to ensure that total micronutrient intake is adequate when using ONS products in a supplementary role as they may not provide sufficient to meet requirements.

Box 25.5 Ethical issues when starting or stopping nutritional support

- Consent must be obtained from the patient if he or she is competent.
- Act in the patient's best interest if he or she is not competent to give consent.
- People receiving nutritional support, and their carers, must be kept informed about their treatment. They should also have access to appropriate information and be given the opportunity to discuss diagnosis and treatment options.
- Provision of nutrition support is not always appropriate, e.g. if detrimental or no benefit is expected from nutritional support, i.e. imminent death,
- Decisions on withholding or withdrawing of nutrition support and hydration require a consideration of both ethical and legal principles (both at common law and statute including the Human Rights Act 1998).

See ➲ Chapter 35, 'Palliative care', and ➲ Chapter 32, 'Mental Capacity Act 2005'.

Next step

If an undernourished patient is unable to achieve an adequate intake orally using the above suggestions and is considered to need additional support, feeding artificially via the gut if it is functioning (see ➲ this Chapter, 'Enteral feeding') or directly into the blood (see ➲ this Chapter, 'Parenteral nutrition') will be required. Ethical issues should be considered when planning nutritional support (Box 25.5).

Enteral feeding: introduction

'Enteral' refers to the GI tract so theoretically, 'enteral feeding' encompasses all nutrition assimilated via the gut, including eating and drinking. However, in clinical practice the term is usually used to describe the administration of nutritional feed into the gut through a tube including via nasogastric, nasojejunal, gastrostomy, and jejunostomy routes. If the gut is accessible and functioning, nutrition should be provided by enteral as opposed to parenteral feeding (Box 25.6).

Enteral feeding is indicated when oral feeding is insufficient or unsafe and it is most commonly used in patients with the following features or disorders:[7]

• unconscious patient;
• neuromuscular swallowing disorders, e.g. stroke;
• physiological anorexia;
• upper GI obstruction, e.g. head and neck or oesophageal tumour;
• GI dysfunction or malabsorption, e.g. GI dysmotility, pancreatitis;
• increased nutrient requirements;
• psychological problems;
• specific treatment, e.g. Crohn's disease.

To undertake enteral feeding, the patient must have some GI tract function.
  ❶ Absolute contraindications include:

• complete obstruction;
• prolonged ileus;
• severe GI tract bleeding (while bleeding is active and patient is
  haemodynamically unstable).

The enteral routes available encompass two main delivery points:

1. Gastric feeding – feed is delivered directly into the stomach via
   orogastric, nasogastric, gastrostomy, or oesophagostomy tube.
2. Post-pyloric feeding – feed is delivered after the stomach directly
   into the bowel via nasoduodenal, nasojejunal, gastrojejunostomy, or
   jejunostomy tube.

Before the insertion of an enteral feeding tube, ethical issues should always be considered. Informed consent must be obtained if the patient has the mental capacity. Whereas offering adequate food and water is seen as a basic duty of care, artificial nutrition support is regarded as medical treatment.

---

7 National Institute for Health and Care Excellence (NICE) (2006). *Nutrition support for adults: Oral nutrition support, enteral tube feeding and parenteral nutrition.* Clinical guideline 32. Available at: ℛ https://www.nice.org.uk/guidance/cg32.

Box 25.6 Advantages of enteral over intravenous feeding
- More physiological than feeding synthetic nutrients into blood
- Absorbed nutrients transported via portal circulation directly to liver to support synthesis and metabolic regulation
- Promotes integrity of GI tract mucosa
- Reduces bacterial translocation, e.g. bacteria migrating from gut lumen into circulation, so associated with lower risk of sepsis and multi-organ failure
- Stimulates gall bladder emptying so reducing risk of gallstone formation
- Provides (usually) all dietary constituents, including some conditionally essential, e.g. glutamine, which may not be added to intravenous formulae
- Provides (usually) dietary fibre which stimulates colonocytes and short chain fatty acid production, optimizing bowel function
- Microbiologically safer than intravenous feeding
- Avoids complications associated with intravenous access including pneumothorax, catheter embolism, etc.
- Cheaper
- Easier (usually) for staff, carers, and patients to manage

Routes for enteral feeding

Nasogastric feeding

Nasogastric (NG) feeding is indicated when:
- the patient is unable to take sufficient nutrition orally;
- the GI tract is functioning normally;
- nutrition support is predicted to be required for <4-6weeks;
- nutrition support likely to be required for >4-6weeks but a gastrostomy tube is contraindicated.

Tubes and placement
- Fine bore tubes (French gauge 6–9) should be used in preference. Wide bore tubes or 'Ryle's' tubes (French gauge 10–18) are associated with ↑ complications, e.g. nasal/oesophageal ulceration and ↓ patient comfort. From 2015, all enteral tubes should have an ENfit connector. There are dual-purpose, wide-bore tubes that have been designed specifically for gastric drainage and short term feeding.
- NG tubes should be placed by healthcare professionals who have relevant training and appropriate skills. A risk assessment should be carried out before insertion and local procedures should be followed.
- Tube should be passed via nose with the help of integral guide wire if possible, ask the patient to sit rather than lie during insertion; swallowing sips of iced water as tube is inserted helps (providing patient is safe to do so). It is important that nothing is administered via the NGT until gastric placement is confirmed and internal stylets/guide wires should not be lubricated before gastric placement is confirmed.[8]
- It is vital to establish that the tube position is in the stomach and not the lungs. Feeding via an incorrectly placed tube may cause death or serious harm. Local policies and procedures must be followed. If there are no local policies and procedures, BAPEN (2012) provides a decision tree to support safe tube insertion.[9] Tube position should be confirmed by:
  - checking aspirate using CE marked pH sticks or paper; pH<5.5 is indicative of gastric placement in adults;
  - X-ray is recommended if there is any doubt about the position of the tube or an aspirate is not obtainable. However, an X-ray only confirms the position of the NGT at the time of X-ray.
- Correct tube position must be confirmed:
  - after initial insertion;
  - before administering each feed and after breaks in feeding;
  - at least once daily during continuous feeding;
  - following episodes of vomiting, retching, and coughing;
  - if evidence of tube displacement, i.e. tape is loose or visual tube is longer;
  - before administering medication;
  - further information on patient safety and risk associated with misplaced tubes is available from NHS (2016).[10]

8 National Patient Safety Agency (NPSA). (2012). Harm from flushing of nasogastric tubes before confirmation of placement. NPSA/2012/RRR001. NPSA, London.

9 BAPEN (2012). Available at: ℛhttps://www.bapen.org.uk/pdfs/decision-trees/naso-gastric-tube-insertion.pdf.

10 NHS (2016). Available at: ℛ https://improvement.nhs.uk/documents/194/Patient_Safety_Alert_Stage_2_-_NG_tube_resource_set.pdf.

Alternative methods for placing and confirming position of nasogastric tubes

Other novel insertion and position-confirming techniques have been established and include:

- electromagnetic sensing devices e.g. Cortrak 2 Enteral Access System™ (Corpak Medsystems);
- integrated real-time imaging system (IRIS) (Covidien Commercial Ltd), which uses a 3-mm camera to visually aid tube placement.

When using tube placement devices, it is vital that correct placement is still checked using pH or X-ray testing.[11]

For what to feed, see ➔ this Chapter, 'Enteral feeding regimes'.

Nasojejunal feeding

Nasojejunal (NJ) feeding enables nutrition to be infused directly into the jejunum. It is the route of choice when feeding is required short term, e.g. <4-6 weeks and the upper GI tract is either dysfunctional or inaccessible, but the GI tract is both functional and accessible distal to the stomach.

Advantages:
- reduces risk of aspirating feed as a result of gastroparesis;
- facilitates early post-operative feeding.

Disadvantages:
- placement of tube is more difficult;
- tubes are more prone to becoming blocked;
- tube may migrate into stomach – risk reduced with placement beyond the ligament of Treitz.

Tubes and placement
- Fine bore tubes of adequate length (100-120 cm) are required.
- Double or triple lumen tubes are available to facilitate simultaneous feeding (post-pylorus), aspiration (gastric) ± pressure regulation.
- To ensure placement in the jejunum, NJ tubes usually require endoscopic insertion or guidance radiologically. As with gastric placement, electromagnetic sensing devices, e.g. Cortrak 2 Enteral Access System™ (Corpak Medsystems) have also been demonstrated to be reliable in ascertaining post-pyloric tube placement.[12]
- Blind placement at the bedside has varying rates of success. Self-advancing tubes, e.g. Tiger 2™ Tube (Cook Medical, USA) have cilia-like flaps that allow peristalsis to pull the tube into the small bowel more effectively.

For what to feed, see ➔ this Chapter, 'Enteral feeding regimes'.

11 NICE (2016). Available at: ℜ https://www.nice.org.uk/advice/mib48/chapter/Summary.

12 Windle, E.M., *et al.* (2010). Implementation of an electromagnetic imaging system to facilitate nasogastric and post-pyloric feeding tube placement in patients with and without critical illness. *J. Hum. Nutr. Diet.* **23**, 61–8.

Gastrostomy feeding

- A feeding gastrostomy is an artificial route made between the stomach and outside the body for feeding when the GI tract between mouth and stomach is inaccessible or unsafe or when long term enteral tube feeding is anticipated. Although this can be made surgically if the patient is undergoing an upper abdominal operation, it is more commonly formed as a percutaneous endoscopic gastrostomy (PEG) or radiologically inserted gastrostomy (RIG).
- There is often confusion and misunderstanding of gastrostomy terminology so it is important that every patient with a gastrostomy has clearly documented in their notes the date of insertion, size, and how it is retained.
- From 2015 all enteral tubes should have an ENfit connector.

Percutaneous endoscopic gastrostomy
Indication
- Patients requiring enteral nutrition support >4-6 weeks.

Contraindications
- Pharyngeal/oesophageal tumour (depending on tumour position).
- Severe obesity.
- Portal hypertension or gastric varices.
- Total or partial gastrectomy.
- Ascites.
- Peritoneal dialysis.
- Coagulopathy.

Advantages
- PEGs can be inserted as a day-care procedure provided appropriate aftercare is available.
- ↓ Inadvertent removal of tube so fewer disruptions to feeding in comparison to nasal tubes.
- ↓ Reflux and aspiration of feed (as tube cannot migrate into the oesophagus), so overnight feeding may be safer.
- Cosmetically more appealing, especially for patients who are 'out and about'.
- Discreet fixation devices (button tubes) are available that facilitate tube detachment and are more practical for active patients, especially children.
- Easily removed when no longer needed, either endoscopically or traction removable if tubes with compressible or deflatable internal bumpers are used. They can also be removed by cutting (internal fixation device passes out through GI tract). A risk assessment and appropriate patient follow-up is recommended as there is a risk of bowel obstruction and perforation

Radiologically inserted gastrostomy
Advantages over PEG:
- More suitable for patients with compromised ventilation if endoscopy sedation is undesirable.
- Insertion success rate is >PEGs.
- Lower risk of tumour seeding in head and neck cancer patients than when an endoscope is used.

Disadvantages
- Longevity of tubes <PEGs (need to plan replacements).
- Greater risk of misplacement than PEGs as normally balloon or 'pig-tail' retained tubes.
- Associated with some post-procedural pain.
- Clearer picture of anatomy allowing tube placement in difficult patients where endoscopic placement may have failed.

Gastrostomy-specific complications
- Rare but serious complications include peritonitis, infection, bowel perforation, haemorrhage, and aspiration pneumonia, but prompt recognition of these with early action reduces the risk of serious harm or death. It is recommended that:[13]
1. Local protocols specify the observations to be taken in the immediate recovery period.
2. Medical notes are marked with a high visibility sticker warning of the possible complications that could occur and the necessary actions.
3. Where patients are discharged within 72 hours of tube insertion, equivalent warnings should be communicated to the GP, community nurses, care home nurses, as well as to the patient and/or carers.
- Tube displacement. Reasonable care is needed to avoid inadvertently removing gastrostomy. Tube length and position of external markers should be checked daily to ensure tube has not migrated into/from the stomach. Those held by an internal balloon device may dislodge if balloon deflates; this should be checked weekly by withdrawing and replacing water contained within. If the tube is inadvertently removed, the tract will remain patent for up to 48 hours. A replacement tube should be inserted as soon as possible if the tract is mature; if no spare tube is available, the tract could be preserved with a *temporary* Foley catheter but not used for feeding and a replacement gastrostomy then inserted when possible.
- Peristomal infection/abscess. This can be ↓ by giving prophylactic antibiotics at insertion and undertaking good clinical practice, e.g. bathe, dry carefully, and check daily for redness, signs of gastric leak.
- Overgranulation. Relatively common but can generally be reduced by correct positioning of the external fixation disc. Topical steroid treatment may be required.
- 'Buried bumper syndrome'. This may occur if the internal fixation plate becomes buried within the abdominal wall as a result of overgrowth. This can be prevented by releasing the tube and rotating it by 360° every week (except in those with jejunal extension). Gastrostomies held in by an internal balloon are not prone to 'buried bumper syndrome'.

Other types of gastrostomy
- A surgical gastrostomy may be placed if an endoscopic insertion is not possible and the patient is undergoing surgery for other reasons. Complications include haemorrhage, skin excoriation from leaking

13 National Patient Safety Agency (NPSA). (2010). Early detection of complications after gastrostomy. Rapid response report NPSA/2010/RRR010. NPSA, London.

gastric fluid, wound dehiscence, and intraperitoneal leakage of gastric contents.

Home enteral feeding
- Patients with an enteral feeding tube may be hospital inpatients, but many manage their own nutrition in the community, either alone or with the help of carers. Advice on management of both feeding and tube care, and practical assistance is vital for this nutrition support to be successful and not become another burden for a chronically ill person. Dietitians and nutrition nurses with expertise in this area have a vital role to play and their valuable input cannot be overemphasized.
- Ongoing supplies of feed and consumable items, 'plastics', required for delivery and tube care need to be organized for patients in the community, along with education for them and their carers about how to manage feeding with maximum care and minimum stress.

For what to feed, see ➲ this Chapter, 'Enteral feeding regimens'.

Further information

National Institute for Health and Care Excellence (NICE) (2006). *Nutrition support for adults: Oral nutrition support, enteral tube feeding and parenteral nutrition.* Clinical guideline 32. Available at: ℘ https://www.nice.org.uk/guidance/cg32.

Jejunostomy feeding

A feeding jejunostomy is an artificial route made between the jejunum and outside the body. It is used when the GI tract between mouth and jejunum is inaccessible, unsafe, or malfunctioning, and when long term enteral tube feeding is anticipated.

The indications are similar to those for gastrostomy, i.e. nutritional support required for >4-6 weeks, but where post-pyloric feeding is required, e.g. in gastric stasis. The contraindications are the same as for gastrostomy. Jejunostomy tubes may be inserted during upper GI surgery as a reliable source of post-operative feeding, even when this feeding method may be anticipated for <4-6 weeks.

Gastrojejunostomy
Involves use of a jejunal extension conversion kit, which can be attached to an existing PEG to deliver feed into the jejunum.

Jejunostomy
Most commonly inserted during upper-GI surgery, although can also be inserted via direct percutaneous puncture in interventional radiology departments that have the appropriate technical skill. There is no internal retention device so these tubes must be secured externally. The tubes used directly puncture the jejunum, although some are designed to be tunnelled under the skin and are held in place using a felt-like cuff under the skin surface.

For what to feed, see ➲ this Chapter, 'Enteral feeding regimens'.

Enteral feeding regimens

- The patient's nutritional requirements should be estimated (see ➲ this Chapter, 'Estimating requirements in disease states'). Energy and protein are very important and usually take priority, but fluid, electrolytes, macro- and micronutrients, and fibre also need consideration.
- The type and amount of feed that will provide the requirements should be calculated: the dietitian is best placed to advise.
  - Most standard feeds = 100 kcal and 4 g protein/100 mL.
  - Most high energy feeds = 150–200 kcal and 6 g protein/100 mL.
- Method and rate of administration should be determined to ensure all feed is given in a way best suited to the patient's preference, convenience, and medication. Options include:
  - *continuous infusion* over 16–24 hours ± regulated by a pump. This should be used for patients in intensive care and for those who have difficulty tolerating large quantities of feed;
  - *intermittent infusion* over 8–20 hours ± regulated by pump. Providing 'rest' periods may facilitate patient activity, eating, and sleeping; alternatively, feeding can be undertaken overnight. Stopping feeding for >4 hours is associated with ↓ gastric pH and ↑ antibacterial effect;
  - *bolus feeding* of approximately 100–500 mL given by gravity feed or syringed in over 10–30 minutes × 4–10 times daily. Time-consuming and may lead to abdominal symptoms especially in sick patients, but is more physiological, e.g. resembles 'meal pattern', so can work well for stable patients.
- Initial administration of feeding needs special consideration:
  - There is little evidence that starter regimens, i.e. diluted feeds or very slow rates of initial delivery, are associated with improved feed tolerance, even with hypertonic feeds, but they will result in delayed administration of the full feed volume. Dilution of ready-to-feed enteral preparations also introduces a risk of contamination.
  - If the patient has been eating relatively normally prior to starting enteral feeding and is reasonably well, then higher rates of feeding should be initiated, i.e. at least 50% of the target volume that will meet requirements. This should be increased to the target volume over the first 24–48 hours according to metabolic and GI tolerance.
- If the patient is deemed at risk of refeeding syndrome, feeding should be initiated according to refeeding guidance, see ➲ this Chapter, 'Refeeding syndrome'.
- It is not necessary to check gastric aspirates in stable patients who tolerate feeding well. For acutely ill patients, i.e. feeding on intensive care or high dependency units, see ➲ this Chapter, 'Critical care'.

Monitoring enteral feeding

- Monitoring the patient on a regular basis will minimize the risk of developing complications and help ensure that the patient's nutritional requirements are met and contribute to the best use of resources.
- Each patient should have an individualized monitoring plan, which should be regularly reviewed.
- Categories of variables for monitoring include:
  - anthropometric;
  - biochemical/laboratory;
  - clinical;
  - dietary/nutritional.
- Deciding which variables and how often to monitor them depends on the clinical and nutritional status of the patient, the disease process, the duration of feeding, and the patient's location. Obviously, a stable patient who has been fed via a PEG for 18 months and lives at home will require less monitoring than a patient receiving NG feeding on an intensive care unit. The guidance in Tables 25.6 and 25.7, drawn from the National Institute for Health and Care Excellence, provide an outline that should be adapted to the needs of individual patients.

Table 25.6 Guidelines for laboratory monitoring of enteral feeding in hospital inpatients*

Variable	Frequency
Na$^+$, K$^+$, urea, creatinine	Baseline, daily until stable, then 1–2 times/week
Blood glucose	Baseline, 1–2 daily (or more if needed) until stable, then weekly
Mg^{++}, PO$_4$	Baseline, daily if risk of refeeding, 3 times/week until stable, then weekly
LFTs, INR	Baseline, twice/week until stable, then weekly
Corrected Ca^{++}, albumin	Baseline, then weekly
C reactive protein	Baseline, then 2–3 times/week until stable
Full blood count, MCV	Baseline, 1–2 times/week until stable, then weekly
Fe^{++}, ferritin	Baseline, then as required
Folate, B$_{12}$	Baseline, then as required

Monitoring of Zn^{++}, Cu^{++}Mn, 25 OH vitamin D, and bone density is rarely needed in patients receiving enteral feeding unless there is cause for concern.

*Source: data from National Institute for Health and Care Excellence (NICE) (2006). *Nutrition support for adults: Oral nutrition support, enteral tube feeding and parenteral nutrition.* Clinical guideline 32. ℘ https://www.nice.org.uk/guidance/cg32.

Table 25.7 Guidelines for nutritional, anthropometric, and clinical monitoring of enteral feeding in hospital inpatients*

Variable	Frequency
Nutrient intake†	Daily
Volume of feed delivered†	Daily
Fluid balance chart	Daily
Weight†	Daily if concerns about fluid balance, otherwise weekly reducing to monthly
BMI†	Start of feeding and then monthly
Mid-upper arm circumference (MUAC)†	Monthly – useful as a surrogate for BMI or to calculate MAMC
Triceps skinfold†	Monthly – indirect measure of body fat and used to calculate MAMC
Mid-arm muscle circumference (MAMC) †	Monthly – assessment of lean body mass (LBM)
Calf circumference†	Monthly – may be a better indicator of LBM than MAMC
Hand grip dynamometry†	Weekly – to assess muscle function/strength
Nausea/vomiting†	Daily initially reducing to twice weekly
Diarrhoea†	Daily initially reducing to twice weekly
Constipation†	Daily initially reducing to twice weekly
Abdominal distension	As necessary
Nasally inserted tubes	
Tube position†	Before each feed begins
Nasal erosion†	Daily
Tube fixation†	Daily
Tube integrity†	Daily
Gastrostomy or jejunostomy tubes	
Stoma site†	Daily
Tube position†	Daily
Tube insertion and rotation†	Weekly
Balloon water volume†	Weekly
General clinical condition†	Daily
Temperature	Daily initially and then as needed
Blood pressure	Daily initially and then as needed
Drug therapy†	Daily initially reducing to monthly when stable
Are goals being met?†	Daily initially, reducing to twice weekly and then progressively to 3–6 months unless clinical condition changes

(Continued)

Table 25.7 (Contd.)

Variable	Frequency
Are goals still appropriate?†	Daily initially, reducing to twice weekly and then progressively to 3–6 months unless clinical condition changes

*Source: data from National Institute for Health and Care Excellence (NICE) (2006). *Nutrition support for adults: Oral nutrition support, enteral tube feeding and parenteral nutrition*. Clinical guideline 32. ℘ https://www.nice.org.uk/guidance/cg32.

†Community: variables that should be monitored in patients on long-term enteral feeding in the community; see ➲ next section for frequency.

Monitoring enteral feeding in stable patients in the community

- Who by? Monitoring should be undertaken by a healthcare professional with relevant training and skills. Some observations may be made by the patient and/or their carers and where possible, training and support should be provided for them, especially in understanding when to report observations and who to.
- Frequency? Every 3–6 months or more frequently if condition changes.
- Which variables? See Table 25.7, variables marked with |. Laboratory tests are rarely needed in stable patients where feeding is successfully established.

Complications of enteral feeding

Tube blockage (nasogastric, nasojejunal, percutaneous endoscopic gastrostomy)

Prevention
- Flush tube with water every 6 hours, and at start and end of rest periods. Follow local policy for the type of water advised. Sterile water is likely to be recommended in immune-compromised or those fed post-pylorically. Use 30–60 mL water in a 60-mL syringe as a minimum.
- Flush the tube before and after the administration of medication and assume medications are given separately and avoiding crushed tablets where possible. (see ➡ this Chapter, 'Enteral feeding and drugs').
- Low pH (associated with gastric aspirates) encourages protein precipitation. Flush tube with water after each aspiration.

Unblocking
- Never use guide wire—it may pierce tube and injure patient.
- Ensure tube is un-kinked and feel external part of tube to identify any lumps. If located, these may be dispersed by squeezing tube gently.
- Use a 60-mL syringe of warm water to apply push/pull pressure
- Progress on to soda water or sodium bicarbonate and leave in the tube for 30 minutes.
- Pancreatic enzymes, and a commercial product, Corflo Clog Zapper (Corpak Medsystems, Gatwick UK) containing papain and amylase have also been shown to be effective.

Aspiration
- ↑ Risk with ↑ age, dementia, disordered swallow, sedation, supine position, ventilation, and low nursing levels.
- Feed may be aspirated into respiratory tract without obvious vomiting.
- Signs include dyspnoea, cyanosis, tachycardia, and hypotension.
- Can lead to pneumonia with associated ↑ morbidity and mortality.
- Prevent by encouraging patients to lie in semi-recumbent position, elevating bed by 30–45° (unless haemodynamically unstable), use iso-osmotic feeds (optimize gastric emptying).
- Review mode/rate of feeding: continuous infusion may inhibit gastric emptying so changing to bolus feeding may ↓ aspiration risk in some patients. However, in gastroparesis, e.g. ventilated patients, bolus feeding may ↑ gastric volume and potential ↑ risk.
- Pro-motility drugs, e.g. metoclopramide, may be of benefit in ventilated patients with gastroparesis. In others, limited benefit and side effects have been reported so this medication is not generally recommended to prevent tube migration[14] and is associated with risk.[15]
- Consider placing tube post-pylorically (see ➡ this Chapter, 'Routes for enteral feeding').

14 EMA (2013). *European Medicines Agency recommends changes to the use of metoclopramide.* European Medicines Agency. Available at: ℘ www.ema.europa.eu.

15 Silva, C.D., et al. (2009). Metoclopramide for migration of naso-enteral tube. *Cochrane Database Syst. Rev.* CD003353.

Diarrhoea
- Common in enterally fed patients.
- Characteristics of faecal output, e.g. frequency and consistency, are useful in identifying potential abnormality and action needed:
  - frequent liquid stools will compromise absorption, cause patient discomfort, and present difficulties in care so will require intervention;
  - occasional semi-formed motions may be tolerated by patient and carers.
- Diarrhoea can have multiple causes and enteral feed should not automatically be blamed and stopped (Table 25.8).

Microbiological contamination
- Enteral feeds provide an ideal environment for bacteria to multiply in; the consequences of contamination are potentially very serious.
- Where possible, use pre-packaged sterile ready-to-use feeds.
- Check packaging and expiry on all feed and equipment used.
- Demonstrate good hand hygiene practice.
- Ensure systems marked single use are only used once. If pre-packaged feeds and giving sets are used, they should be replaced every 24 hours and feeding tubes replaced according to the manufacturer's guidelines.
- Ensure that reusable equipment for single patient use, e.g. community syringes are cleaned, labelled, and stored appropriately.
- The maximum safe hang-time, i.e. duration of administration, will depend on the feed, patient, and location of delivery. All unused feed should be discarded at the end of the maximum feed time and replaced with fresh feed (see Table 25.9).
- Non-sterile feeds, e.g. re-constituted powder, should be prepared with strict attention to hygiene, covered and stored in a refrigerator for <24 hours. Unused feed must be discarded.
- The reservoir of feed (bag, bottle, carton) must not be hung below the level of the patient's stomach.
- Tap water from a main supply, i.e. drinking water, is suitable for tube flushing, unless the patient is immune-compromised or fed post-pylorically. If the tap water comes from a tank or is of uncertain quality, use cooled boiled or sterile water.

Table 25.8 Factors associated with causing diarrhoea and potential solutions

Causes	Potential solutions
Medication, especially antibiotics and sorbitol	Seek expertise from pharmacist to review and modify if possible
↓ Fibre in gut lumen and consequent effect on colonocytes	Consider changing to a fibre-providing feed
↓ or ↑ change in bowel microflora	Send stool specimen, e.g. to check for *Clostridium difficile*, *Escherichia coli*, and treat accordingly Consider probiotics orally or administered by syringe and flush, although evidence remains unclear (do not add to feed or post-pylorus)*
Rate of continuous feeding	Change to bolus regimen if feeding intragastrically, OR ↓ rate if feeding post-pylorus
Hyperosmolar feed	If using high energy feed, consider changing to standard 1 kcal/mL feed and increasing volume. If using peptide or elemental feed, review osmolarity between brands
Contaminated feed	Ensure good clinical practice; see above
Constipation leading to overflow	Check if colon impacted with faeces; if so, prescribe suppository. Change to fibre feed, ensure adequate hydration, encourage mobility if patient able
Malabsorption (rather than directly feed-related)	Especially in patients with pancreatic or small bowel disease. Differentiate from feed-related diarrhoea by history, visual examination of faecal output (i.e. fatty globules) and spot faecal fat. If present, change feed to semi-elemental feed. Prescribe pancreatic enzyme replacement therapy (see ➲ Chapter 27, 'Pancreatic enzyme replacement therapy'). Consider bile salt sequestrants if bile salt malabsorption suspected or diagnosed

*Whelan, K., *et al.* (2010). Safety of probiotics in patients receiving nutritional support: a systematic review of case reports, randomized controlled trials, and nonrandomized trials. *Am. J. Clin. Nutr.* **91**, 687–703.

Table 25.9 Recommended maximum hang-time for enteral feeds*

Sterile feed in a closed system	24 hours
Sterile feed in an open system at home	12 hours
Sterile feed in an open system in hospital	8 hours
Sterile feed in an open system in hospital (neonates)	4 hours
Non-sterile feed, i.e. re-constituted from powder	4 hours
Non-sterile feed, i.e. with additives	4 hours

*Source: data from Bankhead, R., *et al.* (2009). Enteral nutrition practice recommendations. *J. Parent. Enter. Nutr.* **33**, 122–67.

Enteral feeding and drugs

Patients receiving enteral feeding are often unable to take medication orally and ∴ it may need to be administered via the feeding tube. Using this route or crushing tablets or opening capsules is generally outside the drug's product licence, meaning that the prescriber and practitioner accept liability for any adverse effects resulting from their administration. In each case, advice should be sought from a pharmacist and the following considered.

• If the patient can still take the drug orally (and that is the licensed route), this is best.
• Review all medication—is it all still needed?
• Does the tube deliver the drug distal to the site of absorption?
• ❶ Drugs have a notorious reputation for blocking feeding tubes, especially sticky liquids and antacids, so care must be taken at each dosing.
• Should the drug usually be given before/after or with food? This may mean that the feed has to be stopped; the feeding regimen should be amended to take this into consideration so that the patient still receives the total volume prescribed.
• Drugs should not be added to the feed but should be introduced into the tube using a 60-mL syringe (smaller syringes ↑ pressure in tube and may cause it to split).
• Each drug should be administered separately, unless advised by a pharmacist, followed by 10 mL water. A gap may be required between different drugs.
• Wherever possible, prescribe medication in liquid form or as soluble tablets. Crushing tablets and opening capsules should be considered a last resort.
• Soluble tablets should be dissolved in 10–15 mL water before administration.
• Liquids should be diluted with an equal volume of water and mixed well before administration.
• Tablets that have to be crushed should be ground finely using a pestle and mortar or tablet-crusher. Mix with 10–15 mL water to syringe into tube. Rinse crusher and syringe in rinse water to ensure full drug dose is given.
• Do not crush or chew tablets or capsules that are enterically coated, modified, or slow release.
• Staff should wash their hands and wear gloves to minimize exposure to the drugs. Cytotoxic medication and hormones should not be crushed because of the risk associated with staff exposure.

Further reading

British Association of Parenteral and Enteral Nutrition (2004). Administering drugs via enteral feeding tubes. A practical guide. ℘ http://www.bapen.org.uk/pdfs/d_and_e/de_pract_guide.pdf.
White, R., Bradnam, V. (2015), Hand book of drug administration via enteral feeding tubes. 3rd edn. Pharmaceutical Press, London.

Blended enteral feeding

Patient-led feeding using blended (i.e. liquidized or pureed) food via a gastrostomy tube is increasing, especially in those living at home and on long term tube feeding where some clinical benefits have been reported. However, it is not currently recommended as first line treatment[16,17] because of concerns of potential risks associated with:

- micro-organism contamination from non-sterile preparation techniques, which may cause gastrointestinal or systemic infection;
- blocking tubes arising from particle size, which may lead to disruption of feeding and, if efforts to unblock it are unsuccessful, tube replacement;
- nutritional inadequacy as a result of poorly designed feed recipes and/or excessive dilution with low nutrient fluids.

These concerns are difficult to quantify and there is currently limited evidence to define precisely what is or is not safe practice when blended foods are prepared in a domestic setting. In spite of this, patients and carers who wish to explore blended feeding need to be supported and to be helped to make informed decisions about feeding. Guidance about risk assessing individual situations is available to assist dietitians working in this area.[18]

Further reading

The patient-led websites below provide practical and useful information for practitioners wanting to learn more about blended diets; their inclusion does not confer endorsement.

- Feeding Tube Awareness Foundation. Available at: ℘ https://www.feedingtubeawareness.org/tube-feeding-basics/diet-nutrition/blended-diets/
- Real Food for Real People. Available at: ℘ http://www.foodfortubes.org/

16 Breaks, A., et al. (2018). Blended diets for gastrostomy fed children and young people: a scoping review. J. Hum. Nutr. Diet. 31(5), 634-46.

17 British Dietetic Association (2019). The use of blended diet with enteral feeding tubes. Available at: ℘ https://www.bda.uk.com/improvinghealth/healthprofessionals/policy_statements/policy_statement_-_blended_diet

18 British Dietetic Association (2015). Practice toolkit: Liquidised food via gastrostomy tube. Available at: ℘ https://www.bda.uk.com/professional/practice/liquidisedtoolkit.Due for update in 2019.

Parenteral nutrition

Parenteral nutrition (PN) refers to the administration of nutrients via the intravenous route. It is required when a patient has intestinal failure to a degree that prevents adequate absorption of nutrients via the GI tract. Complications associated with the access route and the nutrient formulation can occur with PN, so careful patient selection and monitoring are essential.[19]

Indications

PN should be considered when a patient is malnourished or at risk and has an inadequate or unsafe oral or enteral intake OR a non-functional, inaccessible, or perforated (leaking) gastrointestinal tract.[7] See **➔** Chapter 26 'Gastrointestinal disease' for further indications.

Routes for provision of PN

Patients who require PN in the short term, can be fed continuously, and a regimen of <1200 mOsmol/L may be fed via a peripheral route, e.g. Venflon cannula. The following may minimize the risk of thrombophlebitis:
- access the largest peripheral vein available;
- use a small cannula;
- use a GTN (glyceryl trinitrate) patch distal to the exit site.

Where it is anticipated that patients may require PN for >14 days, are to be fed on a cyclical basis, or require a regimen of >1200 mOsmol/L, central catheter insertion may be appropriate. The tip of the catheter is inserted to lie in the lower portion of the superior vena cava or right atrium to minimize the risk of thrombosis. Examples include:
- single dedicated feeding catheter;
- peripherally inserted central catheter (PICC);
- multi-lumen catheter using one lumen dedicated for PN.

Where PN is anticipated to be required on a more permanent basis, access can be provided by:
- single lumen cuffed catheter;
- implanted port (Portacath).

PN regimens

PN is not an emergency treatment. Before introducing PN, it is important that a full assessment is completed by a suitably trained healthcare professional who is part of a multi-disciplinary nutrition support team. This should include anthropometry, biochemistry, clinical condition, fluid balance, medication, recent oral intake, and risk of refeeding syndrome. From this, the nutritional requirements can be calculated and the appropriate regimen prescribed to minimize metabolic complications.
- To meet a patient's nutritional requirements PN must contain:
  - fluid;
  - nitrogen;

---

19 NCEPOD (2010). A mixed bag: An enquiry into the care of hospital patients receiving parenteral nutrition. Available at: ✍ http://www.ncepod.org.uk/2010report1/downloads/PN_report.pdf.

- source of energy as a combination of carbohydrate and fat;
- electrolytes;
- fat- and water-soluble vitamins;
- trace elements.
- A pharmacy production unit may provide compounded PN or multi-chamber PN.
  - *Advantages of compounded PN*: greater flexibility to meet the needs of complex patients whose individual requirements could not be met with a standardized regimen;
  - *Advantages of multi-chamber PN*: wide range of formulations available, still some flexibility for adding electrolytes, less cost of having a specialized pharmacy production unit.
- Vitamins and trace elements should always be added to ensure PN is complete.

Monitoring parenteral nutrition

Patients receiving PN must be monitored regularly to detect potential complications associated with PN and/or changes to their clinical condition (Tables 25.10 and 25.11).

Complications

See Table 25.12.

Complications related to catheter insertion and access routes can be minimized by robust hospital policies and procedures. Catheter-related bloodstream infections can develop if an aseptic non-touch technique is not used during catheter handling. Hospitals should have policies in place to minimize the risk of catheter-related sepsis occurring as it can be fatal. To minimize the risk of infection, always feed via a dedicated feeding catheter.

Metabolic complications from the PN solution can be minimized if a thorough assessment by a suitably trained professional has been completed. If a lack or an excess of any of the components of PN are provided, then patients may experience complications such as hyperglycaemia, overhydration including oedema, dehydration, and electrolyte abnormalities including refeeding syndrome.[7] Deranged LFTs are common in patients receiving PN and the cause is usually multi-factorial. To address this, efforts should be made to avoid sepsis, minimize hepatotoxic medications, and exclude other causes of liver disease (pancreatitis, gallbladder disease).

Home parenteral nutrition (HPN)

Patients requiring HPN should be cared for by a specialist multi-disciplinary nutrition support team with the experience and skills required to manage HPN.

Table 25.10 Guidelines for clinical monitoring patients on PN*

Type	Rationale
Daily monitoring	
Fluid input and output; patient's weight	To prevent over- or underhydration
Patient's clinical condition; temperature; feeding line; catheter entry site; skin over catheter tip	To observe and act on possible signs of infection
Nutrient intake	To ensure regimen meets nutritional requirements
Nutrient losses; nausea/vomiting; diarrhoea/stoma/fistula losses	To consider losses when ensuring nutritional adequacy
Weekly monitoring	
Anthropometry: BMI; mid-arm muscle; triceps skinfold	To monitor change in nutritional status
Function measures: grip-strength	To monitor change in nutritional status
Variable frequency monitoring	
Are goals being met?	Daily initially, reducing to twice weekly and then progressively to 3–6 months unless clinical condition changes
Are goals still appropriate?	Daily initially, reducing to twice weekly and then progressively to 3–6 months unless clinical condition changes
Bone density	On starting long term PN, then every 2 years

*Source: data from National Institute for Health and Care Excellence (NICE) (2006). *Nutrition support for adults: Oral nutrition support, enteral tube feeding and parenteral nutrition*. Clinical guideline 32. ℬ https://www.nice.org.uk/guidance/cg32.

Table 25.11 Guidelines for laboratory monitoring of patients on PN*

Variable	Frequency
Na^+, K^+, urea, creatinine	Baseline, daily if at risk of refeeding syndrome until stable, then 1–2 times/week
Blood glucose	Baseline, 1–2 daily (or more if needed, e.g. in diabetes) until stable, then weekly
Mg^{2+}, PO_4	Baseline, daily if risk of refeeding, 3 times/week until stable, then weekly
LFTs, INR	Baseline, twice/week until stable, then weekly
Ca^{2+}, albumin	Baseline, then weekly
C reactive protein	Baseline, then 2–3 times/week until stable
Zn^{2+}, Cu^{2+}	Baseline, then every 2–4 weeks depending on results
Se	Baseline if risk of depletion, further tests depending on baseline
Full blood count, MCV	Baseline, 1–2 times/week until stable, then weekly
Fe^{2+}, ferritin	Baseline, then every 3–6 months
Folate, B_{12}	Baseline, then every 2–4 weeks
Mn^{2+}	Every 3–6 months if on long term PN
25 OH vitamin D	Every 6 months if on long term PN

*Source: data from National Institute for Health and Care Excellence (NICE) (2006). *Nutrition support for adults: Oral nutrition support, enteral tube feeding and parenteral nutrition.* Clinical guideline 32. ⌖ https://www.nice.org.uk/guidance/cg32.

Table 25.12 Possible complications associated with PN

Related to	Examples
Catheter insertion	Pneumothorax, haemothorax, air embolism
Access routes	Thrombophlebitis, central vein thrombosis, catheter-related bloodstream infection, catheter occlusion, catheter fracture
PN solution	Fluid and electrolyte imbalance, metabolic disturbances, impaired liver function

Estimating requirements in disease states

Provision of nutritional support to patients requires estimation of their nutritional requirements to avoid both over- and underfeeding.

Energy

Three methods can be used to estimate nutritional energy requirements for patients requiring nutritional support:

1. A factorial method: basal metabolic rate (BMR) estimated using equation developed in healthy populations followed by the addition of an activity factor, stress factor, or allowance for weight gain to estimate total energy requirements (TEE) for the patient's specific disease state. This method was previously recommended.[20]
2. Use of a regression equation such as the Penn State[21] or Swinamer[22] equations. These include patients' physiological parameters such as body temperature and ventilatory requirements, and are primarily designed for use in the critically ill.
3. Energy per kg body weight, e.g. 20-25 kcal/kg for critically ill patients in the catabolic phase.[23] This method is currently recommended.[24]

❶ All three methods should be used with caution because they are poorly validated or applicable to only a narrow group of patients. It is also important to remember that energy expenditure will change during the course of an illness and monitoring of nutritional status is crucial.

❶ BMR equations, such as those by Henry,[25] are intended for healthy populations and their predictive accuracy for patients is questionable.[26]

❶ The method recommended by the British Dietetic Association Parenteral and Enteral Nutrition Group (PENG)[24] for estimating energy requirements for adults changed in 2018 from a factorial method to one where requirements are based on energy values per kg body weight (BW) or per kg fat free mass (FFM) (Box 25.7, Table 25.13).

Protein

Maintenance of nitrogen balance depends on past and recent energy intake, metabolic state and protein intake. Largest protein losses have been

20 Weekes, E., Soulsby, C. (2011). Energy requirements. In: Todorovic, V.E., Micklewright, A. (2011). *A Pocket Guide to Clinical Nutrition*. 4th edn. British Dietetic Association, PENG.

21 Frankenfield, D., *et al.* (2004). Validation of two approaches to predicting resting metabolic rate in critically ill patients. *JPEN* 28, 259–64.

22 Swinamer, D.L., *et al.* (1990). Predictive equations for assessing energy expenditure in mechanically ventilated critically ill patients. *Crit. Care Med.* 18, 657–61.

23 Singer, P. *et al.* (2009). ESPEN guidelines on parenteral nutrition: intensive care. *Clin. Nutr.* 28, 387–400.

24 Todorovic, V.E., Mafrici, B. (2018). *A Pocket Guide to Clinical Nutrition*. 5th edn. British Dietetic Association, PENG.

25 Henry, C.J.K. (2005). Basal metabolic rate studies in humans: measurement and development of new equations. *Public Health Nutr.* 8, 1133–52.

26 Flancbaum, L., *et al.*, (1999) Comparisons of indirect calorimetry, the Fick method and prediction equations in estimating the energy requirements of critically ill patients. *Am. J. Clin. Nutr.* 69, 461–6.

Box 25.7 Summary of the PENG Guidelines for estimating energy requirements[24]

- Resting energy expenditure (REE) is estimated per kg actual BW or per kg FFM where FFM should be measured not estimated.
- Detailed tables[24] based on systematic review of published evidence provide values for REE per kg BW and REE per kg FFM, respectively, for a number of clinical conditions. In the absence of disease-specific data, REE may be estimated using 20-25 kcal per kg BW per day.
- REE is the energy expended lying still, at physical and mental rest after an overnight fast with no stimulants. It is likely to represent the minimum energy requirement for a patient because it does not include diet-induced thermogenesis (DIT) or physical activity (PA) (see ➔ Chapter 5, 'Energy balance').
- Although the terms BMR and REE are often used interchangeably, BMR is a theoretical concept which cannot be easily measured so the term REE is most often used in clinical studies.
- A physical activity level (PAL) which is a combined factor for diet-induced thermogenesis (DIT) and physical activity (PA) is added to the REE.
- The current recommendations were made after completion of a formal guideline development process, including conducting five systematic reviews of clinical studies where resting energy expenditure (REE) was measured in patients with acute or chronic illness, and were developed for adults receiving nutritional support, whether by the oral, enteral, or parenteral route.
- There is a lack of clinical studies investigating the nutritional requirements of patients at the extremes of BMI (<18.5 kg/m^2 or >30kg/m^2) except in intensive care units.
- In obese individuals, the use of actual body weight may overestimate requirements while in underweight individuals, this may result in underestimation of requirements. Regular clinical monitoring is, therefore, essential in these patients.

Table 25.13 Estimating energy requirements in illness and disease*

1	Carry out a clinical assessment (including measurements of actual body weight (BW) or fat free mass (FFM) and determination of BMI):
2a	Estimate resting energy expenditure (REE): REE (kcal/day) = BW × [disease-specific value] kcal/kg BW REE (kcal/day) = FFM × [disease-specific value] kcal/kg FFM • Disease-specific REE values according to clinical condition and age can be obtained from PENG systematic review (Tables 3.1 and 3.2 in reference 24). • If there is clinical evidence of metabolic stress, it may be necessary to use REE figures towards the top of the range of REE values.

(Continued)

Table 25.13 (*Contd.*)

- In the absence of disease-specific data,† REE may be estimated using 20-25 kcal/kg BW/day.
- BMI <18.5 kg/m² in the absence of disease-specific data,† REE may be estimated using 25-30 kcal/kg BW/day.
- BMI <30 kg/m², REE may be estimated using the Mifflin equations (see below) using actual body weight, sex, height, and age.‡

Men: 10 × weight (kg) + 6.25 × height (cm) − 5 × (age) + 5

Women:10 × weight (kg) + 6.25 × height (cm) − 5 × (age) −161

Note. All of the above assume that the patient is not at risk of refeeding syndrome and/or that any refeeding issues have been fully addressed.

3	Estimate total energy expenditure (TEE)

TEE (kcal/day) = REE (kcal/day) × PAL

PAL†	Description	Example
1.00-1.10	In bed and immobile	Acute illness or injury or post-surgery
1.10-1.20	In bed and/or sitting out	Hospital ward, care home, or at home
1.20-1.25	Limited mobility	Hospital ward or at home with full time care
1.25-1.40	Sedentary	Care home or at home

*Source: data from Todorovic, V.E., Mafrici, B. (2018). *A Pocket Guide to Clinical Nutrition*. 5th edn. Birmingham: British Dietetic Association, PENG.

†PENG Requirements Guideline Group consensus 2018.

‡Mifflin, M.D., *et al.* (1990). A new predictive equation for resting energy expenditure in healthy individuals. *Am. J. Clin. Nutr.* **51**, 241–7.

documented in sepsis, major trauma, and burns. In these conditions, nitrogen balance is almost impossible to achieve in the early catabolic phase post injury.[27] The method recommended by the British Dietetic Association Parenteral and Enteral Nutrition Group (PENG) for estimating protein requirements for nutritional support for adult patients with disease (Box 25.8) is based on a review of published guidelines.[24]

Fluid

- Basic requirements are 30-35 mL/kg for enteral nutrition[28] and 25-30 mL/kg for parenteral nutrition.[29]
- Fluid requirements should be considered on an individual basis taking account of losses of body fluids and input from other sources such as intravenous (IV) fluids and medication.

27 Cerra, F., *et al.* (1987). The effect of stress level, amino acid formula and nitrogen dose on nitrogen retention in traumatic and septic stress. *Ann. Surg.* **205**, 282–7.

28 Tyler, D.S. (1989). Chapter 7 pp. 223–50. In: *Handbook of surgical intensive care*. 2nd edn. Ed. HK Lyerly. Year Book Medical Publishers, Chicago.

29 National Institute for Health and Care Excellence (NICE) (2013). *Intravenous fluid therapy in adults in hospital*. Clinical guideline 174. Available at: ℬ https://www.nice.org.uk/guidance/cg174.

Box 25.8 Summary of the PENG Guidelines for estimating protein requirements[24]

- Disease-specific values for estimating protein requirements per kg actual BW for specific clinical conditions are available from PENG review of published guidelines (Table 3.9 in reference 24).
- In the absence of a protein guideline for a specific clinical condition, the PENG Requirements Guideline Group 2018 recommends using 1.0–1.5 g protein per kg actual body weight per day.
- Extremes of BMI: An intake of 1.0–1.5 g protein per kg actual body weight per day is likely to result in underfeeding in the underweight and overfeeding in the overweight. However, the only published guidelines providing evidence-based recommendations on how to adjust intake in these patients recommend high protein hypocaloric feeding.[30]
  - For obese adults requiring nutritional support:
    BMI >30 kg/m^2, use 75% of value estimated using actual weight.
    BMI >50 kg/m^2, use 65% of value estimated using actual weight.
  - For underweight adults requiring nutritional support:
    BMI < 18.5 kg/m^2, start at the upper end of the range (i.e. 1.5 g per kg) as less than this may result in underfeeding.

Electrolytes

Table 25.14 lists the estimated daily requirement for electrolytes.

Table 25.14 Estimated daily requirements for electrolytes *

Electrolyte	Enteral requirement	Parenteral requirement
Sodium	25–70 mmol/day † (1 mmol/kg)	1.0 mmol/kg[26]
Potassium	50–90 mmol/day † (1 mmol/kg)	1.0 mmol/kg In hypokalaemia, additional K$^+$ (mmol) required = (4.0 – actual serum K$^+$) × 0.4 × body weight (kg)
Calcium	10–17.5 mmol/day †	0.1–0.15 mmol/kg
Magnesium	Male: 7.8–12.3 mmol/day Female: 6.2–10.9 mmol/day †	0.1–0.2 mmol/kg
Phosphate		Equimolar with calcium; do not exceed 50 mmol/day in enteral or parenteral feeds

* Source: data from Todorovic, V.E., Mafrici, B. (2018). *A Pocket Guide to Clinical Nutrition*. 5th edn. British Dietetic Association, PENG, Birmingham.

† Ranges given are LRNI – RNI (Department of Health 1991) (see ➲ Chapter 2 'Dietary Reference Values'). The LRNI will meet the requirements of only a few people who have low needs. The RNI will meet the requirements of 97.5% of the population during health and thus should be the target intake. More may be required in patients with poor status, increased losses from diarrhoea, stoma/fistulae, nasogastric aspirates/vomiting or venting gastrostomies, or altered requirements because of disease process.

30 Choban P et al. (2013) ASPEN clinical guidelines: nutrition support of hospitalised adult patients with obesity. *JPEN* 37:714–44.

Example of requirement calculations

Man aged 58 years, weight 81 kg, height 1.72 m, sitting up in bed following haemorrhagic cerebral vascular accident (CVA). He is unable to swallow at present and enteral feed to be started (Box 25.9).

Box 25.9 Example of estimation of requirements[24]

Clinical assessment
- Recent CVA so likely metabolic stress
- BMI = 27 kg/m^2

Energy requirements
- Resting energy expenditure (REE) for haemorrhagic stroke (BMI 18.5-30 kg/m^2, age ≤65 years) is 24 kcal/kg
- Combined factor for physical activity and diet-induced thermogenesis (PAL) is 1.1-1.2. See Table 25.13 for patients who are in bed/sitting out in the hospital setting.

  REE = 24×81 = 1944 kcal/day

  TEE = 1944×PAL (1.1 to 1.2) = 2138 to 2333 kcal/day

- Estimated energy requirements are between approximately 2140 and 2330 kcal/day.

Protein requirements
- There are no specific guidelines for protein requirements in haemorrhagic stroke, therefore use 1.0 to 1.5 g/kg/day.
- Estimated protein requirements are between approximately 81 and 121.5 g/day.

Fluid requirements
- Patient has no significant additional fluid losses.
- Use 30 mL/kg = 2430 mL/day.
- Estimated fluid requirements are approximately 2430 mL/day.

Summary
Patient's nutritional requirements are between approximately 2140 and 2330 kcal, 81 and 122 g protein, and 2500 mL fluid daily.

Further reading

Todorovic, V.E., Mafrici, B. (2018). *A Pocket Guide to Clinical Nutrition*. 5th edn. British Dietetic Association, Birmingham.

Refeeding syndrome

❶ Enthusiasm for nutritional support and a desire to replete very under-nourished patients rapidly can be fatal unless care is taken to avoid refeeding syndrome (RfS). See Box 25.10 for a list of patients potentially at risk and Box 25.11 for the clinical features.

Definition

Severe fluid and electrolyte shifts and related metabolic complications in malnourished patients undergoing refeeding.

Pathophysiology

- In starvation, ↓ intake of energy and particularly carbohydrate → ↓ insulin secretion and ↑ catabolism of fat and protein for energy → ↓ intracellular electrolytes and especially ↓ phosphate (↓ intracellular phosphate co-exists with normal serum phosphate levels).
- Initiating feeding → change from predominantly fat and protein metabolism to carbohydrate with ↑ insulin secretion → stimulation of cellular uptake of phosphate, potassium, and water → hypophosphataemia, hypokalaemia, and hypomagnesaemia → RfS.

Key points for RfS awareness

- Risk of refeeding may occur in response to oral, enteral, or parenteral nutrition support.
- The early features of RfS are non-specific and may not be recognized.
- Awareness and understanding of RfS by clinical staff is limited and serum phosphate is often not routinely measured and the significance of depleted levels is not always appreciated. Dietitians who work in nutrition support have an important role in increasing awareness about RfS.
- Normal serum values *before* feeding starts do not indicate that the patient is at low risk of RfS. In RfS, serum levels only fall *after* feeding starts so this is when monitoring must take place.
- In most cases, RfS can be anticipated and prevented.

Further reading

Boateng, A.A., et al. (2010). Refeeding syndrome: treatment considerations based on collective analysis of literature case reports. *Nutrition* **26**, 156–67.

Stanga, Z., et al. (2008). Nutrition in clinical practice—the re-feeding syndrome: illustrative cases and guidelines for prevention and treatment. *Eur. J. Clin. Nutr.* **62**, 687–94.

Management of RfS

The prescription[7] for people at high risk of developing RfS should consider:

- Start nutrition support at maximum of 10 kcal/kg/d, increasing levels slowly to meet or exceed full needs by 4-7 days.
- Use only 5 kcal/kg/d in extreme cases (e.g. BMI<14 kg/m^2 or negligible intake for >15 days) and monitor cardiac rhythm continually in these and others who already have or develop cardiac arrhythmias.
- Restore circulatory volume and monitor fluid balance and overall clinical status closely.

- Provide immediately before and during the first 10 days of feeding:
  - oral thiamine 200-300 mg/daily (vitamin B co-strong one to two tablets three times daily OR full dose daily intravenous vitamin B preparation);
  - multivitamin and trace element supplement once daily.
- Provide oral, enteral, or intravenous supplements of:
  - potassium (likely requirement 2-4 mmol/kg/d);
  - phosphate (likely requirement 0.3-0.6 mmol/kg/d);
  - magnesium (likely requirement 0.2 mmol/kg/d intravenous OR 0.4 mmol/kg/d oral).

For all electrolyte abnormalities, treat according to local protocols.

Box 25.10 Patients potentially at risk from refeeding syndrome*

At risk
- Any patient who has had little or no nutritional intake for >5 days

High risk
- Any patient with one of the following:
  - Little or no nutritional intake for >10 days
  - BMI <16 kg/m^2
  - Unintentional weight loss >15% within last 3-6 months
  - Low levels of potassium, magnesium, or phosphate before feeding
- Any patient with two of the following:
  - Little or no nutritional intake for >5days
  - BMI <18.5 kg/m^2
  - Unintentional weight loss >10% within last 3-6 months
  - History of alcohol abuse or drugs including insulin, chemotherapy, antacids, diuretics

Extremely high risk
- Little or no nutritional intake for >15 days
- BMI<14 kg/m^2

* Adapted from National Institute for Health and Care Excellence (NICE) (2006). *Nutrition support for adults: Oral nutrition support, enteral tube feeding and parenteral nutrition*. Clinical guideline 32. ℛ https://www.nice.org.uk/guidance/cg32.

Box 25.11 Clinical features of refeeding syndrome
- Rhabdomyolysis, weakness, paralysis
- Leukocyte dysfunction, haemolytic anaemia
- Respiratory depression and failure
- Pulmonary oedema
- Arrhythmias, cardiac arrest, congestive heart failure
- ↓ Glomerular filtration rate
- Liver dysfunction
- Diarrhoea, constipation, ileus
- Seizures, confusion, coma, sudden death

Metabolic response to injury

The term 'metabolic response to injury' describes the biochemical and hormonal consequences of major injury, trauma, surgery ± infection, and the resulting nutritional changes that may have very significant clinical effects. Traditionally, the response has been described as having two phases, known as the ebb and flow (Table 25.15). Recent studies have shown that good acute clinical management may reduce or possibly eliminate the ebb phase, and that it may not be detectable at all in less severe injury.

Overall effects

- Loss of appetite leads to ↓ nutrient intake.
- Disruption of fat and carbohydrate metabolism with apparent inability to use these as metabolic substrates (hence ↑ circulating levels and deposition of lipid in adipose and vital organs). Controlling hyperglycaemia by giving insulin will help ↓ risk of death.
- Lean tissue broken down may provide amino acids required during inflammatory response, e.g. acute phase proteins, lymphocyte proliferation, glutathione synthesis.
- Protein loss—may be substantial and have clinical consequences (see Table 25.16). In context of 'whole body protein', lean tissue contains ~205 g protein/kg and an average 70-kg man comprises ~10 kg protein.

❶ Most of this protein is 'essential' and cannot be lost without functional implications, i.e. ↓ resistance to infection, ↑ muscle weakness (including respiratory and skeletal muscle) leading to ↓ pulmonary function and ↓ physical activity.

Effect of starvation

Although there are some similarities between the metabolic response to injury and starvation, i.e. both lead to depletion, there are important differences (Table 25.17). Starvation may interfere with the metabolic response.

❶ Providing nutritional support to patients after injury will not reverse the biochemical effects observed, during the metabolic response to injury, e.g. nitrogen loss. However, it will help to ameliorate the effects of depletion and limit the clinical consequences (see ➡ this Chapter, 'Undernutrition').

Table 25.15 Simplified model of metabolic response to injury

Metabolic and clinical effects	Ebb phase* (acute)	Flow phase† (hypermetabolic)
Energy expenditure	↓	↑
O₂ consumption	↓	↑
Cardiac output	↓	↑
Body temperature	↓	↑
Circulating levels of		
• Glucose	↑	↑
• Lactate	↑	↔
• Free fatty acids	↑	↑
• Catecholamines	↑	↑
• Glucagon	↑	↑
• Cortisol	↑	↑
• Insulin	↓	Insulin resistance
Urinary nitrogen loss	↑	↑

*Occurring immediately after trauma, the ebb phase is the brief 'shock' phase (lasts ~0–8 hours).

†The flow phase follows the ebb phase and is a longer 'catabolic' phase (lasts ~5–10 days).

Table 25.16 Estimated loss of protein (g) over 10-day period following trauma and untreated infection

	Tissue loss	Blood loss	Protein catabolism
Muscle wound	500–750	150–400	650
35% burn	500	150–400	600
# Femur	–	up to 200	580–860
Gastrectomy	up to 60	20–180	525–650
Typhoid fever	–	–	675

Table 25.17 Differences between the metabolic response to injury and starvation

	Injury	Starvation
Energy expenditure	↑	↓
Nitrogen losses	↑	↓
Plasma insulin and glucose	↑	↓
Plasma free fatty acids	↑ Turnover	↓ Turnover
Plasma clearance of exogenous triglycerides	↑	↓

Critical care

Defined as patients requiring:
- advanced respiratory support alone *or*;
- basic respiratory support together with the support of at least two organ systems;
- includes patients with multi-organ failure.

The aims of nutrition support in critical care (CC) patients are to minimize nutritional losses and provide basic nutrient requirements to sustain life. Repletion of pre-existing undernutrition during a period of critical care is unlikely to be achieved and should not be a goal because of ↑ risk associated with overfeeding. This section is an overview of some of the aspects associated with the provision of nutrition in this environment, as the issues are often complex. It is important to use clinical judgement with evidence-based practice and to work with the multi-disciplinary team (MDT).

Route of feeding

Access to feeding routes may be limited by the patient's condition, but wherever possible, the gut should be used as first choice (see ➋ this chapter, 'Routes for enteral feeding').

Enteral feeding

There is evidence[31] to support early initiation of enteral feeding in haemo-dynamically stable CC patients. The presence of a standard initial regimen is associated with significant improvement in nutrition practices, as this allows clinical staff to begin feeding as soon as possible.[32]
- Measuring gastric residual volumes (GRV) as a means of determining absorption, and thus delivery of enteral feeding, has been questioned,[33] and continues to be researched. Setting the threshold too low can be associated with creating an unnecessary limit on the quantity of feed provided as a result of stopping the feed for aspirate checks and the residual volume not being returned to the stomach. A GRV of up to 500 mL is not associated with adverse effects in GI outcomes or ventilator-associated pneumonia (VAP). Early use of prokinetic agents could also be considered. VAP has primarily been ascribed to leakage around the endotracheal tube cuff of subglottic secretions containing pathogenic microorganisms.[34]

31 Kreymann, K.G., *et al.* (2006). ESPEN guidelines on enteral nutrition: Intensive care. *Clin. Nutr.* **25**, 210–23.

32 Heyland, D.K., *et al.* (2010). Nutrition impact of enteral feeding protocols on enteral nutrition delivery. *J. Parenter. Enteral Nutr.* **34**, 675–84.

33 Hurt, R.T., McClure, S.A. (2010). Gastric residual volumes in critical illness: what do they really mean? *Crit. Care. Clin.* **26**, 481–90.

34 Reigner, J. *et al.* (2013). Effect of not monitoring gastric residual volumes on risk of ventilator associated pneumonia in adults receiving mechanical ventilation and early enteral nutrition: A randomised control trial. *JAMA* **309**, 249–56.

- A single high aspirate measurement should not lead to the cessation of feeding unless there is overt regurgitation or signs that the patient is aspirating fluid into the respiratory tract.
- Risk of aspirating feed can be reduced (see ⊃ this chapter, 'Complications of enteral feeding').
- The quantity of feed provided effects mortality and there is evidence to suggest that frequent interruption of feeding is the cause of less than anticipated calories being delivered. Some centres are moving away from an hourly feeding rate to a volume to be delivered over 24 hours.[35]
- Using enteral nutrition compared to parenteral nutrition has no effect on overall mortality but enteral nutrition is associated with reduced infection complications and length of stay in the CC unit. This has been attributed to reduced macronutrient provision rather than the enteral nutrition itself.[36]
- If absorption is limited and precludes administration of the total volume of enteral feed prescribed to meet requirements, it can be supplemented with parenteral nutrition (see guidance below). This will facilitate an adequate total nutrient intake but continue the physiological benefits of feeding via the gut.
- Immune-modulating formulae should be used with caution in patients in critical care (see ⊃ this chapter 'Clinically functional nutrients'). Read the literature related to the use of a particular supplement in a specific condition to determine if use will enhance the individual patient's recovery.

Parenteral nutrition (see ⊃ this Chapter)

- Parenteral nutrition can play an invaluable role where enteral feeding is not possible or not succeeding. Parenteral nutrition should only be undertaken during the first 7 days if there is a high nutrition risk. Supplementary parenteral nutrition should be delayed until 7-10 days regardless of risk.[37]
- Avoiding overfeeding is important (see Box 25.12).

Nutritional requirements in critical care

- *Energy:* requirements can be estimated by calculation using standard formulae but values provide only an approximation and may need adjusting to suit individual patients. Further reading on requirements for obese patients and those patients at risk of refeeding syndrome is encouraged. Indirect calorimetry is used in some units and this can give a greater guide to energy requirements. Energy requirements are slightly ↓ if patients are ventilated rather than breathing spontaneously, but will ↑ as weaning progresses. Consider the energy contribution of fluids or

35 McClave, S.A., et al. (2015). Volume based feeding in critically ill patients. *J. Parenter. Enteral Nutr.* 39, 707–12.

36 Elke, G., et al. (2016). Enteral vs parenteral nutrition in critically ill patients: An updated systematic review and meta-analysis of randomised control trials. *Crit. Care* 20, 117.

37 McClave, S.A., et al. (2016). Guidelines for the provision and assessment of nutrition support therapy in the adult critically ill patient. *J. Parenter. Enteral Nutr.* 40, 159–211.

Box 25.12 Potential consequences of overfeeding
- ↓ Tolerance of feeding, e.g. diarrhoea
- ↑ Physiological stress
- Metabolic acidosis
- Uraemia
- ↑ Respiratory quotient, i.e. ↑ CO_2 produced so weaning harder
- Hyperglycaemia → impaired wound healing
- Hypercholesterolaemia and hypertriglyceridaemia
- Excess lipid → ↓ reticuloendothelial system → ± immunosuppression
- Hepatic steatosis
- Refeeding syndrome

---

medicines used with the patient, e.g. patients sedated using propofol will receive additional energy from the lipid emulsion it is carried in. When taking account of the energy provision from other sources, aim to ensure that the adequacy of other nutrients is maintained in the remaining energy provided.[37]
- *Protein/nitrogen:* CC patients have ↑ protein turnover and ↑ nitrogen loss as an unavoidable feature of the metabolic response to injury: nutritional support will not reduce this but will help minimize the accompanying depletion. Evidence suggests that providing >0.2 g nitrogen/kg body weight/day has no additional benefit in septic or trauma patients.
- *Carbohydrate:* in critical illness, glucose administration should not exceed the maximum glucose oxidation rate, 4 mg/kg/min. Consider glucose contribution of medication, particularly in patients <45 kg.
- *Lipid:* in critical illness give 0.8–1.0 g/kg/day (see top bullet, this section re. propofol). Approximately 3.0–4.5% total energy should be provided as lipid to prevent essential fatty acid deficiency. Research is ongoing into the use of specific lipid sources within CC.
- *Fluid, electrolytes, micronutrients:* all parenteral nutrition should contain a daily dose of vitamins and trace elements. However, for some conditions, also consider the daily use of fat-soluble vitamins. Fluid and electrolyte requirements need to be assessed on an individual basis, taking account of clinical condition and treatment. The volume of fluid should be agreed by working in the MDT.

Further reading

Dhaliwal, R., et al. (2014). The Canadian critical care nutrition guidelines in 2013: an update on current recommendations and implementation strategies. *Nutr. Clin. Pract.* **29**, 29–43.

Heyland, D.K., et al. (2011). Optimal amounts of calories for critically ill patients: Depends on how you slice the cake! *Crit. Care Med.* **39**, 2619–26.

National Institute for Health and Care Excellence (NICE) (2009). *Rehabilitation after critical illness.* Clinical guideline CG83. ℘ http://www.nice.org.uk/guidance/cg83.

Singer, P., et al. (2009). ESPEN guidelines on parenteral nutrition: Intensive Care. *Clin. Nutr.* **28**, 387–400.

Surgery

Nutritional depletion is associated with ↑ morbidity and mortality following surgery. Surgery itself is associated with ↑ nutritional losses (see ⮞ this Chapter, 'Metabolic response to injury') and nutritional support is not able to prevent these. However, appropriate nutrition support is capable of minimizing the depletion (i.e. loss of lean body mass) accompanying major surgical intervention, and is associated with:

- repletion of lean body mass;
- improved skeletal muscle force;
- ↓ fatigue;
- ↑ ventilatory, cardiac, and gut function;
- ↑ immunity;
- ↑ sense of wellbeing.

There is less evidence that nutrition support has beneficial effects in relatively well-nourished individuals who have undergone minor–moderate surgery indicating that routine nutritional support for all surgical patients is inappropriate, especially considering the potential side effects of feeding and cost implications.

However, it is widely accepted that patients who are critically ill, severely injured, or nutritionally depleted prior to surgery will benefit from nutrition support. This raises two issues:

- identifying patients who will benefit (see ⮞ Chapter 4, 'Individual assessment');
- optimum timing of nutrition support.

Pre-operative nutrition

Feeding undernourished patients 7–10 days prior to surgery is associated with a reduction in non-infectious complications. Shorter periods show no benefit. Obviously, delaying surgery is clinically inappropriate in some patients, but pre-operative feeding should be considered before elective surgery in those who are severely depleted. NICE guidance[7] recommends that malnourished patients who are scheduled to undergo major abdominal surgery and have a functioning GI tract but are unable to take adequate nutrition orally, should be considered for pre-operative enteral tube feeding.

Pre-operative fasting and enhanced recovery after surgery

Overnight fasting prior to surgery is unnecessary,[38] metabolically disadvantageous, and clinically detrimental. Evidence shows that allowing patients to take clear fluids until 2 hours before surgery and solid food until 6 hours before elective surgery is safe.[39] Oral carbohydrate and fluid loading prior to surgery is associated with reduced post-operative insulin resistance and improved clinical outcomes. This is incorporated into protocols for enhanced recovery after surgery (ERAS) which are associated with fewer

---

38 Brady, M.C., et al. (2003). Preoperative fasting for adults to reduce postoperative complications. *Cochrane Database Syst. Rev.* DOI: 10.1002/14651858.CD004423 (reviewed 2010).

39 Gustafsson, U.O., et al. (2012). Guidelines for perioperative care in elective colonic surgery: Enhanced Recovery After Surgery (ERAS®) Society recommendations. *Clin. Nutr.* 31, 783–800.

complications and 30-50% ↓ length of hospital stay.[40] Most studies have been undertaken in colonic surgery but there is increasing evidence in other surgical areas and guidelines are available.[41] There is limited evidence on using ERAS protocols in people with diabetes.[42]

Commercial products to facilitate pre-surgical carbohydrate loading are available (Preload® Vitaflo; PreOp® Nutricia) or 'home made' versions can be mixed at ward level (e.g. equivalent to 50 g complex carbohydrate/ maltodextrins in 400 mL water or see local protocols).

40 Lungqvist, O., et al. (2017). Enhanced Recovery After Surgery: a review. *JAMA Surg.* **152**, 292–8.

41 ERAS Society (2017). List of guidelines. Available at: ℅ http://erassociety.org/guidelines/list-of-guidelines/.

42 Albalawi, Z. et al. (2017). Enhanced Recovery After Surgery (ERAS®) in individuals with diabetes: a systematic review. *World J. Surg.* **41**, 1927–34.

Spinal cord injury

Spinal cord injury (SCI) can result in either temporary or permanent impairment of the normal motor, sensory, or autonomic function.

- *Tetraplegia*: injury to the spinal cord in the cervical region with associated loss of function in all four extremities.
- *Paraplegia*: injury in the thoracic, lumbar, or sacral segments resulting in loss of function in the lower limbs.

Short term nutritional issues (<3 months after injury)

- SCI patients who are undernourished have ↑ risk of adverse clinical outcomes including length of hospital stay and 12-month mortality.[43]
- Patients should undergo assessment to determine their nutritional status as soon as possible after injury. Determining body weight may be difficult; estimating requirements may be inaccurate because of variation in individual needs, other co-existing injuries, and reduced mobility.
- Nutritional support may be required if the patient is unable to eat sufficient food. Adequacy of energy, protein, and all micronutrient intakes should be considered as well as fibre and fluid. Energy requirements should ideally be assessed by indirect calorimetry as there is no evidence that prediction equations provide useful estimates in acute and sub-acute SCI.[44]
- There is no evidence of clinical improvements associated with omega-3 fatty acid supplementation in SCI in humans.
- The effects of very low fat ('ketogenic') diets have been investigated but there is currently insufficient evidence on which to base recommendations.
- Depression, anxiety, and loss of appetite as well as frequent clinical investigations and treatment may limit nutrient intake. Awareness of the importance of good nutrition is needed among the whole multi-disciplinary care team and patients' family and friends. Input from a registered dietitian is needed to optimize nutritional care.

Longer term nutritional issues (>3 months after injury)

- An optimum nutrient intake will help support an active rehabilitation programme. This will include the provision of adequate energy to participate in physiotherapy sessions and sufficient protein and micronutrients to facilitate any continuing healing process and minimize complications associated with limited mobility, e.g. loss of skin integrity.
- Constipation is very common and can have a serious impact on quality of life and long term health. The degree of bowel dysfunction depends on the extent and location of the injury on the spinal cord with complete damage above the 12th thoracic vertebra (T12) associated with loss of anal muscle control. However, in most patients, a high

43 Wong, S., *et al.* (2014). Is undernutrition risk associated with an adverse clinical outcome in spinal cord-injured patients admitted to a spinal centre? *Eur. J. Clin. Nutr.* **68**, 125–30.

44 Nevin, A.N., *et al.* (2016). Investigation of measured and predicted resting energy needs in adults after spinal cord injury: a systematic review. *Spinal Cord* **54**, 248–53.

fibre diet with ↑ intake of fluid (>35 mL/kg/day) will help to regulate bowel movements and reduce risk of constipation. For those previously unfamiliar with a high fibre diet, sources should be introduced slowly over a 6-week period to optimize tolerance (see ➋ Chapter 26, 'Constipation').

- Increasing body weight may become a concern in some people whose level of energy expenditure is curtailed by their lack of mobility. There is also evidence of reduced resting energy expenditure (REE) (↓ ~20%), probably 2° to loss of lean body mass. Excessive weight gain may hamper rehabilitation if wasted muscles are overburdened and ↑ the chance of pressure sores (as does underweight). Increasing energy expenditure through limited activity should be encouraged where possible and dietary energy should be tailored to this. If an energy-restricted diet is required to match limited energy expenditure on a long term basis, care must be taken to ensure that the diet is totally adequate in all other nutrients. A regular review by a dietitian may be appropriate.
- Life expectancy after SCI ranges from 70% to 92% of normal. As a consequence, and because many SCI patients are young adults, the influence of nutrition on the promotion of long term good health and preventing cardiovascular disease is important. Advice should be based on the guidance given in 'The Eatwell Guide' (see ➋ Chapter 2), accompanied by consideration of energy balance to maintain an optimum weight.
- For individuals whose activity and socializing may be curtailed by their injury, food can provide an important pleasure and this should not be subverted because of the therapeutic effects of a healthy diet!

Further information

🕭 http://www.spinal.co.uk/

Head injury

Patients sustaining brain damage through external injury to the head or surgery to treat stroke (see ⮡ Chapter 23, 'Stroke/cerebrovascular accident') will require nutritional support in the short and long term.

Nutrition may not be a priority immediately (<24 hours) after injury as resuscitation and emergency surgery may be required to preserve life.

However, in the following days, patients may become hypermetabolic and hypercatabolic (see ⮡ this chapter, 'Metabolic response to injury'). Requirements should be calculated on an individual basis by a dietitian with experience in caring for the critically ill.

Energy requirements

- REE may ↑ ~40–200% of normal, although this increase may be moderated by pharmaceutical sedation (↓ ~12–32%).
- Energy expended through physical activity is usually minimal.
- Most head injured patients are well-nourished at the time of injury, although this should not be assumed.
- Accompanying injuries, e.g. after a road traffic accident, must be considered and may ↑ energy requirements.
- Prediction equations often provide unreliable estimates of energy expenditure.
- Actual expenditure should be measured using indirect calorimetry if possible.

Protein requirements

- Protein is used as a preferred source of energy and so nitrogen losses increase in the first week post-injury and may remain raised for some weeks.
- Reported N losses vary from 0.29 to 0.73 g/kg body weight/day (≡ 125–300 g protein for a 70-kg man). Negative nitrogen balance results.
- Monitoring N losses will give an indication of requirements, although feeding cannot prevent N loss, it will minimize consequences.
- Providing 0.35 g N/kg body weight is associated with better outcome than lower intakes.

Nutritional support

Systematic review[45] has shown that instigation of early nutrition support (<72 hours) is associated with significantly ↓ risk of death (RR 0.35; 95% CI 0.24–0.50). It also reported a non-significant trend towards parenteral nutrition being associated with a more favourable outcome than enteral, but this may be confounded by the fact that parenteral feeding usually commences earlier (Box 25.13).

---

45 Wang, X., et al. (2013). Nutritional support for patients sustaining traumatic brain injury: a systematic review and meta-analysis of prospective studies. *PLoS One* **8**, e58838.

Box 25.13 Nutrition support in patients with head injury[46]

- Establish nutrition support protocol for patients with head injury.
- If possible, initiate nutrition support <72 hours after injury.
- Enteral feeding into the jejunum is associated with lower risk of pneumonia than nasogastric feeding.
- Feeding using immune-enhancing formulae is associated with lower risk of infection.
- Estimate energy expenditure using indirect calorimetry once or twice weekly or when change in clinical status.
- Assess protein status using urine urea nitrogen twice weekly (not reliable method in renal dysfunction).
- Administer continuous feeding using a pump to control delivery rate.
- Monitor feed tolerance using nutrition support protocol (see ➲ this Chapter, 'Monitoring enteral feeding').

46 Vizzini, A., et al. (2011). Nutritional support in head injury. *Nutrition* **27**, 129–32.

Burn injury

Severity of burn injury is defined by depth and the % of total body surface area (% TBSA) that has been affected. A major burn is considered as > 20% TBSA. Exudate loss and the inflammatory response to damaged tissue results in a bi-phasic physiological and metabolic response to injury. The first 24-48 hours of 'burn shock' is characterized by hypovolemia, low cardiac output, oedema, and hypometabolism. This is followed by a prolonged hypermetabolic, hypercatabolic phase with accelerated proteolysis, lipolysis, and glycogenolysis.

Nutritional requirements

Energy requirements

Adults
Toronto equation:
$-4343 + (10.5 \times \% \text{ TBSA}) + (0.23 \times CI) + (0.84 \times HB) + (114 \times T) - (4.5 \times PBD)$
CI: total kcal intake in previous 24 hours; HB: resting energy requirement calculated by the Harris-Benedict equation; T: maximum core temperature (°C) in previous 24 hours; PBD: days post injury.

Children
Hildreth formulae:
0–1 years $(2100 \times SA) + (1000 \times BSA)$
1–12 years $(1800 \times SA) + (1300 \times BSA)$
>12 years $(1500 \times SA) + (1500 \times BSA)$
SA: body surface area (m^2), calculated by $\sqrt{(\text{height (cm)} \times \text{weight (kg)} \div 3600)}$
BSA: surface area of burn (m^2), calculated by $(SA \times \% \text{ TBSA}) \div 100$

Minor burn injuries
Adults: standard basal metabolic rate predictor e.g. Henry equation (see appendix).
Children: estimated average requirement for age/gender.[47]

Protein requirements
Adults: 1.5-2 g/kg/day
Children: 1.5-3 g/kg/day

Fluid and electrolytes
• Fluid requirements are best managed by the medical team because of complex needs to replace exudate loss and manage ever shifting fluid balance.

---

47 Scientific Advisory Committee on Nutrition (SACN) (2011). Dietary reference values for energy. Available at: ℛ https://www.gov.uk/government/publications/sacn-dietary-reference-values-for-energy.

- Magnesium and phosphate levels require close monitoring and often regular correction because of losses via the exudate.
- High solute loads from medication and aggressive fluid resuscitation commonly result in hypernatremia. Conversely, hyponatremia from fluid overloading and side effects of medication can also be a problem. Again, close monitoring is advised.

Vitamins, minerals, and trace elements
- Zinc, copper, and selenium are important co-factors involved in wound healing and immune function. Depletion is common in burns and correction should be considered when deficiency is identified.
- Patients are at high risk of vitamin D deficiency because of prolonged hospital stay and a life-long need to protect scar tissue from sun exposure. Patients should be screened for deficiency and supplemented when required.

Feeding routes
Oral feeding
A previously well-nourished patient with a minor burn injury (adults <15% TBSA, children <10%) is likely to achieve nutritional requirement from oral intake. Advice on energy dense, high protein options or oral supplements may be required.

Nasogastric feeding
Patients with moderate injury size (adults >15% TBSA, children >10%) or those who are already malnourished may require nasogastric feeding to support wound healing and weight maintenance. Pain and swelling from facial burns can make eating and drinking difficult. In these cases, nasogastric feeding should also be considered.

Nasojejunal feeding
Gastric stasis is common in major burns and it is advisable to opt for post-pyloric feeding.

Other considerations
Feed delivery
- Early enteral feeding has been shown to reduce inflammatory cytokines, reduce bacterial translocation, and improve bowel perfusion. Aim to start feeding within 12 hours.
- Feed delivery can be interrupted by frequent surgery and long dressing changes. It is helpful to learn the daily routine of the patient so feeding plans can incorporate these interruptions. Volume-based feeding and catch up rates may be helpful.

Blood sugars
Stress response to burn injury increases serum glucose levels. Levels consistently >8 mmol/L increase incidence of wound infections and slow healing. Initiation of, or adjustment to, insulin therapy may be required.

Stress ulcers
High prevalence of gastric and duodenal ulcers is common in major burns. As such, prophylactic proton pump inhibitors are recommended.

Oxandrolone

Oxandrolone is an anabolic steroid used in major burns to help increase the rate of wound healing, preserve lean body mass and improve trajectory of growth in children.

Adults: 10 mg b.d.
Children: 0.1 mg/kg b.d.

Propranolol

Propranolol is a beta-blocker used to moderate the hypermetabolic response, reduce lipolysis, and reduce incidence of hepatomegaly.

Adults and children: 2 mg/kg/day (dose to be titrated until heart rate reduced by 15-20%)

Glutamine

Glutamine reduces inflammatory cytokines and improves the immunological and physiological function of the bowel. Avoid with renal insufficiency.

Adults: 0.3-0.5 g/kg/day (enteral)
Children: Insufficient evidence

Further reading

Rousseau, A.F., et al. (2013). ESPEN endorsed recommendations: nutritional therapy in major burns. *Clin. Nutr.* 32, 497–502.

Clinically functional nutrients

Functional foods have been defined as 'foods that by virtue of physiologically active food components provide health benefits beyond basic nutrition' by the International Life Sciences Institute of North America (ILSI 2008) (see ⊙ Chapter 8, 'Functional foods and nutraceuticals'). This section considers nutrients that may have some clinical benefits if consumed in larger than usual intakes in specific medical conditions.

Glutamine

Glutamine (Gln) is a conditionally indispensable amino acid:

- an important source of fuel in rapidly dividing cells, e.g. enterocytes and immune cells;
- precursor for antioxidant glutathione;
- becomes indispensable in stress situations, e.g. catabolic patients, as body pool ↓ rapidly to fuel-stimulated lymphocytes, etc.;
- standard parenteral solutions do not include Gln.

Systematic reviews of glutamine interventions report different conclusions varying with the diagnosis of the participants, their existing glutamine status, and the route of delivery. The most recent of these[48] reports the potential of parenteral Gln supplementation to improve outcomes in critically ill patients with ↓ hospital mortality (RR = 0.55; 95% CI 0.32-0.94). However, routine Gln supplementation of critically ill patients is not recommended because of the possible risk of adverse effects.[37]

Arginine

Arginine (Arg) is a conditionally indispensable amino acid:

- plays a role in transport, storage, and excretion of nitrogen;
- precursor for nitric oxide;
- becomes indispensable in stress situations, e.g. trauma and sepsis, when Arg levels ↓ as it is used for nitric oxide pathways.

Systematic reviews of arginine supplementation report improved clinical outcomes in head and neck cancers[49] and improved immune function.[50] As with Gln, concerns have been raised about adverse effects but feeding regimes containing Arg are recommended in severe trauma, traumatic brain injury, and post-operative patients requiring enteral nutrition but not in patients with sepsis.[37] There is debate about Arg requirements, which ↑ with nitric oxide production, and the optimum route; 15-30 g/day is considered safe.[51]

48 Stehle, P., et al. (2017). Glutamine dipeptide-supplemented parenteral nutrition improves the clinical outcomes of critically ill patients. Clin. Nutr. **17**, 75–85.

49 Vidal-Casariego, A., et al. (2014). Efficacy of arginine-enriched enteral formulas in the reduction of surgical complications in head and neck cancer. Clin. Nutr. **33**, 951–7.

50 Kang, K., et al. (2014). Effect of L-arginine on immune function: a meta-analysis. Asia Pac. J. Clin. Nutr. **23**, 361–9.

51 Patel, J.J., et al. (2016). When is it appropriate to use arginine in critical illness? Nutr. Clin. Pract. **31**, 438–44.

Nutrition in gastrointestinal diseases

Mouth disorders 622
Dental health 624
Oesophageal disorders 628
Stomach disorders 632
Gastrectomy and stomach surgery 636
Small intestine disorders: introduction 640
Malabsorption: introduction 642
Steatorrhoea 644
Lactose intolerance 648
Inflammatory bowel disease 652
Coeliac disease 656
Intestinal failure and short bowel 660
Fistulae 662
Gastrointestinal stoma 664
Intestinal transplantation 666
Irritable bowel syndrome 668
Disorders of the colon 672
Gallbladder disorders 676

Mouth disorders

Injury or disease in the mouth (including lips, oral cavity, tongue, and naso-pharynx) can rapidly compromise nutritional status by inhibiting eating and drinking. To counter this, nutrient intake can be optimized through the modification of food texture or by instigating nutritional support via tube feeding.

Cancer of the mouth and pharynx

Mouth, lip, salivary gland and pharyngeal cancers account for ~4% cancers worldwide (710,000 new cases in 2018) but are more common in developing countries; oral cancer represents about 2-3% of total malignancies in the UK. Associated risk factors include smoking and chewing tobacco, chewing betel nut, alcohol intake (risk trebles with more than three drinks/day), low vegetable and fruit intake, consumption of salted fish, and exposure to sun and human papillomavirus. Treatment includes surgery, chemotherapy, and radiotherapy, which should be undertaken at a specialist centre. Patients' nutritional status and need for tube feeding should be assessed by an experienced dietitian at diagnosis and before treatment, and offered individual dietary advice to help maximize nutrient intake if required (see ➔ Chapter 24, 'Managing nutritional status in cancer').

Further reading

Mouth Cancer Foundation /National Institute for Health and Care Excellence (NICE) (2017). Head and neck cancer QS146. Available at: ꙮ https://www.nice.org.uk/guidance/qs146.

Salivary gland disorders

Disorders include saliva deficiency, inflammation secondary to infection, and calculi. Inflammation can hinder chewing and reduce the flow of saliva, further impeding food intake. Treatment of the underlying condition is required and nutrient intake should be supported by providing moist food that requires little chewing (see ➔ Chapter 23, 'Modification of texture of food and fluid'). Xerostomia (dry mouth) relating to lack of saliva is also associated with Sjögren syndrome, diabetes mellitus, and taking anticholinergic, antihistamine, and decongestant medications, as well as some anticancer treatment. Artificial saliva substitutes are available on prescription as gel, spray, and tablets, and may help both food intake and promote oral hygiene. Dentures incorporating a refillable reservoir have been devised to facilitate delivery of saliva substitutes.

Jaw wiring

Fixation of the maxilla/mandible may be undertaken following a fractured jaw, oral surgery, or (very rarely) in the treatment of obesity. The procedure may accompany complex maxillofacial surgery in the presence of severe trauma or may be relatively straightforward in elective jaw wiring for obesity.

- A liquid or semi-liquid diet is required (Table 26.1). This can be based on a combination of supplemented drinks, both home-made and commercial, that can be sucked through the gaps between the jaws.
- Consideration must be given to the total nutrient intake to ensure adequacy for the duration of the fixation (usually 3–8 weeks following

Table 26.1 Example of liquid diet

	Volume, mL	Energy, kcal	Protein, g
Orange juice	250	110	2
Porridge, pureed with milk and sugar	300	200	7
Milky coffee with sugar	250	180	8
Drinking yogurt	200	190	8
Tomato juice	250	50	2
Proprietary nutrition supplement*	200	200	8
Mug of tea	300	20	—
Ice cream	100	180	4
Creamy lentil soup (lump-free)	200	130	5
Proprietary nutrition supplement*	200	200	8
Pureed fruit with very thin custard	250	220	6
Banana smoothie	250	180	2
Hot chocolate with milk	250	240	10
Approximate total	3000	2100	70

Vitamin and mineral supplementation may be required, depending on the duration of liquid diet and the individual's requirements.

*Volume and composition vary with brand. See Table 25.5 for examples of proprietary oral nutrition supplements.

fracture); a higher protein intake may be required by patients who have suffered a traumatic fracture while energy should be limited in the treatment of obesity.
- Including some soluble fibre, e.g. pureed porridge or lump-free lentil soup, may help alleviate constipation that is common because of the preclusion of most fruit, vegetable, and wholegrain items. Alternatively, the bulk-forming laxative, ispaghula husk, may be given, but care must be taken to ensure an adequate fluid intake.
- Mouth hygiene should be maintained by gently brushing the exterior tooth surfaces and fixtures and using saline or antiseptic mouthwash on waking, before retiring to bed, and after every meal and snack.

Dental health

Healthy teeth and gums contribute to overall health and wellbeing.
- Efficient, pain-free mastication facilitates the intake of a varied and well-balanced diet.
- Good oral hygiene is associated with ↓ risk of cardiovascular disease and ↓ occurrence and progression of respiratory tract infections.
- Complete and decay-free teeth contribute to psychosocial wellbeing by enhancing facial appearance and speech.

Dental caries

Definition

Caries (cavities, tooth decay) are holes in the structure of the tooth.

Prevalence

In the UK, tooth decay has ↓ greatly since the 1970s when fluoride tooth-paste was introduced. The percentage of adults with no teeth of their own fell from 28% in 1978 to 6% in 2009.[1] In 2013, 31% of 5-year-old and 46% of 8-year-old children in England, Wales, and Northern Ireland had experienced decay in their primary teeth while 46% of those aged 15 years had experienced decay in their permanent teeth.[2] Children from lower income families were more likely to have tooth decay than those from other income groups: 21% compared to 11% with severe or extensive decay at 5 years old.[2]

Pathogenesis

Bacteria living in the dental plaque ferment dietary carbohydrate into acid, which demateralizes the tooth enamel, initiating the cariogenic process (see Box 26.1). The pH of the mouth determines the extent of decay; for enamel, the critical pH is ~5.5 and for dentine, ~6.2, and decay will usually occur at lower (more acidic) pH.

Prevention

In addition to reducing plaque bacteria by regular brushing and flossing, and regular dental visits, dietary prevention includes:
- minimizing effects of fermentable carbohydrate;
- maximizing oral pH.

Dental erosion

Definition

Erosion is the acidic destruction of the tooth surface. It does not include the abrasion and attrition associated with normal wear and tear on the biting surface of the teeth.

1 Steele, J. et al. (2011) *Adult dental health survey 2009*. Available at: ℜhttp://content.digital.nhs.uk/pubs/dentalsurveyfullreport09.

2 Health and Social Care Information Centre (2015). *Children's dental health survey*. Available at: ℜ http://content.digital.nhs.uk/catalogue/PUB17137.

Prevalence

In the UK, prevalence is increasing and associated with ↑ consumption of acidic and/or carbonated soft drinks and herbal teas. The risk of erosion is ↑ by consuming carbonated (OR 1.6; 95% CI: 1.3, 2.0) and sports drinks (OR 2.1; 95% CI: 1.0, 4.8) and ↓ by consuming yogurt (OR 0.9; 95% CI: 0.8–1.0) and milk (OR 0.96; 95% CI: 0.91–0.99).[3]

Pathogenesis

In erosion, enamel-eroding acid is not derived from bacterial fermentation of dietary carbohydrate (Box 26.1), but from acidic fluid in the mouth, either from dietary intake or regurgitation of stomach contents (reflux/vomiting). Unlike caries, there is no critical pH as erosion is also influenced by calcium, phosphate, and buffering capacity.

Prevention

This is based on reducing acid contact. Reflux or vomiting (spontaneous or self-induced, e.g. in bulimia nervosa) require investigation. Dietary prevention includes:

- limiting acidic food and drink, including diet drinks, to mealtimes;
- finishing meal with alkaline food, e.g. cheese or milk;
- avoiding acidic food or drink last thing at night;
- drinking acidic drinks through a straw and minimizing sipping, swishing, and frothing in the mouth, including fizzy water;
- beware acidic medication, e.g. chewable vitamin C tablets;
- avoiding brushing teeth immediately after acidic food, ideally wait 1 hour after meals;
- 🔴 using a baby feeder filled with fruit juice or other acidic drink as a comforter leads to prolonged contact with teeth and potentially very severe erosion.

3 Salas, M.M., et al. (2015). Diet influenced tooth erosion prevalence in children and adolescents: Results of a meta-analysis and meta-regression. *J. Dent.* 43, 865–75.

Box 26.1 Fermentable carbohydrate

- *Type of carbohydrate* determines cariogenicity: sucrose > fructose, glucose, maltose > lactose, galactose > maltodextrins, polysaccharide > sorbitol, xylitol.
- *Frequency of exposure:* regular ingestion of small quantities of carbohydrate is more damaging to teeth than one larger intake because repeated exposure prevents oral pH from increasing above the 5.5 threshold, thus perpetuating tooth demineralization.
- *Texture of foods:* sticky/chewy food leaves residue on teeth that prolongs exposure to carbohydrate and leads to a lower oral pH. Toffees and dried fruit have a greater potential to contribute to dental caries than the same quantity of carbohydrate taken as fruit juice which rapidly leaves the mouth.

Maximizing oral pH

- Milk and dairy products are alkaline and contain protein, calcium, and phosphate, which play a role in re-mineralizing dental enamel following acid exposure.
- Saliva can be stimulated by chewing sugar-free gum for 10 min after meals. Freshly secreted saliva has a pH of >6.3, i.e. above critical threshold and therefore protective.
- Using a drinking straw with acidic drinks (fruit juices and carbonated beverages) can reduce the fall in pH compared with drinking from a cup.

Oesophageal disorders

After chewing and swallowing, food is transported via the oesophagus (or gullet) to the stomach. Although food passes rapidly through the oesophagus compared to other parts of the gastrointestinal (GI) tract, disorders that restrict food intake can have a major detrimental influence on nutritional status (see ➔ Chapter 1, 'Digestion').

Achalasia

Achalasia leads to food being retained in the oesophagus as a result of reduced peristalsis and incomplete opening of the lower oesophageal sphincter. Difficulty with swallowing food leads to weight loss in up to 60% of patients, but achalasia also may occur in obesity.

Treatment includes balloon dilatation, surgery, stent insertion, or injection of botulinum toxin to relax the sphincter.

Nutritional management may also help and includes small frequent meals, avoiding foods that exacerbate dyspepsia and very hot or cold foods, taking time over meals and not eating late at night or before lying down. Chewing well and eating in an upright position (rather than reclining or slumped) may facilitate the passage of food into the stomach. Nutritional assessment should be undertaken to ensure that weight loss through an inadequate intake is prevented.

Dysphagia

Dysphagia (discomfort, difficulty, or pain when swallowing) is common in oesophageal disorders. Inflammation or occlusion of the oesophageal lumen impairs the final stage of swallowing as food passes from the pharynx to the stomach by the combined effects of peristalsis and gravity. Patients with oesophageal dysphagia are less at risk from aspirating food or liquid into the respiratory tract than those with dysphagia 2° to stroke where the oral and pharyngeal stages of swallow may also be impaired.

Nutritional management should include assessment of the swallowing problem and an evaluation of the optimum texture of foods and liquids (see in ➔ Chapter 23, 'Modification of texture of food and fluid'). In general, patients with more severe oesophageal disorders will require more liquids and thinner textures than those with milder dysphagia. The nutritional adequacy of the intake should be evaluated and progress monitored in the context of the underlying condition.

Oesophageal cancer

Approximately 8,900 cases are diagnosed in the UK annually, making this the 14th most common malignancy. Worldwide, an estimated 572,000 new cases are diagnosed annually. It is more common in men than women and in people aged >60 years. Smoking, heavy alcohol intake, being overweight, low intake of fruit and vegetables, consuming caustic substances, and a precancerous condition, Barrett's oesophagus, are risk factors.

Treatment may include surgery, chemotherapy, radiotherapy (see ➔ Chapter 24, 'Cancer treatment'), laser treatment, and/or the insertion of a stent (see ➔ this chapter, 'Oesophageal stents').

Nutritional management should include assessment of nutritional status and aim to provide adequate energy and nutrient intake in a format that can be swallowed and is acceptable to the patient (see ➔ Chapter 23, 'Modification of texture of food and fluid'). Patients with oesophageal cancer are often undernourished on diagnosis as a result of an inadequate intake because of symptoms; depletion may be exacerbated by treatment. Even obese patients may be undernourished, i.e. muscle loss but excess fat. Therefore, appropriate nutritional evaluation and support is essential and associated with better tolerance of chemo- and radiotherapy. Oral supplements may help, but post-pyloric tube feeding may be required, particularly if surgery is undertaken and a jejunostomy tube, possibly inserted at theatre, may provide valuable access.

Oesophageal stricture

Strictures may arise from benign causes (e.g. gastro-oesophageal reflux, damage secondary to intubation) or secondary to malignancy, and result in increasing difficulty swallowing.

Treatment is aimed at the underlying cause and attempts to limit the occlusive effects of the stricture include balloon dilatation and stenting.

Nutritional management should ensure an adequate intake. Small, frequent meals comprising moist, semi-solid food and nourishing liquids may be tolerated but, if not, tube feeding should be instigated before severe depletion or dehydration occurs.

Oesophageal varices

See ➔ Chapter 28, 'Oesophageal varices'.

Oesophagitis

Inflammation of the oesophagus is associated with acid reflux from the stomach and hiatus hernia. Prolonged oesophagitis can lead to thickening and hardening of the mucosal cells, known as Barrett's oesophagus, a precancerous risk for developing oesophageal cancer.

Nutritional management See ➔ this chapter 'Indigestion, heartburn, gastro-oesophageal reflux disease (GORD), and hiatus hernia'.

Oesophageal stents

The endoscopic insertion of a self-expanding metal stent (SEMS) into a strictured oesophagus may prevent total occlusion and help the patient to maintain their oral intake. Stents are mainly used as palliation in oesophageal cancer but can also play a role in the management of benign strictures and oesophageal fistulae. Complications include haemorrhage, stent migration, tumour overgrowth, and food-related blockages. SEMS are recommended in preference to plastic as they are associated with fewer blockages.

Nutritional management should include dietary advice about maintaining an adequate energy and nutrient intake and how to minimize the risk of tube blockage (see Box 26.2). Even though this treatment is seen primarily as palliative, 75–90% of patients resume a near-normal diet after stent insertion and improvements in nutritional status and survival have been reported.

Box 26.2 Dietary advice after oesophageal stent placement[4]

Fluids
- Prescribe a fluid-only diet for first 24 hours after insertion.
- Once food is introduced, advise frequent consumption of any type of liquid after eating food to wash away any debris.
- There is no evidence to support the use of fizzy drinks. These may cause problems with acid reflux if stent is placed distally.
- If the stent becomes blocked following eating, drink warm water to flush through.

Food
- Advice given should be modified to take account of the patient's tumour (in oesophageal cancer), their ability to chew, continuing dysphagia, and posture/position.
- Texture modification should reflect individual patient's needs (see ➲ Chapter 23, 'Modification of texture of food and fluid') and appropriate written advice should be given.
- Patients should be advised to:
  - take small mouthfuls and chew all food well;
  - sit upright when eating;
  - eat slowly and without rushing;
  - drink plenty of fluid.
- Patients are often advised to restrict foods considered potentially stent-blocking. However, experimental evidence suggests that few items need to be totally avoided.
  - *Foods causing occlusion:* dry meat, fruit with pith, skins of capsicum peppers and tomatoes, ≥7 sultanas, dried apricots;
  - *Foods able to pass through stent if taken in small mouthfuls and chewed for twice the usual time:* sandwiches, dry toast, apple, tinned pineapple, fresh orange segments with pith removed, ≤6 sultanas, chopped dried apricots, boiled egg, muesli, meat, and poultry;
  - Controversial items such as nuts and vegetables, including lettuce, caused no occlusions.

4 Holdoway, A., *et al.* (2003). Palliation in cancer of the oesophagus—what passes down an oe-sophageal stent? *J. Hum. Nutr. Diet.* **16**, 369–70.

Stomach disorders

Nausea and vomiting

Nausea and vomiting can have a significant effect on nutritional status by greatly reducing intake or preventing the digestion and absorption of food consumed. These symptoms may relate to a GI disorder, food poisoning, or other systemic condition, e.g. uraemia, or treatment, e.g. chemotherapy (see **⮞** Chapter 24, 'Cancer treatment'). Treatment of the underlying cause or self-limitation may bring resolution but, in many cases, managing the situation may help maintain an adequate nutritional intake. For vomiting in children <5 years, see NICE (2009).[5]

Nutritional management in adults
Try:
- chilled foods as these may be more acceptable than hot items;
- plain foods in small quantities may be better tolerated;
- sip drinks throughout the day, but wait for 15 minutes after eating before taking more fluid;
- ginger flavours, mints, and plain biscuits.

Avoid:
- off-putting smells (food or others);
- foods that don't appeal: may include spicy or greasy items;
- lying down after eating: a gentle walk may help;
- extreme hunger by eating small amounts regularly.

In severe cases, dehydration may be a concern and oral rehydration solution or intravenous fluids may be required.

Indigestion, heartburn, gastro-oesophageal reflux disease (GORD), and hiatus hernia

This spectrum of gastric disorders is common with approximately 9-28% of adults in Europe and the USA experiencing symptoms of GORD.[6] Although diet has been implicated in the aetiology (erratic eating habits, obesity, alcohol, and other specific food items), much of this is anecdotal and there is little firm evidence.

Symptoms range from postprandial discomfort to sharp burning pain below the sternum or between the shoulder blades, regurgitation of acidic stomach contents into the oesophagus, and possibly mouth and, in severe cases, mucosal damage.

Nutritional management (in addition to treatment with proton pump inhibitors and H_2 blockers) should include review of diet and lifestyle with the aim of reducing excess body weight and introducing a regular eating pattern

5 National Institute for Health and Care Excellence (NICE) (2009). *Diarrhoea and vomiting caused by gastroenteritis in under 5s: diagnosis and management*. CG84. Available at: ℛ http://www.nice.org.uk/guidance/CG84.

6 Boeckxstaens, G., et al. (2014). Symptomatic reflux disease: the present, the past and the future. *Gut* **63**, 1185–93.

based on the 'Eatwell Guide (see ➔ Chapter 2). Specific dietary advice is mostly anecdotal and not supported by systematic review[7] of limited studies. Practical suggestions that may help include:

- elevating the head-end of the bed to facilitate a semi-upright position while sleeping;
- eating small, regular meals in place of less frequent, but larger meals;
- eating earlier in the evening and avoiding late night meals;
- sitting upright, rather than slumped while eating and avoid bending, lifting, or lying down immediately after meals;
- avoiding foods that are known to cause discomfort to individual.

Gastritis and peptic ulcers

Gastritis is the inflammation of the mucosal surface of the stomach. It can range from a mild, asymptomatic form to severe ulceration, which if untreated may lead to perforation. Peptic ulcers include lesions in the stomach and duodenum. Eighty per cent of gastritis and peptic ulcers are associated with *Helicobacter pylori* infection (see Box 26.3), but a high intake of alcohol and non-steroidal anti-inflammatory drugs is also implicated.

Symptoms include nausea, vomiting (possibly blood-stained), and pain.

Nutritional management In severe cases, patients have no desire to eat and 'resting' the stomach from food for 1–2 days may help alleviate pain; adequate fluid including sugar and electrolytes will minimize risk of dehydration, but clearly are not nutritionally adequate. Nutrient intake should be ↑ over 1–3 days by providing other nourishing fluids and then bland, non-irritating foods that the patient feels able to manage. There is little clinical evidence about specific foods to avoid, but most individuals are aware of items that exacerbate symptoms (often spicy, highly flavoured foods with a high fat content) and thus should decide whether or not to risk eating them (see Box 26.4). Fruit and juice with perceptible acidity have traditionally been avoided on the grounds that these exacerbate gastric pH; there is no evidence for this and the antioxidants provided by these food items play a valuable role in promoting healing so they should not be avoided. Some people may find plain, bland food is tolerated best and that milk and milky foods are most agreeable; again, there is no evidence to support this and patients should be encouraged to eat a wide range of foods. Ultimately, a varied and well-balanced diet that sustains a healthy weight should be the goal.

Stomach cancer

Approximately 7,000 cases are diagnosed in the UK annually, making this the 16th most common cancer. Worldwide, approximately 1,033,000 people are diagnosed annually. It is more common in individuals with *Helicobacter pylori* infection and those eating a high intake of smoked, cured, and salted food. A diet high in fruit and vegetables is protective.

7 Kaltenbach, T., *et al.* (2006). Are lifestyle measures effective in patients with gastroesophageal reflux disease? An evidence-based approach. *Arch. Intern. Med.* **166**, 965–71.

Box 26.3 *Helicobacter pylori*—are there any nutritional implications?

H. pylori is a bacterium commonly found in the stomach. Infection may be asymptomatic, but is associated with gastritis, ulceration, and ↑ risk of stomach cancer. Prevalence of infection ↑ with age and is highest in developing countries and people of lower socio-economic status. In the UK, ~30% of people born in the 1930s are infected compared with <5% born in the 1970s.

- Acquisition of infection is by person-to-person transmission (oral–oral and faecal–oral) and possibly also via food. Overcrowding and poor hygiene practices are implicated. Good personal and food hygiene may ↓ risk of transmission.
- Oral probiotics may act as a beneficial adjunct to antibiotic eradication therapy. Further studies are needed to clarify optimum dose and population.
- A high salt diet and *H. pylori* infection may act synergistically to promote atrophic gastritis.[8] This effect may be partly attenuated by dietary antioxidants, i.e. from fruit and vegetables, and these cellular mechanisms are supported by epidemiological findings.
- Although there is no evidence from dietary trials, it is logical to recommend ↑ fruit and vegetable intake and avoid excessive dietary salt, i.e. a healthy diet, for people with *H. pylori* infection.

Symptoms include heartburn, anorexia and bloating progressing to vomiting (sometimes blood stained), pain on eating, and severe weight loss.

Treatment is surgical resection (see ➔ this chapter, 'Gastrectomy and stomach surgery') if the tumour is operable. Chemotherapy and radiotherapy may be used in conjunction or as alternatives (see ➔ Chapter 24, 'Cancer treatment').

Nutritional management depends on treatment but should aim to maintain an optimum nutritional intake whether by mouth or through artificial nutrition support. Each patient should be individually assessed and their requirements evaluated and nutrition support planned on the basis of these and the access available for feeding. Specific advice is required after surgical resection.

8 Haley, K.P., et al. (2016). Nutrition and helicobacter pylori: Host diet and nutritional immunity influence bacterial virulence and disease outcome. *Gastroenterol. Res. Pract.* **2016**, 3019362.

Box 26.4 Is it necessary for people with stomach disorders to avoid spicy food?

- Studies investigating the clinical effects of spices report different results that vary with the type and quantity of spice eaten and the habitual intake and GI health of consumers:
  - Curcumin, extract of turmeric, is associated with ↓ *H. pylori* effects mediated through antioxidant/anti-inflammatory properties.[9]
  - Capsaicin, extract of chili, can aggravate symptoms in some people with dyspepsia and irritable bowel syndrome, but regular ingestion may ↓ symptoms in GORD and is associated with ↓ incidence of gastric ulcers in epidemiological studies.
  - Garam masala is associated with more rapid gastric emptying in humans.
  - Clove and nutmeg inhibit *H. pylori* growth *in vitro*, possibly explaining low rates of gastric disease in countries like Thailand.
  - Ginger is reported to have anti-emetic and gastro-protective effects mediated through antioxidant effects.[10]
- *Conclusion*: inadequate evidence for advising increased intake of these spices but equally, no evidence to support discouraging intake: more good quality research is required.

9 Sarkar, A., *et al.* (2016). Curcumin as a potential therapeutic candidate for Helicobacter pylori associated diseases. *World J. Gastroenterol.* 7, 2736–48.

10 Haniadka, R., *et al.* (2013). A review of the gastroprotective effects of ginger (Zingiber officinale Roscoe). *Food Funct.* 4, 845–55.

Gastrectomy and stomach surgery

The type of surgical resection of the stomach, e.g. for cancer, perforation following severe ulceration or traumatic injury, varies depending on the degree and position of the lesion to be removed, anatomical reconstruction, and type of procedure (laparoscopic, endoscopic, or open), but can be briefly summarized as follows (see Fig. 26.1):

• *Total gastrectomy:* resection of complete stomach with anastomosis of oesophagus to the small bowel and reconnection of the duodenum to the small bowel (Roux-en-Y reconstruction). Cardiac and pyloric sphincters removed.

• *Partial gastrectomy:* resection of distal (pyloric) end of stomach by anastomosis of remaining part of upper stomach to duodenum or, more commonly, small bowel (Biliroth 2 reconnection). Pyloric sphincter removed.

• *Oesophago-gastrectomy:* resection of proximal (cardiac) end of stomach and lower oesophagus by anastomosis of lower stomach to upper oesophagus. Cardiac sphincter removed.

• *Vagotomy:* cutting the vagus nerve, to reduce acid secretion also causes a decrease in peristalsis and alters the emptying patterns of the stomach. It is often undertaken with gastrectomy or a pyloroplasty, a procedure to widen the outlet from the stomach to the small intestine.

The type of surgery, anastomosis, and removal of sphincter muscles have nutritional relevance because they influence eating-related symptoms after surgery. Meta-analysis[11] of studies of total gastrectomy indicates that surgical formation of a pouch is nutritionally and symptomatically better than reconstruction without a pouch and is associated with similar morbidity and mortality.

Nutritional management

Patients should be offered drink and food on the first post-operative day and advised to begin cautiously and gradually increase intake.[12] Those consuming <60% requirements by the 6th post-op day should be given individualized nutritional support. Food-related complications include the following:

• Feeling full after very small quantities of food is common, particularly following total gastrectomy, so small meals eaten frequently (~ hourly, initially) will help to maximize nutrient intake and thus contribute to healing. Bulky foods and fizzy drinks may be best avoided at first as these may exacerbate feelings of fullness. Drinking separately from eating may also help.

• Dumping syndrome is caused by the rapid movement of dietary sugar/ refined carbohydrate into the intestine. Early postprandial symptoms include dizziness, faintness, sweating, and a sudden drop in blood pressure. Later symptoms can occur ~2 hours after eating including weakness, cold, and faintness associated with hypoglycaemia resulting from excessive release of insulin in response to rapidly absorbed dietary

11 Zong, L., *et al.* (2011). Pouch Roux-en-Y vs no pouch Roux-en-Y following total gastrectomy: a meta-analysis based on 12 studies. *J. Biomed. Res.* **25**, 90–9.

12 Mortensen, K., *et al.* (2014). Consensus guidelines for enhanced recovery after gastrectomy. *Br. J. Surg.* **101**, 1209–29.

carbohydrate. First line treatment for early and late symptoms is dietary modification:[13] eat small meals regularly, limit refined carbohydrate, include high fibre and protein foods, chew well and drink liquids >30 minutes after meals. The intensity of symptoms may resolve within 3 months of surgery.

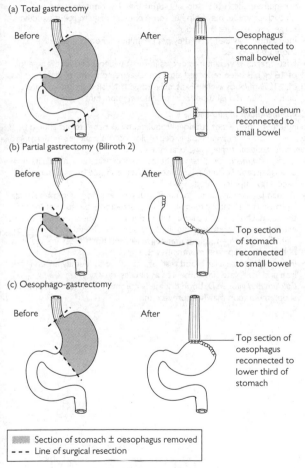

(a) Total gastrectomy

Before　　　　After

Oesophagus reconnected to small bowel

Distal duodenum reconnected to small bowel

(b) Partial gastrectomy (Billroth 2)

Before　　　　After

Top section of stomach reconnected to small bowel

(c) Oesophago-gastrectomy

Before　　　　After

Top section of oesophagus reconnected to lower third of stomach

▨ Section of stomach ± oesophagus removed
- - - Line of surgical resection

Fig. 26.1 Gastrectomy and stomach surgery.

13 van Beek, A.P., et al. (2017). Dumping syndrome after esophageal, gastric or bariatric surgery: pathophysiology, diagnosis, and management. Obes. Rev. 18, 68–85.

- Diarrhoea is relatively common in the first 1–2 months after gastric surgery and can be related to dumping syndrome. If so, the same dietary modification is required. Anti-motility medication, e.g. codeine phosphate or loperamide hydrochloride, may help.
- Vomiting of bile and other digestive juices may occur after partial or total gastrectomy, particularly in the morning. No dietary modification is required; antacids or motility stimulants, e.g. domperidone or metoclopramide, may help but some patients require reconstructive surgery to alleviate the problem.
- Indigestion may be relieved by peppermint oil. Foods that exacerbate should be avoided.
- Post-operative weight loss occurs in most patients and an average loss of 16 kg has been reported after total gastrectomy for malignancy; loss of >10% of body weight is associated with ↑ risk of complications and death.[14] Nutritional support is, therefore, important.

Supplementation of nutrients

Supplementation is not routinely required by all patients but should be determined on an individual basis depending on the patient's underlying disorder, extent of surgery, and oral intake.

- *Energy and macronutrients:* weight loss may indicate an inadequate intake or a recurrence of malignant disease; intake should be assessed and, if necessary, supplemented.
- *Vitamin B_{12}:* prophylactic vitamin B_{12} supplementation by intramuscular injection is mandatory following total gastrectomy because of loss of the stomach-derived intrinsic factor required for absorption. In patients with partial gastrectomy, vitamin B_{12} absorption should be checked to identify requirement. Note that deficiency will not appear immediately but may develop over months/years.
- *Iron and folate:* regular blood tests are required to identify anaemia and iron and/or folate supplemented as necessary.
- *Calcium and vitamin D:* bone disease is common after gastrectomy and supplementation may help prevent this.

14 Ryan, A.M., *et al.* (2007). Short-term nutritional implications of total gastrectomy for malignancy and the impact of parenteral nutrition support. *Clin. Nutr.* **26**, 718–27.

Small intestine disorders: introduction

The small intestine comprises ~7 m of the GI tract running from the pyloric sphincter of the stomach to the ileocaecal valve and comprises:
• duodenum;
• jejunum;
• ileum.

Its main function is to digest and absorb energy, nutrients, and water from the partially digested food passing through its lumen. As a consequence, any disorders of the small intestine that result in impaired function will potentially have a significant influence on absorption and, therefore, also on nutritional status.

Disorders with nutritional implications include:
• malabsorption (including steatorrhoea and lactose intolerance);
• inflammatory bowel disease (Crohn's disease and ulcerative colitis);
• coeliac disease;
• intestinal failure and short bowel syndrome;
• fistulae.

Malabsorption: introduction

Symptoms

Diarrhoea, abdominal distension, flatulence from intestinal gas production, weight loss.

Aetiology

Multifactorial, (see Box 26.5).

Treatment

The underlying cause of malabsorption should be treated wherever possible, e.g. treating infections, prescribing pancreatic lipase in insufficiency, avoiding gluten in coeliac disease. Nutritional management by adapting the diet may also be required.

Nutritional management

- Individual patients should be assessed and advised by a dietitian with expertise in treating patients with malabsorption.
- Consideration must be given to the cause of malabsorption to identify the specific section of the small intestine that is affected and thus which nutrients are likely to be inadequately absorbed, e.g. disaccharides are absorbed in the proximal jejunum, vitamin B_{12} in the ileum (see ➔ Chapter 1, 'Digestion').
- The inadequate absorption of some specific nutrients, e.g. fat and lactose, will result in generalized malabsorption of most other nutrients because of the effect of interaction with other unabsorbed components and\or bacterial action, i.e. 'intestinal hurry' after osmotic effects of unabsorbed food components causing increased luminal fluid.
- In addition to dietary manipulation which may resolve symptoms, consideration must be given to overall nutritional adequacy and, in patients who have become nutritionally depleted by malabsorption, restoration of nutritional status.

Box 26.5 Main causes of malabsorption

Anatomical
- Surgical resection
- Fistulae

Enzyme insufficiency
- Pancreatic insufficiency, e.g. lipase
- Lactase deficiency, 1° or 2°

Mucosal insufficiency
- Villous atrophy
- Coeliac disease
- Crohn's disease
- Radiation enteritis
- Impaired transport
- Lymphangiectasia

Luminal factors
- Altered pH, e.g. neuroendocrine tumours, Zollinger–Ellison syndrome
- Bile acid malabsorption
- Bile salt insufficiency

Systematic conditions
- Scleroderma
- Lymphoma

Infection
- Bacterial overgrowth, e.g. in blind loops
- Parasitic infections

Drugs
- Antibiotics
- Excessive laxative use.

Steatorrhoea

Untreated fat malabsorption is potentially very serious because undigested fat forms complexes within the GI lumen with calcium and other minerals preventing them and a wide range of other nutrients from being absorbed.

If steatorrhoea arises from pancreatic lipase insufficiency, this should be treated with pancreatic enzymes, rather than dietary fat restriction (see ⊃ Chapter 27, 'Pancreatic enzyme replacement therapy'). However, steatorrhoea caused by bile insufficiency cannot be so readily treated and a low fat diet may be required.

Low fat diet

The amount of fat tolerated varies between individuals and it is suggested that a very low fat diet of ~20 g/day (Table 26.2) is instigated temporarily (days only) until symptoms resolve and then small amounts of additional dietary fat are added to the diet to tolerance. Most patients with malabsorption can tolerate a diet providing ± 40 g fat and there is no benefit from advising a lower level of restriction than one that ameliorates symptoms. Attention must be given to the following:

- Total energy content of the diet. 40 g fat provides <20% of the energy requirements of most adults (in a healthy diet, fat provides 30–35% of energy) so the deficit must be made up by ↑ carbohydrate ± protein intake or by supplementing with medium chain triglycerides (see Box 26.6).
- Fat-soluble vitamins, A, D, E, and K. If absorption is in doubt, vitamin status should be assessed. Supplements can be given orally or by intramuscular injection depending on the degree of malabsorption. Dose of A, D, E, and K supplementation in patients with cystic fibrosis is given in Table 30.1, p. 742. Studies are required to identify optimum dose in other patients with steatorrhoea.
- Calcium. Supplements, e.g. 1600 mg/40 mmol daily, should be given if steatorrhoea is prolonged or there is evidence of bone thinning.
- Essential fatty acids. The limited dietary fat consumed should include some linolenic and linoleic fatty acids.

Table 26.2 Sample menu for temporary very low fat diet (20 g)*

	Weight, g	Energy, kcal	Fat, g
Orange juice	250	110	—
Cereal with sugar (not muesli/granola)	55	210	0.5
Skimmed milk for whole day	600	210	0.6
Toast, two slices	75	180	1.7
Marmalade	20	50	—
Coffee with skimmed milk + sugar	250	40	—
Low fat yogurt	150	170	1.7
Dates	40	120	0.2
Sandwich, four slices bread	140	330	2.2
½ tsp polyunsaturated margarine†	3	20	2.4
Lean ham	80	80	2.2
Sliced tomatoes	60	10	—
Banana	110	90	0.4
Tea with skimmed milk + sugar	250	40	—
Toasted tea cake with honey	45	120	0.9
Roast chicken, no skin	120	120	3.7
Boiled potatoes, large serving	200	170	0.2
Carrots and peas	200	60	0.4
Gravy made without fat	80	—	—
Tinned fruit in syrup	100	70	—
Low fat custard	75	70	1.1
Low fat chocolate drink	250	40	1.4
Marshmallow or jelly sweets	30	90	—
Approximate total	—	2400	19.6

Fat intake should be ↑ to tolerance according to individual needs (most patients will tolerate ~40g/day).

*Supplementary fat-soluble vitamins ± calcium supplements should be prescribed.

†Source of essential fatty acids.

Box 26.6 Medium chain triglycerides

- Medium chain triglycerides (MCT) comprise fatty acids with 6-12 carbon atoms (long chain triglycerides [LCT] have fatty acids with >12 carbons).
- Partially water-mixable so more easily emulsified than LCT; useful in bile insufficiency.
- More easily hydrolysed than LCT; useful in lipase insufficiency.
- Absorbed directly into portal circulation; chylomicron transport via lymph not required.
- Provide 855 kcal/100 mL (approximately 8.4 kcal/g compared with 9.0 kcal/g with LCT); a useful source of energy if ordinary fat cannot be taken.
- Available as:
  - oil (MCT oil, Nutricia);
  - emulsion (Liquigen®, Nutricia);
  - powder with carbohydrate (MCT Duocal®, SHS);
  - powder with carbohydrate and protein (MCTprocal®, Vitaflo);
  - complete or partially complete feeds (Nutrison MCT, Nutricia; Peptamen® HN, Nestlé).
- Indications include steatorrhoea, lymphangiectasia, and ketogenic diets for epilepsy.
- As a result of partial solubility, MCT in oil have an osmotic effect so this should be introduced into the diet gradually (<15 mL oil per dose) to avoid diarrhoea.
- In cooking, the oil has a low flash point so using very high temperatures can give food a burnt taste.
- Emulsion can be added to low fat milkshakes to increase energy.

Lactose intolerance

Insufficiency of lactase is the most common cause of carbohydrate-related malabsorption (sucrase and maltase deficiency is very rare except in Greenland). The term 'lactose intolerance' is used to describe the symptoms associated with this form of malabsorption that depend on (1) the quantity of lactose ingested and (2) the degree of lactase deficiency. This can be categorized as:

- 1° as a result of autosomal recessive disorder where lactase production is ± normal in children <4 years but declines in older children and adults leading to lactose intolerance. Prevalence varies with ethnicity: African-Caribbean >80%, Indian >50%, White Europeans <10%. 1° lactose intolerance may also occur at birth (but is rare) from a hereditary total lactase deficiency.
- 2° as a result of ↓ lactase production from intestinal villi damage typically after GI infection. This is usually temporary (~weeks) and lactase production may slowly resume spontaneously as damage resolves.

Nutritional management

This is based on a low lactose diet (Table 26.3). This is relatively straight forward in adults and older children providing that the rest of the diet includes sufficient variety to meet all nutrient requirements including calcium. However, expertise is required to plan a regime for infants and younger children, because of the important nutritional role milk usually plays, to ensure that their intake is sufficiently low in lactose and yet remains otherwise nutritionally adequate: seek advice from a paediatric dietitian. In particular, care is needed with substitute milks (e.g. rice, oat, coconut) because many contain substantially less protein and micronutrients than cow's milk.

Diet for lactose intolerance

Individuals vary in the amount of lactose they can tolerate without experiencing symptoms of malabsorption (diarrhoea, bloating, and discomfort). There is no benefit in avoiding more lactose than is necessary to control symptoms. Systematic review[15] has indicated that 12 g of lactose as a single dose of milk (i.e. ~240 mL) is tolerated by most people with lactose intolerance (15 g if consumed with other nutrients), whereas doses of 24 g are associated with substantial symptoms.

There is insufficient evidence[15] to support adaptation of the colon to small doses of lactose or of benefit from lactose-reduced milk, lactase supplements taken with milk, probiotics, or treatment with rifaximin.

Dietary calcium intake may be compromised in individuals avoiding milk and other dairy products. This is particularly a concern for children, teenagers, pregnant women, and those with a family history of osteoporosis. Good sources of non-milk calcium include oily fish, e.g. sardines, white or brown bread, calcium-fortified soya drinks (see ➡ Chapter 6, 'Calcium' and discussion of calcium in ➡ Chapter 16, 'Vegetarians').

---

15 Shaukat, A., et al. (2010). Systematic review: Effective management strategies for lactose intolerance. *Ann. Intern. Med.* **152**, 797–803.

Table 26.3 Foods that are usually lactose-free and those that contain lactose

Foods usually free from lactose	Foods containing lactose*
Soya milks	Milk: skimmed, semi-skimmed, and whole (cow's, goat's, sheep's)
Rice milk drinks	
Non-dairy creamers (check label)	Cheese spread, cream, and cottage cheese
Most hard cheese contains very little lactose so is well tolerated, e.g. cheddar, Brie, Edam	Cream and sour cream
	Evaporated and condensed milk
	Yogurt
Breads made without milk	Breakfast cereal with milk
Breakfast cereals made without milk	Instant mashed potato mixes
Pasta, noodles, macaroni	Prepared breads, muffins, biscuits, or rolls made with milk
Potatoes, rice, other cooked grains	
Rice cakes	Pancakes or batter made with milk
Margarine without whey (check label)	Butter
Non-dairy creamers (check label)	Margarines with butter or milk
Oils	
Some salad dressings (check label)	
All fresh fruits and vegetables	Creamed vegetables, e.g. mashed potato
Cooked fruit or vegetables made without milk products	Fruit smoothies made with yogurt
Fruit and vegetable juices	Fruits or vegetables cooked with milk
	Vegetables coated in batter
All fresh cooked, plain meat, and fish	Breaded or battered meat or fish
Cooked dried peas and beans	Main dishes with white sauce such as macaroni cheese, fish in parsley sauce
Eggs cooked without milk	
Peanut butter, nuts, and seeds	Meats in cream sauces
Soya cheese and tofu products	Omelette or soufflés with milk
Broth, bouillon, consommé	Cream soups
Vegetable or meat soups without milk	Soup mixes with milk products
Gravies made with water	White sauces and gravies
Plain herbs and spices	
Fruit ices and sorbets	Custard or sauce made from milk
Honey, sugar, syrups, molasses, and powdered sweeteners	Cream or cheese filled cake or pastries
Jellies, jams, preserves	Fudge, coated candies, and chocolates
Pies and other baked foods without milk	Ice cream unless lactose-free
	Toffee, butterscotch, or caramels

* Many people with lactose intolerance can eat some of these foods and a very strict, lactose-free diet is required by very few individuals. It is recommended that very intolerant individuals and carers of small children check labels of food products and proceed with caution if the following ingredients are listed: milk powder, milk protein, milk solids, non-fat milk solids, whey, whey solids, or protein.

Infants and children <5 years with confirmed lactose intolerance should be given an appropriate lactose-free milk substitute (e.g. Enfamil® O-Lac, Nutramigen; Galactomin 17, SHS, Nutricia; SMA® LF, SMA Nutrition) under the advice of a paediatric dietitian.

❶ A diet for lactose intolerance is not the same as a milk-free diet which is required for cow's milk allergy (see ➲ Chapter 37, 'Food hypersensitivity').

Inflammatory bowel disease

Inflammatory bowel disease (IBD) comprises Crohn's disease (CD) and ulcerative colitis (UC), which are characterized by relapsing and remitting chronic gastrointestinal inflammation. IBD should not be confused with irritable bowel syndrome (IBS).

At least 300,000 people in the UK have IBD and millions of people are affected across the world. It is less common in Africa, Asia, and Central and South America. All ages can be affected but diagnosis is most frequent in children and young adults.

The cause of IBD is not fully understood but it involves a genetic predisposition, environmental triggers, and immune dysfunction alongside a complex interaction with the gut microbiome.

In CD, patchy inflammation can affect anywhere from the mouth to the anus, but is most common in the ileocaecal region. Abdominal pain, diarrhoea, and weight loss feature. Recurrent episodes of inflammation lead to deep ulceration, strictures, and fistulae; surgical resection may be required, sometimes repeatedly.

In UC, inflammation is continuous and affects the mucosal lining. It is confined to the colon and rectum; it can be rectal sparing and may extend continuously towards the caecum. Abdominal pain, diarrhoea (with blood and mucus), and anaemia feature, and acute episodes may occur. Complications include perforation and toxic megacolon. Surgical resection may be required, leading to the formation of a colostomy or ileo-anal pouch.

Undernutrition occurs in 20-85% of patients with IBD because of the complex interaction between the altered metabolism, reduced dietary intake, increased nutritional requirements, and increased GI losses. Undernutrition includes energy and protein depletion and, in some patients, specific micronutrient deficiencies. Loss of >5% body weight at diagnosis is independently associated with development of severe disease.

Severe nutritional depletion is usually less of a problem in UC compared with those with CD, probably as a result of inflammation affecting areas of the gut distal to the site of absorption of most nutrients. IBD patients frequently have a poor appetite or consume a restricted diet in an effort to relieve their symptoms, and poor nutritional status is common.

Patients with IBD should have support from a care team made up of a range of different healthcare professionals, including a dietitian for nutritional assessment and dietary management.

Nutritional assessment and monitoring
- Weight and BMI (and height in children and adolescents) should be monitored and documented at all outpatient appointments and weekly during admissions.
- Unplanned weight loss should be noted and if >10% in the previous 3-6 months, initiate appropriate dietary management in accordance with local guidance (see ➔ Chapter 25, 'Treatment of undernutrition).
- Assess vitamin D status and supplement if required (see ➔ Chapter 6, 'Vitamin D').
- Vitamin B$_{12}$ status should be measured annually in patients with ileal CD.
- Assess patients for iron deficiency, with or without anaemia. Oral or intravenous supplementation may be required, check with local guidance.

- Calcium intake, vitamin D status, and bone density should be monitored, especially in those receiving corticosteroids for more severe disease, and supplements may be required.

Preventing/treating undernutrition
- Providing nutritional support is a high priority and should be an integral part of management. The form/degree of support will depend on current severity, i.e. in exacerbation or remission, and part of GI tract affected.
- Those most likely to require nutritional support include children and adolescents (who are still growing), patients with existing undernutrition, and those with an exacerbation of symptoms, partial obstruction, and requiring or recovering from surgery.
- Although patients may avoid specific foods, wherever possible restricted items should be minimized and a 'normal' diet encouraged including energy and protein dense foods, i.e. there is no proven specific diet for CD or UC.
- In CD, patients with strictures or partial obstruction should avoid fibrous foods that may cause pain and/or lead to an obstruction, e.g. stringy beans, citrus fruit pith, meat gristle, nuts.
- No dietary restrictions should be routinely advised; there is no evidence to support the use of low residue diets.
- Patients should be encouraged to eat as normally as possible.
- If they are unable to consume an adequate intake orally, enteral nutrition should be considered. This is preferable to parenteral as it is associated with significantly fewer complications. Using parenteral nutrition to 'rest the bowel' does not alter clinical outcome.
- In proven fat malabsorption, limiting dietary fat (~40 g/day or to tolerance) may help. However, this should *not* be routinely advised because of the concentrated energy provided by dietary fat and its potential therapeutic effects mediated via rate of apoptosis in inflammatory cells.
- The anti-inflammatory effects of *n*-3 fatty acids (i.e. from oily fish, see Box 23.3) on remission in IBD have been investigated. Studies to date have provided inconsistent results and there is insufficient evidence to support recommending omega-3 supplementation.
- Oral nutritional supplements should be offered if insufficient food is consumed (see ➔ Chapter 25, 'Treatment of undernutrition'). Most commercial products (except powders that are mixed with milk) are low in lactose so acceptable even if 2° lactose intolerance is suspected (see ➔ this Chapter, 'Lactose intolerance').
- Enteral feeding is the preferred route if oral intake is inadequate and should be considered early before nutritional depletion is allowed to progress. Enteral nutrition should not be offered to maintain remission after surgery.[16]

---

16 National Institute for Health and Care Excellence (NICE) (2012). *Crohn's disease. Management in adults, children and young people.* CG152. Available at: ℗ http://www.nice.org.uk/Guidance/CG152.

- Total parenteral nutrition (see ➡ Chapter 25, 'Parenteral nutrition') is an appropriate adjunctive therapy in patients with fistulae if an adequate nutritional intake cannot be achieved enterally.
- Standard micronutrient supplementation should be given if oral intake is inadequate or absorption compromised.
- Calcium and vitamin D supplementation should be considered in all patients receiving corticosteroids. CD is the cause of 2° osteoporosis.
- There is insufficient advice to recommend probiotics as beneficial in maintaining remission in CD.

Dietary management of active CD

- In children and young people, exclusive enteral nutrition is used as first line therapy[16] to facilitate growth and development. In adults, exclusive enteral nutrition is usually adjunctive, i.e. to address undernutrition, in pre-surgical optimization and prevent or ameliorate malnutrition rather than primary treatment, where it might be used where other primary treatments are not possible (e.g. immunosuppressive agents, biological therapy, or corticosteroids) or it is the patient's choice.
- The optimum treatment duration for exclusive enteral nutrition is unknown, a clinical response can be achieved in 10 days but mucosal healing can take up to 8 weeks.
- Elemental (amino acid-based) or polymeric (containing whole protein) enteral feeds are equally as effective as each other, but less effective than corticosteroids in the treatment of active CD in adults. Elemental enteral feeds are less palatable and more expensive than polymeric and consideration should be given to compliance if patients are advised to consume these over a long period.

Dietary management of UC

- There is no evidence that either elemental or other dietary interventions have a specific therapeutic impact on the condition although maintaining nutritional status is important, particularly if surgery is anticipated.
- Patients undergoing colectomy may benefit from specific advice about their food intake after surgery.
- Patients with UC have ↑ risk of colon cancer and, to minimize this, those in remission should be advised to eat a healthy diet along the lines of the 'Eatwell Guide' (see ➡ Chapter 2).

Dietary management of functional GI symptoms in IBD

Approximately 39% of patients with IBD have functional GI symptoms and dietary management of these is effective using strategies similar to those described for irritable bowel syndrome, e.g. a low FODMAP diet (see ➡ this Chapter, 'Low FODMAP diet'). It is important that active disease is ruled out as a cause for symptoms before initiation of dietary intervention. In clinical practice, disease activity can be assessed by physician global assessment and biomarkers (e.g. faecal calprotectin, C reactive protein) and discussed with the IBD team on whether it is appropriate to try dietary approaches to manage functional GI symptoms. A low FODMAP diet reduces the prebiotic content of the diet so it is important that strict FODMAP restriction should only last up to 8 weeks. Patients should be encouraged to reintroduce high FODMAP foods to personal tolerance after this time.

Education on the low FODMAP diet should be provided by a dietitian experienced in this dietary intervention.

Further reading

Dignass, A., et al. (2010). The second European evidence-based consensus on the diagnosis and management of Crohn's disease: Current management. J. Crohn's Colitis 4, 28–62.

Forbes, A., et al. (2017). ESPEN guideline: Clinical nutrition in inflammatory bowel disease. Clin. Nutr. 36, 321–47.

National Institute for Health and Care Excellence (NICE) (2012). Crohn's disease. Management in adults, children and young people. CG152. Available at: ℜ http://www.nice.org.uk/Guidance/CG152.

National Institute for Health and Care Excellence (NICE) (2015). Inflammatory bowel disease. QS81. Available at: ℜ http://www.nice.org.uk/Guidance/qs81.

Travis, S.P.L., et al. (2008). European evidence-based consensus on the management of ulcerative colitis: Current management. J. Crohn's Colitis 2, 24–62.

Coeliac disease

Coeliac disease (CoD) is an autoimmune condition resulting in mucosal damage of the small intestine. It is caused by the ingestion of 'gluten', a generic term for specific proteins (prolamines) found in the endosperm of certain cereals including wheat (gliadins), rye (secalins), and barley (horedins). Up to 1% of the UK population is affected by CoD, although delayed and late diagnosis is common. Worldwide prevalence is estimated at between 0.5% and 2%.

Coeliac disease can present at any age and has a wide range of symptoms. Some affect the gut and include bloating, constipation, or diarrhoea, excessive wind, nausea, and vomiting (with or without unintentional weight loss). Other symptoms include tiredness, recurrent mouth ulcers, anaemia (deficiency of any one or combination of iron, folic acid, or vitamin B_{12}), osteoporosis, joint or bone pain, dermatitis herpetiformis (DHp), depression, alopecia, infertility, repeated miscarriage, and neurological symptoms such as peripheral neuropathy, ataxia, and cognitive deficits.

Diagnosis

This is a two-stage process:[17] first, a serological test measuring total IgA level and IgA tissue transglutaminase (tTGA). Both antibody tests are highly sensitive and specific to coeliac disease but may fail to diagnose up to 10% of cases. The second step is a duodenal biopsy, which is considered to be the 'gold standard' diagnostic test. It is essential that anyone being tested for CoD continues to eat a normal gluten-containing diet, as avoiding gluten beforehand can cause false negative results. In patients who are antibody-negative, but where there is still clinical suspicion of CoD (e.g. based on symptoms or positive family history), a duodenal biopsy should still be undertaken, ensuring that the patient is not on a self-imposed gluten-free (GF) diet.

Treatment

The only treatment for CoD is the life-long exclusion of gluten from the diet. This is a major task and should always involve expert dietetic counselling; an annual dietetic review for all patients with CoD is also recommended,[17] and should include monitoring of weight, symptoms, diet, and need for nutritional advice.

The GF diet

Foods can be categorized into three groups:
• Foods and ingredients that are naturally GF, including rice, corn (maize), potato, polenta, quinoa, milk, cheese, eggs, fresh fruit and vegetables, fresh meats including poultry, fresh fish, and seafood, pulses, butter, margarine, cooking oils.
• Foods that contain obvious sources of gluten (e.g. made with gluten-containing cereals), such as bread, pasta, wheat-based breakfast cereals, cakes, and biscuits.

17 National Institute for Health and Care Excellence (NICE) (2015). *Coeliac disease: Recognition, assessment and management.* NG20. Available at: ℘ https://www.nice.org.uk/guidance/ng20.

- Foods that may include a gluten-containing cereal as an ingredient, e.g. used as a thickener, filler, or carrier for flavours. These include many manufactured soups, sauces, sausages, and ready meals.

Special GF products

A wide range of specially manufactured GF products is produced as substitutes for foods that usually contain gluten. The range includes staples such as breads, pasta, and flours, and luxury items such as biscuits, cakes, and ready meals. At present, some of the GF staple items are prescribable for people with medically diagnosed CoD, but the type and quantity that can be prescribed varies geographically and the system is currently under review. Luxury GF foods are generally not prescribable. An increasing number of GF products is available for purchase in supermarkets, on the Internet, or in health food shops. A list of prescribable GF foods is available in:

- Monthly Index of Medical Specialties (MIMS);
- British National Formulary (BNF);
- Drug Tariff;
- Coeliac UK's Food and Drink Directory.

Guidelines are available to assist healthcare professionals on adequate amounts to prescribe.[18]

Food labelling

It is essential that people with CoD understand food labels, so they know how to check that a food is suitable. All pre-packaged foods bought in the UK must comply with EU allergen labelling legislation. If an ingredient containing gluten is deliberately used in any pre-packed food (regardless of the amount), it must be stated on the ingredients list. Manufacturers must name the gluten-containing grain such as, 'wheat', 'rye', 'barley', 'oats'. Some will also include the word 'gluten', e.g. 'wheat gluten'.

In July 2016, regulations for GF labelling were revised:[19]

- Foods that contain < 20 ppm of gluten can be labelled 'gluten-free'. This includes naturally gluten-free foods, specialist substitute products, and pure, uncontaminated oats and oat products.
- Products that contain between 21 and 100 ppm gluten can be labelled 'very low gluten'. This will include specialist substitute products (mainly obtained on prescription).

Crossed Grain symbol

Some GF manufactured products are identified using the Crossed Grain symbol, which is used under licence from the charity, Coeliac UK. Some supermarkets have their own symbol which shows that the food is GF.

Contamination

People with CoD should be advised to avoid contamination with gluten. It is important when at home to use a separate toaster (or use toaster bags)

---

18 Coeliac UK (2019). *National prescribing guidelines*. Available at: ℘ https://www.coeliac.org.uk/information-and-support/coeliac-disease/once-diagnosed/prescriptions/national-prescribing-guidelines/.

19 Food Standards Agency (2016). *Labelling of 'gluten-free' foods*. Available at: ℘ https://www.food.gov.uk/business-industry/allergy-guide/labelling-of-gluten-free-foods.

to prepare gluten-free toast, as well as separate bread boards and spread containers to prevent contamination with breadcrumbs. Sometimes even naturally gluten-free grains (such as buckwheat) can be contaminated during milling or processing. Manufacturers may issue voluntary guidance on food labels that state the product 'may contain' a gluten cereal, which means they have identified a risk that the product may be contaminated.

Other sources of gluten
- The Medicines and Healthcare products Regulatory Agency (MHRA) advise that listed prescribed medications in MIMS and BNF are gluten-free; people with CoD should discuss with their doctor any unexpected side effects.
- Wine, cider, liqueurs, and spirits (including malt whisky) are gluten-free, but beer, lager, stout, and ales may not be so should be avoided. Specially manufactured gluten-free ales and beers are available.
- Most traditional communion wafers are made from wheat flour. Specially manufactured very low gluten wafers are available
- Coeliac UK produces a regularly updated list,[20] giving details of GF status of many manufactured products.

Oats
There is limited good quality evidence that adults with CoD can tolerate the gluten-like protein found in oats (avenins). However, most oats and oat products are often contaminated with other sources of gluten during milling, which makes them unsuitable for someone with CoD. Anyone with CoD wanting to eat oats must make sure that they are pure and uncontaminated,[20] as well as receiving follow-up from their healthcare team.

Adherence to GF diet
Everyone with CoD is advised to follow a strict life-long GF diet. Evidence suggests that adherence varies between 45% and 94%, and that non-adherence is associated with greater health risk of ↓ bone mineral density (osteopenia), osteoporosis, and a modestly ↑ risk of malignancy. The reasons for non-adherence are numerous and varied including:
- Restrictions to everyday lifestyle.
- Difficulties maintaining a strict diet when eating out, at school, while travelling, or when on holiday.
- Longer food preparation and cooking.
- Some patients can feel well and lack symptoms so perceive little benefit from following a GF diet.

Other dietary factors to consider
Calcium
Adults with CoD are recommended to ↑ calcium intake to optimize their bone health. The requirement for younger adults with CoD is 1000 mg/day and for men aged ≥55 years and post-menopausal women is 1200 mg/day. In some cases, supplements may be required, which should be determined on individual basis. There is no increased calcium requirement for children.

20 Coeliac UK (2019). *Food and drink information*. Available at: ℅ https://www.coeliac.org.uk/information-and-support/your-gluten-free-hub/food-and-drink-information/.

Healthy eating

At diagnosis of CoD, most adults have a normal BMI or are overweight. In addition, weight gain after starting a GF diet is common. Once established on a GF diet, people with CoD should be advised to combine this with healthy eating (see ➲ Chapter 2, 'Eatwell Guide') and healthy weight recommendations for the general population (see 'Adult BMI ready reckoner' inside front cover).

Gluten sensitivity

CoD has been described as part of a wider spectrum of gluten sensitivity,[21] which includes both GI and extra-intestinal including neurological symptoms. It is now clear that some people who do not have CoD benefit from excluding dietary gluten. Terms defining this spectrum have been published.[22]

Other reasons for avoiding gluten

Recent public interest in healthy and asymptomatic people following a GF diet has arisen in response to perceived health and performance advantages. There is limited robust evidence for avoiding gluten in the absence of CoD or other gluten sensitivity. Excluding dietary gluten limits foods like wholegrain that contribute positively to a well-balanced healthy diet and there is concern that this may have long-term health consequences.[23] As a result, the promotion of GF diets to asymptomatic people without CoD is not recommended.

Further information

Coeliac UK. Available at: ℅ www.coeliac.org.uk Helpline 0333 332 2033.

Ludvigsson, J.F. et al (2014), Diagnosis and management of adult coeliac disease: guidelines from the British Society of Gastroenterology. *Gut* **63**, 1210–28. Available at: ℅ http://www.bsg.org.uk/images/stories/docs/clinical/guidelines/sbn/bsg_coeliac_14.pdf.

National Institute for Health and Care Excellence (NICE) (2015). Coeliac disease: Recognition, assessment and management. NG20. Available at: ℅ https://www.nice.org.uk/guidance/ng20.

21 Aziz, I., et al. (2012). Does gluten sensitivity in the absence of coeliac disease exist? *BMJ* 345, e7907.

22 Ludvigsson, J.G., et al. (2013). The Oslo definition for coeliac disease and related terms *Gut* **62**, 43-52.

23 Lebwohl, B., et al. (2017). Long term gluten consumption in adults without celiac disease and risk of coronary heart disease: a prospective cohort study. *BMJ* **357**, j1892.

Intestinal failure and short bowel

Patients with intestinal failure (IF) require specialized nutritional support which is integral to their medical management. European guidelines[24] classify IF into five pathophysiological conditions:

- short bowel;
- intestinal fistula;
- intestinal dysmotility;
- mechanical obstruction;
- extensive small bowel mucosal disease.

Nutritional implications

- IF depends on the degree and site of intestinal disease or resection and whether there is continuity with the rest of the gut or a high output stoma or fistula.
- Parenteral support will usually be required in individuals with short bowel with:
  - <100 cm of jejunum (fluid ± electrolytes only);
  - <75 cm of jejunum (parenteral nutrition);
  - <50 cm of jejunum + colon intact (parenteral nutrition).
- The remnant gut may be able to adapt and increase absorptive capacity (depending on underlying condition) over a period of up to 2 years and allow the withdrawal of parenteral support. Dietary modification and hormonal stimulation can help to optimize this.
- Most patients are treated at specialist centres where relevant expertise is available. Each patient must be individually assessed and advised by a registered dietitian with experience in managing IF. Patients are frequently malnourished because of their underlying condition and interruptions in nutrition support.

The long-term dietary management is shown in Table 26.4. Requirements are higher because of the malabsorption that occurs from reduced absorptive capacity and rapid transit. Regular monitoring of nutritional status is an essential component of ongoing medical care which will facilitate optimum oral intake and thus ↓ dependency on parenteral nutrition.[25]

Diet in short bowel—jejunostomy

Hypotonic drinks should be avoided because fluids providing <90 mmol Na+/L will result in sodium secretion into the lumen leading to ↑ fluid loss. A high salt intake is recommended because of high sodium losses from the jejunum and patients will benefit from an oral rehydration solution containing a minimum of 90 mmol Na+/L.

Diet in short bowel—jejunocolic anastomosis

A high carbohydrate (60% energy), low fat (20% energy) diet is associated with reduced faecal weight and ↑ water absorption. Increasing CHO intake

24 Pironi, L., et al. (2016). ESPEN guidelines on chronic intestinal failure in adults. *Clin. Nutr.* **35**, 247–307.

25 Culkin, A., et al. (2009). Improving clinical outcome in patients with intestinal failure using individualised nutritional advice. *J. Hum. Nutr. Diet.* **22**, 290–8.

Table 26.4 Long-term nutritional management of short bowel

Nutrients	Jejunostomy	Jejunocolic anastomosis
Energy	High	High
Protein	High	High
Fat	High	Low to moderate and MCT
Carbohydrate	Low to moderate	High
Salt	Added required	Normal
Fluid	Restricted, ORS required	No restriction usually required
Oxalate	No restriction	Low

MCT, medium chain triglyceride; ORS, oral rehydration solution.

is important as colonic bacteria will convert it to short chain fatty acids, which will be readily absorbed in the colon therefore contributing significantly to energy balance. Reducing fat intake is essential to help decrease steatorrhoea and thus maximize absorption of other nutrients, although restrictions should be minimized to those needed to control symptoms because fat is a good source of energy. Medium chain triglycerides may be used to provide additional energy (see Box 26.6). Fat soluble vitamins should be supplemented or status monitored. Oxalate intake should be minimized because of ↑ risk of calcium oxalate renal stones (ideally avoid rhubarb, spinach, beetroot, peanuts, and excessive tea).

Further reading

Culkin, A. (2014). Intestinal failure and nutrition. In: *Advanced nutrition and dietetics in gastroenterology.* Ed: M Lomer, p. 210. Wiley Blackwell, Oxford.

Fistulae

Gastrointestinal fistulae are abnormal holes in the gut allowing the contents (partially digested food, secretions, water, and electrolytes) to escape either into another part of the thoracic or abdominal cavities or to the outside. Most (~80%) arise as a complication of surgery, while some occur spontaneously in inflammatory bowel disease, diverticular disease, and radiation enteritis, or as a result of trauma. The mortality, morbidity, and nutritional consequences are significant. Established high output enterocutaneous fistulae should be managed in the same way as other high output stomas. (See ➔ this chapter, 'Gastrointestinal stoma').

Nutritional implications

- Patients with fistulae are often undernourished because of their underlying disease and the consequences of nutrient loss via the fistula. Impaired nutritional status will adversely affect closure, whether surgical or spontaneous.
- Previous practice was to advise patients to consume nil by mouth and start parenteral nutrition in an attempt to heal the fistula despite limited evidence of efficacy. There is no evidence that parenteral nutrition is superior to feeding via the enteral route, and it is reasonable to allow patients oral intake with an established fistula. Current practice in specialist units is to allow all patients to eat, if they are able to, regardless of the fistula output unless there is intra-abdominal sepsis which is exacerbated by using the enteral route. In these patients, parenteral nutrition may be required (see ➔ Chapter 25, 'Parenteral nutrition'). This should take account of the individual's losses via the fistula and, depending on the site, additional fluid and electrolytes may be required to replace losses.
- Fistuloclysis, enteral feeding via the fistula, may be possible and desirable in some patients. If achieved, this avoids the complications associated with parenteral nutrition.[26] Nutrition support can be provided by accessing the GI tract distally to the fistula if high, e.g. oesophageal, gastric, jejunal. A minimum length of 75 cm of small bowel distal to the fistula is required to achieve independence from parenteral nutrition. The reinfusion of chyme from the proximal GI limb is recommended if acceptable to the patient. Evaluation of fistula losses is required to facilitate adequate replacement of nutrients, fluid, and electrolytes and, in some patients, enteral feeding proximal to a fistula may increase output. Enteral feeding should not be automatically discounted in fistula patients because of its advantages associated with lower rates of infection and maintaining GI integrity.

26 Teubner, A., et al. (2004). Fistuloclysis can successfully replace parenteral feeding in the nutritional support of patients with enterocutaneous fistula. *Br. J. Surg.* **91**, 625–31.

Gastrointestinal stoma

Stoma differ from GI fistulae in that access to the GI tract is deliberate and aims to facilitate either:

- *Input* = nutrient intake into the stomach (feeding gastrostomy) or jejunum (feeding jejunostomy), (see ➜ Chapter 25, 'Routes for enteral feeding').
- *Output* = effluent from the jejunum (jejunostomy), ileum (ileostomy), or colon (colostomy).

Jejunostomy

See ➜ this chapter, 'Intestinal failure and short bowel syndrome'.

Ileostomy

Usually formed after resection in inflammatory bowel disease. Although most patients eat a normal diet, depending on the length of remaining ileum, attention must be given to the fluid and electrolytes lost from the ileostomy effluent. Losses >1500 mL/day will require additional fluid and salt. If severe, IV support may be required. Dehydration from a high output stoma is a common cause of readmission, and patients will benefit from an oral rehydration solution. Vitamin B_{12} is absorbed at the distal end of the ileum so patients with ileocaecal resection will require supplementation, e.g. intramuscular injection 1 mg hydroxocobalamin every 3 months.

Some patients prefer to avoid specific foods if they experience unacceptable symptoms (see Box 26.7). The identification of recognizable food remains, e.g. pips, skins, grain husks, in the effluent may concern some patients. Providing this is not associated with a high output or other symptoms, reassurance should be given and patients advised to chew their food well.

Colostomy

Like ileostomy, a colostomy is often formed after resection in inflammatory bowel disease, bowel cancer or diverticular disease. As effluent leaves the GI tract distally to the ileum, there is less concern with fluid and electrolyte losses. Patients should, therefore, eat as normally as possible but avoid specific foods that cause unacceptable symptoms (see Box 26.7). Patients with a colostomy may experience constipation and should be encouraged to increase their intake of fluid, fruit and vegetables, and wholegrain cereals (see ➜ this chapter, 'Constipation'). Diarrhoea should be investigated if prolonged and exceeding 1,000 g/day.

Box 26.7 Reported effects of foods in some people with a gastrointestinal stoma

- ↑ *Output:* high fibre foods, fruits and vegetables, spicy foods, alcohol, fruit juice, beans;
- *Flatus-producing:* onions, peas, beans, carbonated drinks, spicy foods, beer, milk, cabbage, garlic;
- *Offensive odour:* fish, onions, leeks, garlic, eggs.

Further reading

Culkin, A. (2014). Stomas and nutrition. In: *Advanced nutrition and dietetics in gastroenterology.* Ed: M Lomer, p. 218. Wiley Blackwell, Oxford.

Intestinal transplantation

Transplantation (Tx) of the intestine (small bowel) may be undertaken singly or in conjunction with other abdominal organs, including the liver and pancreas. Approximately 170 intestinal transplants were undertaken in the UK between 2006 and 2016; just over half of these were in children; in the USA, ~150 are undertaken annually.

Indications include irreversible intestinal failure with impaired venous access, intestinal failure-associated liver disease, life-threatening episodes of catheter-related sepsis and/or inadequate maintenance on parenteral nutrition.

Long-term follow-up studies (up to 10 years) show that surviving patients can be sustained independently of parenteral nutrition and that growth velocity in children can be maintained, although catch-up growth is rare. Successful post Tx pregnancy has been reported.

Nutritional management

Goals include:
- reducing the risk of graft rejection;
- improving gut trophicity, i.e. maximizing function, which may be acquiescent;
- optimizing nutritional status.

Feeding route

There are no studies to indicate optimum post-transplant nutritional management, but parenteral nutrition, which is usually essential *before* surgery, is required in the early post-operative period. Parenteral nutrition is usually gradually ↓ and stopped within 2 weeks in adults and usually between 30 and 85 days in children depending on individual needs. Enteral nutrition is theoretically well-placed to improve gut trophicity, optimize absorptive function and prevent bacterial translocation. Although tolerance of enteral feeds may be limited after surgery by ischaemia-reperfusion injury, denervation, and absence of lymphatic drainage of the graft, feeding into the gut should commence as soon as possible and ideally within 5–7 days.[27]

Access

Some centres feed into the stomach and others into the jejunum via either a jejunostomy or gastro-jejunostomy because of delayed gastric emptying.

Feed

Practice varies between centres, with elemental feeds commonly used and some evidence that peptide-based formulae are tolerated. Diluted feeds are used in some centres, whereas others use full strength from initiation. Clearly, studies are needed to identify best practice. Energy requirements are elevated[28] because of hypermetabolism associated with surgery and less than complete absorption[29] of enteral nutrition

27 Columb, V. et al. (2009). Nutrition support after intestinal transplantation: how important is enteral feeding? *Curr. Opin. Clin. Nutr. Metab. Care* **12**, 186–9.

28 Matthé, S., et al. (2016). Energy expenditure and growth failure after intestinal transplantation. *Pediatr. Transplant.* **20**, 162-7.

29 Ordonez, F. et al. (2013). Intestinal absorption rate in children after small intestinal transplantation. *Am. J. Clin. Nutr.* **97**, 743-9.

Short-term dietary restrictions

Limiting fat intake (if malabsorption or chylous ascites are present) and avoiding dairy products (because of possible lactose intolerance) may be appropriate in the post-operative period but can often be relaxed if these are tolerated.

Long-term

Most adult patients lose weight in the first year after Tx, some as much as 25% in spite of nutrition support. However, most are able to transfer to an oral intake and maintain an adequate nutritional status after transplantation, although ~10% will require continued nutritional support.[30] Absorption of lipids and fat-soluble vitamins may remain below normal in some patients and is probably associated with an inadequate post-surgical lymphatic circulation. Monitoring of fat-soluble vitamin status is, therefore, required. Long-term morbidities[30] include dysmotility (59%), hypertension (37%), osteoporosis (22%), and diabetes (11%), indicating that dietary advice should progress with post-Tx recovery and move towards a healthy, well-balanced diet for optimum long-term health (see ➔ Chapter 2, 'Eatwell Guide').

30 Abu-Elmagd, K.M., et al. (2012). Long-term survival, nutritional autonomy and quality of life after intestinal and multivisceral transplantation. *Ann. Surg.* **256**, 494-508.

Irritable bowel syndrome

Irritable bowel syndrome (IBS) is a common, chronic GI disorder of gut-brain interaction with no identified structural pathology and a symptom-based diagnosis (Box 26.8). It affects all races and ages, although prevalence decreases with increasing age and onset of new symptoms after the age of 50 years is uncommon. Estimated prevalence in the UK general population is 6–21%. More women than men are affected (odds ratio of 1.67), and health-related quality of life is worse than in diabetes and end-stage renal disease. Symptoms may overlap with other GI disorders, e.g. dyspepsia, coeliac disease, IBD, and include:

A—abdominal pain or discomfort;

B—bloating or abdominal distension;

C—change in bowel habit (constipation/diarrhoea).

Aetiology

Understanding of the multiple pathophysiological processes that determine IBS symptoms is evolving, and these include motility disturbance, visceral hypersensitivity, altered mucosal and immune function, altered GI microbiota, and altered CNS processing. Stress is reported as a triggering factor in ~50% of sufferers. The majority of IBS sufferers associate eating a meal with their symptoms. Although food intolerance is not implicated in the pathogenesis, dietary metabolites contribute to symptoms, and hypersensitivity to visceral and colonic distension may underpin sensitivity to carbohydrate fermentation.

Box 26.8 Diagnosis of IBS[31]

A positive diagnosis of IBS should be considered if a person has abdominal pain or discomfort for at least 6 months that is:

- either relieved by defaecation or associated with altered bowel frequency or stool form *and*
- has at least two of the following symptoms:
  - altered stool passage (straining, urgency, incomplete evacuation;
  - abdominal bloating;
  - symptoms made worse by eating;
  - passage of mucus.

Supporting diagnosis: lethargy, nausea, backache, bladder symptoms.

Dietary and lifestyle advice

People with IBS should be offered information explaining about the importance of self-help in managing their condition and including advice about diet and general lifestyle, physical activity, relaxation, and symptom-targeted medication.

- Encourage regular meals and take time to eat.
- Avoid missing meals or leaving long gaps between eating.

---

31 National Institute for Health and Care Excellence (NICE) (2017). *Irritable bowel syndrome in adults: diagnosis and management.* CG61. Available at: ℜ http://www.nice.org.uk/guidance/CG61.

- Drink at least eight cups/day, especially water or other non-caffeinated drinks.
- Restrict tea and coffee to three or fewer cups/day.
- Reduce intake of alcohol and fizzy drinks.
- Consider limiting intake of wholemeal or high-fibre wheat flour and breads, cereals high in wheat bran.
- Discourage use of added bran.
- Limit fresh fruit to three portions daily (a portion ≈ 80 g).
- Avoid sorbitol, an artificial sweetener found in sugar-free sweets, chewing gum, and drinks.
- Oats and linseeds (up to one tablespoon/day) may help.
- If probiotics are tried, it is advisable to take for at least 4 weeks at the dose recommended by the manufacturer while monitoring the effect.
- Discourage use of aloe vera.
- There is insufficient evidence to support use of herbal remedies in IBS.

If, after following the above advice, food intake is still considered to be adversely associated with IBS symptoms, a referral to a registered dietitian for further advice should be offered. This may include single food avoidance or an exclusion diet (e.g. a low FODMAP [fermentable oligosaccharides, disaccharides, monosaccharides, and polyols] diet),[32] using evidence-based practice guidelines.[33]

Low FODMAP diet

This complex second-line dietary intervention involves reducing intake of short chain fructans, galactans, polyols, fructose, and lactose for 3-6 weeks,[32,33] with education delivered by a dietitian with expertise in FODMAP education to ensure successful adherence and symptom management and a nutritionally adequate diet.[33] Mechanisms explaining symptom generation involve delivery of water to the small intestine by their osmotic activity and colonic gas production causing luminal colonic distension.[34,35] If effective, it should be followed by systematic reintroduction of individual FODMAPs to tolerance, supporting long-term IBS symptom self-management and dietary variety. If ineffective, the intervention should be terminated, a normal, healthy diet advised and other therapeutic options considered.

32 National Institute for Health and Care Excellence (NICE) (2015). *Irritable bowel syndrome in adults: Diagnosis and management of irritable bowel syndrome in primary care.* CG61 addendum. Available at: ℅ https://www.nice.org.uk/guidance/cg61

33 McKenzie, Y.A., *et al.* (2016). British Dietetic Association systematic review and evidence-based practice guidelines for the dietary management of irritable bowel syndrome in adults (2016 update). *J. Hum. Nutr. Diet* **29**, 549-75.

34 Staudacher, H.M., *et al.* (2014). Mechanisms and efficacy of dietary FODMAP restriction in IBS. *Nat. Rev. Gastroenterol. Hepatol.* **11**, 256-66.

35 Murray, K., *et al.* (2014). Differential effects of FODMAPs (fermentable oligo-, di-, mono-saccharides and polyols) on small and large intestinal contents in healthy subjects shown by MRI. *Am. J. Gastroenterol.* **109**, 110-19.

Further information

McKenzie, Y.A., *et al.* (2016). British Dietetic Association systematic review and evidence-based practice guidelines for the dietary management of irritable bowel syndrome in adults (2016 update).
J. Hum. Nutr. Diet. **29**, 549–75.

National Institute for Health and Care Excellence (NICE) (2016). *Irritable bowel syndrome in adults.*
QS114. Available at: ℅ https://www.nice.org.uk/guidance/qs114.

National Institute for Health and Care Excellence (NICE) (2017). *Irritable bowel syndrome in
adults: diagnosis and management.* CG61. Available at: ℅ https://www.nice.org.uk/guidance/
CG61.

Resources

BDA Key fact sheet: describes the role of the dietitian in the treatment of IBS (2015). Available at: ℅
https://www.bda.uk.com/improvinghealth/healthprofessionals/keyfacts/ibstrustadietitian.

First-line information on IBS and diet, endorsed by NICE (2016). Available at: ℅ https://www.nice.org.
uk/guidance/cg61/resources/endorsed-resource-british-dietetic-association-bda-2546534989.

IBS Network. Available at: ℅ www.ibsnetwork.org.

Disorders of the colon

Constipation

Constipation is a significant health problem in the UK and most high income countries and is associated with a high number of medical consultations and expenditure on laxatives, especially in older people. Worldwide prevalence in children varies between 1% and 80%.

Intractable and severe constipation requires investigation and treatment of any specific underlying pathology. However, in many cases, a regular and more frequent bowel habit can be achieved by simple dietary measures, although dietary interventions alone should not be used as first-line treatment in idiopathic constipation in children.[36]

Nutritional management is compatible with ➜ Chapter 2, 'Eatwell Guide', and is based on increasing dietary fibre (see ➜ Chapter 5 'Carbohydrate') and taking an adequate fluid intake. For adults, this could include:

- Change to wholegrain bread and gradually increase daily intake to 200 g (six to seven average slices).
- Eat a large bowlful (50 g) of wholegrain cereal daily.
- Increase fruit and vegetable intake to 400 g/day. This is equivalent to five portions per day.
- Try wholegrain rice and pasta as alternative to white varieties.
- Include nuts, beans, and pulses.

Other measures include the following:

- To be effective in increasing faecal bulk and promoting bowel activity, cereal fibre must be able to absorb fluid. To do this, there must be sufficient fluid in the colon. In adults, fluid intake should be a minimum of 35 mL/kg/day (i.e. ~2.5 L for a 70-kg man) and should lead to passing of pale, straw-coloured urine. For children, see Table 13.1, p. 259.
- People with a very low fibre diet should be advised to increase their intake of fibre gradually to help the GI tract adapt and to avoid possible side effects of abdominal distension and ↑ flatus. If these symptoms occur, they are often self-limiting and resolve spontaneously. If they do not, selecting different fibre-containing foods may help identify those that cause less difficulty, but are still effective at promoting bowel evacuation.
- A high intake of cereal bran is not recommended as a first-line treatment in constipation because of the potential for sequestering micronutrients and thus ↓ their absorption. Its effects are variable, rapid in some people but less effective in others. In addition, bran has been associated with bloating and flatulence and, in elderly people with a low fluid intake, bowel impaction. If bran is used, it should be introduced slowly into the diet and limited quantities (<10 g/day) taken in conjunction with plenty of fluid and a well-balanced diet.

---

36 National Institute for Health and Care Excellence (NICE) (2017). *Constipation in children and young people: diagnosis and management.* CG 99. Available at: ℛhttps://www.nice.org.uk/guidance/cg99.

- Prunes and prune juice are often used to treat constipation and are probably effective because of their sorbitol and phenolic compounds.[37]

Diverticular disease (diverticulosis)

Diverticula are blind pouches found in the intestinal wall, particularly in older people. Traditionally, this has been attributed to ↑ intraluminal pressure as a result of constipation and a low fibre diet, but age, diet, inflammation, and genetics may all contribute to diverticular formation.[38] In themselves, diverticula are not considered pathological, but may become inflamed and infected resulting in diverticulitis. This is manifest as colicky pain with diarrhoea and/or constipation; bleeding, abscesses, and perforation may complicate. An acute episode requires treatment with antibiotics and surgery in severe cases. On recovery, a healthy diet including fibre and an adequate fluid intake is advisable (see ➡ Chapter 2, 'Eatwell Guide', and this chapter, 'Constipation'). There is no evidence that nuts cause or exacerbate diverticulitis.[39] Systematic review of the role of probiotics in the management of diverticular disease is inconclusive.

Haemorrhoids

Haemorrhoids (or piles) are swollen and inflamed blood vessels in the rectum and anus. They arise after prolonged constipation when pressure in the distended colon is combined with straining to evacuate the bowel, and are most common in older adults and during/after pregnancy. Patients presenting with internal (non-prolapsing) haemorrhoids should be advised to increase their fibre and fluid intake. Others should be referred to a colorectal surgeon and may benefit from advice to ↑ fibre and fluid intake after treatment.

Increasing fibre intake is useful for softening faeces, relieving constipation, and thus reducing straining. Fibre supplementation reduces episodes of bleeding and discomfort in patients with internal haemorrhoids, although this may take up to 6 weeks; it does not improve external (prolapsed) haemorrhoids. Cereal fibre is most effective in increasing stool weight (see ➡ this Chapter, 'Constipation') and bulk-forming laxative, ispaghula husk, may help.

Cancer of the colon and rectum (bowel)

The incidence of bowel cancer in the UK is approximately 42,000 new cases annually, making this one of the four most common cancers. Worldwide, it is estimated that 1.8 million new cases were diagnosed in 2018. It is more common in men, especially if deprived, and in people aged ≥85 years. Nutritional factors contribute to risk (Table 26.5).

37 Lever, E., *et al.* (2013). Systematic review: the effect of prunes on gastrointestinal function. *Aliment. Pharmacol. Ther.* **40**, 750-8.

38 Commane, D.M., *et al.* (2009). Diet, ageing and genetic factors in the pathogenesis of diverticular disease. *World J. Gastroenterol.* **15**, 2479–88.

39 Peery, A.F., *et al.* (2013). Diverticular disease: reconsidering conventional wisdom. *Clin. Gastroenterol. Hepatol.* **11**, 1532-7.

Table 26.5 Nutritional factors associated with convincing or probable risk of colorectal cancer[40]

Factors associated with ↑ risk	Factors associated with ↓ risk
Red and processed meat	Dietary fibre
Obesity	Physical activity
Abdominal fatness	
Alcohol	

Treatment

Usually includes surgery (colectomy with or without formation of a temporary or permanent colostomy; see ➜ this chapter 'Gastrointestinal stoma'), and sometimes chemotherapy and/or radiotherapy (see ➜ Chapter 24, 'Cancer treatment').

Nutritional management

Enhanced recovery protocols for colorectal cancer surgery are associated with improved clinical outcome[41] (see ➜ Chapter 25, 'Pre-operative fasting and enhanced recovery after surgery'). Robust evidence that dietary or lifestyle interventions can influence remission or survival is lacking but as colorectal cancer is prevalent and survival is improving, many people are living with this condition and might benefit from appropriate advice. It is reasonable to encourage regular exercise and limiting of refined carbohydrate, sugar-sweetened beverages, and red and processed meat in those who make a good recovery after surgery. Maintaining an adequate and well-balanced intake can help to optimize the patient's nutritional status and ability to withstand future treatment. Patients may seek dietary advice relating to a colostomy (see ➜ this chapter, 'Gastrointestinal stoma') or may benefit from guidance if the tumour or treatment is compromising nutritional intake. Depending on the stage of the tumour at diagnosis, long-term dietary advice compatible with the Eatwell Guide (see ➜ Chapter 2) may be appropriate, whereas for others, nutrition support to counter weight loss (see ➜ Chapter 25, 'Treatment of undernutrition') or a more palliative approach to eating (see ➜ Chapter 35) should be considered.

---

40 Cancer Research UK (2019). Bowel cancer risk. Available at: ⌖ https://www.cancerresearchuk. org/health-professional/cancer-statistics/statistics-by-cancer-type/bowel-cancer/risk-factors.

41 Pędziwiatr, M., *et al.* (2016). Is ERAS in laparoscopic surgery for colorectal cancer changing risk factors for delayed recovery? *Med. Oncol.* **33**, 25.

Gallbladder disorders

Gallstones

Gallstones are relatively common in populations consuming a 'Western-type' diet and it is estimated that ~10% of adults in the UK have gallstones, two-thirds of whom are asymptomatic. The prevalence increases with age and is more common in women. Most gallstones in the UK (~80%) are composed of predominantly cholesterol, whereas others have a higher proportion of bilirubin, calcium, and pigments. Cholesterol precipitates into stones when bile becomes (1) supersaturated and (2) gallbladder emptying is reduced. See Box 26.9 for the risk factors for cholesterol gallstones.

Preventing gallstones

No dietary intervention studies have been undertaken to prevent gallstones but based on epidemiological evidence, it is reasonable to advise:

- Meals compatible with the 'Eatwell Guide' (see ➔ Chapter 2).
- Reducing excess body weight using modest energy restriction <1.5 kg/week (very low calorie diets may exacerbate bile cholesterol saturation).
- Eating regularly to minimize bile stasis, which accompanies fasting.
- Eating breakfast on rising (cholesterol concentrations are highest in bile produced overnight).
- Taking regular exercise.

Box 26.9 Risk factors for cholesterol gallstones

- Age >40 years
- Female
- Genetic variation
- ↑ Dietary fat
- ↑ Dietary refined carbohydrate
- ↓ Dietary fibre
- Obesity
- Yo-yo dieting (repeated cycles of losing and re-gaining weight)
- Hyperlipidaemia
- Pregnancy
- Diabetes mellitus and insulin resistance
- Liver disease
- Cystic fibrosis
- Gallbladder dysmotility
- Bile salt loss (ileal disease ± resection)
- Nil enterally (fasting or parenteral nutrition)
- ↓ Physical activity.

Cholecystitis

Approximately 1–4% of people with gallstones develop symptoms each year including pain (epigastric, upper or lower abdominal), nausea and vomiting; generally, these symptoms are non-specific. Acute cholecystitis features prolonged severe pain (right subcostal) and fever. Management is usually surgical and most often via laparoscopic cholecystectomy. Approximately 9% of people experience bile acid malabsorption after cholecystectomy (see ➲ this chapter, page 642).

Dietary management of cholecystitis

Historically, a low fat diet was advocated on the basis that restricting fat intake reduced gallbladder contractions and reduced pain but there is a lack of evidence to underpin this.[42] The gallbladder is known to contract in response to the oral intake of most nutrients and also in anticipation of intake and, therefore, limiting dietary fat may not improve symptoms. If a stone obstructs the hepatic or common bile duct, preventing bile from reaching the GI tract, it may lead to jaundice, nausea, and steatorrhoea (see ➲ this Chapter, 'Steatorrhoea'). This is relatively uncommon and requires medical intervention. If a patient is well enough to eat, s/he should be advised to only avoid specific foods associated with triggering their symptoms.[42]

Gallbladder cancer

Approximately 1,000 people in the UK are diagnosed annually, i.e. <1% of total new cancer cases. It is more common in women and in those aged >75 years. Worldwide, approximately 219,000 people were diagnosed with cancer of the gallbladder or extrahepatic ducts in 2018. Increasing BMI and high intake of sugar-sweetened beverages are risk factors.[43,44] There is no evidence to support specific dietary advice in gallbladder cancer but nutrition support may be required for those undergoing surgery or other treatment (see ➲ Chapter 25, 'Treatment of undernutrition' and ➲ Chapter 24, 'Cancer treatment').

Cholecystosteatosis

Similar to, but very much less common than non-alcoholic steatohepatitis (NASH), which affects the liver (see ➲ Chapter 28, 'Liver disease'), cholecystosteatosis is fatty infiltration of the gallbladder accompanied by chronic infiltration and antioxidant tissue damage. This results in ↓ contractility and thus bile stasis, which ↑ risk of gallstone formation. Although associated with dietary carbohydrate, the pathogenesis, prognosis, and role of nutrition in management is unknown.

42 National Institute for Health and Care Excellence (NICE) (2014). Gallstone disease: diagnosis and management. CG188. Available at: ℜ https://www.nice.org.uk/guidance/cg188.

43 Borena, W., et al. (2014). A prospective study on metabolic risk factors and gallbladder cancer in the metabolic syndrome and cancer (Me-Can) collaborative study. PLoS One **9**, e89368.

44 Larsson, S.C., et al. (2016). Sweetened beverage consumption and risk of biliary tract and gallbladder cancer in a prospective study. J. Natl. Cancer Inst. **108**, djw125.

Pancreatic disease

Pancreatic function *680*
Chronic pancreatitis *682*
Acute pancreatitis *684*
Pancreatic cancer *685*
Pancreatic enzyme replacement therapy *686*

Pancreatic function

The pancreas has both exocrine and endocrine functions (Table 27.1).

Table 27.1 Synthetic functions of the pancreas and consequences of impairment

Exocrine functions	Endocrine functions
Pancreatic lipase	Insulin
Pancreatic proteases	Glucagon
Pancreatic amylase	Somatostatin

Inability to digest macronutrients leading to malabsorption and undernutrition. Maldigestion of fat results in fat-soluble vitamin malabsorption.	Type 3c diabetes is more likely to occur in disease to the tail of the pancreas. Lack of glucagon can result in significant hypoglycaemia

Chronic pancreatitis

Annual incidence in the UK is 40–70 per 100,000, with men approximately four times more likely to be affected than women.

Aetiology includes excessive alcohol intake (60–80% of cases in populations with 'Western lifestyle'), idiopathic (20% of cases). Other causes include biliary tract disease, duct obstruction, smoking, and trauma. Chronic pancreatitis (CP) can develop following repeated episodes of acute pancreatitis.

Symptoms/complications include severe abdominal pain, malabsorption, diabetes, and malnutrition. Malnutrition is frequently reported and arises because of poor intake 2° to pain, malabsorption, hypermetabolism, hyperglycaemia, and failure to provide nutrition support.

Nutritional management of chronic pancreatitis, (Box 27.1)
- *Poor intake 2° to pain:*
  - Surgical procedures to relieve obstruction of the pancreatic duct.
  - Pancreatic enzyme replacement therapy (PERT) may help, but more evidence needed.[1]
  - Mixed antioxidant supplements may help but data are not conclusive.[2]
  - Distal jejunal feeding and restriction of oral intake can improve symptoms prior to definitive treatment.
  - Give analgesia before meals.
  - Liquid meals may be better tolerated than solid food.
- *Malabsorption:*
  - Fat, protein, and carbohydrate malabsorption occur. This causes ↓ transit time and ↑ faecal loss of energy, protein, vitamins A, D, E, K, thiamine, folic acid, Ca, Mg, and Zn.
  - Prescribe PERT and advise about dosage in relation to food.
  - Dietary fat intake ~30–40% of energy is usually well tolerated.
- *Hypermetabolism:*
  - Limited data suggest that 30–50% of CP patients have raised resting energy expenditure (~110% of predicted values) even when expressed per kg fat free mass, i.e. taking account of malnutrition.
  - In the absence of individual measurements, base energy requirements on predicted value +10%.
- *Hyperglycaemia:*
  - Type 3c diabetes is common and more likely to occur as the disease progresses. This type of diabetes is often described as brittle, with rapid changes in blood glucose levels.[3]
  - Management is similar to type 1 diabetes with low threshold for insulin therapy.

---

1 Yaghoobi, M., *et al.* (2016). Pancreatic enzyme supplements are not effective for relieving abdominal pain in patients with chronic pancreatitis: Meta-analysis and systematic review of randomized controlled trials. *Can. J. Gastroenterol. Hepatol.* **2016**, 8541839.

2 Zhou, D., *et al.* (2015). Antioxidant therapy for patients with chronic pancreatitis: A systematic review and meta-analysis. *Clin. Nutr.* **34**, 627-34.

3 Duggan, S.N., *et al.* (2017). The nutritional management of type 3c (pancreatogenic) diabetes in chronic pancreatitis. *Eur. J. Clin. Nutr.* **71**, 3-8.

Box 27.1 Key points for nutrition support in CP

- Patients with CP do not normally require any dietary restrictions.
- Endocrine and exocrine failure are usually progressive, so patients require long-term follow-up.
- Patients who are well-nourished should be encouraged to follow healthy eating advice, avoiding alcohol and smoking. Weight bearing exercise and safe sunlight exposure should be encouraged to help reduce the risk of osteoporosis.
- Patients with more advanced CP are often underweight and frail ∴ providing adequate nutritional support is paramount but may be confounded by the symptoms and complications described above.
- Input from a dietitian with pancreatic expertise area is required.

Key points for dietary advice

- Patients with a poor appetite may benefit from practical advice about increasing oral intake (see ➜ Chapter 25 'Treatment of undernutrition').
- If malabsorption is present, advice should be given about pancreatic enzyme replacement (see ➜ this chapter, 'Pancreatic enzyme replacement therapy').
- Low fat diets have no role to play in the treatment of pancreatitis as they will exacerbate low energy intake and can mask the onset of steatorrhoea.
- A compromise should be reached between dietary advice to optimize blood sugar if hyperglycaemia develops (see ➜ Chapter 22, 'Goals and principles of dietary management') and to enhance intake to maintain body weight or reverse weight loss.
- Abstaining from alcohol is highly advisable as continuing alcohol intake is associated with ↑ morbidity and mortality. Smoking increases the risk of pancreatic cancer and worsens pain. Consequently, smoking cessation should be encouraged.
- Successful long-term enteral nutrition support provided by elemental feeding via an endoscopically placed naso-jejunal tube associated with relief of pain has been reported.[4]
- Micronutrient status should be assessed.

---

4 Skipworth, J.R., et al. (2011). The use of nasojejunal nutrition in patients with chronic pancreatitis. *JOP* **12**, 574-80.

Acute pancreatitis

Annual incidence internationally is 5-80 in 100,000.

Aetiology includes gallstones (~40% of cases in populations with 'Western lifestyle'), excessive alcohol intake (~35% of cases), idiopathic (15% of cases). Repeated acute episodes can lead to CP.

Symptoms/complications include severe pain, nausea, vomiting, pseudo-cysts, fistulae, shock, and multi-organ failure.

Management should include nutrition support (Box 27.2).

Box 27.2 Key points for nutrition support in acute pancreatitis

- Meta-analysis[5] shows better clinical outcomes are associated with:
  - enteral feeding rather than starvation (one study showing 78% ↓ mortality risk, $p = 0.01$);
  - enteral, rather than parenteral nutrition (10 studies, relative risk of infective complications, 0.41 (95% CI: 0.30, 0.57), $p = 0.00001$; relative risk of mortality, 0.60 (0.32, 1.14), $p = 0.12$).
- Meta-analysis[6] in severe acute pancreatitis (SAP) shows enteral nutrition is associated with more diarrhoea than parenteral (29% vs. 7%), but less hyperglycaemia (11% vs. 29%).
- Enteral feeding should commence early in the disease.[7]
- SAP patients are at high risk of delayed gastric emptying because of extrinsic compression of the duodenum, and early placement of naso-jejunal feeding tubes should occur where there is extensive disease in the head of the pancreas.
- Naso-gastric feeding may be tolerated, but naso-jejunal feeding is safe and also well-tolerated.
- Parenteral nutrition is preferable to no nutrient intake where enteral feeding cannot be undertaken, e.g. ileus >5 days.

---

5 Marik, P.E., et al. (2004). Meta-analysis of parenteral nutrition versus enteral nutrition in patients with acute pancreatitis. *BMJ*. **328**, 1407.

6 Petrov, M.S., et al. (2010). Comparison of complications attributable to enteral and parenteral nutrition in predicted severe acute pancreatitis: a systematic review and meta-analysis. *Brit. J. Nutr.* **103**, 1287-95.

7 Petrov, M.S., et al. (2009). A systematic review on the timing of artificial nutrition in acute pancreatitis. *Brit. J. Nutr.* **101**, 787-93.

Pancreatic cancer

Cancer of the pancreas is the 11th most common malignancy diagnosed in the UK (~10,000 new cases per year). It is equally common in men and women but more likely to occur in people aged >50 years. Body fatness, smoking, and a history of pancreatitis are risk factors. Long-term outcomes remain poor.

Treatment may include surgery, chemotherapy, radiotherapy, or palliative care depending on the stage of the tumour at diagnosis (see ➜ Chapter 24, 'Cancer treatment' and ➜ Chapter 35, 'Palliative Care').

Pancreatic cancer can cause obstruction of the biliary tree (causing jaundice) and/or obstruction of the duodenum. Duodenal stenting and liquid diets may be needed if gastric outflow obstruction occurs.

Nutritional management should include assessment of nutritional status and aim to provide adequate energy and nutrient intake in a format that can be tolerated by the patient. Patients with pancreatic cancer are often undernourished on diagnosis as a result of poor intake and severe pain; depletion may be exacerbated by treatment. Appropriate nutritional support is ∴ essential, but depends on the treatment given and overall prognosis.

- Dietary restrictions are not usually needed.
- Nutritional support, preferably via the enteral route, may improve wellbeing.
- Malnutrition and sarcopenia worsen surgical outcomes in patients undergoing potentially curative surgery.
- After pancreatico-duodenectomy, enteral (not parenteral) nutrition is preferable in the post-operative period.
- Pancreatic enzymes should be used to treat malabsorption, improve nutrition through adequate digestion and absorption, and to help control pain (even if steatorrhoea is absent).
- Supplementation with n-3 fatty acids may be associated with weight gain (including lean tissue) and improved quality of life.
- Bile acid malabsorption and bacterial overgrowth can occur after pancreatico-duodenectomy.

Further information

Gianotti, L., et al. (2009). ESPEN guidelines on parenteral nutrition: Pancreas. Clin. Nutr. 28, 428–35.
Meier, R., et al. (2006). ESPEN guidelines on enteral nutrition: Pancreas. Clin. Nutr. 25, 275–84.

Pancreatic enzyme replacement therapy

Pancreatic enzymes include lipase, amylase, and proteases, which contribute to the digestion of fat, carbohydrate, and protein, respectively. Their insufficiency can result in malabsorption but this can be treated effectively with pancreatic enzyme replacement therapy (PERT) where combined enzymes are provided as capsules, granules, or tablets (Table 27.2). Patients require advice about the use of PERT to optimize the effects of therapy.

- The dose prescribed may need to be adjusted to resolve malabsorption and should be varied depending on what is eaten. Larger meals will require higher doses. Specific advice should be given to individual patients by healthcare professionals with expertise in using PERT.
- Enzymes should be taken with all foods containing fat, protein, or starchy carbohydrate, e.g. meals and snacks. Sugary foods containing no fat and protein do not require PERT.
- Enzyme doses should be spread out throughout the meal/snack. with the first capsule taken at the beginning and further capsules spread out throughout the meal/snack.
- Enzymes are deactivated by heat so should not be mixed with hot food or drinks or stored above 25°C.
- Enzymes are also deactivated by acidity (pH<4). Capsules containing enterically coated microtablets should be swallowed whole or, if opened, swallowed without chewing the contents as this will expose the enzymes to the denaturing effects of gastric acid.
- Proton pump inhibitors/H_2 antagonists may be prescribed to reduce gastric secretions and maximize the effects of PERT.
- Skin or oral mucosa contact with enzymes taken as powder/granules may cause irritation or ulceration and should be avoided.
- High strength preparations are available. Reports have associated these with the rare development of large bowel strictures when taken by children with cystic fibrosis (CF). As a result, daily dose in CF is recommended as not exceeding 10,000 units lipase/kg body weight/day,[8] and adequate hydration should be ensured. New or changing abdominal symptoms should be investigated.

8 Munck, A. (2010). Nutritional considerations in patients with cystic fibrosis. *Expert Rev. Resp. Med.* **41**, 47-56.

Table 27.2 Examples of pancreatic enzyme replacements available in the UK

Brand name (manufacturer)	Enzyme content (BP units/capsule*)		
	Lipase	Protease	Amylase
NutriZym® 22 (Merck Serono)	22,000	1,100	19,800
Pancrease™ HL (Janssen)	25,000	1,250	22,500
Creon® 25,000 (Mylan)	25,000	1,000	18,000
Creon® 40,000 (Mylan)**	40,000	1,600	25,000
Low strength preparations			
Creon® Micro (Mylan)	5,000	200	3,600
Pancrex (Essential)	5,000	300	4,000
Creon® 10,000 (Mylan)	10,000	600	8,000

* Except for Creon® Micro (gastro-resistant granules, enzyme content in BP units/100 mg) and Pancrex (granules, enzyme content in BP units/g).

** Limited availability in the UK

Liver disease

Introduction and nutritional assessment 690
Non-alcoholic fatty liver and non-alcoholic steatohepatitis 692
Hepatitis and cirrhosis 694
Ascites and oedema 696
Hepatic encephalopathy 698
Steatorrhoea and oesophageal varices 699
Liver transplantation 700

Introduction and nutritional assessment

Nutrition-related functions of the liver include:

- protein metabolism (synthesis and regulation of amino acids);
- carbohydrate metabolism (maintain blood glucose, store glycogen);
- lipid metabolism (production of triglycerides and lipoprotein);
- emulsification of dietary fat by bile prior to digestion;
- micronutrients (storage of vitamins A, B_2, B_3, B_6, B_{12}, K, folate).

In liver disease, these functions are often impaired and this, combined with poor nutrient intake, leads to many patients with liver disease becoming undernourished and requiring nutrition support. In turn, this increases risk of poor clinical outcomes including ↑ mortality. In addition, overnutrition leading to obesity is associated with increasing prevalence of non-alcoholic fatty liver disease and non-alcoholic steatohepatitis. Therefore, screening for both undernutrition and over-nutrition and assessing nutritional status are essential parts of management.

Nutritional screening

The Royal Free Hospital Nutrition Prioritization Tool is designed to be used by nurses or other clinical staff to identify patients with cirrhosis who are at high risk of malnutrition. It can be completed within 3 minutes and is validated with 100% sensitivity and 73% specificity.[1]

Nutritional assessment

Assessment of nutritional status is difficult in patients with liver disorders because standard methods are confounded by the disease process, e.g. fluid retention distorts body weight (see this chapter, 'Ascites and oedema'), ↓ liver function precludes use of most biochemical markers, e.g. baseline CRP is raised in cirrhosis and further increases with infection, are limited in severe disease. The Royal Free Hospital Global Assessment, designed to be used by dietitians and nutrition-trained health professionals, overcomes these challenges and provides a reliable evaluation of nutritional status which has prognostic and construct validity[2] (see Box 28.1 and Fig. 28.1).

1 Arora, S., et al. (2012). PMO-040 The development and validation of a nutritional prioritising tool for use in patients with chronic liver disease. Available at: ℅ http://gut.bmj.com/content/gutjnl/61/Suppl_2/A90.1.full.pdf.

2 Morgan, M.Y. et al. (2016). Derivation and validation of a new global method for assessing nutritional status in patients with cirrhosis. *Hepatology* 44, 823-35.

Box 28.1 Assessing global nutritional status in patients with liver disease[2]

- Determine body mass index (derived from estimated dry weight, see Table 28.2) relative to 20 kg/m^2
- Determine mid-arm muscle circumference (MAMC) relative to the 5th percentile of gender- and age-matched reference values (Bishop's 1981 standards; see Appendix 2)
- Estimate adequacy of recent energy intake relative to estimated requirements (see ⊃ Table 28.1 and Chapter 25, 'Estimating requirements in disease states')
- Follow algorithm (Fig. 28.1), using additional factors likely to impair nutritional status (e.g. ascites, malabsorption) if present to subjectively override final category of nutrition

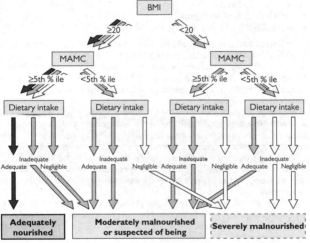

Subjectively override using additional factors likely to impair nutritional status.

Fig. 28.1 Algorithm for assessing nutritional status in patients with liver disease.

Non-alcoholic fatty liver and non-alcoholic steatohepatitis

Although many people with liver disease are undernourished, overnutrition is also associated with ↓ liver function. Fatty liver and steatohepatitis are part of a progressive spectrum of conditions, although progression is not inevitable:

Non-alcoholic fatty liver (NAFLD) → Non-alcoholic steatohepatitis (NASH) → Fibrosis → Cirrhosis → Hepatocellular carcinoma.

Pathogenesis is poorly understood, but relates to ↑ insulin resistance → peripheral lipolysis →↑ free fatty acids → hepatic de novo synthesis of triglycerides → deposits of lipid in hepatocytes. A putative *HFE* gene mutation may mediate effects of obesity as many, but not all, patients with NAFLD are obese and only a proportion of obese people develop NAFLD.

Prevalence depends on diagnostic method and population, but is currently rising with increasing rates of obesity and potentially exceeds prevalence of viral hepatitis:

- *NAFLD*: 7–35% of adult population.
- *NASH*: 2.5–6% of adult population.

Definition and co-morbidities NAFLD occurs when lipid deposits occur in >5% of hepatocytes in the absence of significant alcohol intake (>20 g/d in men; >10 g/d in women), viral or other cause of liver disease. NASH occurs when inflammation occurs 2° to NAFLD. Co-morbidities include diabetes (40-50%), hyperlipidaemia (20-80%), and hypertension (70%), i.e. cardiovascular risk factors.

Prognosis for patients with NASH, survival is ~95%, ~90%, and ~84% at 1, 3, and 10 years, respectively but varies with genetic and environmental factors. Deteriorating health associated with NASH represents a considerable health burden because of ↑ prevalence associated with obesity.[3]

Treatment options include sequentially, depending on the stage of progression:[3] lifestyle modification, addressing components of metabolic syndrome, liver-targeted pharmacotherapy, and management of complications of cirrhosis.

Lifestyle intervention focuses on weight reduction in obesity and overweight and, if successful, can reverse NAFLD progression with reduction in liver fat, inflammation, and fibrosis.[4] Rapid weight loss >1 kg/week should be discouraged. NICE guidelines advise:[5]

- Offer advice on physical activity and diet to people with NAFLD who are overweight/obese, in line with NICE obesity guidelines.

3 Dyson, J.K., *et al.* (2015). Non-alcoholic fatty liver disease: a practical approach to treatment. *Postgrad. Med. J.* **91**, 92–101.

4 Wong, V.W., *et al.* (2013). Community-based lifestyle modification programme for non-alcoholic fatty liver disease: a randomized controlled trial. *J. Hepatol.* **59**, 536-42.

5 National Institute for Health and Care Excellence (NICE) (2016). *Non-alcoholic fatty liver disease (NAFLD): assessment and management.* NICE guideline 49. Available at: ℜ https://www.nice.org.uk/guidance/NG49/chapter/Recommendations#lifestyle-modifications-for-nafld.

- Explain to people with NAFLD that there is some evidence that exercise reduces liver fat content.
- Consider lifestyle interventions in NICE obesity guideline for people with NAFLD regardless of BMI.
- Do not offer omega-3 fatty acids to adults with NAFLD because there is not enough evidence to recommend use.
- Explain to people with NAFLD who drink alcohol the importance of staying within the national recommended limits for alcohol consumption.

Most trials in NAFLD and NASH have focused on pharmacological rather than lifestyle interventions and robust evidence about specific dietary advice is limited,[6] although a Mediterranean-type diet has been recommended (see Box 28.2).

Box 28.2 Lifestyle advice and areas of uncertainty in NAFLD[7,8]

- Weight loss: 3–5% improves steatosis; 7% NASH; 10% fibrosis
- Energy restriction: 500 kcal/day deficit
- Macronutrients: follow Mediterranean diet
- Physical activity: increase; ≥6 physical activity ratio for 75 min/week
- MUFA: no data
- PUFA: insufficient data
- Fructose: restriction might be beneficial
- Vitamin E: may be beneficial in non-DM
- Antioxidants: insufficient data
- Coffee: may reduce fibrosis
- Probiotics: insufficient data

6 Zivkovic, A.M. et al. (2007). Comparative review of diets for the metabolic syndrome: Implications for non-alcoholic fatty liver disease. Am. J. Clin. Nutr. 86, 285–300.

7 Hannah, W.N., et al. (2016). Lifestyle and dietary interventions in the management of nonalcoholic fatty liver disease. Dig. Dis. Sci. 61, 1365–74.

8 EASL, EASD, EASO (2016). EASL-EASD-EASO Clinical Practice Guidelines for the management of non-alcoholic fatty liver disease. J. Hepatol. 64, 1388–402.

Hepatitis and cirrhosis

Hepatitis—acute and chronic

Hepatitis is an inflammation of the liver and can arise from (i) a viral infection, e.g. hepatitis A, B, C, D, E, or G, (ii) an auto-immune response, or (iii) from other damage, e.g. alcoholic hepatitis. The nutritional implications vary depending on the severity and duration of the condition. See Box 28.3 for implications for mothers with viral hepatitis who wish to breastfeed.

Acute hepatitis In general, patients with acute hepatitis are very ill, have a poor appetite, and eat very little. No dietary restrictions should be imposed and patients should be encouraged to eat what they can. Small frequent snacks and nourishing drinks may be better tolerated than large meals. Fat restrictions used in the past are not evidence-based and dietary fat will not exacerbate the condition but will provide valuable calories if the patient is able to eat it. Severe undernutrition may accompany acute alcoholic hepatitis and instigating early nutrition support, usually through enteral feeding, is recommended.

Chronic hepatitis Nutritional status of people with chronic hepatitis may vary from those who are very undernourished following prolonged illness and poor intake to those who are obese, either incidentally or secondary to long-term treatment with steroids. Individual assessment is required and nutritional advice tailored accordingly.

Nutritional management

Appropriate nutritional management is important and influences prognosis.
- Undernourished patients who go on to liver transplantation have a greater risk of complications than those who are better nourished.
- Obesity is a risk factor for development and progression of chronic liver disease and is associated with poor response to antiviral therapy.

Box 28.3 Is it safe for women with viral hepatitis to breastfeed?

- *Hepatitis B:* Yes. Transmission of hepatitis B via breastmilk has not been reported. Infants should receive hepatitis B immunoglobulin and the first dose of hepatitis B vaccine within 12 hours of birth followed by completion of the vaccination series. Breastfeeding should not be delayed until the infant is fully immunized. Mothers are advised to take care of their nipples to avoid cracking and bleeding.
- *Hepatitis C:* Yes. There is no documented evidence that breastfeeding spreads hepatitis C. However, it is spread by blood so it is advisable to temporarily stop feeding if nipples become cracked and bleed. ℰ https://www.cdc.gov/breastfeeding/disease/hepatitis.htm.

Cirrhosis

Cirrhosis is irreversible damage of the hepatocytes. People with cirrhosis are often undernourished (prevalence between 10% and 100% depending on population), ∴ require nutritional support. Dietary restrictions should not be routinely imposed. Complications arising from cirrhosis, including ascites, oedema, encephalopathy, and steatorrhoea, may benefit from dietary modification providing it is undertaken within a context of nutritional adequacy, i.e. feed first, restrict second, and only if this does not compromise overall nutrient intake.

Energy: approximately 30% of patients with cirrhosis are hypermetabolic and therefore have ↑ energy requirements. About 50% are normometabolic and the remainder have ↓ energy expenditure. It is not possible to identify energy requirements without measuring using indirect calorimetry. Estimated energy requirements are provided in Table 28.1.

Protein: requirements are usually ↑ in cirrhosis and reflect impaired hepatic synthetic function (Table 28.1).

Carbohydrate: intake is important as hepatic glycogen stores are limited in cirrhosis leading to preferential metabolism of body fat and protein stores. Regular intake of carbohydrate, four to six times daily and a 50 g evening snack[9] is recommended. In hyperglycaemia, unrefined carbohydrate should not be restricted but taken in preference to sugary foods with insulin or oral hypoglycaemic agents as indicated.

Fat: provides a useful dietary energy and is usually well-tolerated except in some patients with cirrhosis 2° to cholestatic disease.

Table 28.1 Estimated energy and protein requirements* recommended by the European Society for Parenteral and Enteral Nutrition (ESPEN) Consensus Group**

	Non-protein energy, kcal/kg/day	Protein, g/kg/day
Cirrhosis	35–40	1.2–1.5

*Guidance is not explicit about whether these values are based on actual or ideal weight and whether modification is required if a patient has considerable fluid retention.

Source: data from Plauth, M., et al. (2006). ESPEN guidelines on enteral nutrition: liver disease. Clin Nutr. **25, 284–94.

9 Yamanaka-Okumura, H., et al. (2006). Effect of late evening snack with rice ball on energy metabolism in liver cirrhosis. Eur. J. Clin. Nutr. **60**, 1067–72.

Ascites and oedema

Fluid retention is common in cirrhosis and end-stage liver disease, and has relevance to nutrition.

- Abdominal distension can ↓ food intake leading to impaired nutritional status. Discomfort can be extreme and breathing impaired.
- Energy expenditure increases because of exertion of carrying additional weight.
- Negative nitrogen balance can be induced by repeated large volume paracentesis, even if intravenous albumin infused.
- Limiting dietary sodium can help reduce or control the degree of fluid retention, and thus improve symptoms but care is needed to ensure dietary intake remains otherwise adequate.

Nutritional management of ascites and oedema

- Assess nutritional status including estimating body weight without excess fluid (Table 28.2). Body weight is used to monitor fluid status but not nutritional status; regular monitoring of MAMC and triceps skinfold thickness is needed to assess lean tissue and body fat.
- Patients should be encouraged to eat as much as they are able and be tempted with tasty food.
- Small, frequent meals with snacks every 1–2 hours may optimize intake.
- The energy density of foods may be ↑ by the addition of concentrated sources, e.g. sugar, honey, double cream, oil, and salt-free butter.
- Fat should not be restricted unless the patient finds it unpalatable or has clinically diagnosed steatorrhoea.
- Decisions about whether to restrict sodium intake must balance the potential benefits against the risk of reducing nutrient intake. Patients should be advised individually by a registered dietitian with experience in this area.

Low sodium diets for ascites and oedema

Patients are usually prescribed diuretics that ↑ urinary Na^+ output and ∴ induce negative Na^+ balance and fluid loss. Limiting dietary Na^+ intake will facilitate this and → a more rapid resolution, ↓ doses of diuretics being prescribed, and fewer associated complications. However, these advantages must be balanced against the detrimental effect that a low Na^+ diet may have on total nutrient intake. A no-added salt diet (80–100 mmol Na^+/day) is usually advised and lower restrictions avoided because they are unpalatable.

No-added salt diet

- Avoid salt at the table.
- Keep salt in cooking to minimum.
- Avoid high salt foods including most preserved or tinned items, such as bacon, ham, sausages, tinned and packet soups, stock cubes, tinned vegetables, meats and fish, crisps and similar savoury snacks.
- Cheese (cheddar-type) should be limited to 100 g/week.
- Fast foods and ready-meals should be avoided unless they are known to provide <30 mmol Na^+ (700 mg Na/1750 mg NaCl) per portion.

Practical advice about using pepper, vinegar, spices, herbs, and lemon or frying food to add flavour may help adherence and encourage nutrient intake.

Other sources of sodium
- Antacids.
- Some antibiotics—check with pharmacist for suitable alternatives.
- Salt substitutes—most contain K^+ salts, but some also contain Na^+.
- Sodium bicarbonate.

1 mmol Na^+ = 23 mg Na^+ = 58.5 mg NaCl (salt)
100 mmol Na^+ = 585 mg NaCl = 5.9 g salt

Table 28.2 Guidelines for estimating fluid weight (kg) in patients with ascites and peripheral oedema*

	Ascites	Oedema
Minimal	2.2	1.0
Moderate	6.0	5.0
Severe	14.0	10.0

*Source: data from Mendenhall, C.L. (1992). Protein-calorie malnutrition in alcoholic liver disease. In: Watson, R.R. and Watzl, B. eds. *Nutrition and alcohol*. Boca Raton, FL: CRC Press pp. 363–84.

Hepatic encephalopathy

There is no good evidence to support dietary protein restriction in the treatment of hepatic encephalopathy (HE), although this was previously used. Limiting protein intake may exacerbate encephalopathy[10] and lead to rapid deterioration in nutritional status because protein requirements are increased in chronic liver disease. There is evidence[11] that 1.2 g/kg protein daily is well-tolerated by patients with HE.

Nutritional management of HE

- Sufficient protein to meet the estimated requirements should be provided (ESPEN recommendation in cirrhosis is 1.2–1.5 g/kg/day, see Table 28.1).
- Protein is best tolerated if spread out across the day. Eating several smaller meals and a bedtime snack is preferable to fewer large meals.
- Vegetable and dairy protein may be better tolerated than protein from meat and fish but acceptability depends on individual patients' preference.
- A high fibre diet, if acceptable, can contribute to a shorter gastrointestinal transit time, minimizing the opportunity for absorbing unwanted nitrogenous compounds of potential concern in HE. However, this may not be suitable for those with a small appetite who require more energy dense foods.
- Enteral feeding may be required if oral intake is inadequate.
- A recent of several meta-analyses of the effects of branched chain amino acids (BCAA) reported improvements in HE but no impact on nutritional status, mortality, or quality of life.[12] An optimum dose has not been defined but it is recommended that BCAA are taken at night to maximize their protein effects rather than being used solely as an energy source.
- There is limited evidence of benefit from probiotics.[13]

10 Merli, M., et al. (2009). Dietary and nutritional indications in hepatic encephalopathy. Metab. Brain Dis. 24, 211–21.

11 Córdoba, J., et al. (2004). Normal protein diet for episodic hepatic encephalopathy: results of a randomized study. J. Hepatol. 41, 38-43.

12 Gluud, L.L., et al. (2017). Branched-chain amino acids for people with hepatic encephalopathy. Cochrane Database Syst. Rev. 5, CD001939. DOI: 10.1002/14651858.CD001939.pub4.

13 Dalal, R., et al. (2017). Probiotics for people with hepatic encephalopathy. Cochrane Database Syst. Rev. 2, CD008716. DOI: 10.1002/14651858.CD008716.pub3.

Steatorrhoea and oesophageal varices

Steatorrhoea

Although ≥50% of patients with chronic liver disease have ↑ faecal fat excretion, relatively few have steatorrhoea. Those who do predominantly have cholestatic liver disease (e.g. primary biliary cholangitis or primary sclerosing cholangitis) rather than parenchymal disease (e.g. 2° to alcoholic or viral damage). Restricting dietary fat intake has the potential to ↓ steatorrhoea (see ➔ 'Low fat diet' Chapter 26).

Dietary fat contributes to the palatability of food and also provides:

- energy;
- fat-soluble vitamins;
- essential fatty acids.

A low fat diet, i.e. <30% of dietary energy, is not recommended unless the symptoms of steatorrhoea are jeopardizing nutritional status or quality of life. Dietary fat should only be reduced to a level that helps manage steatorrhoea, and never advised prophylactically. Advice may be needed to ensure that the diet remains adequate in all other nutrients:

- energy: ↑ carbohydrate, including sugar, and protein; medium chain triglyceride (MCT) supplements do not require bile for emulsification and are an additional source of energy (see Box 26.6);
- fat-soluble vitamins: supplements are required—follow local policy;
- essential fatty acids: include small amounts of PUFA within the limited amounts of fat tolerated.

Steatorrhoea caused by bile insufficiency cannot be treated with pancreatic enzyme replacement therapy. However, liver patients who also have pancreatic insufficiency may require these (see ➔ Chapter 27, p. 686).

Oesophageal varices

Bleeding oesophageal or gastric varices are a life threatening complication of chronic liver disease. Patients remain 'nil by mouth' during active bleeding and until their condition stabilizes. Nutritional implications arise if the patient's intake remains inadequate for prolonged periods, either because s/he is 'nil by mouth' or because of fear of eating.

There is no evidence that eating rough food, e.g. toast or crisps, increases the incidence of re-bleeding, although some patients may prefer to take softer foods temporarily, particularly if they have undergone repeated endoscopic treatment. Feeding via a naso-enteric tube is recommended if oral intake is inadequate even in the presence of oesophageal varices and is not associated with ↑ incidence of re-bleeding or mortality or ↑ length of hospital stay.[14,15] Gastrostomy feeding is not recommended.[15]

14 Cabré, E., et al. (2007). Reply to Dr Andus' letter. *Clin. Nutr.* 26, 273-4.

15 Plauth M et al. (2006). ESPEN guidelines on enteral nutrition: liver disease. *Clin. Nutr.* 25, 284–94..

Liver transplantation

Approximately 950 liver transplants are undertaken annually in the UK and 8,000 in the USA.

Pre-operatively

Patients being worked up for transplantation should undergo a detailed nutritional assessment (Box 28.1) to establish their nutritional status and identify scope for nutritional support. Undernourished patients have a significantly greater risk of increased morbidity and mortality after surgery so implementing early pre-surgery nutritional support is vital.[16]

Immediately post-operatively

Post-operative nutrition support varies from centre to centre and there is no clear evidence of best practice.[17] Early feeding via a naso-jejunal tube has been shown to be a safe and effective method of feeding post-transplant patients associated with reduced infections. Naso-gastric feeding may also be used. Parenteral nutrition is only indicated if the GI tract cannot be used for >5 days and, wherever possible, attempts should be made to feed via the gut.

Short-term recovery

When oral intake resumes, patients should be encouraged to eat an unrestricted diet; transient hyperglycaemia from medication does not require dietary intervention, but insulin may be needed. Food safety advice[18] is important because of immunosuppression, although practice varies between centres with some advising the avoidance of high risk foods, e.g. unpasteurized dairy products and shellfish, whereas others advise no restrictions. The effects of immunosuppressive drugs, e.g. ciclosporin and tacrolimus, can be potentiated by consumption of large quantities of grapefruit[19] with serious adverse consequences. However, these effects vary with format of grapefruit, i.e. fresh, juice, concentrate etc., and as a result, total avoidance is advised by some centres (see ➔ Chapter 38 'Drug-nutrient interactions').

Medium- to long-term

Following liver transplantation, most patients gain weight, especially in the first 6 months. This is appropriate if correcting pre-transplant undernutrition. However, ~40% patients become obese at 3 years after surgery and 40-70% go on to develop diabetes, dyslipidaemia, or hypertension. As a result,

16 Kalafateli, M., *et al.* (2017). Malnutrition and sarcopenia predict post-liver transplantation outcomes independently of the Model for End-stage Liver Disease score. *J. Cachexia Sarcopenia Muscle* **8**, 113-21.

17 Langer, G., *et al.* (2012). Nutritional interventions for liver-transplanted patients. *Cochrane Database Syst. Rev.* **8**, CD007605. DOI: 10.1002/14651858.CD007605.pub2.

18 NHS (2017). *How to prepare and cook food safely*. Available at: https://www.nhs.uk/live-well/eat-well/how-to-prepare-and-cook-food-safely/.

19 Peynaud, D., *et al.* (2007). Tacrolimus severe overdosage after intake of masked grapefruit in orange marmalade. *Eur. J. Clin. Pharmacol.* **63**, 721-2.

long-term cardiovascular risk is a major cause of post-transplant death. In addition, excessive weight gain after transplantation is associated with development of *de novo* non-alcoholic fatty liver disease in the graft with associated morbidity (see earlier pages in this chapter).

Healthy lifestyle advice, e.g. the 'Eatwell Guide (see ➲ Chapter 2), and physical activity guidelines should be provided to patients within the first 6 months and support given in transferring from a high energy, high protein intake pre-transplant to healthy eating after recovery from surgery. Regular monitoring of body mass index and serum lipids is used to identify those who need more specific guidance. Appropriate advice about increasing energy expenditure should also be included and statins may be routinely prescribed to help manage hyperlipidaemia.

Further information

British Liver Trust (2018). *Diet and liver disease*. Available at: ℬ https://britishlivertrust.org.uk/information-and-support/living-with-a-liver-condition/diet-and-liver-disease/.

Kidney disease

Introduction 704
Nutritional assessment 706
Nutrition in chronic kidney disease stages 1-3 710
Nutrition in chronic kidney disease stages 4-5 712
Malnutrition in kidney disease 716
Nutritional considerations in chronic kidney disease 718
Nephrotic syndrome 722
Nutritional requirements in dialysis 724
Renal transplantation 728
Nutrition in AKI 730
Kidney stones 732
Useful websites 734

Introduction

Classification

- *Chronic kidney disease (CKD)*: abnormality of the structure or function of kidneys, lasting >3 months; often progressive. Has been classified into stages 1–5 (Fig. 29.1).
- *Established stage 5 CKD*: a description of those who have reached stage 5 CKD and require renal replacement therapy (dialysis, transplantation) or conservative management.
- *Acute kidney injury (AKI)*: sudden, rapid deterioration of kidney function caused by injury or illness; often reversible.

CKD is categorized into stages according to glomerular filtration rate (GFR) and albumin creatinine ratio (ACR) (Fig. 29.1). AKI is categorized into stages according to serum creatinine and urine output (Table 29.1).

Prevalence of chronic kidney disease

The prevalence of CKD continues to rise in association with the world-wide increase in obesity and diabetes. Figures from the UK estimate that

GFR and ACR categories and risk of adverse outcomes			ACR categories (mg/mmol), description and range		
			<3 Normal to mildly increased	3–30 Moderately increased	>30 Severely increased
			A1	A2	A3
GFR categories (mL/min/1.73²), description and range	≥90 Normal and high	G1	No CKD in the absence of markers of kidney damage		
	60–89 Mild reduction related to normal range for a young adult	G2			
	45–59 Mild–moderate reduction	G3a¹			
	30–44 Moderate–severe reduction	G3b			
	15–29 Severe reduction	G4			
	<15 Kidney failure	G5			

Increasing risk →

Fig. 29.1 Classification of CKD using GFR and ACR categories

Adapted with permission from Kidney Disease: Improving Global Outcomes CKD Work Group (2013). Updated reference: KDIGO (2017). Clinical practice guideline update for the diagnosis, evaluation, prevention, and treatment of chronic kidney disease: Mineral and bone disorder (CKD-MBD). *Kidney Int. Suppl.* **7**, 1–59.

the prevalence of CKD stages 3–4 was approximately 13% but only 2% progress onto stage 5 (2013/2014 data). Increasing prevalence and incidence of CKD is also a particular problem in the developing world, and for individuals of ethnic minorities (e.g. South East Asian and Chinese populations) residing in developed countries.

Contributing causes of kidney disease
See Box 29.1.

Table 29.1 Classification of AKI

Stage	Serum creatinine	Urine output
Stage 1	1.5–1.9 × baseline OR ≥0.3 mg/dL (≥26.5 µmol/L) increase	<0.5 mL/kg/h for 6–12 hours
Stage 2	2.0–2.9 × baseline	<0.5 mL/kg/h for ≥12 hours
Stage 3	3.0 × baseline OR Increase in serum creatinine to ≥4.0 mg/dL (≥352.6 µmol/L) OR Initiation of renal replacement therapy OR In patients <18 years, decrease in eGFR to <35 mL/min per 1.73m^2	<0.3 mL/kg/h for ≥24 hours OR Anuria for ≥ 12 hours

---

Box 29.1 Contributing causes

Chronic kidney disease
- Diabetic nephropathy
- Hypertension
- Infection, e.g. chronic pyelonephritis or sepsis from severe urinary tract infection
- Nephrotic syndrome
- Polycystic kidney disease
- Tumour, e.g. multiple myeloma, amyloidosis
- Familial, e.g. Alport's syndrome
- Unknown reasons

Acute kidney injury
- Hypovolaemia (shock)
- Heart failure
- Sepsis, multi-organ failure
- Acute glomerulonephritis
- Toxic reaction, e.g. drugs, poison
- Obstruction of urinary output, e.g. tumour, kidney stone

Nutritional assessment

Nutritional assessment on an individual basis should be carried out to allow a holistic assessment of nutritional status and needs. This includes:

- Anthropometrics: weight and BMI should be interpreted with caution in view of potential fluid balance abnormalities and oedema in patients with kidney disease. It is important to collect anthropometric data that will allow assessment of alterations in lean body mass that can otherwise be masked by fluid shifts and changing fat mass over time. Handgrip strength, mid-arm muscle circumference, skinfold thickness, and bioelectrical impedance analysis (see ➜ Chapter 4, 'Body composition') have all been employed to monitor patients with CKD, particularly those on dialysis. Waist circumference can be useful for assessing cardiovascular risk (see Table 21.2, p. 471).
- Biochemical and haematological data: examples of interpretation of these results are shown in Table 29.2.
- Medical history including duration of diagnosis of CKD, clinical signs and symptoms, drug history, and all other co-morbidities.
- Diet history (see ➜ Chapter 4, 'Individual assessment').
- Environmental and psychosocial factors: in addition to the usual psychosocial influences on diet (housing, family, support networks, financial situation, and ability to cook), dialysis patients often suffer from loss of independence, depression, and anxiety associated with chronic illness. Assessing a patient's knowledge together with their motivation and confidence to change is important as nutritional treatment can be complex.
- Physical activity level, functional ability, and physical examination (see ➜ Chapter 4, 'Individual assessment').
- Fluid status and fluid balance.
- Subjective global assessment (SGA) has been found to be a useful adjunct to evaluate the nutritional status in patients with CKD. The results have been found to be reproducible and a number of formats are available online. Factors including weight change, dietary intake and gastrointestinal (GI) side effects, physical examination, and fluid status are rated against a 3- or 7-point scale, to formulate a SGA score.

Table 29.2 Interpretation of biochemical and haematological data

Blood result (normal range)	Importance
Potassium (K⁺) 3.5–5.0 mmol/L	Hyperkalaemia may be related to an excessive dietary K⁺ intake or other factors. It can result in cardiac arrhythmia or cardiac arrest. ↓ values may result in general muscle weakness. Low levels in patients on dialysis may indicate poor nutritional intake as K⁺ is found in most foods
Sodium (Na⁺) 136–146 mmol/L	Critical for blood pressure control, muscle and neurological function. Not a direct indicator of salt dietary intake. Most often associated with fluid status
Urea (Ur) 2.7–7.5 mmol/L	Derived from protein degradation, influenced by diet, hydration, and urine production. Urea is influenced by type of protein consumed, degree of anabolism, and dialysis adequacy. Data from urea kinetic modelling can be used indirectly to estimate the protein intake in dialysis
Creatinine (Cr) 55–110 mmol/L	Normal waste product of muscle breakdown, not usually affected by dietary protein. Normally ↑ in CKD. Used to calculate estimated GFR
Albumin (Alb) 35–50 g/L	Has been found to be a good predictor of mortality in CKD; however, requires careful interpretation: can be influenced by fluid imbalance or an acute phase response as indicated by ↑ CRP levels (trauma, surgery, or infection). The large body pool and long half-life (14–20 days) renders albumin relatively insensitive to immediate changes in nutritional status
Pro-albumin 18–38 mg/L	Shorter half-life and smaller body pool than albumin, is influenced by the acute phase response and anaemia
Bicarbonate (HCO₃) 22–29 mmol/L	Reflects the degree of acidosis or alkalosis in the body. In later stages of CKD, kidneys are unable to maintain normal acid-base balance and HCO₃ may ↓, leading to metabolic acidosis. May also ↓ with diabetic keto-acidosis, diarrhoea, fever, or starvation. Low serum bicarbonate levels in CKD often lead to hyperkalaemia and are usually treated with sodium bicarbonate
C-reactive protein (CRP) <8 g/L	A non-specific positive acute phase protein that can be used to diagnose infectious and inflammatory diseases, associated with mortality in CKD. ↑CRP is an indicator of inflammation and can result in ↓ albumin
Protein catabolic rate (PCR)—calculated	In steady state, PCR correlates well with dietary protein intake. However, in catabolic patients, urea generated by muscle breakdown far exceeds that derived from diet. Conversely, anabolism may produce false ↓ PCR. As PCR is usually normalized for actual body weight, extremes in weight will affect nPCR

(Continued.)

Table 29.2 (*Contd.*)

Blood result (normal range)	Importance
Calcium (Ca^{++}) 2.2–2.6 mmol/L	Often corrected for albumin as albumin carries half the calcium in the blood. ↑ levels may cause confusion and forgetfulness, depression, fatigue, muscle spasms, and cramps. Raised calcium levels are often seen in later stages of CKD mineral and bone disorders. ↓ levels may be seen after a surgical parathyroidectomy and may cause numbness and muscle spasms
Phosphate (PO_4) 0.8–1.50 mmol/L	↓ levels may indicate poor food intake or may result as part of the metabolic imbalances associated with refeeding syndrome. Low levels are frequent post renal transplant and in those receiving frequent haemodialysis/ haemofiltration ↑ levels are problematic in CKD (see ➔ this chapter, 'Mineral and bone disorder')
Haemoglobin (Hb)	↓ levels cause anaemia, ↓ quality of life with effects on mental function, exercise tolerance, fatigue, appetite, and sleep patterns (see ➔ Chapter 6, 'Iron')
Lipid profile	↓ total plasma cholesterol levels are associated with ↑ mortality, possibly as an indicator of ↓ nutritional intakes. ↑ cholesterol and ↑ triglycerides are often found in patients with CKD and post kidney transplant See ➔ Chapter 23, 'Cardiovascular disease'

Normal levels can differ between both laboratories and hospitals. ➔ Target ranges for many blood results for CKD patients can be controversial, you may want to check recent guidelines and local practice patterns for target ranges.

Nutrition in chronic kidney disease stages 1–3

Medical management of CKD mainly consists of interventions to slow the rate of decline in renal function and limit any associated complications, such as cardiovascular disease (CVD).

Nutritional management should include reduction of all modifiable cardiovascular risk factors including:

- hypertension (limiting salt intake to 5-6 g/day);
- managing glucose level in diabetes;
- achieving a healthy weight (BMI 20–25 kg/m^2);
- lipid lowering;
- smoking cessation if appropriate;
- regular exercise;
- limiting alcohol intake (<14 units a week).

Nutrition in chronic kidney disease stages 4-5

- Disease progression in CKD is extremely variable, with some individuals suffering rapid progression, whereas others maintain stable renal function for several years.
- A patient with progressing CKD (stage 4 CKD onwards) must be referred to a specialist renal dietitian for nutritional assessment.
- Nutritional advice should be tailored to the specific needs of the individual with a view to minimizing the risk of potential disease progression and related risk factors (e.g. CVD).

Nutritional requirements

- *Energy* requirements are between 30 and 40 kcal/kg ideal body weight (IBW)/day depending on age and level of physical activity. This may be reduced in overweight and obese individuals
- *Protein* an intake of 0.8-1.0 g/kg IBW/day is recommended (a mild degree of restriction), especially in patients consuming excessive protein or for the short-term management of uraemic patients awaiting the start of dialysis. Limiting protein intake <0.75 g/kg IBW/day is not recommended, because although this is thought to ↓ uraemic symptoms and ↓ rate of decline in renal function, benefits are marginal when compared with ↑ risk of malnutrition. Protein intake may ↓ spontaneously as the GFR ↓, particularly if GFR is <25 mL/min. It is more likely that patients nearing stage 5 CKD will require nutrition support to achieve an adequate intake, rather than dietary restrictions. Timely initiations of dialysis will ↓ extent of malnutrition. Protein provision should not be >1.3g protein/kg IBW/day in these patients.
- *Phosphorus:* Current evidence does not support early restriction. In practice, dietary restriction may be used if phosphate level increases and/or patients become symptomatic. Phosphorus-containing foods are shown in Table 29.3. Advice should be given to reduce intake of foods high in phosphorus while ensuring adequate dietary protein intake. Foods high in phosphorus should be substituted with nutritionally equivalent foods that are lower in bioavailable phosphorus (this requires renal dietetic expertise). Some patients require phosphate binders in addition to dietetic advice if hyperphosphataemia persists, rather than risk malnutrition related to inadequate dietary protein intake.
- *Potassium:* restriction is required if consecutive K⁺ levels are >5.5 mmol/L as is often the case with the use of ACE (angiotensin converting enzyme) inhibitors or ARBs (angiotensin receptor blockers) which reduce renal potassium excretion. Non-dietary causes of hyperkalaemia are shown in Table 29.4. Strategies for limiting dietary K⁺ are described in Box 29.2.
- *Salt intake:* intake should be limited to 5-6 g/day: see ➲ Chapter 28, 'Ascites and oedema'). This is particularly important in alleviating thirst for those who require fluid restriction.
- *Fluid:* restrictions are usually only required in CKD if there is a marked ↓ urine output (<1000 mL/day), severe oedema, or a history of heart failure. For people with diabetes requiring fluid restriction, attention should be paid to glycaemic control to avoid thirst.

Table 29.3 Examples of foods high in phosphorus

Drinks	Dark carbonated drinks, hot chocolate, milk shakes, milk and other milky drinks.
Dairy products	Processed and hard cheeses, custard, milky puddings, ice cream, and yogurt
	Milk contains phosphorus but up to half pint/day is recommended as part of a balanced diet
Meat/fish and eggs	All meat, fish, and eggs contain some phosphorus but are necessary to meet protein requirements
	Processed foods containing these foods often contain phosphate additives which are more readily absorbed sources of phosphorus
Other	In plant foods, much of the phosphorus is bound to phytates, leading to ↓ phosphorus absorption in the GI tract
	These include beans, peas, seeds, nuts, and wholegrain foods
	Cooking may increase phosphorus availability
	In summary, the phosphorus absorption rate of these foods is variable but a diet containing wholegrains may have lower net phosphorus absorption than a more refined diet
	Peanut butter, chocolate, baking powder
Phosphorus additives	Additives containing phosphorus have 100% bioavailability. These are added to a variety of commonly used foods including cola, processed meat, fish and cheese, freeze dried foods, bakery products and beverages. Phosphorus is not reported in the nutritional information, but is listed in the ingredients list
	Additives containing phosphorus include: E101, E106, E339-343, E450-452, E540-545, E1410, E1412, E1414, and E1442

Chronic kidney disease in the older person

Nephron mass and GFR deteriorates with normal aging. Many older individuals in whom CKD is diagnosed may never require dialysis. This should be taken into account before advising overzealous dietary restrictions, particularly in the very old.

Table 29.4 Non-dietary causes of hyperkalaemia

Metabolic factors	Acidosis, insulin insufficiency, infection/sepsis, rapid catabolism
Drugs	K⁺-containing drugs, e.g. iatrogenic (oral/IV potassium replacement)
	Drugs affecting K⁺ excretion, e.g. ACE inhibitors (e.g. ramipril, captopril, lisinopril), ARBs (e.g. candesartan, losartan, valsartan), β-blockers, non-steroidal anti-inflammatory drugs
	K⁺-sparing diuretics, e.g. amiloride, spironolactone
	Immunosuppressant medication, e.g. tacrolimus
Cellular trauma	Haemolysed blood sample, blood transfusion, infection, gastrointestinal haemorrhage, rhabdomyolysis, crush injuries, burns, gangrene, some solid tumours, tumour lysis, hypoaldosteronism
Constipation	Reduced gut excretion
Dialysis	Inadequate dialysis or missing dialysis sessions
Others	Extreme exercise

Box 29.2 Strategies for limiting K⁺ intake

The following foods are high in potassium—use very sparingly.

• *Fruits:* Banana, avocado, all dried fruit. Limit all other fruit to three 80 g servings per day.
• *Potatoes:* Jacket potatoes, chips, potato crisps. Limit boiled potatoes to one serving per day.
• *Vegetables:* Beetroot, sun-dried tomatoes, tomato puree. Limit all other vegetables to two to three 80 g servings per day.
• *Pulses:* Baked beans, kidney beans, lentils, other beans and pulses (these are also sources of protein hence a detailed renal dietetic assessment is required before advising patient to limit pulses).
• *Drinks:* Fresh fruit juices, coffee, drinking chocolate, malted drinks.
• *Other:* Salt substitutes (e.g. LoSalt), hummus, nuts, peanut butter, chocolate, milk, yogurt, evaporated and condensed milk, yeast extract, liquorice.

Alter cooking methods (K⁺ is very water soluble):

• Boil potatoes and vegetables in plenty of water (do not boil twice as the second boil does not remove significant additional amounts of K⁺ but reduces palatability).
• Chop potatoes and other large vegetables into small chunks to increase the surface area for K⁺ removal.
• Parboil vegetables before adding them to stews, soups, etc.
• Avoid pressure cooker and microwave cooking for cooking potatoes and vegetables.
• Limit portion size and quantities of fruit and vegetables high in potassium but ensure patient has an adequate intake of lower potassium fruit and vegetables.

Malnutrition in kidney disease

- Malnutrition in CKD is referred to as protein energy wasting (PEW).
- PEW describes the multiple nutritional and catabolic alterations that occur in kidney disease and is associated with ↑ risk of hospital admission, morbidity, mortality, and ↓ quality of life.
- An estimated 20–60% of all patients with CKD (including dialysis) are at risk of PEW. These figures vary depending on the stage of CKD and method used to assess PEW.
- Poor nutritional status prior to initiation of dialysis is associated with poorer outcomes on dialysis.
- Despite its limitations as an indicator of nutritional status, low serum albumin levels are independently associated with ↑ risk of death in patients on haemodialysis (HD), peritoneal dialysis (PD), and after kidney transplant.
- Insufficient oral intake because of poor appetite is often problematic but not the only cause of PEW. Other contributory factors include chronic inflammation, co-morbidities, metabolic acidosis, and accumulation of uraemic toxins resulting in increased muscle catabolism, polypharmacy, and appetite suppression.
- Dialysis treatment may interfere with meal patterns, leading to a reduced intake and increased risk of PEW.

Nutrition support

Patients with kidney disease who are at increased risk of malnutrition should be assessed by a renal dietitian and advised to supplement their oral intake with high energy and/or high protein foods (food fortification) or nutritional supplements (see ➲ Chapter 25, 'Treatment of undernutrition'). Where oral intake alone is insufficient to meet needs, nutrition support in the form of enteral tube feeding or parenteral nutrition support should be considered (see ➲ Chapter 25, 'Enteral feeding' and 'Parenteral nutrition').

- A range of oral supplements exist including, nutrient dense supplement drinks and energy and protein modules. The choice of nutritional supplements should be based on patients' preference, nutritional requirements, electrolyte levels, and fluid status.
- Specifically formulated renal supplements or enteral feeds, which are low in K^+ and/or phosphorus and nutrient dense may be required if K^+ or phosphate levels are elevated or fluid restriction is required.
- Powdered milkshake style products may not be appropriate because of higher electrolyte and fluid content.
- Fluids from supplements or feeds contribute to the daily fluid allowance. If artificial nutrition support is required, attention must be given to the total fluid intake. Patients may need a review of their dialysis prescription (e.g. increased frequency of HD) to facilitate increased fluid removal.
- Parenteral nutrition should be considered for patients with a non-functioning or inaccessible gastrointestinal tract.
- Intradialytic nutrition:
  - *Intradialytic parenteral nutrition (IDPN)* can be used to supplement energy and protein intakes during each HD session. Although it is

expensive, it has the advantage of providing nutrients with minimal additional fluid and ensuring patient compliance. Short-term evaluation of IDPN suggests it may be of benefit in some patients, but few studies have evaluated the long-term benefits. Metabolic studies suggest that IDPN may be able to switch a patient from a catabolic to an anabolic state, and can ↑ serum albumin, dry weight, muscle strength. In principle, it can only provide up to 1100 kcal and 8 g of nitrogen per session. However, in practice some of the nutrition will be lost in the dialysate fluid. Close nutritional monitoring, including blood glucose, GI symptoms, and biochemistry is required. Patients with diabetes may also require adjustment to insulin dosage.

- *Intra-peritoneal amino acids (IPAA)* were used in continuous ambulatory peritoneal dialysis patients in the past as a method to promote nitrogen uptake and improve nutritional status. However, studies have failed to show these benefits. Instead, IPAA is often used in patients with diabetes to reduce their glucose load. The exchange must be done at the same time as a meal to enhance amino acid uptake.

Nutritional considerations in chronic kidney disease

CKD-mineral and bone disorder

As GFR falls <30 mL/min, the kidney's ability to adequately regulate calcium and phosphate homeostasis is also reduced. A chain of inter-related biochemical abnormalities occurs in CKD mineral and bone disorder (Table 29.5). In the long-term, this can result in 2° hyperparathyroidism, renal bone disease, and vascular and soft tissue calcification, known collectively as CKD-mineral and bone disorder (CKD-MBD). This is associated with ↑ prevalence of cardiovascular disease and ↑ mortality.

Management of CKD-MBD

Management intensifies with ↑ stages of CKD.

- *Phosphorus* intake may need to be restricted to 800–1000 mg/day. Emphasis should be placed on reducing phosphorus from foods with low nutrient density e.g. cola drinks, processed cheese, products containing baking powder (e.g. scones), and food with phosphorus-containing additives. Many foods high in phosphorus are also good protein sources, so care should be taken to ensure that dietary protein intake is adequate for the stage of CKD.
- *Phosphate binders* can be used when it is not possible to control the phosphate with diet alone. Binders are usually classified into two groups; calcium based and non-calcium-based. They work by binding with phosphorus in the GI tract to prevent systemic absorption and exert variable efficacy and GI side effects.
- *Vitamin D* deficiency is prevalent in the general population as well as in CKD. Controversy exists over the best type of vitamin D to prescribe. Either 25 vitamin D, 1,25 vitamin D, or a precursor to 1,25 vitamin D can be used in CKD.
- *Calcimimetic agents* increase the sensitivity of calcium-sensing receptors in the parathyroid gland, thereby inhibiting PTH secretion. These are used in patients with uncontrolled PTH levels for whom parathyroidectomy is contraindicated.

Cardiovascular risk

CVD accounts for up to 50% of deaths in CKD. An individual with kidney disease is more likely to die of CVD than reach the stage of requiring dialysis. Traditional CVD risk factors account for only part of this ↑ risk. CVD risk can be ↓ by a combination of changes in diet, lifestyle, and physical activity.

Traditional modifiable CVD risk factors in CKD

- *Hypertension*: in addition to medical management, a no-added-salt diet (5-6 g/day) is beneficial (see ➔ Chapter 28, 'Ascites and oedema').
- *Hyperlipidaemia*: ↑ cholesterol and ↑ triglycerides are frequently found in patients with CKD and post kidney transplant.
- *Weight management*: see ➔ this chapter 'Weight management'.
- *Lifestyle choices*: particularly smoking and low physical activity levels, see ➔ this chapter 'Exercise'.
- *Diabetes*: see ➔ this chapter 'Diabetes'.

Table 29.5 Abnormalities of mineral bone metabolism in CKD

Blood result	Abnormality in CKD
Phosphate	Inability to remove sufficient phosphate begins early in CKD, although serum phosphate levels are maintained in the 'normal' range until CKD stage 4 (GFR<30 mL/min)
Calcium	Calcium may ↓ with decreased absorption caused by a fall in vitamin D status
Parathyroid hormone (PTH)	PTH ↑ gradually when GFR <60 mL/min, initially as a response to ↓ calcium and vitamin D levels as well as ↑ phosphate
Vitamin D	Reduced conversion of 25 vitamin D into its active form 1,25 vitamin D, begins when GFR <60 mL/min
Fibroblast growth factor 23 (FGF23)	FGF23 decreases the reabsorption and ↑ excretion of phosphate. Levels are ↑ in CKD (even before PTH levels start to ↑). FGF23 levels are not usually measured in practice but used predominantly in research

CKD-specific modifiable CVD risk factors
- *Deranged mineral bone metabolism* (as described above) is associated with vascular and soft tissue calcification.
- *Anaemia* can contribute to left ventricular hypertrophy; see ➋ this chapter 'Anaemia'.
- *Other* volume-overload, chronic inflammation, and malnutrition.

Anaemia
Anaemia is common in CKD, because of iron deficiency and/or a relative lack of erythropoietin, which develops when GFR <60 mL/min, and should be investigated if Hb <130 g/L (♂ and post-menopausal ♀) and <120 g/l (pre-menopausal ♀). Intravenous or oral iron can be given as first-line treatment. Ferritin levels should not be >800 ng/mL. Epoetin, synthetic erythropoietin which stimulates erythropoiesis, can be used to maintain Hb levels between 105 and 125 g/L.

Diabetes
Diabetes is the cause of kidney disease in approximately 40% of CKD patients. Nutritional priorities in patients with diabetes and CKD are:
- Optimize glycaemic control (HbA1c <53 mmol/mol or <7.0%)*.
- Optimize management of blood pressure and proteinuria.
- Emphasis on management of modifiable CVD risks.
- Weight management.

*However, once on haemodialysis, HbA1c targets should be individualized; if the patient is on a hypoglycaemia-inducing treatment, the aim should be between 58 and 68 mmol/mol (7.5–8.5%).[1]

1 Joint British Diabetes Society for Inpatient Care (JBDS-IC) (2016). *Management of adults with diabetes on the haemodialysis unit*. Available at: ℘ http://www.diabetologists-abcd.org.uk/JBDS/JBDS_RenalGuide_2016.pdf.

Weight management

Where possible, obese patients (BMI >30 kg/m^2) should be encouraged to ↓ body weight through diet, healthy eating, and exercise. Weight loss goals should be realistic and tailored to the individual patient.

Reasons for weight management in CKD

- Weight loss has been shown to ↓ proteinuria, blood pressure, and insulin resistance in patients with CKD.
- BMI >35 kg/m^2 with co-morbidities is likely to ↓ the chance of being accepted for kidney transplant.
- Increased risk of CVD, diabetes, hypertension, and some cancers.
- Excess weight may impair mobility and independence.

Exercise

Patients at all stages of CKD should be encouraged to take regular exercise. Specialist input from exercise professionals, such as physiotherapists, may be useful in providing support to those with ↑ levels of frailty or physical disability.

Nephrotic syndrome

Characterized by proteinuria >3 g/day, hypoalbuminaemia, and generalized oedema. Hyperlipidaemia, clotting problems, and hypertension are also often observed. There are a number of causes (Box 29.3).

Treatment

Aims to control oedema, ↓ proteinuria, and treat complications, e.g. infections, hyperlipidaemia, and clotting problems. Immunosuppression therapy is often used. Diet therapy has a role to play (Box 29.4).

Oedema Limiting salt intake to 5-6 g/day can potentiate the antihypertensive and antiproteinuric effects of ACE inhibitors. Fluid restriction may be necessary, depending on the response to diuretics and other treatments such as albumin infusions. Oedema can mask PEW.

Proteinuria/hypoalbuminaemia 0.8-1 g protein/kg ideal body weight/day is recommended. Proteinuria is targeted with ACE inhibitors, strict blood pressure control, and good diabetes control. A high protein diet is not advised as this causes ↑ permeability and hyperfiltration in the glomerular basement membrane, which could exacerbate proteinuria. There is very limited evidence to recommend a low protein diet (<0.8 g protein/kg IBW/day).

Hyperlipidaemia Incidence of myocardial infarction is five to six times greater in nephrotic syndrome (NS). In addition to dietary intervention, lipid-lowering drugs are used to control cholesterol and triglycerides.

Thromboembolism 10–30% of adults with NS develop emboli, a ↓ protein diet has been shown to improve fibrinogen levels.

Box 29.3 Causes of nephrotic syndrome

- Focal segmental glomerulosclerosis 30%
- Membranous nephropathy 25%
- Diabetes 20%
- Minimal change nephropathy 10%
- Amyloidosis 4-10%
- Others include systemic lupus erythematosus, IgA nephropathy, toxic glomerulopathy, e.g. caused by gold or penicillamine.

Box 29.4 Summary of dietary considerations in nephrotic syndrome

- *Energy:* 'normal requirements', i.e. 30–35 kcal/kg IBW/day
- *Protein:* 0.8–1 g/kg ideal body weight per day
- *Lipids:* within healthy recommendations
- *Micronutrients:* ensure adequate intake, including vitamin D
- *Salt:* limited to 5-6 g/day
- *Potassium:* monitor as serum levels may ↑ with ACE inhibitors

Nutritional requirements in dialysis

Dialysis is usually initiated once GFR falls to <10 mL/min or the patient has uraemic symptoms. If a patient chooses conservative care rather than dialysis, their nutritional goals should be re-assessed to take this into account. Appetite and food intake often improve gradually once dialysis has begun and uraemic symptoms are alleviated. Nutritional requirements for dialysis are shown in Table 29.6. Where possible, general healthy eating guidelines are recommended, e.g. 50% total energy from complex carbohydrates, high fibre and 30–35% energy from fat (predominantly poly- and monounsaturated fatty acid sources with low saturated fats). If intake is poor, healthy eating guidelines should be relaxed to help achieve nutritional adequacy.

Nutritional requirements in peritoneal dialysis

Energy 30-35 kcal/kg/IBW. Overweight patients may require energy restriction to compensate for the additional glucose absorbed from dialysate. Initial advice should concentrate on ↓ excessive intake of fat and sugar. High use of hypertonic dialysate to control fluid balance will ↑ energy provision. Fluid management together with limiting salt intake should be emphasized.

Protein requirements are increased in PD; a minimum of 1.1-1.2 g/kg IBW is recommended because of dialysate losses. High protein requirements may be difficult to achieve by diet alone, particularly in those with poor appetite or during and after peritonitis. Specific targets for protein-rich foods and snacks, and use of prescribed protein supplements may be required.

Phosphorus restrictions and phosphate binders are often required based on blood results.

Potassium dietary restriction is rarely needed in PD because of continuous, daily clearance.

Fluid Ultrafiltration (UF) volume can vary depending on the glucose concentration of dialysate used. UF volume may be added to the daily fluid intake allowance. Long-term use of hypertonic solutions may cause damage to the peritoneal membrane, producing hyperpermeability, loss of peritoneal integrity and ↑ weight. Use of higher glucose concentration dialysate should be minimized especially in obese patients, those with diabetes or hypertriglyceridaemia, and are seldom used. These patients need more stringent Na^+ and fluid restrictions.

Fibre A high intake of soluble fibre is of particular importance in PD (see ➲ Chapter 5, 'Carbohydrate'). Preventing constipation is important for optimal functioning of PD and laxatives are used daily.

Table 29.6 Daily nutritional guidelines for patients on PD and HD

	PD	HD	Main food sources
Energy	30–35 kcal/kg IBW (including glucose absorbed from dialysate)	30–40 kcal/kg IBW	Starchy foods e.g. cereals, bread, rice, pasta, potato Sugars and fats
Protein	Minimum 1.0–1.2 g/kg IBW	Minimum 1.1 g/kg IBW Maximum 1.4g/kg IBW	Meat, fish, eggs, pulses, nuts, dairy foods
Potassium	Not limited unless hyperkalaemic	1 mmol/kg IBW	Potatoes, fruit and vegetables, fruit juice, nuts, crisps, coffee, chocolate
Phosphorus	Limit phosphorus intake If phosphorus or PTH levels raised, limit intake of food additives Ensure adequate protein intake		Processed foods and drinks, e.g. sausages, ham, pizza, cake mixes, frozen desserts, cola drink
Salt	5-6 g salt	5-6 g salt	Table salt, processed foods, e.g. smoked/cured foods, tinned and packet foods, ready meals
Fluid	500-750 mL + previous day urine output + ultrafiltration (usually residual renal function present)	500-750 mL + previous day urine output	Drinks, gravies, sauces, soups, jelly, yogurt

Table 29.7 Strategies for limiting fluid intake

Limit fluid intake	Use small-volume cup for drinks Suck ice cubes and ice lollies Take tablets with food (unless otherwise directed)
↑ Awareness	Education about fluid content of certain foods, e.g. jelly, custard, soup, ice-cream, yogurt, dhal Measuring jug tally, e.g. fluid intake is monitored by taking required liquid throughout the day from a jug/bottle initially containing the desired daily volume
Thirst prevention	Limit salt intake Maintain blood glucose within range if patient has diabetes
Techniques	Take sugar-free sweets or chew gum Fruit may also be refreshing (within K+ allowance if applicable)
Regular mouth care	Rinse mouth with water regularly, lip salves, etc.

Nutritional requirements in haemodialysis

Energy 30–40 kcal/kg IBW. Some patients have difficulty achieving recommended intakes ∴ will need advice aimed at ↑ energy intake using energy-rich foods and/or prescribed supplements.

Protein 1.1–1.4 g/kg/IBW.[2] Protein requirements are ↑ because of disturbed metabolic status and loss of amino acids through dialysis. Nutritional supplementation of protein and/or energy may be required to achieve requirements where appetite and dietary intake is ↓.

Fluid restriction is required, limiting intake to daily urine volume +500 mL (i.e. to meet insensible losses). Anuric patients will require more severe restriction. Advice varies between renal units, i.e. some advise 500 mL/d, others 1000 mL/d). Advice should be provided to help adherence to fluid allowance (Table 29.7). Interdialytic fluid gain should be monitored by measuring body weight and aiming for a maximum gain of 2 kg or 3% dry body weight between HD sessions.

Salt intake should be limited to 5–6 g/day. Patients should be educated about salt being the major drive to thirst, as limiting salt intake is likely to lead to better fluid (and blood pressure) control than attempting to limit fluid intake alone.

Phosphate clearance is not particularly effective with conventional HD. Nocturnal dialysis achieves significantly better phosphate clearance, enabling some patients to relax their dietary restrictions and usually avoiding the need for phosphate binders. Patients on nocturnal HD may experience hypophosphatemia and require ↑ phosphorus intake.

Potassium Advice to reduce potassium intake may be required, this is partly dependent on residual renal function. Non-dietary causes of hyperkalaemia (Table 29.4) should be excluded. Limiting dietary K^+ intake is generally staged following ongoing review of blood levels. Strategies for limiting K^+ intake are shown in Box 29.2.

Vitamin deficiencies can occur in HD because of dialysate losses, abnormal metabolism and dietary restrictions. Overt deficiency is rare. Some renal units routinely prescribe a water-soluble vitamin supplement containing B vitamins, vitamin C, and folate. Vitamin A is not routinely prescribed because of high levels of retinol binding protein. Supplementation of water-soluble vitamins may be considered in those undergoing >15 hours HD/week as they are more likely to have more significant losses.

Minerals and trace elements Of 14 essential minerals and trace elements (see ⮕ Chapter 6, 'Minerals and trace elements'), deficiencies in Zn, Cu, Mn, and Cr have been reported in CKD, mostly because of dietary restriction and drug interactions. Deficiency should be confirmed before starting supplementation. Catabolism and inflammatory response can influence interpretation of serum trace elements.

---

2 Naylor, H.L., *et al.* (2013). Renal Nutrition Group of the British Dietetic Association; British Dietetic Association evidence-based guidelines for the protein requirements of adults undergoing maintenance haemodialysis or peritoneal dialysis. *J. Hum. Nutr. Diet.* 26, 315-28.

Renal transplantation

Renal transplantation is considered to offer many patients with kidney failure the best chance of rehabilitation and optimal quality of life. A patient may have spent a prolonged length of time at the pre-dialysis stage and then some time on dialysis before receiving a transplant or may be able to receive a kidney transplant before starting dialysis. Those on long-term dialysis are likely to have established metabolic effects of CKD, including:

- anaemia;
- mineral and bone disorder;
- protein energy wasting;
- cardiovascular disease.

Immunosuppressive therapy, used to prolong the life of the transplanted kidney, can exacerbate all of the above conditions as well as creating additional problems (see Box 29.5).

Immediately post-transplant

Nutritional care should be the same as for any other post-surgical patient: monitoring blood biochemistry and urine volume, ensuring the return of normal gut function and appetite and meeting requirements with supplements if necessary. The rate at which biochemistry and urine volume return to normal can vary (from a couple of days after surgery to several weeks) and needs to be monitored closely. Treatment varies accordingly from fluid and electrolyte (Na^+, K^+, Mg^{++} and PO_4^-) restrictions to intravenous support if urine output is excessive and serum electrolyte levels drop below normal. This is often seen within the first 3 months after transplant and hypophosphatemia may persist.

❶ Dehydration at this stage can damage the new kidney.

As the patient is more susceptible to infection, some advice on food safety is also useful.[3] Food safety advice is particularly important at this stage because of the high dose of immunosuppressants and hence a reduced immune response to food borne micro-organisms.

Once kidney function has stabilized

The main aims of dietary therapy are to encourage a healthy balanced diet and ↓ risk factors for cardiovascular disease. The risk of obesity ↑ post-transplantation and dietary advice should be given to the patient prior to hospital discharge, with regular follow-up in outpatient clinics to prevent excessive weight gain. Advice should include healthy eating, exercise, and other lifestyle improvements including stress management, avoidance of smoking, and excessive sun exposure. Barriers to eating a healthy diet may result from habits formed while adhering to pre-transplant dietary restrictions. Steroid use, ↑ appetite, and ↑ dietary freedom can result in excessive food intake that contributes to rapid ↑ body fat.

3 For information on food safety, see NHS Choices available at: ℞ https://www.nhs.uk/live-well/eat-well/how-to-store-food-and-leftovers/.

Box 29.5 Side effects of immunosuppressive treatment

- Protein hypercatabolism
- ↑ appetite leading to obesity
- Hyperlipidaemia
- Glucose intolerance and ↑ risk of diabetes
- Hypertension
- Hyperkalaemia
- Interference with vitamin D metabolism
- ↑ cancer risk
- ↑ infection risk (opportunistic viral and bacterial infections that may ↓ appetite and ↑ nutrient requirements)
- Gum hypertrophy

Box 29.6 Summary of nutritional management in kidney transplantation

- Educate patient regarding food safety
- Monitor biochemistry, especially cholesterol, triglycerides, glucose, K^+, PO_4^-, Ca^{++}, PTH, haemoglobin
- Monitor blood pressure control
- Aim for healthy body mass index
- 'The Eatwell Guide' is an appropriate food model to use
- Encourage a variety of fruit and vegetables and five portions/day
- Encourage high fibre foods
- Encourage fish particularly oily fish, lean meats, and pulses
- Foods high in sugar, saturated fat, and salt should be eaten sparingly
- Encourage ↓ fat dairy products
- Ensure Ca^{++} requirements are met
- Advise alcohol within usual safe drinking limits
- Encourage physical activity and regular exercise
- Avoid smoking
- Avoid excessive sun exposure

Longer-term

Weight management and improvement in lipid levels have been achieved with diet and exercise interventions. These interventions help ↓ risk of metabolic syndrome or diabetes, although many patients also need medication to control blood lipids. Improved muscle and bone strength may also result from diet and exercise advice but vitamin D and calcium supplements may also be required (Box 29.6).

Nutrition in AKI

Nutritional status in AKI is influenced by the underlying aetiology of disease, pre-existing malnutrition, degree of catabolism, and length of hospitalization. Patients with AKI and hypercatabolism require prompt nutritional support.

Continuous renal replacement therapy (CRRT)

Severe AKI can be treated with intermittent haemodialysis (IHD) or CRRT. CRRT is often used in intensive care to treat critically ill, unstable patients with AKI who might be adversely affected by blood pressure changes and fluid restrictions associated with IHD. This slow, continuous dialysis therapy removes fluid and metabolites via diffusion and/or convection over a 24 hour period.

Nutritional requirements in AKI

- *Energy:* Similar to healthy individuals in non-septic patients. In sepsis, the BMR may be # by up to 30%. Some authors suggest 20–30 kcal/kg body weight (BW)/d. Others suggest 25–35 kcal/kg BW/d.[4]
- *Protein:* Patients with AKI but no additional catabolic stress are usually able to maintain neutral or positive nitrogen balance at 0.8-1 g/kg/ BW/d. Dialysis-dependent patients require additional protein to replace losses during dialysis. Estimated losses during dialysis:

  HD: 1–1.5 g nitrogen (6 – 9 g protein)/session;

  CRRT: 1.5 – 2.0 g nitrogen (9 – 12.5 g protein)/24 hours.

  Those with sepsis, trauma, inflammation, or multiple organ failure have ↑ protein requirements (1.2-1.7 g/kg/BW/d with some authors suggesting up to 2.5 g/kg/BW/d).[5] Patients in a catabolic state may have a marked rise in blood urea nitrogen as nitrogen balance becomes negative. Urea nitrogen appearance can be measured to estimate total nitrogen balance.
- *Electrolytes and minerals:* Some patients may require temporary dietary restriction of K^+ and/or Na^+. However, because of the risk of malnutrition, non-dietary contributors to hyperkalaemia should be considered before restricting dietary intake. Dietary phosphorus restriction is usually not a priority in AKI. Patients undergoing CRRT do not usually require dietary restrictions and many need full nutrition support. Patients receiving CRRT may develop hypokalaemia, hypophosphataemia, and hypomagnesaemia, and require

4 McClave SA et al. (2016). Guidelines for the provision and assessment of nutrition support herapy in the adult critically ill patient American Society for Parenteral and Enteral Nutrition and American Society for Critical Care Medicine (ASPEN - SCCM) *J. Parenter. Enteral Nutr.* **40**:159–211.

5 Patel JJ et al. (2017) Protein requirements for critically ill patients with renal and liver failure. *Nutr. Clin. Pract.* **32**:101S–111S.

supplementation. These are important metabolic derangements, especially in ventilated patients, as electrolyte depletion can lead to increasing muscle weakness, alterations in acid–base balance, and to further nephrotoxicity (especially tubular damage). Daily monitoring is necessary. At different stages of AKI, supplementation or restriction may be necessary, often determined by the catabolic state of the patient and the modality of dialysis (e.g. intermittent or continuous).

- *Fluid:* Not normally restricted on CRRT. Restrictions may be necessary if the patient is receiving IHD.

Kidney stones

Incidence
Kidney stones (nephrolithiasis or renal calculi) affect ~10% of men and ~5% of women in their lifetime. Significant differences in incidence are seen in different populations, suggesting genetic and/or environmental influences such as diet and climate. Populations of the developed world are more at risk with ↑ incidence seen in White > Asian and Hispanic > Black populations.

Stone formation
- Stone formation can occur anywhere in the kidney, ureter, or bladder.
- The size of stone can vary from microscopic to large 'staghorn' calculi and can lead to kidney failure if the kidney or urinary tract becomes obstructed.
- Stones vary in composition (Table 29.8).
- ↑ Urinary concentration of Ca^{++}, Na^+, oxalate, urate, and citrate promote stone formation and ↑ urinary concentration of Mg^{++}, pyrophosphate, citrate, and nephrocalcin inhibit stone formation.
- Stone formation can also be linked to congenital kidney abnormalities, short bowel syndrome or recurrent infection with urease positive organisms.
- About 50% of stone formers excrete ↑ urinary Ca^{++}, >7.5 mmol/day in men or >6.2 mmol/day in women. Hypercalciuria may be a result of ↑ absorption of Ca^{++} from the gut, Ca^{++} resorption from the bone, or ↓ ability of the kidney to reabsorb Ca^{++}.
- Stone formation is exacerbated by ↓ urine output volume because of low fluid intake or ↑ losses from the GI tract, e.g. intestinal failure.

Dietary treatment of kidney stones
The diet of people in the affluent world has been scrutinized with respect to intake of animal protein, Na^+, Ca^{++}, oxalate and purine. It appears that even with identical dietary intakes, people with a tendency to form stones will form larger crystals than non-stone formers.
- *Fluid:* 2–3 L/day (250 mL every 4 waking hours + 250 mL at meals).
- *Protein:* 1 g protein/kg ideal body weight.
- *Calcium:* restriction is not advised, 700–800 mg/day; hypercalciuria can be ↓ by ↑ alkali load (i.e. fruit/vegetables), dietary fibre, K^+, and PO_4;
- *Salt:* limit to <6 g/day.
- *Oxalates:* only 10–15% of urinary oxalate is derived from dietary intake while the rest is formed endogenously (from vitamin C and glycine metabolism); if 24 hour urinary oxalate is >440 mmol, check for ↑ oxalate foods (Table 29.9) and megadose intakes of vitamin C; pyridoxine supplements may ↑ stone formation.
- *Purines:* if 24 hour urinary uric acid is >4 mmol check for ↑ purine-containing foods (Table 29.10); orange juice may help prevent formation of uric acid stones as it is high in citrate without containing high oxalate.
- *Other:* ↑ intake of K^+, Mg^+, fibre, fruit, and vegetables is associated with ↓ stone risk; ↑ refined carbohydrate may ↑ risk.

Table 29.8 Main types of renal stone disease

Composition	Incidence (%)	Possible causes
Calcium oxalate: up to 50% may contain calcium hydroxyl phosphate	75	Idiopathic hypercalciuria 1° Hyperparathyroidism ↓ Urine citrate Hyperoxaluria Hyperuricosuria
Magnesium ammonium phosphate (struvite or triple phosphate)	10–20	Bacterial infection
Uric acid	5	Low urine pH Hyperuricosuria
Cystine	1–2	Cysteinuria

Table 29.9 Oxalate-rich foods*

Drinks	Beer, black tea, cocoa, juices from high oxalate fruits, instant coffee powder, Ovaltine
Fruit	Blackberries, blueberries, gooseberries, kiwi, raspberries, rhubarb, strawberries, tangerines
Vegetables	Beetroot, celery, green beans, leeks, okra, parsley, runner beans, spinach, sweet potato, watercress, yam
Legumes	Baked beans, soy products, e.g. tofu
Grains	Wheat germ, bran
Nuts and seeds	Almonds, cashews, peanuts, pecans, sesame seeds, sunflower seeds
Other	Plain chocolate, soy sauce

*Bioavailability varies.

Table 29.10 Purine-rich foods

Meat	Offal—liver and kidneys, heart and sweet-breads Game—pheasant, rabbit, venison
Fish	Anchovies, herring, mackerel, sardines, sprats, whitebait, trout, seafood, especially mussels, crab, shrimps and other shellfish, fish roe, caviar
Other	Meat and yeast extracts, e.g. Bovril, Marmite, commercial gravy, beer, alcohol

Useful websites

Guidelines

Joint British Diabetes Society for Inpatient Care (JBDS-IC) (2016). Available at: ℘ http://www.diabetologists-abcd.org.uk/JBDS/JBDS_RenalGuide_2016.pdf.

The Renal Association clinical guidelines. Available at: ℘ http://www.renal.org/guidelines/Introduction#sthash.CeOVQN4J.dpbs.

Department of Health (2004). National Service Framework for Renal Services. Available at: ℘ https://www.gov.uk/government/publications/national-service-framework-kidney-disease.

National Kidney Foundation—Kidney Disease Outcomes Quality Initiative (KDOQI). Available at: ℘ http://www.ajkd.org/content/kdoqiguidelines.

NICE (2015). Chronic kidney disease in adults: assessment and management. Available at: ℘ https://www.nice.org.uk/guidance/cg182.

Patient information

Kidney Research UK. Available at: ℘ http://www.kidneyresearchuk.org/health-information.

The Kidney Patient Guide. Available at: ℘ http://www.kidneypatientguide.org.uk/site/contents.php.

The Blood Pressure Association (includes information on exercise for those with ↓ mobility). Available at: ℘ http://bpa.jamkit.com/Home.

Respiratory disease and cystic fibrosis

Asthma 736
Chronic obstructive pulmonary disease 737
Other respiratory conditions 738
Cystic fibrosis 740

Asthma

The prevalence, morbidity, and mortality associated with asthma has increased worldwide over the last few decades. Rates in the UK are stable but approximately 5.4 million people currently receive treatment for asthma and ~1,500 people died from the condition in 2017. Asthma is associated with various non-dietary causes; diet may contribute in some people but is not a predominant cause. A healthy diet that is compatible with the Eatwell Guide (see ⊃ Chapter 2) is recommended. In addition, these dietary factors are relevant:

Fruit and vegetables A high intake is associated with ↓ risk of developing asthma and ↓ wheeze in children and adults with the condition.[1] Overall diet quality, including adequate fruit and vegetables, is associated with improved asthma symptoms in adults and this is independent of body mass index (BMI).[2] There is also evidence that following a Mediterranean-style diet is associated with lower risk of asthma-related outcomes in children.[3] These effects are probably mediated through adequate intakes of antioxidant micronutrients. There is no evidence that antioxidant supplements are beneficial.

Obesity Excess body weight, especially central obesity, is associated with ↑ risk of asthma, probably mediated through systemic and airway oxidative stress. Weight loss has been shown to ↓ respiratory symptoms in overweight people (see ⊃ Chapter 21, 'Weight management').

Salt A high intake of salt has been implicated in adversely effecting airway reactivity, but there is no evidence that reducing salt intake improves symptoms.[4] A healthy diet should provide <6 g total salt intake daily, including salt added to processed foods.

Food hypersensitivity

Cow's milk has been linked anecdotally to asthma but objective testing indicates that diet and food hypersensitivity is important in only a minority of individuals; in these, food avoidance can improve symptoms and ↓ drug therapy and hospital admission (see ⊃ Chapter 37 'Food hypersensitivity'). There is no evidence that feeding infants soya-based, rather than cow's milk, formula reduces the risk of having asthma; breastfeeding is recommended for at least the first 6 months of life and is associated with ↓ risk of asthma in children[5] (see ⊃ Chapter 13 'Breast versus bottle feeding', p. 262).

1 Seyedrezazadeh, E., et al. (2014). Fruit and vegetable intake and risk of wheezing and asthma: a systematic review and meta-analysis. *Nutr. Rev.* **72**, 411-28.

2 Li, Z., et al. (2017). Longitudinal study of diet quality and change in asthma symptoms in adults, according to smoking status. *Br. J. Nutr.* **117**, 562-71.

3 Garcia-Marcos, L., et al. (2013). Influence of Mediterranean diet on asthma in children: a systematic review and meta-analysis. *Pediatr. Allergy Immunol.* **24**, 330-8.

4 Pogson, Z., et al. (2011). Dietary sodium manipulation and asthma. *Cochrane Database Syst. Rev.* **3**, CD000436.

5 Lodge, C.J., et al. (2015). Breastfeeding and asthma and allergies: a systematic review and meta-analysis. *Acta Paediatr.* **104**, 38-53.

Chronic obstructive pulmonary disease

An estimated 1.2 million people in UK are living with diagnosed chronic obstructive pulmonary disease (COPD) and approximately 57,000 died from bronchitis, emphysema and other COPD in England and Wales in 2017. Non-dietary causes of COPD, especially smoking, are primarily implicated in the pathogenesis but overall diet score also contributes to risk of developing the condition.[6] In addition, both undernutrition and excessive body weight are adversely associated with clinical outcomes in COPD.

Undernutrition People with COPD are frequently malnourished (prevalence 10-60%) and this is associated with poor respiratory function, ↑ susceptibility to infection, and poor prognosis (relative risk for low BMI compared with high in people with severe COPD is 7.1 [95% CI: 3.0, 17.1]). Systematic review of studies evaluating nutritional support (dietary advice/ oral nutrition supplements) indicates that this is associated with improvement in anthropometric measures and grip strength.[7]

Obesity Some people with COPD are also obese, although the proportion varies with the population studies. They experience worse respiratory symptoms (dyspnoea and exercise limitation) and higher mortality[8,9] than healthy weight COPD sufferers, which may be mediated through ↑ inflammatory status. There is no evidence yet about the benefits of weight reduction in this population but it is reasonable to advise a nutritious diet without excessive energy.

Current clinical guidance[10] based on grade D evidence (non-analytical studies and expert opinion) advises that:
- BMI should be calculated in patients with COPD.
- Patients with BMI <20 or >25 kg/m² should be referred to a dietitian.
- If BMI is <20 kg/m², patients should be given nutritional supplements to ↑ energy intake and be encouraged to take exercise.
- In older patients, attention should also be paid to changes in weight, particularly if the change is more than 3 kg.

6 Varraso, R., *et al.* (2015). Alternate Healthy Eating Index 2010 and risk of chronic obstructive pulmonary disease among US women and men: prospective study. *BMJ* **350**, h286.

7 Collins, P.F., *et al.* (2012). Nutritional support in chronic obstructive pulmonary disease: a systematic review and meta-analysis. *Am. J. Clin. Nutr.* **95**, 1385-95.

8 Hanson, C., *et al.* (2014). Influence of diet and obesity on COPD development and outcomes. *Int. J. Chron. Obstruct. Pulmon. Dis.* **9**, 723-33.

9 Lambert, A.A., *et al.* (2017). Obesity is associated with increased morbidity in moderate to severe COPD. *Chest* **151**, 68-77.

10 National Institute for Health and Care Excellence (NICE) (2019). *Chronic obstructive pulmonary disease in over 16's: diagnosis and management.* NICE guideline 115. Available at: ℞ https://www.nice.org.uk/guidance/NG115.

Other respiratory conditions

Lung cancer

Lung cancer is the third most common cancer in the UK with approximately 47,000 new cases and 35,000 deaths per year. Worldwide, it is estimated that there are ~1.8 million new cases per year. Smoking contributes to 86% of cases. A higher intake of fruit and vegetables has a protective effect, which may be associated with their antioxidant content. However, trials of antioxidants vitamin A and β-carotene supplements do not yield the same benefits and are, in fact, associated with ↑ incidence of lung cancer and ↑ mortality so should be discouraged.[11] Eating fruit and vegetables, rather than taking supplements, is thus recommended (see ➔ Chapter 2 'Eatwell Guide').

Patients with lung cancer are often undernourished, especially in later stages. Nutrition support should be considered in the context of their treatment and prognosis (see ➔ Chapter 24 'Cancer').

Lung transplantation

Approximately 210 lung and heart-lung transplants are undertaken in the UK and 2,300 in the USA each year. Post-transplant risk of death is higher in underweight patients (↑ 15% [95% CI: 3%, 28%]) and in those who are overweight (↑ 15% [5%, 39%]) than those with a healthy weight.[12] Pre-surgical nutritional support has been shown to be effective in increasing body weight in underweight patients; nutritional assessment and advice before transplant may help improve outcome. Diabetes and osteoporosis are common problems following transplantation and pre-emptive dietary advice may help manage these (for comparable advice, see ➔ Chapter 28 'Liver transplantation', p. 700).

Tuberculosis

Worldwide, approximately 10 million people became ill with tuberculosis (TB) in 2018 and 1.5 million people died. In the UK in 2018, there were approximately 4,700 cases. Undernutrition is a risk factor for developing TB and weight loss is regarded as a classic symptom. Patients who are malnourished are at greater risk of dying than those who are not. Vitamin D influences immune response and deficiency is associated with ↑ risk.[13] Nutrition interventions may ↑ body weight but evidence of improved clinical outcomes is lacking at present.[14] People with TB and those at risk do not require a special diet, but are likely to benefit from an adequate and well-balanced intake.

11 Cranganu, A., et al. (2009). Nutrition aspects of lung cancer. Nutr. Clin. Pract. 24, 688–700.

12 Lederer, D.J., et al. Obesity and underweight are associated with an increased risk of death after lung transplantation. Am J. Respir. Crit. Care Med. 180, 887-95.

13 Huang, S.L., et al. (2016). Vitamin D deficiency and the risk of tuberculosis: a meta-analysis. Drug Des. Devel. Ther. 11, 91-102.

14 Grobler, L., et al. (2016). Nutritional supplements for people being treated for active tuberculosis. Cochrane Database Syst. Rev. 6, CD006086.

Cystic fibrosis

Approximately 70,000 people worldwide and 11,000 people in the UK have cystic fibrosis (CF), an autosomal recessively inherited disorder that affects the exocrine glands leading to pancreatic insufficiency and chronic lung disease. Weight loss and undernutrition are common problems and are associated with a worse clinical outcome. Recent advances in drug therapy have improved clinical outcomes; however, some older children and adults with CF have gained excess weight, requiring healthy eating guidance.

Causes of weight loss and undernutrition in CF

Impaired nutrient absorption Malabsorption occurs in ~85% of people with CF, i.e. 'pancreatic insufficient'. Inadequate secretion of pancreatic enzymes should be treated by replacement therapy but not dietary fat restriction (see ➔ Chapter 27, 'Pancreatic enzyme replacement therapy', p. 686). If adequate pancreatic enzymes are taken, a normal to high fat diet can be tolerated by almost all patients. ❶ Fat restriction is potentially harmful because it is associated with restricted energy intake. However, in a very small minority of cases where steatorrhoea cannot be controlled adequately in spite of appropriately taken high dose pancreatic supplements, a modest fat restriction should be tried *providing* that an adequate energy intake is maintained and the patient is closely monitored. People with CF who are 'pancreatic sufficient' tend to have fewer nutritional problems as absorption is not impaired.

Increased requirements Energy needs increase as a result of fat malabsorption and ↑ costs of respiration. It is estimated that energy requirements are 110–200% of those of healthy people.[15] Protein requirements are also likely to be ↑ as a result of ↑ nitrogen losses via the gut and sputum; there are no current guidelines for protein intake but intake should at least meet the reference nutrient intake (see Appendix 6, 'Dietary reference values'). Therefore, most people with CF need to consume ↑ energy, ↑ fat, ↑ protein intake plus micronutrient supplementation, see ➔ this chapter 'Nutritional management'.

Poor food intake Appetite may be poor as a result of tiredness and repeated chest infections. ↑ respiratory tract secretions may limit consumption of some supplement drinks. The nutrient density of the diet should be considered to ensure that requirements are met within the limited quantity of foods consumed. Encouraging positive eating behaviour can help improve intake.[16]

15 Cystic Fibrosis Trust (2016). Nutritional management of cystic fibrosis, 2nd edn. Available at: ℔ https://www.cysticfibrosis.org.uk/~/media/documents/the-work-we-do/care/consensus-documents-with-old-address/nutritional-management-of-cystic-fibrosis-sep-16.ashx?la=en.

16 Stark, L.J. et al. (2011). The effects of an intensive behavior and nutrition intervention compared to standard of care on weight outcomes in CF. *Pediatr. Pulmonol.* 46, 31–5.

Nutritional management

- All people with CF should have their nutritional status reviewed annually by an experienced CF dietitian and if admitted to hospital, should be reviewed by a CF dietitian at least twice per week or more frequently if appropriate.[15] Nutrient intake is significantly greater in CF patients when they are reviewed at least annually by a dietitian.
- Oral supplements. Although some patients may be able to consume sufficient ordinary food to meet their needs, others will benefit from home-made or commercial supplements (➔ Chapter 25 'Treatment of undernutrition', p. 568). However, these are not essential, and dietary advice and monitoring are equally important.[17]
- Enteral tube feeding. Supplementary or total enteral feeding may be needed for patients who are unable to maintain an adequate oral intake in the long-term or for shorter periods following an exacerbation of respiratory problems. It is particularly beneficial in children, in whom overnight feeding for 6 months is associated with improved nutritional status and catch-up growth.
  - Feeding can either be via nasogastric (tubes can be passed nightly) or gastrostomy (see ➔ Chapter 25 'Routes for enteral feeding', p. 574). Feeding regimens should take account of the higher requirements in CF and if supplementary feeding, aim to provide 30–50% of energy needs (but check that oral intake is able to provide the rest).
  - Energy dense feeds may be useful, i.e. 1.5-2.4 kcal/mL, but otherwise general feeding guidelines relevant to the age of the patient should be followed.
  - Pancreatic enzyme replacement may be given orally before feeding commences, but fat content is often tolerated well because the feed is delivered slowly over several hours. If enzymes are required but cannot be taken orally, seek expert advice.
  - Insulin may be required if feeding results in hyperglycaemia.
  - Encouraging intake during the day, i.e. between overnight feeds, helps ↑ resumption of oral intake and social aspects of feeding.
- Fat soluble vitamin status should be checked at least annually in all patients, i.e. plasma levels of vitamins A, D, and E plus prothrombin time to assess adequacy of vitamin K. Most patients are considered to require supplementation, especially in pancreatic insufficiency (Table 30.1), although five recent Cochrane systematic reviews (2014-17) of supplementation with vitamins A, D, E, and K and antioxidants in CF have not identified clinical benefit or harm.

17 Smyth, R.L. et al. (2012). Oral calorie supplements for cystic fibrosis. *Cochrane Database Syst. Rev.* **10**, CD000406.

Table 30.1 Recommendations for daily intake and monitoring of fat-soluble vitamins in cystic fibrosis

Vitamin	Age	Intake/day[15]	Monitoring[18]
A mg [IU]	1–12 months	0.45 [<1,500]	Serum retinol (deficiency <20 µg/dL)
	>1 year	0.45–3.0 [1,500–10,000]	Retinol binding protein
			Zinc level
D µg [IU]	0–12 months	10–50 [400–2,000]	Serum 25 (OH) vitamin D in late autumn/winter
	>1 year	10–125 [400–5,000]	
E IU	0–12 months	40–80	Serum α-tocopherol
	1–3 years	50–150	
	4–7 years	150–300	
	>8 years/adult	150–500	
K	<2 years	300 µg/kg	Prothrombin time
	2–7 years	5 mg	Protein induced by vitamin K absence or antagonist II (PIVKA II)
	>7 years/adult	5–10 mg	

Infants with CF

- Ideally, CF babies should be breastfed (associated with better pulmonary function if ≥4 months breastfeeding). Those with pancreatic insufficiency (PI) require pancreatic enzymes with each feed. Enzyme dose should be adjusted individually to optimize absorption.
- If breastfeeding is not possible/preferred, regular infant formulae can be given, again with pancreatic enzymes in PI.
- Pancreatic enzymes as microspheres should be mixed with a little breastmilk or formula and given to the infant on a spoon. For larger feeds, split the dose and give at start and during feed; check that microspheres do not remain in the mouth after feeding. Enzymes should not be given with formula milk in a bottle or feeder.
- Sodium supplements may be required because of ↑ losses. Requirements should be assessed on an individual basis taking into account Na⁺ loss from the GI tract.
- Some infants with higher energy requirements may need additional supplementation. This should be undertaken with the advice of a registered dietitian with paediatric CF experience.

18 Munck, A. (2010). Nutritional considerations in patients with cystic fibrosis. *Expert Rev. Resp. Med.* **41**, 47–56.

Complicating factors

CF and diabetes mellitus

Approximately 20% of adolescents and up to 50% of adults with CF develop diabetes, and dietary advice for the two conditions needs to be combined with individualized dietary education. It is imperative to maintain an adequate energy intake so fat should not be restricted (unless overweight) but some saturated fat can be replaced by monounsaturates. As a bulky, ↑ carbohydrate diet may not be practical for those with a small appetite, foods contributing refined carbohydrate should not be restricted but eaten in conjunction with other items to dissipate the glycaemic effect and insulin prescribed if necessary.

CF and liver disease

Hepatic steatosis occurs in 25-75% of CF patients but is considered a relatively benign condition. However, it progresses to cirrhosis in approximately 5-15% of cases and in these, malnutrition is a frequent problem. Energy requirements increase by an additional 20-40%. Additional problems with malabsorption may occur if bile composition is altered or output is ↓ and this cannot be remedied by ↑ pancreatic enzyme supplementation. If it becomes necessary to ↓ fat intake (and this should be avoided if possible), then an adequate energy intake must be maintained using carbohydrate and protein sources. Liver transplantation may be necessary and usually leads to an improvement in pulmonary function, as well as restoration of liver function.

Further information

Cystic Fibrosis Trust (2016) Nutritional management of cystic fibrosis, 2nd edn. Available at: ℬ https://www.cysticfibrosis.org.uk/~/media/documents/the-work-we-do/care/consensus-documents-with-old-address/nutritional-management-of-cystic-fibrosis-sep-16.ashx?la=en.

Morton, A.M. (2009). The nutritional challenges of the young adult with cystic fibrosis: transition. Proc. Nutr. Soc. 68, 430–40.

Munck, A. (2010). Nutritional considerations in patients with cystic fibrosis. Expert Rev. Resp. Med. 41, 47–56.

Human immunodeficiency virus (HIV) infection

Introduction, nutritional goals, and assessment 746
Unintentional weight and lean tissue loss 748
Cardiovascular risk and complications associated with HIV
    disease and treatment 749
Additional dietary issues 750

Introduction, nutritional goals, and assessment

Introduction

Untreated human immunodeficiency virus (HIV) infection leads to progressive suppression of immune function, eventually rendering the body susceptible to opportunistic infections and tumours. Although there is no cure, antiretroviral therapy (ART) is highly effective in suppressing HIV replication. HIV disease is now a chronic condition, and typical cause of death in this population has shifted from traditional AIDS(Acquired Immune Deficiency Syndrome)-related illnesses to non-AIDS events, the most common being atherosclerotic cardiovascular disease, liver disease, end-stage renal disease, and non-AIDS-defining malignancies. There is a diverse range of nutritional conditions associated with HIV, reflecting the complexity of the disease, pharmacological management, and an emerging burden of co-morbidities as people living with HIV grow older. Indeed, in well-resourced countries the majority of people living with HIV are now overweight or obese.

- Malnutrition and HIV have similar deleterious effects on immune function (such as reduced CD4 and CD8 lymphocyte cells).
- Decreased nutritional status in people with HIV infection is associated with disease progression, increased morbidity, and reduced survival independent of immunodeficiency and viral load.
- Weight loss, specifically wasting, is an important predictor of HIV progression to AIDS and to death.
- Optimal intake of energy, protein, and micronutrients may help augment immune function.
- At present, there is no evidence of benefit from nutrition interventions because of the limited studies undertaken.[1]
- In people living with HIV, treatment of metabolic co-morbidities may be more challenging, therefore risk assessment and prevention measures should be undertaken

Nutritional goals

- Prevent and treat unintentional weight and lean tissue loss.
- Manage symptoms and complications associated with HIV disease and treatment.
- Promote good health, adherence to treatment, and prevent nutritional deficiencies.
- Reduce risk for or treat metabolic co-morbidities including cardiovascular disease, type 2 diabetes, and loss of bone mineral density.

1 Grobler, L., et al. (2013). Nutritional interventions for reducing morbidity and mortality in people with HIV. *Cochrane Database Syst. Rev.* **2**, CD004536. DOI: 10.1002/14651858.CD004536.pub3.

Nutritional assessment

This should be undertaken regularly including:

- Detailed diet history. Extending the diet history to include patterns and timing of intake can identify challenges associated with adherence to antiretroviral therapy regimens.
- Check for intake of nutritional supplements and complementary or alternative medicines as these have potential to interfere with antiretroviral metabolism.
- Height.
- Weight.
- Body mass index (BMI).
- Skin-fold measurements and circumferences (see ➲ Chapter 4, 'Anthropometry', p. 54) are useful to monitor body composition and shape changes linked to HIV disease and ART, i.e. HIV-associated lipodystrophy syndrome.
- Head circumference (infants and children under 2 years).

Unintentional weight and lean tissue loss

This remains a significant complication in the era of effective ART. The aetiology is multifactorial, with the main precipitating factors being:
- reduced nutritional intake;
- altered metabolic requirements;
- malabsorption.

Management

Optimization of ART and treatment of underlying conditions and opportunistic infections are priorities. Nutritional status and requirements should be assessed using standard methods, adjusting for HIV and any opportunistic infections.
- Aim to ↑ energy and protein intake.
- Encourage small, frequent, nutritious meals, snacks, and drinks.
- Appropriate use of proprietary energy and protein supplements.
- Symptoms such as nausea, vomiting, diarrhoea, taste changes, and anorexia must be identified and treated (see ➲ Chapter 24, 'Cancer treatment', p. 546).
- Artificial nutrition support should be considered if nutritional needs are not met orally despite intervention.
- Nasogastric for short-term support.
- Percutaneous endoscopic gastrostomy (PEG) for longer term intervention (see ➲ Chapter 25, 'Routes for enteral feeding', p. 574).
- Parenteral nutrition is indicated in cases where it is not possible to feed via the gastrointestinal tract (see ➲ Chapter 25, 'Parenteral nutrition', p. 594).
- Resistance exercise has been successfully used as a safe, cost-effective method of promoting lean body mass, resulting in gains equal to those achieved through administration of anabolic steroids ± testosterone supplements.

Cardiovascular risk and complications associated with HIV disease and treatment

A higher prevalence of ↓ bone mineral density, vitamin D deficiency, insulin resistance, hypertension, hepatic steatosis, and ↑ cardiovascular risk has been reported in HIV positive people compared to individuals who are HIV negative.

Known metabolic and morphological disturbances associated with HIV infection and treatment may include:

- *Dyslipidaemia:* ↑ total and LDL cholesterol and triglycerides, ↓ HDL cholesterol.
- Insulin resistance, hyperglycaemia, and poorer outcomes in diabetes management.
- Bone demineralization.
- Visceral, breast, and dorso-cervical fat accumulation.
- Lipoatrophy: loss of subcutaneous fat from limbs, buttocks, and face.

Management

Careful choice of ART, nutritional screening and assessment, and appropriate nutritional advice may help prevent long-term complications.

- There is an association between excessive weight gain when initiating ART and later development of metabolic co-morbidities. Those initiating ART should receive dietetic monitoring and intervention.
- Patients should have regular physical, biochemical, and detailed monitoring of dietary intake for signs of development of metabolic side effects and for risk of developing coronary heart, disease, diabetes, and bone demineralization.
- Advice should be based on the 'Eatwell Guide' (➲ Chapter 2, p. 27).
- Those with hyperlipidaemia or ↑ risk of CVD, diabetes, or osteoporosis should receive more intensive dietary advice.
- Exercise should be encouraged as it may benefit metabolic variables and abdominal shape.
- Limited evidence suggests that ↑ fibre diets are associated with a ↓ risk of developing central fat deposition.
- Additional modifiable risk factors to address include smoking, hypertension, and obesity.
- Dietary treatment of diabetes should follow current guidelines (see ➲ Chapter 22, 'Goals and principles of dietary management', p. 502). Note: HbA1c may be underestimated in those prescribed ART.
- Weight-reducing advice may help reduce visceral adiposity.

Achieving good health and nutritional status

Good dietary intake and a healthy lifestyle may be particularly important for people living with HIV as they have a higher risk of ill-health compared to those not infected. Good nutrition and a regular meal pattern may help maintain a healthy body weight, avoid long-term complications, and promote good adherence to treatment.

Additional dietary issues

Prevention of mother-to-child transmission of HIV

Most children become infected with HIV through mother-to-child transmission during pregnancy, delivery, or breastfeeding. Prevention of mother-to-child-transmission programmes have significantly reduced this to <1%.

In the UK and other well-resourced countries, where there is access to safe, clean water and where milk substitutes are affordable and easily available, avoidance of breastfeeding by women living with HIV is recommended to prevent transmission of HIV via this route (see ➜ Chapter 13, 'Contraindications to breastfeeding', p. 263).

❶ This advice does not apply in countries where there is no uninterrupted access to infant formula milk and clean water and where other specific conditions are not met. According to WHO Guidelines:

- Exclusive breastfeeding is recommended for infants born to women living with HIV for the first 6 months of life.
- Complementary foods should be introduced at age 6 months and breastfeeding should continue for 12 months in environments where replacement feeding is not appropriate.
- Breastfeeding should only stop when a nutritionally adequate and safe diet can be provided without breastmilk.

Children living with human immune virus

In children, HIV disease has a more rapid progression to AIDS compared to adults, and their immature immune systems make them more vulnerable to opportunistic infections. Children infected with HIV may have increased energy requirements of around 10% and while recovering from illness this may increase by 50–100% above requirements of healthy, uninfected children. Conversely, others may be well-nourished and at risk of becoming obese.

Maintaining adequate growth is a priority. Nutritional screening and assessment, including height, weight, anthropometry, and blood lipids, should be part of routine care, and care plans should include the following considerations:

- Encourage healthy eating appropriate to age and nutritional status.
- Medication, including drug interactions with food.
- Disease state.
- Growth and development.
- Activity level.
- Social and financial aspects including housing, cooking facilities.
- Physical and mental health of other family members.
- Confidentiality issues that may prevent families from making use of local health services.
- Cultural background, including traditional foods.

A multi-disciplinary approach to care planning is essential.

Food and drug interactions

Presence or absence of food in the gut may affect drug absorption or modify risk of side effects. Some ART regimens involve food restrictions and requirements. It is important to refer to the manufacturer's current information. See also ➲ Chapter 38, 'Drug–nutrient interactions' and ➲ this chapter, 'Further reading'.

Alternative therapies and drug interactions

Although the majority of alternative treatments are generally safe, there are potential interactions between some herbal and botanical products with ART and other medications that may have serious consequences for treatment success. Clinicians should routinely ask patients about their use of herbal remedies, vitamins and minerals, and alternative treatments.

Food and water safety

Food and water-borne infection is more common in the immunocompromised host. Good food hygiene[2] and avoidance of high-risk foods (e.g. raw/undercooked eggs, unpasteurized milk products, raw/undercooked meat and fish) are advisable.

When food and water-borne infections do occur, it is important that patients see a health worker without delay to minimize illness and avoid weight loss and nutritional impairment.

Further reading

Pribram, V. (2010). *Nutrition and HIV*. Wiley-Blackwell, Oxford.

University of Liverpool (2020) HIV drug interaction checker. Available at: ℘ http://www.hiv-druginteractions.org/.

2 For further information on food hygiene, see resources available from NHS. ℘ https://www.nhs.uk/conditions/food-poisoning/.

Nutrition in mental health

Introduction 754
Pharmacotherapy in mental health 756
Who can contribute to nutritional care in mental health? 758
Nutrition in specific mental health conditions 760
Developmental disorders 764
Eating disorders 768
Dementia 774
Mental Capacity Act (MCA) 2005 778

Introduction

Nutrition interacts with and influences mental health in a comparable way to physical health: a 'healthy and varied diet' can help promote mental wellbeing while an inadequate or excessive intake of food or specific nutrients can have a detrimental effect on mental health (Fig. 32.1). The duration and impact of nutritional effects vary depending on the life stage.

The Community Mental Health Survey (2018) reports that one in six adults has experiences a mental health condition in any given year. The interrelationship between mental health and nutrition includes a diverse range of topics ranging from those close to 'normal' healthy behaviour to the 'extremes' of mental ill health (see Table 32.1).

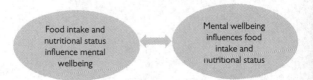

Food intake and nutritional status influence mental wellbeing

Mental wellbeing influences food intake and nutritional status

Fig. 32.1 Relationship between wellbeing and nutritional status.

Table 32.1 Relationship between mood and eating*

Mood disorder and symptoms	Potential nutrition consequences
Depression	
Loss of appetite	Inadequate/inappropriate intake
Anhedonia, apathy, and disinterest in food	Compromised nutritional status
	Weight loss/gain
Altered sleep patterns, inadequate or excessive sleeping, including during the day	Tiredness/lack of concentration
	Dehydration
	Constipation
Tiredness—unable to cook	
Loss of thirst sensation	
Food craving/erratic eating habits	
Comfort eating	
Anxiety	
Restlessness/hyperactivity	↑ Energy expenditure
Dry mouth	Inadequate/excessive intake
Nausea, vomiting, diarrhoea	Difficulty chewing and swallowing
Loss of appetite	Compromised nutritional status
Food refusal	Weight loss/gain
Comfort eating	Tiredness/lack of concentration

* Note. Many of the nutritional consequences will contribute to the symptoms and potentially exacerbate them, e.g. tiredness in depression is associated with poor food intake → inadequate ingestion of energy and nutrients → further tiredness.

Pharmacotherapy in mental health

Drugs used in treating mental health problems may influence food intake and/or nutritional status. It should not be assumed that every patient taking medication will experience any or all of the side effects associated with specific drugs. When side effects arise, they are sometimes managed by adjusting the dose or changing prescription to a similar preparation that may be better tolerated. However, as some pharmacotherapy is long-term, e.g. taken for many years, there may be nutritional implications that require intervention (see Box 32.1).

Box 32.1 Examples of possible nutrition-related side effects associated with selected drugs used to treat mental illness

Antidepressants
- Tricyclic antidepressants, e.g. dosulepin, → dry mouth, sour metallic taste, constipation.
- Selective serotonin re-uptake inhibitors (SSRIs) (5-hydroxy-tryptamine, 5-HT), e.g. fluoxetine, → dose-related side effects including diarrhoea, constipation, dyspepsia, abdominal pain, nausea, vomiting.
- Monoamine oxidase inhibitors (MAOI), e.g. phenelzine, → patients taking these drugs should avoid foods containing high levels of tyramine, e.g. mature cheese, yeast extracts, soya bean products, pickled herring, and certain wines (see ⮕ Chapter 38, 'Drug–nutrient interactions').

Antipsychotics
- Atypical antipsychotics, e.g. clozapine, olanzapine, → ↑ appetite, ↓ satiety, weight gain, hyperglycaemia, diabetes, dyslipidaemia (hypercholesterolaemia; hypertriglyceridaemia), drowsiness, dry mouth, constipation. Clozapine side effects include hypersalivation, impairment of intestinal peristalsis, including constipation, intestinal obstruction, faecal impaction, and paralytic ileus (including fatal cases) reported.
- Thioxanthenes, e.g. flupentixol decanoate (used as depot injection), → ↑ appetite, weight gain, hyperglycaemia, dry mouth, constipation, drowsiness.

Mood stabilizers
- Lithium salts, e.g. lithium carbonate, → nausea, dry mouth, dysgeusia, metallic taste (~ mild, controlled by adjusting dose); electrolyte imbalance: serum electrolytes must be checked (see ⮕ Chapter 38, 'Drug–nutrient interactions'), oedema, weight changes, including weight gain.

Anticonvulsants
- Sodium valproate → sleepiness, increased appetite and weight gain, nausea.
- Carbamazepine → tiredness, abdominal pain, nausea, diarrhoea, constipation.
- Barbiturates, e.g. phenobarbital*, → ↓ vitamin D levels, ↓ folate levels; e.g. phenytoin* → ↓ vitamin D absorption, ↑ turnover, and ↓ absorption of folate

* No longer first choice of treatment but many patients continue to take it.

Who can contribute to nutritional care in mental health?

The vast majority of people with mental health problems live in the community, some autonomously and others requiring considerable support. Obtaining, preparing, and eating a well-balanced diet can be a challenge, and poor diet can exacerbate both short-term symptoms and the risk of chronic health problems associated with mental illness. It is well-documented that people with serious mental illness (SMI), including schizophrenia, bipolar disorder, and major depression, die 10-15 years earlier than the general population. This is largely a result of cardiovascular disease, including heart disease, heart attack, and stroke. A meta-analysis[1] of SMI and cardiovascular disease, which included >3.2 million patients and >113 million people from the general population, reported that the risk of dying from cardiovascular disease was 85% higher in people with SMI than people of a similar age in the general population. Underlying causes may be multiple and include long-term antipsychotic use, adverse lifestyle choices such as smoking, poor diet, and physical inactivity and obesity.

In addition to family, carers, health professionals in primary care, and the community mental health team should be aware of nutritional risk and needs and plan care to manage nutritional concerns. Health professionals should receive training in up-to-date evidenced-based healthy eating and use a motivational approach and appropriate goal setting to help ensure that people with mental illness are given the best support possible with regards to their nutritional care. Dietitians are well-placed to guide other healthcare professionals and support workers with appropriate nutrition training and use of supporting resources to optimize their clients' nutritional status. Referral to dietetic services is required for therapeutic dietary management of physical health co-morbidities, e.g. undernutrition, nutritional deficiencies (i.e. anaemia), overweight, obesity, diabetes, dyslipidaemia, and metabolic syndrome. In addition to considering the health benefits associated with the nutrients supplied by food, the pleasure of eating and the empowerment associated with preparing an edible meal can also make a valuable contribution. Occupational therapists are trained to assess life skills and to provide support with budgeting, shopping and cooking.

1 Correll, C.U., *et al.* (2017). Prevalence, incidence and mortality from cardiovascular disease in patients with pooled and specific severe mental illness: a large-scale meta-analysis of 3,211,768 patients and 113,383,368 controls. *World Psychiatry* 16, 163–180.

Nutrition in specific mental health conditions

Depression

Depression, or major depressive disorder, can be termed mild, moderate, or severe and may include feelings of anxiety. A person may comfort eat, which can lead to unhealthy weight gain or they may experience a loss of appetite with associated weight loss. When severely depressed, most people eat and drink poorly and are at risk of weight loss, becoming underweight, undernourished, and at risk of dehydration.

- Low levels of neurotransmitters, e.g. serotonin, dopamine, noradrenaline, and γ-amino butyric acid (GABA), are observed in depression. Dietary sources of neurotransmitter-precursors, e.g. tryptophan, tyrosine, and phenylalanine may facilitate transmitter production with antidepressant effects. Systematic review[2] indicates that supplements of 5-hydroxy tryptophan or tryptophan are better than placebos at alleviating depression, but insufficient evidence is available to recommend supplementation. Eating a 'normal' varied diet will provide physiological doses.
- Omega-3 fatty acids may also play a role in neurotransmission via their conversion into prostaglandins and leukotrienes or through affecting signal transduction in brain cells. A meta-analysis[3] has found evidence of benefit from omega-3 supplementation (daily doses ~0.1–6.0 g of n-3) in people diagnosed with depression. The benefits seem greater when supplementing higher doses of eicosapentaenoic acid (EPA) and when given as an adjunct therapy together with antidepressants. High doses of EPA will require use of omega-3 supplements without vitamin A and D added to avoid potential toxic intakes of these vitamins.
- People with depression are more likely to have a ↓ intake and ↓ plasma markers of B vitamins. This may be a consequence of poor intake 2° to depressed appetite or co-morbidities rather than causative. Intervention studies are required to identify any potential benefit from supplements.
- Existing evidence suggests that a combination of healthful dietary practices may reduce the risk of developing depression.[4]
- An RCT of an adjunctive dietary intervention was used in treatment of moderate to severe depression using healthy eating guidelines and the Mediterranean diet. The dietary support group showed significantly greater improvement in depression symptoms than the control group and 32% achieved remission compared to 8% in the controls.[5]

2 Shaw, K.A., *et al.* (2009). Tryptophan and 5-hydroxytryptophan for depression. *Cochrane Database Syst. Rev.* CD003198.

3 Appleton, K.M., *et al.* (2010). Updated systematic review and meta-analysis of the effects of n-3 long-chain polyunsaturated fatty acids on depressed mood. *Am. J. Clin. Nutr.* 91, 757–70.

4 Opie, R.S., *et al.* (2016). Dietary recommendations for the prevention of depression. *Nutr. Neurosci.* 20, 161-71.

5 Jacka, F.N. *et al.* (2017). A randomised controlled trial of dietary improvement for adults with major depression (the 'SMILES' trial). *BMC Med.* 15, 23.

Bipolar affective disorder

Bipolar is a complex psychiatric disorder usually treated with mood-stabilizing medication.

- Omega-3 fatty acids play a key role in maintaining 'fluidity' of cell membranes, which influences neurotransmitter receptor function. Addressing relative depletion of omega-3s has been investigated as a potential treatment for bipolar disorder. Systematic review[6] of clinical trials has indicated that omega-3 supplementation is safe and may be useful as adjunctive therapy for depressive but not for manic symptoms. Further studies are required before recommendations can be made.
- A number of studies have investigated the effects of a range of water-soluble vitamins and amino acid supplements in bipolar disorder but without definitive evidence.

Schizophrenia

Patients with schizophrenia usually suffer from hallucinations, paranoia, delusions, and malfunctioning speech or thought.

- Impaired amino acid metabolism, and specifically reduced serotonin synthesis, has been associated with the pathophysiology. Limited evidence indicates that amino acid supplements may reduce some schizophrenic symptoms without adverse effects.
- Several studies have investigated the effects of omega-3 fatty acids in patients with schizophrenia, but systematic review[7] of these has concluded that there is still insufficient good quality and independent evidence on which to base recommendations for supplementation.
- Patients with psychotic disorders, including schizophrenia, have significantly lower levels of vitamin D compared to healthy controls with >50% deficient in vitamin D. Research findings suggest an association between vitamin D and psychotic disorders. However, the relevance of this deficiency remains unclear.[8]
- Weight gain is associated with antipsychotic drugs prescribed for schizophrenia (see ➲ this chapter 'Pharmacotherapy in mental health'. NICE guidance[9,10] recommends that nutritional assessment, including weight, waist circumference, diet, and physical activity, should be evaluated before commencing antipsychotic medication. NICE endorses the Lester UK Adaptation: Positive Cardiometabolic Health Resource developed by the Royal College of Psychiatrists, which is an intervention

6 Montgomery, P., Richardson, A.J. (2009). Omega-3 fatty acids for bipolar disorder. *Cochrane Database Syst. Rev.* CD005169.

7 Irving, C., *et al.* (2010). Polyunsaturated fatty acid supplementation for schizophrenia. *Cochrane Database Syst. Rev.*, CD001257.

8 Adamson, J., *et al.* (2017). Correlates of vitamin D in psychotic disorders: A comprehensive systematic review. *Psychiatry Res.* 249, 78–85.

9 National Institute for Health and Care Excellence (NICE) (2014). *Psychosis and schizophrenia in adults: prevention and management.* Available at: ℛ http://www.nice.org.uk/guidance/cg178.

10 National Institute for Health and Care Excellence (NICE) (2013). *Psychosis and schizophrenia in children and young people: recognition and management.* Available at: ℛ https://www.nice.org.uk/guidance/cg155.

framework for people experiencing psychosis and schizophrenia.[11] It highlights the need to not only screen for cardiometabolic risk but also to intervene and monitor to manage identified risks where indicated.

- Constipation is a common and notable side effect 2° to antipsychotic use and is often unreported by patients unless prompted. Severity can range from mild constipation to fatal bowel obstruction. Constipation has been found in up to 80% of patients taking clozapine and 50% of patients taking other antipsychotics.[12]

Obsessive compulsive disorder (OCD)

OCD is an anxiety disorder and a common mental health condition. About 1.2% of the population have OCD at some point in their lives. It is estimated that there are ~750,000 people living with OCD at any one time in the UK, with half being categorized as severe cases. OCD affects men, women, and children, and can develop at any age.

A person with OCD experiences re-occurring obsessive thoughts, which can be distressing and cause the person to feel anxious. These are followed by related compulsive behaviours to try to manage these thoughts and reduce anxiety levels. These repetitive behaviours can become time-consuming and all-encompassing, and adversely affect the life of the sufferer and their loved ones.

In general, a person's OCD will fall into one of the four main categories:

- checking;
- contamination/mental contamination;
- hoarding;
- ruminations/intrusive thoughts.

Nutritional impact of OCD

- Underweight, undernutrition, and specific nutritional deficiencies can develop e.g. anaemia because of low iron, folate, and/or vitamin B_{12}. This can result from difficulties obtaining food, i.e. going out shopping, food handling, preparation, and cooking (because of contamination concerns, rituals involving preparing food); rituals around eating are time-consuming and take priority over eating; avoidance of foods considered at risk of contamination or only consuming pre-packaged/sealed items drinks.
- Complaints of gastrointestinal (GI) disturbance are likely to be associated with anxiety but can include diagnosis of irritable bowel syndrome; may lead to avoiding many foods fearing an adverse gut reaction leading to inadequate nutrition.
- Co-morbid conditions can add additional nutritional challenges, i.e. eating disorders (restricting calories and food variety), depression (loss of appetite or comfort eating which can lead to overweight), and autistic spectrum disorder (limited array of foods eaten).

11 Available at: ℛhttps://www.nice.org.uk/guidance/cg178/resources/endorsed-resources-lester-uk-adaptation-positive-cardiometabolic-health-resource-556234093.

12 Every-Palmer, S., et al. (2016). Clozapine-treated patients have marked gastrointestinal hypomotility, the probable basis of life-threatening gastrointestinal complications: A cross sectional study. *EBioMedicine* 5, 125-34.

Treatment of OCD

- Cognitive behavioural therapy (CBT) with exposure and response prevention.
- Selective serotonin re-uptake inhibitors (SSRIs) provide effective pharmacological treatment of OCD. Therefore, in theory, foods which ↑ serotonin levels may also provide some benefit. There is no evidence to support this at present.
- NICE guidance for OCD includes body dysmorphic disorder but does not refer to diet, nutrition, or food.[13]

13 National Institute for Health and Care Excellence (NICE) (2005). *Obsessive-compulsive disorder and body dysmorphic disorder: treatment.* Available at: ℛhttp://www.nice.org.uk/guidance/CG31.

Developmental disorders

Autism spectrum disorders

There are around 700,000 people on the autistic spectrum in the UK which is >1 in 100. It is diagnosed in more men than women.

People with autism spectrum disorders (ASD) can have an intellectual ability ranging from a severe learning disability to being academically 'mainstream'; ~10% may also have special skills or abilities. Asperger's syndrome is used to describe those with ASD who have an ability to function at a higher level. The characteristics of the conditions vary between individuals and with time, but can be summarized as:

- difficulties with communication;
- difficulties with social interaction;
- difficulties with behaviour, interests, and activities.

Common co-morbidities include anxiety disorders, OCD, depression, GI disorders, sleep disorders, epilepsy, other neurological conditions, and allergies.

Pathogenesis

The exact cause of ASD is unknown, but a combination of genetic and environmental factors is thought to contribute to changes in brain development. It is unknown whether nutrition is causally implicated.

Common eating/food-related challenges in ASD

- Mealtimes can be stressful because of hypersensitivity to noise, smells, or bright lights. Eating with others may be difficult for some, whereas others may find company at mealtimes helpful. Eating with the TV or radio on, and having set eating times and visual timetables can be helpful.
- Eating a very limited range of foods can potentially lead to nutritional deficiencies and, in young people, to poor bone health and faltering growth. Food colour may influence its acceptability.
- Foods which are predictably the same, e.g. baked beans, are commonly selected and choices may be brand-specific. Some foods are rejected because of their texture or serving with sauce. There may be 'rules' around eating, e.g. different foods must not touch on the plate.
- Sensitive, graded exposure to different foods as well as treatment for related anxiety disorders affecting eating can be helpful.
- Adverse gut symptoms such as constipation, diarrhoea, and stomach bloating may be experienced. Promoting high fibre foods, wholegrains, fruits and vegetables, drinking enough fluid, and being active can help.

Nutrition as treatment

Diet has been investigated as a possible treatment of ASD, particularly as nutritional status plays a vital role in normal brain development.[14]

14 National Institute for Health and Care Excellence (NICE) (2016). *Autism spectrum disorder in adults: diagnosis and management.* Available at: ℜ https://www.nice.org.uk/guidance/cg142.

- *Micronutrient supplementation:* the potential benefits of vitamin B_6 and magnesium supplements have been investigated in 33 trials. However, systematic review[15] has concluded that these do not provide sufficient evidence on which to base recommendations and that further large, well-designed studies are needed.
- *Diets focusing on possible GI co-morbidity:* links between GI tract symptoms and autism have led to evaluation of diets that might alleviate these including gluten- and casein-free diets and food elimination diets. Although there is some evidence[16,17] to support a link between GI epithelial changes and altered immune response in ASD, the dietary benefits are predominantly anecdotal or from small or methodologically limited studies. NICE guidance recommends that exclusion diets, e.g. gluten- or casein-free, should not be used in autism.[18] This is important because some people with ASD may already eat a limited range of foods so further restricting their diet potentially increases the risk of nutritional deficiencies, which could lead to severe weight loss and, in young people, adversely affect growth.
- *Omega-3 fatty acids:* on the basis of their role in brain development and contribution to cell membrane integrity, >100 studies have investigated the role of omega-3s in ASD. However, on systematic review,[19] this number was reduced to one randomized controlled trial that showed a small, but non-significant improvement associated with ~1.5 g/day over 6 weeks. NICE guidance recommends that omega-3 fatty acids are not used to manage sleep problems in autism.[18]

Further reading

Dietitians in Autism: ℘ http://www.dietitiansmentalhealthgroup.org.uk/autism
Food and Behaviour Research: ℘ www.fabresearch.org
National Autistic Society: ℘ www.autism.org.uk
Research Autism: ℘ www.researchautism.net

Attention deficit hyperactivity disorder (ADHD)

ADHD, or hyperkinetic disorder, is a syndrome characterized by hyperactivity, impulsivity, and inattention. People with ADHD may exhibit all of these symptoms or predominantly more of one and less of another. Symptoms vary in severity and only those with significant impairment meet criteria for a diagnosis of ADHD. Symptoms of ADHD can overlap with symptoms of other related disorders.

15 Nye, C., Brice, A. (2009). Combined vitamin B6-magnesium treatment in autism spectrum disorder. *Cochrane Database Syst. Rev.*, CD003497.pub2.

16 Isherwood, E., Thomas, K. (2011). *Dietary management of autism spectrum disorder: Professional consensus statement.* British Dietetic Association, Birmingham.

17 Srinivasan, P. (2009). A review of dietary interventions in autism. *Ann. Clin. Psychol.* **21**, 237–47.

18 National Institute for Health and Care Excellence (NICE) (2013). *Autism spectrum disorder in under 19s: support and management.* Available at: ℘ http://www.nice.org.uk/guidance/cg170.

19 Bent, S., *et al.* (2009). Omega-3 fatty acids for autistic spectrum disorder: A systematic review. *J. Autism Dev. Disord.* **39**, 1145–54.

Pathogenesis

The exact cause of ADHD is unclear but a combination of genetic and environmental factors is thought to contribute to changes in brain development. High coffee intake *in utero* has been suggested as a contributory cause, but epidemiological studies have not identified this as an independent risk factor.

Nutrition as treatment

The role of diet has been investigated as a possible treatment of ADHD with little success:

- *Artificial colouring and additives:* many studies have investigated the benefits of eliminating these from the diet. Current guidance recommends that this should not be a routine treatment.[20] However, clinical assessment should include questions about food and drink and possible links to behaviour. If these are reported, an intake/behaviour diary should be kept, and then, if necessary, a referral made to a dietitian. Further dietary management, e.g. specific dietary elimination, should be jointly managed by a dietitian, mental health specialist/ paediatrician, and patient/carer and young person.
- *Omega-3 (and other) fatty acids:* have been investigated in ADHD because of their role in brain development and contribution to cell membrane integrity. Although some studies have reported improvements in behaviour, the consensus[21] is that there remains insufficient evidence to support supplementation and that further well-designed and long-term studies are needed.
- *Weight loss or poor weight gain:* may arise in adults and children with ADHD if food intake is poor, hyperactivity results in energy expenditure exceeding intake or in association with some medication, e.g. methylphenidate, atomoxetine, or dexamfetamine. Routine monitoring of weight and, in children, plotting height, weight, and BMI on growth charts is required. Taking medication with or after food or changing mealtime to avoid peak drug-action may also help.

20 National Institute for Health and Care Excellence (NICE) (2016). *Attention deficit hyperactivity disorder: diagnosis and management.* Available at: ℜ http://www.nice.org.uk/guidance/CG72.

21 Gadoth, N. (2008). On fish oil and omega-3 supplementation in children: The role of such supplementation on attention and cognitive dysfunction. *Brain Devel.* 30, 309-20.

Eating disorders

- Defined as persistent disturbance of eating (± behaviour) that impairs physical health or psychosocial functioning or both and that is not 2° to any other medical or psychiatric disorder.
- Includes anorexia nervosa (AN), binge eating disorder (BED), and bulimia nervosa (BN).
- Individuals who do not fall within strict diagnostic criteria are described as having other specified feeding or eating disorder (OSFED) and should be treated according to the guidelines that their condition most closely resembles.

Pathogenesis includes

- *Genetic factors:* estimated hereditability 50–83%.
- *Biological factors:* starvation impacts directly on brain and is associated with behavioural and psychosocial impairment. Complex integration of appetite control, motivation to seek food and eat, and self-regulation may also contribute.
- *Environmental factors:* may include events from conception onwards (stress in pregnancy, prenatal complications, prematurity) to societal pressures and concepts of 'fatness' and 'thinness'.

Statistics for eating disorders

BEAT,[22] the UK's eating disorders charity, estimates that ~1.25 million people suffer from eating disorders in the UK and 20% of these are male. The age group most likely to be affected by an eating disorder is those aged 14-25 years, while 1 in 100 women aged 15-30 years are affected by anorexia

General principles of care[23]

- Improving access to services for all people regardless of background and especially where stigma or shame may deter people from seeking help.
- Optimizing communication, including with family members where appropriate, but recognizing the need for confidentiality and consent. Show empathy, compassion, and respect, and being sensitive when discussing a person's weight and appearance.
- Providing good information and support including assessing the impact on home, education, work, and the wider social environment including the Internet and social media.
- Co-ordinating care between health professionals, different services, and in different settings where staff should be appropriately trained to work with the relevant age group.

Identification and assessment

People with eating disorders should be assessed and receive treatment at the earliest opportunity. Those with or at risk of severe emaciation, should

22 Beat (2018). Available at: ℅ https://www.beateatingdisorders.org.uk/.

23 National Institute for Health and Care Excellence (NICE) (2017). *Eating disorders: recognition and treatment*. Available at: ℅ https://www.nice.org.uk/guidance/ng69.

be prioritised. A screening tool alone is not recommended as a sole method of determining whether or not people have an eating disorder. Do not use single measures such as BMI or duration of illness to determine whether to offer treatment for an eating disorder.

When assessing for an eating disorder or deciding whether to refer people for assessment, take into account any of the following:

- Unusually low or high BMI or body weight for their age
- Rapid weight loss
- Dieting or restrictive eating practices when underweight
- Disproportionate concern about their weight or shape
- Family or carers reporting a change in eating behaviour
- Social withdrawal, particularly from situations that involve food
- Other mental health concerns e.g. depression, anxiety, self-harm, OCD
- Problems managing a chronic illness that affects diet, such as diabetes or coeliac disease
- Menstrual or other endocrine disturbances, or unexplained GI symptoms
- Physical signs of:
  - malnutrition, including poor circulation, dizziness, palpitations, fainting, or pallor
  - compensatory behaviours, including laxative or diet pill misuse, vomiting, or excessive exercise
- Abdominal pain that is associated with vomiting or restrictions in diet and that cannot be fully explained by a medical condition
- Unexplained electrolyte imbalance or hypoglycaemia
- Atypical dental wear (such as erosion)
- Taking part in activities associated with a high risk of eating disorders e.g. professional sport, dance, fashion, or modelling.

In addition, be aware in children and young people an eating disorder may also present with faltering growth or delayed puberty.

▶ If an eating disorder is suspected after an initial assessment, refer immediately to a community-based, age-appropriate eating disorder service for further assessment or treatment.

Anorexia nervosa

ICD-10 descriptor: AN is characterized by deliberate weight loss, induced and sustained by the patient. It occurs most commonly in adolescent girls and young women, but adolescent boys and young men may also be affected, as may children who are approaching puberty and older women. It is associated with a specific psychopathology whereby a dread of fatness and flabbiness of body contour persists as an intrusive, overvalued idea, and the patients impose a low weight threshold on themselves. There is usually undernutrition of varying severity with secondary endocrine and metabolic changes and disturbances of bodily function. The symptoms include restricted dietary calories and variety, excessive exercise, micro-exercising, purging by self-induced vomiting, use of laxatives, diuretics, diet pills, and appetite suppressants, including amphetamines. The lifetime prevalence is 0.9% for women and 0.3% for men.

Management[23]
- Support should:
  - include psychoeducation about the disorder;
  - include monitoring of weight, mental, and physical health, and any risk factors;
  - be multi-disciplinary and co-ordinated between services;
  - involve the person's family members or carers if appropriate.
- When treating AN, be aware that:
  - helping people to reach a healthy body weight or BMI for their age is a key goal;
  - weight gain is key in supporting other psychological, physical, and quality of life changes that are needed for improvement or recovery.
- When weighing people with AN, consider sharing the results with them and family members or carers if appropriate.

Psychological treatment in AN

NICE guidelines[23] define approaches for adults and for children and young adults. For adults, these include individual eating disorder focused cognitive behavioural therapy (CBT-ED), the Maudsley Anorexia Nervosa Treatment for Adults (MANTRA), and specialist supportive clinical management. For children and young people, consider AN-focused family therapy delivered as a single-family therapy or combined with multi-family therapy. If AN-focused family therapy is unacceptable, contraindicated, or ineffective, consider individual CBT-ED or adolescent-focused psychotherapy for anorexia nervosa.

Dietary advice in AN
- Dietary counselling should only be offered as part of a multi-disciplinary approach.
- Encouragement should be given to take an age-appropriate oral multi-vitamin and multi-mineral supplement until the patient's diet includes enough to meet the dietary reference values.
- Include family members or carers (as appropriate) in any dietary education or meal planning for children and young people with AN who are having therapy on their own.
- Offer supplementary dietary advice to children and young people with AN and their family or carers (as appropriate) to help them meet their dietary needs for growth and development (particularly during puberty).

Inpatient care
- Admission should not be based on a specific weight or BMI threshold but whether the patient can be safely managed in daycare services, e.g. weight loss >1 kg/week or medical need, e.g. bradycardia.
- Staff should be aware of the risk of refeeding syndrome and how to manage it (see ➔ Chapter 25 'Refeeding syndrome', p. 602).

- Guidelines for the Management of Really Sick Patients with Anorexia Nervosa (MARSIPAN) are available for adults[24] and those aged <18 years (Junior MARSIPAN).[25]
- Feeding without consent should only be undertaken by competent multi-disciplinary teams and using the framework of the Mental Capacity Act 2005 (see ➔ this chapter).
- Post-hospitalization, ongoing care should be planned.
- Medication should not be offered as the sole treatment in AN.

Binge eating disorder

ICD-10 descriptor: BED involves regularly eating very large amounts of food over a short period of time, often in an uncontrolled way. Bingeing can occur when not hungry, when alone, or in secret. Eating can continue until feeling uncomfortably full and may be followed by feelings of upset, shame, and guilt. BED includes some of the features of BN but the overall clinical picture does not justify diagnosis, e.g. there may be recurrent bouts of over-eating and overuse of purgatives without significant weight change or the typical over-concern about body shape and weight may be absent. Lifetime prevalence is 3.5% for women and 2.0% for men.

Management for adults, children, and young people[23]
- Inform patients that all psychological treatments for BED have limited effect on body weight and that weight loss is not the goal of treatment.
- As a first step, encourage the patient to follow an evidence-based BED self-help programme supported by healthcare professionals.
- If this not acceptable, contraindicated or ineffective after 4 weeks, offer specifically adapted group CBT-ED.
- If this is not available or declined, offer individual CBT-ED.
- Medication should not be offered as the sole treatment of BED.
- Dietary and eating-related recommendations from NICE guidelines[23] include:
  - advise people to eat regular meals and snacks to avoid feeling hungry;
  - address emotional triggers for binge eating, using cognitive restructuring, behavioural experiments, and exposure;
  - monitor weekly binge eating behaviours, dietary intake, and weight, sharing the weight record with the patient;
  - advise not to diet as likely to trigger binge eating;
  - aim does not include weight loss, although explain that stopping bingeing is likely to aid weight management in the longer term;
  - body image issues to be addressed.

24 Royal Colleges of Psychiatrists, Physicians and Pathologists (2014). *MARSIPAN: Management of really sick patients with anorexia nervosa.* Available at: ℜ https://www.rcpsych.ac.uk/docs/default-source/improving-care/better-mh-policy/college-reports/college-report-cr189.pdf?sfvrsn=6c2e7ada_2.

25 Royal College of Psychiatrists (2012). *Junior MARSIPAN: Management of really sick patients under 18 with anorexia nervosa.* Available at: ℜ https://www.rcpsych.ac.uk/docs/default-source/improving-care/better-mh-policy/college-reports/college-report-cr168.pdf?sfvrsn=e38d0c3b_2.

Bulimia nervosa

ICD-10 descriptor: BN is characterized by a pattern of overeating (binge eating) followed by purging, which can include self-induced vomiting, taking laxatives, diuretics, diet pills, amphetamines, or excessively exercising ('exercise debting'). This is to compensate for the excess calories eaten during the binge to prevent weight gain. This disorder shares many psychological features with AN, including over-concern with body shape and weight. Repeated vomiting is likely to give rise to disturbances of electrolytes and physical complications, e.g. stomach acid causing erosion of teeth enamel, oesophageal tears. Excessive laxative misuse can cause constipation. Lifetime prevalence is 1.5% for women and 0.5% for men.

Management
- Inform patients that all psychological treatments for BN have limited effect on body weight.
- In adults, as a first step, encourage use of a BN-focused self-help CBT programme, supplemented by brief supported sessions with a healthcare professional.
- If this not acceptable, contraindicated or ineffective after 4 weeks, offer individual CBT-ED.
- In children and young people, offer BN-focused family therapy.
- If this not acceptable, contraindicated, or ineffective, offer individual CBT-ED.
- Medication should not be offered as the sole treatment of BN.

Treating OSFED

For people with OSFED, consider using the treatments for the eating disorder it most closely resembles.

Physical and mental health co-morbidities
Eating disorder specialists are advised to collaborate with other healthcare teams to support effective treatment of physical or mental health co-morbidities in people with an eating disorder. Outcome measures for both the eating disorder and the physical and mental health co-morbidities should be used to monitor the effectiveness of the treatments for each condition and the potential impact they have on one another. Common mental health co-morbidities seen in eating disorders can include:
- Depression
- Panic and anxiety disorders (including generalized, social anxiety)
- Post-traumatic stress disorder
- Obsessive compulsive disorder
- Obsessive compulsive personality disorder
- Emotionally unstable personality disorder
- Sleep disorders
- Substance abuse or dependence.

Diabetes and eating disorders

For people with an eating disorder and diabetes, the eating disorder and diabetes teams should:

- Work in partnership to explain the importance of physical health monitoring to the person.
- Agree who will take responsibility for monitoring physical health.
- Collaborate on managing mental and physical health co-morbidities.
- Use a low threshold for monitoring blood glucose and blood ketones.
- Use outcome measurements for each condition to monitor individual treatment efficacy as well as any possible impact they may have on one another.

If misusing insulin, the recommended treatment plan is:

- A gradual increase in the amount of dietary carbohydrate (if medically safe), so that insulin can be started at a lower dose.
- A gradual increase in insulin dose to avoid a rapid ↓ blood glucose levels, which can ↑ the risk of retinopathy and neuropathy.
- Adjusted total glycaemic load and carbohydrate distribution to meet their individual needs and prevent rapid weight gain.
- Psychoeducation regarding the physical health problems that result from misuse of diabetes medication.
- Diabetes educational intervention if the person has any gaps in their knowledge of diabetes.
- When diabetes control is challenging to manage, do not stop insulin altogether, as this puts the person at high risk of diabetic ketoacidosis.

Further reading

BMJ (2017) Eating disorders. https://www.bmj.com/content/bmj/suppl/2017/12/07/bmj.j5245. DC1/eating_disorders_v18_web.pdf

Dementia

See Box 32.2 for factors influencing eating and drinking in dementia.

Dementia prevalence[26]

- 850,000 people in the UK are living with dementia.
- 7% of people aged >65 years.
- 42,000 people in the UK aged <65 years.
- Prevalence increases with age.

Causes of dementia

- Alzheimer's disease;
- Vascular disease;
- Lewy body disease;
- Huntington's disease;
- AIDS;
- Head injury;
- Prion disease (e.g. CJD);
- Multiple sclerosis;
- Wernicke–Korsakoff syndrome;
- Syphilis.

Box 32.2 Factors influencing eating and drinking in dementia

- Poor memory: forgetting to eat or that they have eaten, forgetting to shop or the names of foods to buy
- Poor co-ordination: inability to put food onto cutlery, move food into the mouth, peel or unwrap food
- Inability to sequence activities needed to prepare meals
- Drug side effects: dry mouth, drowsiness, constipation, dysphagia
- Poor concentration: easily distracted from meals by noise and other activity
- Tremor: spilling drinks, food
- Eating slowly: food becomes unappetizing or removed by carer
- Poor vision/confusion: food not recognized
- Agitation and restlessness: increases energy requirements while reducing opportunities to eat and drink
- Hallucinations: reluctance or refusal to eat food that appears to contain foreign bodies
- Tooth/mouth problems: pain or discomfort, ill-fitting dentures, tooth decay, altered taste
- Choking/swallowing problems: food may be hoarded in the mouth, spat out, taken out or aspirated causing chest infections
- 'Sun-downing': reduced cognitive function in the late afternoon/early evening so meals at this time may not be eaten
- Depression: a common additional diagnosis causing poor appetite and reluctance to eat
- Professional and lay carers may restrict diets because of additional diagnoses, e.g. diabetes, high cholesterol, diverticulitis, or obesity. This may or may not be appropriate

---

26 Alzheimer's Society (2020). Available at: ℬ http://www.alzheimers.org.uk.

Improving nutrition

- Screening for nutritional risk, e.g. using MUST (see ➲ Chapter 25 'Malnutrition universal screening tool', p. 560) or a locally developed nutrition risk screening tool for use within a mental health setting.
- Monitoring weight routinely; thinness is common in dementia because food intake is low, not because it is part of the illness.
- Where there are concerns regarding weight and nutritional intake, including hydration, monitoring food and fluid intake using daily input and output record charts, which are to be reviewed and escalation procedures followed when indicated.
- Maintaining physical activity to help promote appetite and intake.
- Tailoring support to what the individual needs: help with shopping, cooking, company at mealtimes, verbal or physical prompts.
- Using soft and texture-modified foods only when really necessary.
- Asking family carers for advice and information.
- Maintaining independence by offering help not interference.
- Offering snacks: some older people develop a 'grazing habit'. Ensuring snacks are nutritious so that total intake is not compromised.
- Providing choice by allowing people to select from plates of food that can be eaten immediately.
- Avoiding patterned crockery, tablecloths, etc., which may cause visual confusion at mealtimes and distract from the food.
- Putting drinks into clear glasses to make them easier to see.
- Allowing time for meals: hurried meals may cause agitation and distress.
- Limiting noise, distractions, and other activities at mealtimes.
- Ensuring adequate lighting so that food can be seen properly.
- Talking about food and encouraging eating by chatting about the meal.
- Ensuring adequate resources for catering services in institutional settings and in social care packages for people at home.
- Ensuring appropriate training for all staff involved in dementia care.

Increasing nutrient intake

- Using whole milk or Channel Island milk (approximately 5% fat) rather than skimmed or semi-skimmed milk in cooking and for drinks.
- Using sugar (rather than artificial sweeteners) in cooking and drinks.
- Making a cooked breakfast available. People with dementia may eat better early in the day.
- Including fried foods, cakes, and traditional puddings on menus.
- Using alcohol in moderation to stimulate the appetite. This may be offered on its own or added to other drinks before meals.
- Making food available at night for those who sleep poorly.
- Adding butter, margarine, or grated cheese to mashed potato or other vegetables.
- Adding cream, white sauce, butter, or margarine (rather than water or gravy) to food that needs to be pureed.
- Offering high energy snacks and drinks between meals (e.g. cake, biscuits, ice cream, instant desserts, trifle, chocolate, sandwiches).

Finger foods

Finger foods (see Table 32.2) may help people who cannot remember how to use cutlery. They may help people maintain independence and dignity by allowing people to feed themselves and the greater interaction with food may increase intake. Finger food menus must be analysed for nutritional adequacy.

Soft foods and modified-texture diets

If a person with dementia has difficulty chewing or swallowing they require assessment by a speech and language therapist to ascertain safe food and fluid textures for the individual as per the International Dysphagia Diet Standardization Initiative 🔊 http://iddsi.org/framework/.

Care should be taken to ensure that food provided supplies an adequate energy, protein, and micronutrient intake (see ➔ Chapter 23, 'Dysphagia', p. 535). Simply liquidizing ordinary food is rarely adequate and oral nutrition supplements should be considered (see Table 25.5, p. 570).

Tube feeding

Enteral nutritional support should be considered for individuals when in-adequate intake and/or dysphagia are considered to be transient (see ➔ Chapter 25). It is not recommended for those with severe dementia when disinclination to eat is a sign of the gravity of the condition. Decisions to withhold or withdraw nutrition support must be based on ethical and legal principles (see ➔ Chapter 35, 'Palliative care').[27]

Table 32.2 Examples of finger foods

Starchy and cereal	Protein-rich	Dairy	Fruit and vegetables	Energy dense
Buttered rolls	Chicken nuggets	Cheese cubes	Apple slices	Biscuits
Chips	Fish cakes	Sliced cheese	Banana pieces	Chocolate
Crumpets	Fish fingers	Yogurt-covered raisins	Carrot sticks	Crisps
Potato cakes	Hard-boiled egg		Celery sticks	Ice cream cones
Roast potatoes	Meatballs		Cherry tomatoes	Jam tarts
Tea cakes	Samosas		Grapes	Slices of cake
Toast fingers	Sandwiches		Orange segments	
	Sausages			

27 National Institute for Health and Care Excellence (NICE) (2016). *Dementia: supporting people with dementia and their carers in health and social care.* Available at: 🔊 http://www.nice.org.uk/guidance/cg42.

Mental Capacity Act (MCA) 2005

Overview

This Act provides a framework to empower and protect people with limited or no ability to make decisions for themselves. Inability to make a decision may be a result of dementia, mental health issues, learning disabilities, brain injury, a stroke, alcohol or drug misuse, the side effects of medical treatment or other illnesses, or disability. The Act provides guidance and describes duties for people who care for and treat people over the age of 16 years. It defines who can make decisions for them and in which situations, and also describes the process of how this should be done. It facilitates forward planning by allowing people with capacity to anticipate a future time when they are not able to make decisions. The Act covers major decisions such as property and affairs, healthcare, and where they live, as well as day-to-day decisions about what to eat and personal care. It also provides guidance on the use of a Lasting Power of Attorney, Independent Mental Capacity Advocate, and advance decisions concerning life-sustaining treatments. The MCA gives clear guidance regarding:

- Helping someone to make their own decisions.
- Working out if someone is able to make their own decisions.
- Actions to take if someone cannot make decisions.

Deprivation of Liberty Safeguards (DOLS) are a supplement to the MCA. Hospital, residential, and care home staff must understand how people lacking capacity may be deprived of their liberty.

Five key MCA principles

- Every adult has the right to make his or her own decisions and must be assumed to have capacity to make them unless it is proved otherwise.
- A person must be given all practicable steps to help themselves and these steps must be shown not to work before anyone treats them as not being able to make their own decisions.
- Just because an individual makes what might be seen as an unwise decision, they should not be treated as lacking capacity to make that decision.
- Anything done or any decision made on behalf of a person who lacks capacity must be done in their best interests.
- Anything done for or on behalf of a person who lacks capacity should be the least restrictive of their basic rights and freedoms.

The Act contains a two-stage test of capacity. There are two questions that need to be asked in turn:

1. Is there an impairment of, or disturbance in, the functioning of the person's mind or brain? This can be temporary or permanent.
   - If 'No', the person is judged to have capacity.
   - If 'Yes' then the second question to follow is …
2. Does this impairment or disturbance mean that the person lacks capacity at this particular time to make a particular decision?

To answer this, a four-stage assessment is used and a person needs to pass each stage to be deemed to have capacity:

1. Do they understand the information relevant to the decision?
2. Are they able to retain this information for long enough to make the decision?
3. Are they able to use or weigh up the pros and cons of the relevant options?
4. Are they able to communicate the decision by any means including non-verbal?

If a person fails the four-stage test, this must be deemed to result from mental impairment for them to be regarded as lacking in capacity.

Care Act 2014

This Act consolidates previous health and social care legislation and guidance with the aim of providing a consistent approach to adult social care. It covers the wellbeing of the person needing support and their carer. This Act states that it is the duty of local authorities to promote physical and mental wellbeing, and it focuses on the provision of person-centred care, preventative support, and integrated services. The act provides a statutory framework for safeguarding adults in England.

Further reading

℞ https://www.gov.uk/government/collections/mental-capacity-act-making-decisions
℞ http://www.legislation.gov.uk/ukpga/2005/9/contents

Nutrition in neurological conditions

Multiple sclerosis 782
Motor neurone disease 786
Parkinson's disease 788
Alzheimer's disease 790
Ketogenic therapy for epilepsy 792

Multiple sclerosis

Multiple sclerosis (MS) is an autoimmune disorder of the central nervous system. Worldwide, approximately 2.5 million people have MS, with prevalence increasing in northern areas of the northern hemisphere. Prevalence in the UK is estimated at 108,000 people, i.e. 1.3-2.0 per 1,000 varying with location and is higher in women than men. Damage is caused to the myelin sheath surrounding nerves, thus impairing the conduction of impulses. The condition varies from a relapsing/remitting pattern (~85% patients) to a primary progressive form. Nutritional considerations relate to:

• the cause of the condition;
• possible effects on its progression;
• specific nutritional concerns that might arise in some people with MS.

Pathogenesis

Genetic susceptibility and environmental factors have been implicated. A number of dietary factors have been investigated:

• Low vitamin D levels (i.e. resulting from ↓ dietary vitamin D intake or ↓ exposure to sunlight) are associated with ↑ risk of MS.[1]
• Obesity in childhood and adolescence is also associated with higher risk,[2] probably mediated through ↑ inflammation.

Disease progression

Dietary modification and/or supplementation is often considered to help slow MS progress or manage MS symptoms. However, there is no conclusive evidence of sufficient benefit to support definitive dietary guidelines. Areas of potential interest include:

Polyunsaturated fatty acids (PUFA): systematic review[3] of six studies concluded that PUFA have no effect on disease progression, but have a tendency to reduce relapses over 24 months.

Low fat, plant-based diet: a single RCT[4] of a diet providing 15% of energy as fat showed no effect on progression or disability but was associated with less fatigue. This is interesting but requires further investigation before translating to advice for people with MS.

NICE guidelines advise against using PUFA and vitamin D supplements for the treatment of MS.[5] However, vitamin D supplements are recommended

1 Duan, S., et al. (2014). Vitamin D status and the risk of multiple sclerosis: a systematic review and meta-analysis. *Neurosci. Lett.* **570**, 108-13.

2 Hedström, A.K., et al. (2014). Interaction between adolescent obesity and HLA risk genes in the etiology of multiple sclerosis. *Neurology* **82**, 865-72.

3 Farinotti, M., et al. (2012). Dietary interventions for multiple sclerosis. *Cochrane Database Syst. Rev.* **12**, CD004192. DOI: 10.1002/14651858.CD004192.pub3.

4 Yadav, V., et al. (2017). Low-fat, plant-based diet in multiple sclerosis: a randomised controlled trial. *Mult. Scler. Relat. Disord.* **9**, 80-90.

5 National Institute for Health and Care Excellence (NICE) (2019). *Multiple sclerosis in adults: management.* CG186. Available at: ℘ https://www.nice.org.uk/guidance/cg186.

for the general population in the UK in autumn and winter,[6] so it would be reasonable for people with MS to consider taking these for general health. In view of limited evidence, it is reasonable to advise people with MS to follow national dietary guidelines and eat a variety of foods from the major food groups in quantities to maintain a healthy weight (see ➔ Chapter 2, 'The Eatwell Guide', p. 27). Individuals with particular symptoms or weight changes may need more specific advice so consider referral to a registered dietitian.

Specific nutritional concerns

Fatigue, loss of balance, weakness, numbness, tingling, and bladder problems are among the most common symptoms experienced by people with MS. Difficulty in swallowing occurs in >30% of cases, mainly in the late stages, and can have a profound impact on food intake and nutritional status.

- Routine nutritional assessment will help to identify patients whose nutritional intake is suboptimum before depletion results in clinical impairment. Regular (3–6 monthly) monitoring of weight and BMI will be sufficient in most cases but should be reviewed in relapse.
- Practical support, e.g. help with shopping or meal preparation, may be sufficient to help some patients 'normalize' their intake.
- Nutritional supplements may help to increase nutrient intake where sufficient food cannot be consumed (see ➔ Chapter 25, 'Treatment of undernutrition', p. 568).
- Overweight and obesity is common, ~40% of patients diagnosed for 10–13 years, and is related to ↑ co-morbidities. A moderate energy-restricted diet that provides all other nutrient requirements is advisable (see ➔ Chapter 21, 'Weight management: overview', p. 477).
- Constipation, reported in ~40%, may be alleviated by ↑ fibre intake and drinking sufficient fluid, >2 L/day (see ➔ Chapter 26, 'Constipation', p. 672).
- Swallowing difficulties should be evaluated by a speech and language therapist and dietitian with expertise in this area (see ➔ Chapter 23, 'Dysphagia', p. 535).
- If an adequate nutritional intake cannot be maintained orally, feeding via gastrostomy may help improve quality of life (see ➔ Chapter 25. 'Routes for enteral feeding', p. 574). If adequacy of intake is a concern, early intervention may help avert complications associated with under nutrition.

Alternative diets and MS

- Many adults with MS report interest in modifying their diet to help their condition, with approximately 17% currently following a diet.
- A variety of allegedly therapeutic diets for MS are available through the Internet and other media.

6 Public Health England (2016). *PHE publishes new advice on vitamin D*. Available at: ℘ https://www.gov.uk/government/news/phe-publishes-new-advice-on-vitamin-d.

- Some include specific dietary restrictions that may compromise the adequacy of their nutrient intake.
- Other regimes involve the purchase of specific food items or supplements that are not prescribable and often expensive.
- At present, there is little evidence to support dietary manipulation other than that described in 'Specific nutritional concerns' above.
- Some people may need advice about the potential harms and benefits associated with some alternative diets (Box 33.1).

> **Box 33.1 Questions to ask about alternative diets for MS**
> - Is it based on scientific evidence or just promoted by enthusiasts?
> - Will the diet be worse than the symptoms?
> - Is the diet nutritionally adequate?
> - Are the ingredients easily available to buy?
> - How much does it cost?
> - Will it be difficult to prepare or cook the food?
> - Is it recommended by neurologists and dietitians?

Further reading

British Dietetic Association (2015). *Use of alternative diets and supplementation in the management of multiple sclerosis*. Available at: ℞ https://www.bda.uk.com/improvinghealth/healthprofessionals/ms_management.

Habek, M., et al. (2010). Nutrition in multiple sclerosis. *Clin. Neurol. Neurosurg.* 112, 616–20.

Multiple Sclerosis Society (2016). *Diet and nutrition*. Available at: ℞ https://mss-cdn.azureedge.net/-/media/35efd6e20e1f42dcaa04b6e68ffe20a6.pdf?sc_revision=b6991633d48e48988c8d9bafabe689a5.

Motor neurone disease

Motor neurone disease (MND), or amyotrophic lateral sclerosis, is a group of related progressive disorders involving degeneration of the motor neurones leading to muscle weakness and wasting. Sensory neurones, e.g. taste, are not affected, but difficulty chewing and swallowing may arise. The UK prevalence is ~7 in 100,000, with approximately 5,000 adults affected. Worldwide, prevalence varies between ~1 and 11 per 100,00 (median 5.4). Approximately 30% of people with MND die within 1 year of diagnosis and >50% within 2 years.

Undernutrition

Inadequate nutrient intake often leads to poor nutritional status (~20%). This may further impair muscle function and is associated with ↓ survival.

Factors contributing to undernutrition in MND

- Dysphagia: lip and tongue dysfunction, impaired swallow reflex, pharyngeal weakness, and reduced laryngeal elevation.
- Arm weakness: dependence on others to be fed.
- Social consequences: difficulty in eating and excessive salivation may inhibit eating with other people.

Nutritional management[7]

- Assessment of nutritional status by a dietitian (see ⮞ Chapter 4, 'Nutrition assessment', p. 38).
- Evaluation of swallow and advice about an appropriately textured diet from a speech and language therapist and a dietitian: good co-ordination is essential (see ⮞ Chapter 23, 'Dysphagia', p. 535).
- Oral nutrition supplements may help achieve an adequate intake but consistency and texture of food and drink need to be considered.
- Positioning during eating, assistive utensils, and appropriate help may help increase intake.
- Gastrostomy insertion can relieve pressure to eat and should be discussed early. Attention to feed delivery time is required to minimize disruption to sleep and feeding in public.[8] Insertion is recommended if:
  - >10% loss of body weight despite supplementation;
  - unsafe swallow or bulbar symptoms;
  - life expectancy >3 months;
  - able to provide consent and manage feeding process (or carer who can do this).

Systematic review of studies of gastrostomy feeding indicates that this is associated with a tentative survival advantage.[9]

7 National Institute for Health and Care Excellence (NICE) (2016). Motor neurone disease: assessment and management. NG42. Available at: 🔗 https://www.nice.org.uk/guidance/ng42.

8 Rio, A., et al. (2010). Nutritional factors associated with survival following enteral tube feeding in patients with motor neurone disease. *J. Hum. Nutr. Diet.* **23**, 408–15.

9 Katzberg, H.D., et al. (2011). Enteral tube feeding for amyotrophic lateral sclerosis/motor neuron disease. *Cochrane Database Syst. Rev.* 1, CD004030. DOI:10.1002/14651858.CD004030.pub3.

Antioxidants

The role of antioxidants in treating MND, i.e. to combat the oxidative stress contributing to disease progression, has been examined in a number of studies, but systematic review[10] revealed no significant benefits or contra-indications. Although there is no specific evidence to support the use of supplements, diets of altered texture that are provided to patients with swallowing difficulties are often relatively ↓ in antioxidants and this could be addressed by the inclusion of suitably prepared (i.e. fresh and not over-cooked) fruit and vegetables.

Resources

Motor Neurone Association (2017). *Transforming MND care audit tool.* ℰ https://www.mndassociation.org/forprofessionals/transforming-mnd-care/

10 Orrell, R.W., *et al.* (2008). Antioxidant treatment for amyotrophic lateral sclerosis or motor neurone disease. *Cochrane Database Syst. Rev.* 1, CD002829 DOI:10.1002/14651858.CD002829.pub4.

Parkinson's disease

Parkinson's disease (PDis) is a chronic progressive neurological condition with a worldwide prevalence increasing with age from ~40 per 100,000 in those aged 40-49 years to ~1,800 per 100,000 in those aged ≥80 years. Symptoms including hypokinesis (reduced movement and fatigue), rigidity, tremor, and depression can contribute to a poor food intake and impair nutritional status, particularly in the later stages.

Pathogenesis

The causes of PDis are still unclear, although probably include a genetic component with possible environmental influences. Cellular degeneration leads to dopamine insufficiency leading to symptoms of tremor, bradykinesia (slow movement), and rigidity. There is no good evidence that diet or nutritional intake is associated with risk of PDis.

Nutritional management of symptoms

- *Referral to a dietitian* should be considered so that people with PDis can access specialist advice as recommended by NICE.[11]
- *Swallowing difficulties* are common and occur in up to 80% of patients, although in most they are relatively mild and do not impair food intake until a later stage. The patient's ability to swallow should be evaluated by a speech and language therapist and dietitian with expertise in this area to co-ordinate advice and an appropriately textured diet (see ➡ Chapter 23, 'Dysphagia', p. 535).
- *Constipation* is the second most common non-motor symptom and is reported by ~50% of people with PDis. It may arise from a poor overall food intake, ↓ fibre diet as a result of texture modification, or as a side effect of medication. Increasing dietary fibre and an adequate fluid intake (>2 L/day) is advisable. Fibre can be provided for patients requiring a soft/puree diet as oat porridge, pureed/mashed fruits including bananas, prunes, and dates, and thickened lentil-type soups.
- *Weight loss* is associated with ↓ health-related quality of life and reported in ~44% of people with PDis. It results from an inadequate intake possibly as a result of declining ability to shop or prepare food, increasing tremor that makes self-feeding difficult or swallowing difficulties. Energy requirements may be ↑ because of motor symptoms in later stages. An evaluation of the patient's physical status and nutritional needs will help identify how to best address undernutrition (see ➡ Chapter 25, 'Undernutrition', p. 564).
- *Dry mouth* may arise as a side effect of medication. Moist meals served with appropriate sauce may help. Sharp flavour, e.g. lemon and grapefruit, may stimulate saliva.
- *Physical difficulties* in eating, including spillages, may limit intake. Occupational therapist assessment may identify helpful approaches, including the use of non-slip mats, assistive cutlery, two-handled cups, and stay-warm plates if mealtimes are prolonged. Finger foods may also help (see ➡ Chapter 32, 'Dementia', p. 776).

11 National Institute for Health and Care Excellence (NICE) (2017). Parkinson's disease in adults. NG71. Available at: ✆ https://www.nice.org.uk/guidance/ng71.

Other nutritional management

Protein restriction Potential competition between circulating amino acids and PDis medication, levodopa, led to investigation of diets providing ↓ protein (<10 g/day) during the day. Reducing protein intake in older people who are at risk of weight loss raises concern. Following a review of evidence, NICE[11] recommend:

- Advise people with Parkinson's disease to avoid a reduction in their total daily protein consumption.
- Discuss a diet in which most of the protein is eaten in the final main meal of the day for people with PDis on levodopa who experience motor fluctuations.

Antioxidants Free radicals are implicated in the neurological damage of PDis, which has generated interest in the therapeutic value of antioxidants as 'neuroprotective agents' that might slow disease progression. No studies have been undertaken with vitamin C, but evidence from vitamin E studies indicates no benefit and NICE[11] does not recommend vitamin E supplements. A well-balanced diet including five portions of fruit and vegetables per day will help provide a good baseline intake of dietary antioxidants.

Vitamin D There is evidence that vitamin D status is associated with risk of PDis and low serum level increases risk of ↓ motor function.[12] As a result, NICE[11] recommend:

- Advise people with Parkinson's disease to take a vitamin D supplement.

Creatine plays a role in mitochondrial function so supplements have been suggested to help ↓ PDis progression. There is no good evidence to support this and creatine supplements are not recommended.[13]

Caffeine There is insufficient evidence on which to recommend increasing or restricting caffeine intake.

Resources

Parkinson's UK (2016). *Diet and Parkinson's*. ⅏ https://www.parkinsons.org.uk/information-and-support/diet

12 Rimmelzwaan, L.M., *et al.* (2016). Systematic review of relationship between vitamin D and Parkinson's disease. *J. Parkinsons Dis.* **6**, 29-37.

13 Xiao, Y., *et al.* (2014). Creatine for Parkinson's disease. *Cochrane Database Syst. Rev.* **6**, CD009646. DOI: 10.1002/14651858.CD009646.pub2.

Alzheimer's disease

Alzheimer's disease (AD) is the most common form of dementia and affects <0.5 million people in the UK. Worldwide, it is estimated that 50 million people are living with dementia. This section provides a very brief summary of the limited nutrition and dietary-related evidence in the prevention and treatment of AD. See ➜ Chapter 32, 'Dementia', p. 774, for practical advice about supporting people with AD.

- *Aluminium:* a recent meta-analysis[14] of eight studies indicates that chronic exposure to Al is associated with higher risk of AD, but this included occupational exposure to dust as well as ingested Al so it is not possible to extrapolate to dietary intake alone. UK water supply regulations of maximum Al concentration (0.2 mg/L) are comparable with World Health Organization recommendations.[15]
- *B vitamins:* a systematic review[16] concluded that there is no evidence to support vitamin B supplementation in preventing or treating AD.
- *Unsaturated fatty acids and omega-3:* a systematic review[17] concluded that there is insufficient evidence to support supplementation of diet with unsaturated fatty acids in treating AD.
- *Vitamin E:* a systematic review[18] concluded that although there is no evidence that vitamin E supplementation prevents progression or slows cognitive decline in mild cognitive impairment, there is moderate quality evidence that it is associated with slowing functional decline in AD and had no adverse effects. Good dietary sources of vitamin are listed in Box 6.2, p. 107.

So, what is the optimum diet in AD?

Rather than considering individual nutrients separately, a 'whole-diet approach' may have more benefits in AD, e.g. a Mediterranean-type diet is associated with ↓ risk of developing AD and progression of cognitive symptoms[19] (see ➜ Box 23.2 for 'Mediterranean diet', p. 526). In addition, the practical aspects of food provision play an important role in optimizing nutrient intake in AD (see ➜ Chapter 32, 'Dementia', p. 774).

---

14 Wang, Z., et al. (2016). Chronic exposure to aluminum and risk of Alzheimer's disease: A meta-analysis. *Neurosci. Lett.* 610, 200-6.

15 World Health Organization (2010). Aluminium in drinking-water. Available at: ℬ http://www.who.int/water_sanitation_health/publications/aluminium/en/.

16 Dangour, A.D., et al. (2010). B-vitamins and fatty acids in the prevention and treatment of Alzheimer's disease and dementia: a systematic review. *J. Alzheimers Dis.* 22, 205-24.

17 Burckhardt, M., et al. (2016). Omega-3 fatty acid for the prevention of dementia. *Cochrane Database Syst. Rev* 4, CD009002. DOI: 10.1002/14651858.CD009002.pub3.

18 Farina, N., et al. (2017). Vitamin E for Alzheimer's dementia and mild cognitive impairment. *Cochrane Database Syst. Rev* 4, CD002854. DOI: 10.1002/14651858.CD002854.pub4.

19 Singh, B., et al. (2014). Association of Mediterranean diet with mild cognitive impairment and Alzheimer's disease: a systematic review and meta-analysis. *J. Alzheimers Dis.* 39, 271-82.

Ketogenic therapy for epilepsy

The ketogenic diet (KD) is a high fat, restricted carbohydrate regime used to treat epilepsy. It is designed to mimic fasting-induced metabolic changes with ketone bodies, acetoacetate, and β-hydroxybutyrate, becoming the 1° energy substrate for brain and metabolically active tissues in the absence of adequate glucose. Research into the mechanism of action is ongoing, with evidence suggesting carbohydrate restriction and ↑ ketone body and free fatty acid supply will ↓ neuronal excitability via multiple mechanistic pathways beyond simple direct anticonvulsant effects of ketone bodies.

Ketogenic therapy—the dietary variants

Traditional KDs

- *Classical KD*: This original diet is based on a ratio of ketone-producing foods in the diet (fat) to foods that mitigate ketone production (carbohydrate and protein), usually 3:1-4:1 (87-90% energy as fat). Fat is mainly from foods, e.g. cream, butter, oil. Carbohydrate is usually limited to controlled portions of vegetables and/or fruits. Protein is based on minimum requirements for growth and high biological value sources are encouraged. All meals and snacks are prescribed at the correct ketogenic ratio; food must be weighed to ensure dietary accuracy.
- *Medium chain triglyceride (MCT) KD*: Developed in the 1970s, the addition of MCT (usually 30-60% energy depending on tolerance and ketosis) as a replacement for some of the fat from foods will increase ketosis, allowing more carbohydrate and protein. MCT is included at meals or snacks using an oil or emulsion, which are available on medical prescription. Food is weighed but choice lists rather than recipes are often used.

Modified KDs

- *Modified Atkins Diet (MAD)*: Initially based on the Atkins weight loss regime, this restricts carbohydrates and encourages high fat foods but does not limit protein or total calories, or weigh food.
- *Low glycaemic index treatment (LGIT)*: This is more generous in carbohydrates but only those with a glycaemic index of <50 are allowed. Protein, fat, and calories are monitored but not as strictly as a traditional KD. Food is not weighed but based on portion sizes.
- *Modified ketogenic diet*: A UK variant similar to MAD but with a more generous initial carbohydrate allowance and prescribed fat intake using food choice lists.

❶ Note: An individual ketogenic prescription is calculated by the dietitian for both traditional and modified dietary variants.

Efficacy

Many prospective and retrospective studies report reduced seizure frequency and severity on the KD diet. Cognitive and behavioural benefits are also seen with ↓ dependence on anti-epilepsy drugs (AEDs) and improvement in quality of life for many patients and families. Two randomized trials of ketogenic therapy in children reported seizure frequency to be significantly ↓ in diet-treated groups compared with controls. Although adult data are more limited, good outcomes are also being reported in this group.

Indications and contraindications

Ketogenic therapy can benefit all seizure types and syndromes, although it may be particularly helpful in myoclonic epilepsies but is not generally used until more than two appropriate AEDs have failed. NICE recommends that children and young people with epilepsy whose seizures do not respond to AEDs should be referred to a 3° specialist for consideration of the use of a KD.[20] Ketogenic therapy is first-line treatment for the neurometabolic diseases glucose transporter type 1 deficiency syndrome and pyruvate dehydrogenase deficiency. It is mainly used in childhood epilepsy but can also be very successful in infants who require a more cautious approach to initiation and monitoring; the stricter classical KD is advised in this group. The MAD or LGIT may be more suitable for older children and adults and those who prefer a less restrictive diet.

Contraindications include disorders of fatty acid metabolism or those requiring treatment with high carbohydrate intake, history of hyperlipidaemia, or renal calculi and other medical exclusions. Diets should be used with caution if also taking medications that increase risk of acidosis. Compliance of parent and/or caregiver must be considered. Concurrent dietary restrictions because of physical/behavioural feeding difficulties or food intolerances will make implementation more challenging but dairy- or gluten-free diets are possible. The classical KD can easily be given via enteral feeding tube using specialist medical formula.

Implementation

- *Initiation*—Can be started at home without initial fast if carefully monitored by ketogenic team (including dietitian and neurologist) with regular communication, especially during the first few weeks. Exceptions are the very young or medically fragile. Adverse effects on initiation could include excess ketosis, acidosis, hypoglycaemia, vomiting, diarrhoea, and food refusal. Tolerance to KD is built up gradually by starting at a lower ratio (classical diet) or reduced MCT dose (MCT diet); a full diet can be achieved within 1-2 weeks.
- *Supplementation*—Vitamin, mineral, and trace element supplementation is needed to avoid nutritional deficiencies. Requirements are assessed on an individual basis.
- *Monitoring*—Home ketone monitoring by either urine dipstick (acetoacetate) or finger-prick blood test (β-hydroxybutyrate) is initially recommended twice daily but can ↓ once the diet is established especially on modified protocols. Some centres monitor blood glucose during KD initiation and fine-tuning. Regular home weighing is advised. Clinic follow-up will include ketogenic blood monitoring every 3-6 month, including plasma lipids, nutritional indices, and carnitine; urine is

20 National Institute of Health and Care Excellence (NICE) (2016). *Epilepsies: Diagnosis and management*. CG137. Available at: ℘ http://www.nice.org.uk/guidance/cg137.

tested for haematuria and calcium-creatinine ratio. Weight and height are measured to ensure adequate growth and renal ultrasound may be needed if calculi are suspected.

- *Fine-tuning*—Ketogenic therapy is an individual diet prescription that requires regular dietetic review, enabling dietary fine-tuning to achieve ideal ketosis for optimal seizure control without compromising nutrition and growth.
- *Adverse effects*—Gastrointestinal symptoms (commonly constipation and occasionally vomiting, diarrhoea, and abdominal pain), renal calculi (reported in 5-8% on KD), hyperlipidaemia (although no evidence for long-term adverse effects on vascular function) and slowing of linear growth, especially in younger children. Other reported, but less common, complications include decline in whole body and spine bone mineral content with increased fracture risk, infection, bleeding abnormalities, bruising, cardiac complications, hypoproteinaemia, and pancreatitis.
- *Duration and discontinuation*—A 3-month trial is recommended (<3-months in young infants), after which ketogenic therapy can be discontinued if there is no improvement despite appropriate fine-tuning. If a diet is successful it will usually be continued for at least 2 years, but this period of time is individualized based on patient response, not specific guidelines. Discontinuation of ketogenic therapy will be a stepwise process which may take weeks or months; the longer it has been used and the more successful it has been, the more gradual should be the change back to normal diet.

Availability and support

Demand for ketogenic therapy is growing, but availability is variable with limited specialized dietetic resources both nationally and worldwide. Research and clinical interest is now extending beyond epilepsy to possible application of the KD to other conditions such as brain cancer and neurodegeneration. Support groups such as Matthew's Friends (UK) and Charlie Foundation (USA) have facilitated global and local scientific conferences and parent information events, and are an invaluable resource for dietary implementation with family support and sharing of recipes and practical ideas.

Further reading and useful websites

Charlie Foundation for ketogenic therapies. Available at: ℜ https://www.charliefoundation.org/.

Matthew's Friends ketogenic dietary therapies. Available at: ℜ http://www.matthewsfriends.org/.

Martin, K., et al. (2016). Ketogenic diet and other dietary treatments for epilepsy. *Cochrane Database Syst. Rev.* **2**, CD001903.

National Institute of Health and Care Excellence (NICE) (2016). *Epilepsies: Diagnosis and management.* CG137. Available at: ℜ http://www.nice.org.uk/guidance/cg137.

Neal, E.G. (2012). *Dietary Treatment of Epilepsy: Practical Implementation of Ketogenic Therapy.* John Wiley & Sons, Oxford.

Rheumatology, dermatology, and bone health

Osteoarthritis 796
Rheumatoid arthritis 798
Gout 800
Systemic lupus erythematosus 802
Atopic eczema 803
Epidermolysis bullosa 804
Osteoporosis 806

Osteoarthritis

It is estimated that ~8.8 million people in the UK are affected by osteo-arthritis (OA), a progressive, degenerative joint disease. This is the most common reason (91%) for the ~84,000 primary hip replacements undertaken annually. These numbers are likely to ↑ as the population ages, as this condition primarily affects people aged >40 years. The knees, hips, neck, back, hands, and feet are most commonly affected.

Nutritional risk factors

- Obesity is the most important, potentially modifiable risk factor for developing OA in weight-bearing joints, e.g. BMI ≥30 kg/m² is associated with ↑ relative risk of knee OA of 4.6 (95% CI: 2.9, 7.1). Non-weight bearing joints are also affected by obesity, mediated by inflammatory factors secreted by adipose tissue.

Nutritional advice

- Robust evidence does not support any special diet[1] in OA and a varied intake compatible with the 'Eatwell Guide (see ➋ Chapter 2, p. 27) is advisable.
- Weight loss is recommended for those with a BMI ≥25 kg/m². Wherever possible, dietary advice should be combined with exercise (see ➋ Chapter 21 'Obesity', p. 469), which is considered the single most important intervention in OA.[1]
- Glucosamine (glucose with an amino group) and chondroitin (sulphated glycosaminoglycan) are marketed as 'nutritional supplements' for use in OA. Neither is recommended by NICE.[1]

Nutrients of potential future interest

It is estimated that ~31% of people with OA either modify their diet or take nutritional supplements to assist with their condition. The effects of several nutrients, foods, and eating patterns on OA have been considered of potential interest.[2] In most cases, intervention evidence is limited at present:

- Vitamins C and E: insufficient evidence in humans;
- Vitamin D: supplements possibly beneficial only in progressive OA knee;[3]
- Unsaturated fatty acids and omega-3: fish oil supplements associated with ↓ pain and ↑ function in people with OA knee;[4]
- Flavonoids and polyphenols: insufficient evidence in humans;

---

1 National Institute for Health and Care Excellence (NICE) (2014). Osteoarthritis: care and management. CG 177. Available at: ℜ https://www.nice.org.uk/guidance/cg177.

2 Green, J.A., et al. (2014). The potential for dietary factors to prevent or treat osteoarthritis. *Proc. Nutr. Soc.* **73**, 278-88.

3 Bergink, A.P., et al. (2016). 25-Hydroxyvitamin D and osteoarthritis: A meta-analysis including new data. *Semin. Arthritis Rheum.* **45**, 539-46.

4 Hill, C.L. (2016). Fish oil in knee osteoarthritis: a randomised clinical trial of low dose versus high dose. *Ann. Rheum. Dis.* **75**, 23-9.

- Mediterranean diet: associated with better quality of life and ↓ symptoms in OA;[5]
- Ginger: associated with ↓ standardized mean pain −0.3 (95% CI: −0.5, −0.1);[6]
- Vegan diet: no evidence;
- Fasting: no evidence;
- Citrus, honey, vinegar: no evidence.

The practical aspects of eating are also important. Patients with advanced OA may have difficulty in shopping or preparing food and as a result their intake and nutritional status may fall. Appropriate support is required.

Further information

Arthritis Research UK (2014). *Diet and arthritis*. Available at: ℘ https://www.versusarthritis.org/media/1328/diet-and-arthritis-information-booklet.pdf.

Green, J.A., et al. (2014). The potential for dietary factors to prevent or treat osteoarthritis. *Proc. Nutr. Soc.* **73**, 278–88.

5 Veronese, N., et al. (2016). Adherence to the Mediterranean diet is associated with better quality of life: data from the Osteoarthritis Initiative. *Am. J. Clin. Nutr.* **104**, 1043-9.

6 Bartels, E.M., et al. (2015). Efficacy and safety of ginger in osteoarthritis patients: a meta-analysis of randomized placebo-controlled trials. *Osteoarthritis Cartilage* **23**, 13-21.

Rheumatoid arthritis

This chronic, autoimmune condition affects ~400,000 people in the UK, with prevalence worldwide between 0.3% and 1%. The condition is more common in women than men. Joint inflammation causes swelling, pain, muscle weakness, and functional impairment with ~30% of sufferers stopping work <2 years after onset. Rheumatoid arthritis (RA) is associated with a increased risk of cardiovascular and lung disease.

Nutritional risk factors

- Obesity is a risk factor for developing RA with relative risk (RR) of 1.21 (95% CI: 1.02, 1.44)[7] associated with BMI ≥30 kg/m². Risk increases by 13% with each BMI increase of 5 kg/m².
- The Mediterranean diet has been recommended[8] but no association with RA risk was identified in the Nurses' Health Studies of >170,000 women, hazard ratio 0.98 (95% CI: 0.80, 1.20) between the top and bottom quartiles of Mediterranean diet score.[9]
- Coffee has been evaluated as a possible risk: a meta-analysis[10] of five cohort/case-control studies reported an association between high intake and ↑ risk RR = 1.22 (95% CI: 1.08, 1.37).

Nutritional issues

- Some patients with RA have poor nutritional intake 2° to loss of appetite and difficulty in preparing food, especially during periods of inflammatory exacerbation.
- Total energy expenditure in RA is lower than in matched controls, mainly because of a reduction in energy expended through physical activity. Basal metabolic rate may increase during inflammatory exacerbations but only if expressed per kg lean body mass.

Nutritional advice

- Patients with RA do not need a special or restricted diet,[11] but should aim to eat a nutritionally adequate intake, e.g. including all food groups in the 'Eatwell Guide' (see ➔ Chapter 2, p. 27) and consider following a Mediterranean-type diet (see ➔ Box 23.2, p. 526).

7 Feng, J., et al. (2016). Body Mass Index and Risk of Rheumatoid Arthritis: A meta-analysis of observational studies. *Medicine (Baltimore)* **95**, e2859.

8 National Collaborating Centre for Chronic Conditions (2009). *Rheumatoid arthritis: national clinical guideline for management and treatment in adults.* Royal College of Physicians, London. Available at: ℛ https://www.nice.org.uk/guidance/cg79/evidence.

9 Hu, Y., et al. (2015). Mediterranean diet and incidence of rheumatoid arthritis in women. *Arthritis Care Res.* **67**, 597-606.

10 Lee, Y.H., et al. (2014). Coffee or tea consumption and the risk of rheumatoid arthritis: a meta-analysis. *Clin. Rheumatol.* **33**, 1575-83. See erratum in **34**, 403-5.

11 Cramp, F., et al. (2013). Non-pharmacological interventions for fatigue in rheumatoid arthritis. *Cochrane Database Syst. Rev.* **8**, CD008322. DOI: 10.1002/14651858.CD008322.pub2.

- Overweight and obesity are associated with ↑ RA disease activity so attempts should be made to optimize weight by gentle reduction (see ➔ Chapter 21, 'Weight management', p. 477)
- Underweight is associated with ↓ physical function in RA and nutrition support may be required (see ➔ Chapter 25, 'Treatment of undernutrition', p. 568).
- Fish oil supplements are associated with ↓ pain in RA. Meta-analysis[12] of 22 trials reported significant mean reduction of -0.21 (95% CI: -0.42, -0.004). Products with EPA/DHA ratio >1.5 are suitable and not associated with adverse effects.
- Antioxidants are considered to be important but there is no evidence that supplements improve clinical outcomes. Dietary sources have not been evaluated, but it seems reasonable to recommend a diet that provides good food sources of antioxidant micronutrients, not least because of their other health benefits. Five portions of fruit and vegetables daily will provide this.
- Folic acid supplementation (<7 mg/week) is beneficial[13] in patients treated with folate antagonist, methotrexate. Vitamin B_{12} status should be checked before starting.
- Calcium and vitamin D status. Corticosteroids are an effective treatment for RA but patients are susceptible to steroid-induced bone disease (vertebral bone density 85–95% of control values). Good sources of calcium should be consumed daily and a vitamin D supplement considered.[14]
- Exclusion/allergy diets are often followed by RA patients. These may include eliminating meat, dairy products, or 'acidic' foods, or periods of fasting. Evaluative studies, mostly of limited quality, have reported mixed results, but provide inconclusive evidence. Patients should be advised to eat a well-balanced diet that provides good sources of the micronutrients described above, and only restrict their intake if there is evidence of benefit. Review by a registered dietitian will help ensure that nutritional adequacy is maintained.
- Difficulties in obtaining, preparing, and eating food should not be underestimated in patients whose hands or jaws are affected as this may have an adverse effect on intake. Advice and practical support from an occupational therapist and dietitian may help overcome this.

12 Senftleber, N.K., et al. (2017). Marine oil supplements for arthritic pain: a systematic review and meta-analysis of randomised trials. Nutrients 9, pii.42.

13 Shea, B., et al. (2013). Folic acid and folinic acid for reducing side effects in patients receiving methotrexate for rheumatoid arthritis (Review). Cochrane Database Syst. Rev. 5, CD000951. DOI: 10.1002/14651858.CD000951.pub2.

14 Franco, A.S., et al. (2017). Vitamin D supplementation and disease activity in patients with immune-mediated rheumatic diseases: A systematic review and meta-analysis. Medicine (Baltimore) 96, e7024.

Gout

Gout is a metabolic disorder manifest as acute joint disease. It is caused by the deposition of urate crystals in the joints, tendons, and tissues leading to inflammation and severe pain. Prevalence in the UK is ~2.5% and world-wide varies between <1% and 6%; it is more common in Western developed countries and in men.

Pathogenesis and nutritional issues

- High serum urate levels are associated with ↑ urate deposition, but do not always lead to gout. They may arise from:
  - metabolism from endogenous purines;
  - metabolism from dietary purines, e.g. from offal meat, fish, yeast extract, beer, and some vegetables;
  - reduced urinary excretion.
- Obesity and excessive alcohol intake (acute and chronic) is associated with ↑ endogenous urate production and ↓ urinary excretion. Men with BMI >27.5 kg/m² are 16 times more like to report gout than those <20 kg/m².
- Red meat, seafood, and sugar-sweetened beverages are known dietary risk factors.
- 25–60% of patients with gout also have hyperlipidaemia.
- 95% of patients with gout also have hyperinsulinaemia.
- Raised serum urate levels are considered a marker of insulin resistance.

Nutritional advice

- Losing excess body weight is the first priority.[15] This should be undertaken by a modest ↓ dietary energy and ↑ exercise. Aim for a reduction of 0.5–1.0 kg/week.
- Saturated fat should be replaced by mono- or polyunsaturates, especially if hyperlipidaemia is present.
- Alcohol intake, especially from beer and spirits, should be reduced to moderate levels (see ➲ Chapter 9 'Alcohol', p. 206).
- Beef, pork, lamb, and seafood are associated with ↑ serum uric acid so intake should be limited to <100-150 g per day during flare up.[16]
- Although pulses and nuts contain purine, ↑ intake is not associated with ↑ gout risk so their intake should be encouraged.
- Sugar-sweetened soft drinks should be ↓ as fructose content is associated with ↑ serum uric acid. Added fructose should be avoided but not fructose occurring naturally in fruit and vegetables because of the other health benefits associated with these foods.
- Coffee consumption may have some benefit. However, introduction of coffee in large quantities (>6 cups) may trigger an attack (similar to introduction of allopurinol) so care is advisable initially[16].

15 Zhu, Y., et al. (2010). The serum urate-lowering impact of weight loss among men with a high cardiovascular risk profile: The Multiple Risk Factor Intervention Trial. *Rheumatology* **49**, 2391-9.

16 Beyl, R.N. Jr, et al. (2016). Update on importance of diet in gout. *Am. J. Med.* **129**, 1153-8.

- Low fat dairy products are associated with ↓ serum uric acid levels and ↓ gout risk as well as contributing to a healthy-heart diet (see ➲ Chapter 23, 'Cardioprotective diet', p. 524).
- Vitamin C supplements are associated with ↓ serum uric acid. Dietary sources from fruits and vegetables may also be protective. There is no evidence that other antioxidant supplements are beneficial.
- There is no good evidence that omega-3 or omega-6 fatty acid supplements yield any benefit in gout.

Further information

Beyl, R.N., Jr et al. (2016). Update on importance of diet in gout. *Am. J. Med.* **129**, 1153–8.

Dalbeth, N., et al. (2016). Gout. *Lancet* **388**, 2039–52.

UK Gout Society. *All about gout and diet.* Available at: ◈ http://www.ukgoutsociety.org/PDFs/goutsociety-allaboutgoutanddiet-0917.pdf

Systemic lupus erythematosus

Systemic lupus erythematosus (SLE) is a chronic autoimmune condition in which antibodies attack the connective tissues. People of all ages can be affected but it is most common in women of child-bearing age, and has a higher incidence in Black and Asian than in White women.

Nutritional issues and advice

- There is no good evidence that nutrition is implicated in the pathogenesis of SLE or that any special diet is required to reduce symptoms or slow progression.
- SLE is associated with ↑ risk of cardiovascular disease.
  A cardioprotective diet of low saturated fat, avoiding excessive salt, and with ↑ fruit and vegetables is recommended to patients who are well and have a good appetite (see ➜ Chapter 23, 'Cardioprotective diet', p. 524). Cardioprotective exercise is also associated with ↓ depression and ↑ quality of life in SLE.
- Studies evaluating the anti-inflammatory effects of omega-3 fatty acids have reached different conclusions. One trial of dietary supplementation with ≡ 500 mg eicosapentaenoic acid and 350 mg decosahexaenoic acid is associated with a significant ↓ in systemic lupus activity measure.[17] This is equivalent to eating oily fish twice per week, e.g. 2 × 170 g (6 oz) fresh salmon/mackerel.
- Corticosteroids may be used in long-term treatment and SLE patients taking them have ↑ risk of osteoporosis. They should be advised to consume an adequate intake of dietary calcium and vitamin D and increase weight-bearing exercise. One pint (600 mL) of semi-skimmed/whole milk provides the reference nutrient intake for women aged 19–50 years, e.g. 700 mg Ca.
- Some people with SLE develop renal failure and will need referral to a renal dietitian for specific individual dietary modification.
- The health of patients with SLE can vary from relatively well to an acutely ill, hypercatabolic state. Nutritional support may be required if food intake is compromised and should be instigated promptly because poor nutritional status is associated with a worse outcome (↑ in systemic lupus activity measure).
- In people with SLE who are overweight, weight reducing diets can ↓ weight even during corticosteroid treatment and this is associated with ↓ fatigue but no ↑ in disease activity[18].

Further information

Lupus UK (2015). *Lupus and healthy eating.* Available at: ℛ http://www.lupusuk.org.uk/wp-content/uploads/2015/10/Lupus-Healthy-Eating.pdf.

17 Duffy, E.M., *et al.* (2004). The clinical effect of dietary supplementation with omega-3 fish oils and/or copper in systematic lupus erythematosus. *J. Rheumatol.* **31**, 1551–6.

18 Davies, R.J., *et al.* (2012). Weight loss and improvements in fatigue in systemic lupus erythematosus: a controlled trial of a low glycaemic index diet versus a calorie restricted diet in patients treated with corticosteroids. *Lupus* **21**, 649-55.

Atopic eczema

Atopic eczema is a chronic inflammatory itchy skin condition which usually arises in childhood and in most cases, follows a pattern of flares and remission. It is often associated with asthma and allergic rhinitis. A diagnosis of food allergy should be considered in children with atopic eczema who have reacted to a food with symptoms or when symptoms are not controlled by optimum management, especially if associated with GI tract symptoms, e.g. colic, vomiting, and altered bowel habits. A diet history and details of dietary modification should be included in diagnostic investigations.

NICE guidance[19] includes specific direction about diet:

- A trial replacement of cow's milk formula should be offered to infants with moderate-severe eczema which is not controlled by emollients and mild topical corticosteroids. This should be replaced by either extensively hydrolysed protein formula or amino acid formula for 6–8 weeks.
- Children who follow a cow's milk-free diet for longer than 8 weeks should be referred to a dietitian.
- Children with suspected cow's milk allergy should not be given milk from other animals, i.e. goats or sheep, or partially unhydrolysed protein formulae.
- Soya protein should be used as an alternative to cow's milk only in infants aged >6 months.
- The potential effect of maternal diet on eczema in breastfed infants is unknown. However, there is some evidence that breastfeeding protects against eczema in infants for up to 2 years.[20]
- If food allergy is strongly suspected, an exclusion diet should be carried out with advice from a registered dietitian.

In addition,

- Infants with suspected egg allergy who have positive specific IgE to eggs may benefit from an egg-free diet.[21] See ➔ Chapter 37 'Food hypersensitivity', p. 825.
- There is no evidence of benefit in eczema from treatment with supplements including vitamins D and E, selenium, and fish oil.[22]
- Probiotics taken by a mother in pregnancy or during breastfeeding or given to an infant may reduce the infant's risk of eczema.[23] Further research is needed to evaluate possible adverse effects.

19 National Collaborating Centre for Women's and Children's Health (2007). *Atopic eczema in children*. RCOG Press, London. Available at: ℗ https://www.nice.org.uk/guidance/cg57 (no dietary updates 2019).

20 Lodge, C.J., *et al.* (2015). Breastfeeding and asthma and allergies: a systematic review and meta-analysis. *Acta Paediatr.* **104**, 38-53.

21 Bath-Hextall, F.J., *et al.* (2008). Dietary exclusions for established atopic eczema. *Cochrane Database Syst. Rev.* **1**, CD005203. DOI: 10.1002/14651858.CD005203.pub2.

22 Bath-Hextall, F.J., *et al.* (2012). Dietary supplements for established atopic eczema. *Cochrane Database Syst. Rev.* **2**, CD005205. DOI: 10.1002/14651858.CD005205.pub3.

23 Cuella-Garcia, C.A., *et al.* (2015). Probiotics for the prevention of allergy: A systematic review and meta-analysis of randomised controlled trials. *J. Allergy Clin. Immunol.* **136**, 952-61.

Epidermolysis bullosa

Epidermolysis bullosa (EB) is a rare genetic condition that causes severe blistering of fragile skin resulting in wounds, disability, and a heightened risk of skin cancer. It is estimated that >5,000 people in the UK and 500,000 people worldwide have EB. There are different forms with varying severity of symptoms and these may include damage to GI tract membranes resulting in difficulty eating, strictures, and subsequent poor nutritional status and restricted growth (see Box 34.1).

Requirements

- Nutrient requirements may be ↑ to:
  - compensate for nutrient loss via open wounds;
  - optimize healing of skin lesions;
  - support the immune system in combating infection via broken skin;
  - assist in normal GI tract function and ↓ constipation.
- Energy requirements may be ↓ if physical activity/mobility is low.
- ↑ Fluid may be required because of ↑ losses via skin.

Box 34.1 Practical aspects of nutrition and food in EB

- Encourage breastfeeding in infants.
- Normal food is appropriate providing that it can be eaten and sufficient quantity consumed.
- Nutrient dense foods may help meet requirements if intake is poor.
- If activity/mobility is limited, reduce excessive energy that might lead to undesirable weight gain but, if intake is poor, energy dense food may be needed.
- Ensure adequate fluid and fibre intake to minimize constipation, which may damage fragile anal skin (be aware that fibre-rich foods may be filling and limit other intake).
- Spicy, crunchy, and acidic foods may be painful to eat while smooth, cool/warm foods may be more acceptable.
- If pureed foods are needed, ensure they are freshly prepared to minimize nutrient losses and that nutrient density is not compromised by addition of excessive fluid when processed.
- Micronutrient supplementation may be required if intake is poor but limited information is available on requirements.
- Height/length and weight should be monitored on nationally appropriate growth charts, taking account of the individual child's illness.
- Tube feeding, via gastrostomy or nasogastric tube, can be used either as supplementary or total nutrition if insufficient food is taken orally.
- Infants and children should be referred to a paediatric dietitian for individual advice within the context of a multi-disciplinary healthcare team.

Further information

Haynes, L. (2010). Nutrition for children with epidermolysis bullosa. *Dermatol. Clin.* 28, 289–301.

Debra (2008). Nutrition for babies with epidermolysis bullosa https://www.debra.org.uk/downloads/community-support/nutrition-for-babies-with-eb.pdf

Debra (2008). Nutrition in epidermolysis bullosa in children over 1 year of age https://www.debra.org.uk/downloads/community-support/nutrition-for-over-ones.pdf

Osteoporosis

Osteoporosis, thinning of the bones, affects ~3.2 million people in the UK and ~200 million worldwide and is associated with ~300,000 bone fractures annually in the UK.

Nutritional risk factors

- Body mass index <19 kg/m^2.
- High alcohol intake.
- Malabsorption, e.g. coeliac disease, Crohn's disease.
- Generally poor diet, including inadequate calcium and vitamin D intake.

However, most risk factors are not nutrition-related and mostly not modifiable: age >50 years, being female, Asian or White, early menopause, family history, treatment with corticosteroids, smoking, and immobility.

Prevention through an optimum diet

- Peak bone mass is reached in adolescence and young adulthood, i.e. decades before most people are concerned about osteoporosis. It cannot be ↑ in later life so good early bone health is essential.[24]
- Calcium intake for males and females of all ages should meet reference nutrient intakes (RNI) see Table 34.1. Many children in the UK, USA, and Australia do not achieve these intakes and the proportion failing to do so increases with age thus reducing their chance of achieving peak bone mass (see ➔ Chapter 14 'Nutrient deficiencies in children', p. 312). In addition, approximately 16% of women have a Ca intake <400 mg/day (i.e. <57% of the RNI). An inadequate dietary intake will accelerate age-related bone loss and contribute to osteoporosis. See Table 34.2 for good dietary sources of calcium.
- Vitamin D is required in Ca metabolism. It is obtained from:
  - Adequate exposure to sunlight, e.g. face and arms, 10 minutes once or twice daily between April and September (but avoid sunburn). People who spend little time outside, wear clothing that covers most of their skin or have darker skin may not synthesize sufficient vitamin D, and this may result in poor vitamin D status.
  - Dietary sources: the RNI of vitamin D from food sources, fortified foods and supplements for people aged ≥4 years, including women who are pregnant or lactating, is 10 µg or 400 IU daily.[25] It is recognized that it is hard to achieve this intake from food sources alone so a vitamin D supplement of 10 µg/d should be considered by at risk groups (see [26]) and, between October and March, by others.
  - For good food sources, see Table 34.3.

24 Weaver, C.M., et al. (2016). The National Osteoporosis Foundation's position statement on peak bone mass development and lifestyle factors: a systematic review and implementation recommendations. *Osteoporosis Int.* 27, 1281-6.

25 Scientific Advisory Committee on Nutrition (SACN) (2016). *Vitamin D and health*. Available at: ℜ https://www.gov.uk/government/publications/sacn-vitamin-d-and-health-report.

26 Available at: ℜhttps://www.gov.uk/government/publications/vitamin-d-advice-on-supplements-for-at-risk-groups.

- Excessive alcohol intake should be avoided. Lower risk drinking for men and women is ≤14 units/week spread out over several days with a couple of alcohol-free days per week.
- Regular exercise is recommended; children ~60 minutes of moderate intensity exercise daily; adults ~150 minutes of moderate exercise per week plus muscle strengthening exercise on ≥2 days/week.[27]
- Recent studies have suggested that a low vitamin K intake and high salt, protein, and vitamin A intakes are detrimental to bone health. These issues are complex and at present there is insufficient information on which to base recommendations. A varied diet based on the 'Eatwell Guide' (see ➲ Chapter 2, p. 27) is likely to be safe and contribute to good bone health as well as good overall nutrition.
- Maternal nutrition influences the bone health of the next generation and, therefore, prevention of osteoporosis requires long-term public health strategies.

Table 34.1 Reference nutrient intakes (mg/day) of calcium[28*†]

Age	Male	Female
7–10 years	550	550
11–18 years	1000	800
>18 years	700	700

* For younger children, see ➲ Appendix 6, p. 881.

† Source: data from Department of Health (1991). *Dietary reference values for food energy and nutrients for the United Kingdom*. HMSO, London.

Table 34.2 Sources of calcium

Providing ~200 mg Ca		Providing ~50 mg Ca	
Source	Weight (g)	Source	Weight (g)
Milk*, cupful	170	White bread	30
Yogurt, small carton	130	Wholemeal bread	50
Cheese, e.g. cheddar	30	Baked beans	100
Cheese spread	40	Muesli, Swiss	50
Sardines, canned w bones	40	Spinach	30
Sesame seeds	30	Orange	100

* Whole, semi-skimmed, or skimmed.

Whole milk and full-fat cheese contribute saturated fat so selecting a lower fat alternative would provide a healthier option.

27 NHS (2019). *Physical activity guidelines for adults aged 19-64*. Available at: ℘ https://www.nhs.uk/live-well/exercise/.

28 Department of Health (1991). Dietary reference values for food energy and nutrients for the United Kingdom. HMSO, London.

Table 34.3 Dietary sources of vitamin D providing 5 µg

Healthier sources		Other/less healthy sources*	
Source	Weight, g	Source	Weight, g
Cod liver oil	2	Ghee	260
Herring, grilled	30	Pork chop, grilled	450
Salmon, tinned/steamed	50	Butter	550
Pilchards, tinned	60	Whole egg	600
Margarine (all types)	60	Lamb, roasted	650
Egg yolk	100	Beef, roasted	700

*The right-hand column shows quantities >> normal portions and are provided for comparison, not recommended for intake because of the high quantity of associated saturated fat.

Nutritional management

- When osteoporosis is diagnosed, management should include review of dietary adequacy.
- Supplementation with calcium and vitamin D has varying effects, with meta-analyses reaching different conclusions[29] probably because of variation in adherence to long-term supplementation (Ca <10% adherence at 1 year) and different effects on patients who are replete/deplete. In addition, one meta-analysis[30] raised concern about cardiovascular events associated with supplements; this requires clarification. Achieving an adequate Ca intake from dietary sources is safe providing that food sources are not also high in saturated fat and use of a calcium intake calculator is recommended.[31]
- If a calcium intake of 700 mg is not achieved and if osteoporosis medication is prescribed, a supplement of 1000 mg daily is recommended either with or without vitamin D:[32]
  - Ca is available as tablets, effervescent tablets, chewable tablets, granules, and syrup. As the required dose is large, the tablets are usually of considerable size. Major side effects are rare but some gastrointestinal symptoms may occur. Splitting the daily dose into smaller quantities and altering the time of dosing, e.g. before or after food, may help.

29 Rizzoli, R., et al. (2009). Management of osteoporosis in the elderly. *Curr. Med. Res. Opin.* **25**, 2373–87.

30 Bolland, M.J., et al. (2010). Effect of calcium supplements on risk of myocardial infarction and cardiovascular events: meta-analysis. *BMJ* **341**, c3691.

31 National Osteoporosis Society (2013). Vitamin D and bone health: A practical clinical guideline for patient management. Available at: ℘ https://nos.org.uk/media/2073/vitamin-d-and-bone-health-adults.pdf.

32 National Osteoporosis Society (2016). All about osteoporosis and bone health. Available at: ℘ https://nos.org.uk/media/1622/all-about-osteoporosis-august-2016.pdf.

- • Dietary Ca absorption is enhanced by lactose and casein phospholipids which are present in milk. Oxalic acid (i.e. from rhubarb and spinach) and phytate (i.e. from the husk of grains, nuts and seeds), impair calcium absorption.
- Vitamin D status should be monitored if there is a concern about deficiency or non-compliance but is not routinely necessary.[33]
- Protein supplements should be provided for older patients with fractures who are undernourished.[34] Although concern had been raised about possible detrimental effect of protein intake, meta-analysis of 36 studies has found no adverse effects of higher protein diets.[35]
- Recent studies indicate that vitamin K supplementation is associated with ↓ urinary Ca so may provide a future treatment option.[36]

33 Aspray, T.J. et al. (2014). National Osteoporosis Society vitamin D guideline summary. *Age Ageing* **43**, 592-5.

34 Farl, S., et al. (2010). Dietary management of osteoporosis throughout the life course. *Proc. Nutr. Soc.* **69**, 25–33.

35 Shams-White, M.M. et al. (2017) Dietary protein and bone health: a systematic review and meta-analysis from the National Osteoporosis Foundation. *Amer. J. Clin. Nutr.* **105**, 1528-43.

36 Huang, Z.B., et al. (2015). Does vitamin K2 play a role in the prevention and treatment of osteoporosis for post-menopausal women: a meta-analysis of randomised controlled trials. *Osteoporosis Int.* **26**, 1175-86.

Palliative care

Palliative care *812*

Palliative care

Palliative care is the approach taken to provide comfort and quality of life to people with a life-limiting illness and their families. When curative treatment is not possible, palliative care should be integrated at an early stage. The aim is to alleviate symptoms and to support physical, emotional, spiritual, and cultural needs. Although palliative care encompasses end of life care, it should be noted that many people live with an incurable condition for many months or years. Throughout this time, optimizing an individual's nutritional status is essential if physical function and quality of life are to be maintained.

Factors contributing to nutritional risk

Although not everyone with a life-limiting condition will experience deterioration in their nutritional status, undernutrition is common in people receiving palliative care. Reasons for this are often multi-dimensional. Factors which can contribute include:

- *Disease process:* certain diseases such as cancer, motor neurone disease, and end-stage liver failure can alter the body's metabolism, resulting in an increase in nutritional requirements.
- *Symptom burden:* adverse physical symptoms such as nausea, early satiety, dysphagia, taste changes, pain, and weakness can impact greatly on appetite and enjoyment of food. As a consequence, oral intake is decreased and nutritional requirements for macronutrients and micronutrients are not met.
- *Treatment:* treatments such as surgery, chemotherapy, and radiotherapy may be given to palliate the disease. The side effects of these treatments often affect oral intake (see ⟹ Chapter 24, 'Cancer treatment', p. 546). In addition, prescribed medication and poly-pharmacy can also influence appetite and intake.
- *Psychosocial implications:* for the patient and their family, the psychosocial impact of being diagnosed with an incurable condition is significant. Psychological symptoms such as anxiety and depression may directly influence appetite. In addition, financial pressures, isolation, or a loss of independence around activities of daily living may lead to practical difficulties associated with access to food.

For the individual, the physical and psychosocial consequences of nutritional requirements not being met most likely manifest as weight loss and malnutrition. The implications of this are described in ⟹ Chapter 25, 'Undernutrition', p. 564. The clinical and economic pressures in terms of increased morbidity, poorer treatment outcomes, and longer hospital stays must also be considered.

Nutritional management in palliative care

An appropriately validated nutrition screening tool should be used to identify people receiving palliative care who are at nutritional risk. In those susceptible to malnutrition, a comprehensive nutritional assessment should be completed to determine the appropriate management strategy. It must be emphasized that the benefits and burden of nutritional support should be considered on a case-by-case basis where malnutrition has been identified as a concern. In some circumstances, for example end of life care, nutritional intervention may not be deemed appropriate.

Consideration should also be given to those individuals who, although they are not malnourished, have nutritional concerns related to their condition. This may result from, for example, distressing gastrointestinal symptoms or weight gain possibly as a consequence of treatment and medication. As use of complementary diets and nutritional or herbal supplements is common in people living with a diagnosis of incurable disease, this should be addressed as part of the nutritional assessment process.

Oral nutrition support

Oral nutrition, with the appropriate practical assistance to enable feeding, should be the first stage of providing nutritional support. Provision of food and fluids is a basic duty of care and, unless identified as unsafe, should be continued to the end of life. Points to consider include the following:

- Correct the correctable. Underlying symptoms or psychosocial issues which could be improved should be addressed.
- Advice regarding food fortification, meal pattern, and the use of sip feeds and modular nutritional supplements should be discussed and prescribed on an individual basis.
- Previously imposed dietary restrictions, for example to treat dyslipidaemia or diabetes, may need to be relaxed.
- Good oral hygiene and mouth care is important and can help to reduce the risk of infections.
- Supportive care should be provided for the family and carers who may be struggling to understand and accept the difficulties and challenges around eating and mealtimes.
- A balance between encouragement and acceptance of the individual's inability to eat and drink is important.
- In some cases, a reduction in oral intake may be a natural part of the dying process.

Artificial nutrition support

Where nutritional requirements fail to be met orally, consideration should be given to the initiation of artificial nutrition support. A discussion and decision should be based on the likely prognosis, treatment plan, and, where known, the patient's wishes. Both enteral and parenteral feeding have potential complications that need to be considered and weighed up against the likely benefits of feeding. In some cases, it may be appropriate to consider a time-limited trial where outcomes, ideally based on the patient's wishes, should be set and monitored to inform continuation of feeding.

Healthcare ethics

The ethical considerations of the provision of artificial nutrition support in patients receiving palliative care continue to be an area of much debate. In healthcare ethics, four key principles exist which together form a framework within which ethical dilemmas should be discussed. These four key principles are:

- *Autonomy:* a patient's right to self-determination.
- *Non-maleficence:* avoidance of doing harm.
- *Beneficence:* providing benefit.
- *Justice:* fair and equal treatment for all.

When a decision is to be made regarding the use of artificial nutrition support, the following points should also be considered:

- In law, artificial nutritional support is viewed as a medical treatment and as such, can be withheld, given, or withdrawn.
- In patients whose future remains uncertain, a time-limited trial to determine the benefits of feeding may be appropriate.
- Decisions should be made in a timely manner to avoid an irreversible deterioration in nutritional status.
- Informed consent must be obtained from the patient.

The Mental Capacity Act (2005)

Some patients, for example those who are unconscious or with conditions that cause confusion or drowsiness, may lack the capacity to make an informed decision regarding aspects of their healthcare treatment, including the provision of artificial nutrition support. The Mental Capacity Act (2005) for England and Wales provides a legal framework for people aged ≥16 years to protect and empower them in this decision-making process. It also provides guidance on the use of a Lasting Power of Attorney, Independent Mental Capacity Advocate, and advance decisions concerning life-sustaining treatments. Further details are described in ➋ Chapter 32, 'Nutrition in mental health', p. 778.

Palliative care summary

In all cases, nutritional care and support should be considered and provided on an individual basis. To ensure effective outcomes, good communication, multi-professional working, and ongoing support and monitoring are essential.

Further information

Arends, J. et al. (2017). ESPEN guidelines on nutrition in cancer patients. *Clin. Nutr.* **36**, 11–48.

Druml, C. et al. (2016). ESPEN guideline on ethical aspects of artificial nutrition and hydration. *Clin. Nutr.* **35**, 545–56.

European Association for Palliative Care. Available at: ℘ http://www.eapcnet.eu/.

National Institute of Health and Care Excellence (NICE) (2004). Improving supportive and palliative care for adults with cancer. Available at: ℘ http://www.nice.org.uk/csgsp.

Office of the Public Guardian (2016). The Mental Capacity Act Code of Practice. Available at: ℘ https://www.gov.uk/government/publications/mental-capacity-act-code-of-practice

Inherited metabolic disorders

Definitions and management *816*
Emergency regimens for IMD *820*
Phenylketonuria *822*
Refsum's disease *824*

Definitions and management

Definitions
- *Metabolism*: cellular biochemical reactions that occur within the body. This involves the breakdown (catabolism) and formation (anabolism) of chemical compounds.
- *Metabolic pathways*: sequence of chemical reactions of metabolism.
- *Enzymes*: proteins that control the chemical reactions (or steps) in a metabolic pathway.
- *Cofactors*: 'helper molecules' that assist the protein in the biochemical reaction. These are often vitamins.

Inherited metabolic disorders (IMD) are caused by deficient activity of an enzyme (or occasionally multiple enzymes) in a metabolic pathway. The deficiency 'blocks' the metabolic pathway and the clinical consequences of this arise because:
- substrates prior to the 'block' accumulate and can be toxic;
- essential products beyond the 'block' are not formed;
- other compounds may be formed via alternative pathways which may be toxic.

Patients can present at any age: as neonates, throughout childhood, and in adulthood. The severity of the disorder may vary widely depending on the degree of enzyme deficiency. IMD occur in many pathways of amino acid, carbohydrate, lipid, and vitamin metabolism.

Treatment
Based on an understanding of the biochemistry. The mainstays of therapy are:
- Therapeutic diet (see Table 36.1) to:
  - limit the intake of substrate that cannot be catabolized;
  - provide the product that cannot be formed.
- Large doses of cofactor vitamins.
- Medicines that conjugate with toxic metabolites so that the product is excreted in urine.
- Enzyme replacement therapy is possible in a few disorders.
- Liver transplant for some disorders.

IMD are rare and complex so it is essential that patients are managed in a specialist metabolic centre by a multi-disciplinary team including metabolic consultants, dietitians, and nurses, with supporting specialized laboratory services.

Newborn screening for IMD
England screens newborns for six IMDs using dried blood spots:
- Phenylketonuria (since 1969)
- Medium chain acyl-CoA dehydrogenase deficiency (MCADD) in England since 2004, and Northern Ireland, 2009
- Maple syrup urine disease (MSUD) since 2015
- Isovaleric acidaemia (IVA) since 2015
- Glutaric aciduria Type 1 (GA1) since 2015
- Homocystinuria—pyridoxine unresponsive (HCU) since 2015

Table 36.1 Summary of dietary management of some inherited metabolic disorders

Disorder	Dietary management
Amino acid disorders	
Classical phenylketonuria (PKU)	Low phenylalanine diet + phenylalanine-free amino acid supplement
Maple syrup urine disease (MSUD)*	Low leucine, isoleucine, valine diet + leucine, isoleucine, valine-free amino acid supplement
	Isoleucine and valine supplements may be needed
	Give an emergency regimen during illness containing suitable amino acid supplement + valine/isoleucine + glucose polymer*
Tyrosinaemia (TYR) type I and II	Low tyrosine and phenylalanine diet + tyrosine, phenylalanine-free amino acid supplement
	Type 1 also requires medication called nitisinone
Classical homocystinuria (HCU)	Low methionine diet + methionine-free amino acid supplement. Cystine supplements may be necessary
Organic acidaemias*	
Methylmalonic acidaemia (MMA)* Propionic acidaemia (PA)*	Low protein diet (to limit methionine, threonine, valine, isoleucine intake). A methionine, threonine, valine, isoleucine-free amino acid supplement may be recommended if natural protein intake is below safe limits. Tube feeding is often required
Isovaleric acidaemia (IVA)*	Low protein diet (to limit isoleucine intake)
Glutaric aciduria type I (GA1) *	Low lysine or low protein diet (to limit lysine intake) + lysine-free, tryptophan-reduced amino acids before 6 years. Minimum safe protein diet post 6 years
	Give an emergency regimen during illness containing suitable amino acid supplement + glucose polymer*
Urea cycle disorders*	
Ornithine carbamoyl transferase deficiency over the counter (OTC)* Citrullinaemia* Argininosuccinic aciduria (ASA)* Carbamoyl phosphate synthase deficiency (CPS 1 def)* N-acetyl glutamate synthase deficiency (NAGS)*	Low protein diet (to limit waste nitrogen for excretion) + L-arginine supplements. Essential amino acid supplements may be needed if natural protein intake is below safe limits

(Continued)

Table 36.1 (Contd.)

Disorder	Dietary management
Carbohydrate disorders	
Classical galactosaemia	Minimal galactose and lactose diet. Infant soya milk substitute. Calcium and vitamin D supplements may be needed.
Glycogen storage disease (GSD) type I* and type III*	Frequent supply of exogenous glucose, provided as continuous overnight tube feeds or uncooked cornstarch before bed and 2-4 hourly daytime feeds or uncooked cornstarch
	Type III: use of uncooked cornstarch and consider high protein diet
Fatty acid oxidation disorders*	
Very long chain acyl-CoA dehydrogenase deficiency (VLCAD)* Long chain 3-hydroxyacyl-CoA dehydrogenase deficiency (LCHAD)*	Minimal long chain fat, ↑ CHO diet and medium chain triglyceride supplements. Frequent daytime feeding and continuous overnight tube feeds or uncooked cornstarch
	Treatment of later presentation of VLCAD will be based on severity
Medium chain acyl-CoA dehydrogenase deficiency (MCADD)*	Normal diet, avoidance of MCT products. Emergency regimen during illness. Base maximum fasting time on age: • 0-4 m: 6 h • 5-8 m: 8 h • 9-12 m: 10 h • >12 m: 12 h
Lipid disorders	
Familial hypercholesterolaemia	Healthy eating, restricted saturated fat, replace with poly- and monounsaturated fat
Type I hyperlipidaemia	Very low long chain fat diet (to tolerance). Medium chain triglycerides can be given
Abetalipoproteinaemia	Very low long chain fat diet. Vitamin A and E supplements. Medium chain triglycerides not recommended

*Disorders requiring emergency regimen during metabolic stress such as intercurrent illnesses, e.g. diarrhoea, vomiting, ear infections, etc. (see ➲ this chapter 'Emergency regimens for IMD', p. 820, for more detailed information).

Emergency regimens for IMD

Metabolic stress, e.g. intercurrent infections combined with poor oral intake and fasting, anaesthesia, or surgery, can precipitate severe metabolic decompensation in some IMD. Decompensation is caused by catabolism with concomitant ↑ production of toxic metabolites. An emergency regimen (ER) of glucose polymer solution is given to provide energy and help minimize the effects of catabolism. The basic ER can be started at home and is similar for all disorders:

- Glucose polymer solution is given orally 2–3-hourly day and night or continuously via a tube.
- Carbohydrate concentration of solution and volume given depends on age and weight (see Table 36.2).
- Glucose polymers can be flavoured to improve palatability.
- If an oral rehydration solution is prescribed for treatment of gastroenteritis, additional glucose polymer needs to be added to provide a final concentration of 10–12% carbohydrate. More concentrated solutions may exacerbate diarrhoea.
- For some disorders, additional specific therapy is given such as drugs to promote excretion of toxic metabolites or amino acids to promote anabolism.
- Patients and carers should be advised to call the metabolic team for advice if they start the ER.
- If the ER is not tolerated, admission to the local hospital for tube feeding of ER or stabilization with IV fluids (10% dextrose) is often necessary.
- Patients and/or carers should be given explicit, hand-held, written ER instructions that explain the disorder, hospital management, and provide contact details for the specialist metabolic centre.
- For detailed information on emergency regimen protocols for use in hospital see: ℘ http://www.bimdg.org.uk.
- ER solutions are not nutritionally complete and prolonged use can result in protein malnutrition. The patient's usual diet should at least start to be reintroduced after 24-48 hours of ER.

Table 36.2 Emergency regimens—composition and fluid volume for age

Age	Glucose polymer concentration, % CHO	Energy, kcal/100 mL	Suggested daily fluid volume given as 2–3-hourly drinks/ tube feeds
0–6 m	10	40	150 mL/kg up to 1,200 mL/day maximum
7–12 m	10	40	120-150 mL/kg up to 1,200 mL/day maximum
1–2 y	15	60	*11–20 kg:*
2–10 y	20	80	100 mL/kg for first 10 kg + 50 mL/kg for next 10 kg
>10 y	25	100	*≥20 kg:* 100 mL/kg for first 10 kg + 50 mL/kg for next 10 kg + 25 mL/ kg thereafter up to 2,500 mL/day maximum
Adults	25	100	35 mL/kg up to 2,500 mL/day maximum

Phenylketonuria

Phenylketonuria (PKU) is caused by a deficiency of the enzyme phenyl-alanine hydroxylase that converts the essential amino acid phenylalanine to tyrosine. Phenylalanine (Phe) accumulates in plasma and is neurotoxic. Tyrosine, which is essential for the synthesis of protein and the catechol-amine neurotransmitters, becomes deficient. Untreated, patients will develop severe mental retardation. Newborn screening for PKU was established in the UK in 1969. Patients are treated with a low Phe diet that is continued throughout childhood and into adulthood (diet for life is recommended). If an adult chooses to come off the low Phe diet, then dietary adequacy must be ensured. During preconception and pregnancy in women with PKU, a low Phe diet is essential to prevent damage to the unborn baby.

Low Phe diet—main principles

- Restrict intake of dietary protein to maintain plasma Phe concentrations within recommended reference range for age (Table 36.3).
- Give a Phe-free amino acid supplement (protein substitute). This is essential because Phe restriction limits natural protein intake to below that needed for normal growth:
  - Generous intakes of Phe-free amino acids are recommended: 0–2 years = 3.0 g/kg body weight/d; 3–10 years = 2.0 g/kg/d; >10 years = 1g/kg/d; maximum 80 g. Amino acid supplement is given three to four times throughout the day, combined with some measured Phe foods.
  - A range of age-dependent prescribable amino acid supplements is available. These vary in nutrient composition and presentation, e.g. infant formula, gels, juice, or milk-type drinks which need reconstitution, ready-made drinks, tablets, capsules (see ➋ Chapter 38, 'Prescription of nutritional products' and *British National Formulary*).
  - Flavourings need to be added to improve palatability/acceptability of some, particularly older formulations.
- Give a vitamin and mineral supplement to meet normal dietary requirements if not added to amino acid supplement or if taking inadequate amounts of amino acid supplement.
- Provide daily Phe allowance. Daily Phe intake varies between patients and depends on the level of enzyme activity:
  - Phe prescribed is based on plasma Phe concentrations;
  - Phe intake is measured using a system of 50 mg Phe exchanges or 1 g protein exchanges if Phe content of food is unknown;
  - Phe is provided in breastmilk/infant formula for babies or low protein foods, e.g. potato, peas, sweetcorn, cereal, for older infants, children and adults;
  - Phe intake is divided evenly across the day.
- Provide adequate energy intake for growth in children and adolescence from a combination of:
  - naturally very ↓ protein foods (e.g. pure fats, sugar, fruit, some vegetables);
  - special ↓ protein, prescribed manufactured foods, e.g. bread and flour mixes, pasta, rice, biscuits, crackers, chocolate, snack pots, cereals, burger and sausage mix.

Table 36.3 Recommended reference ranges for plasma Phe concentrations and frequency of Phe monitoring in PKU*

Age, years	Plasma Phe, μmol/L	Minimum frequency of monitoring
0–11	120–360	0-1 years weekly
		1-11 years fortnightly
>12	120–600	Monthly
Preconception and pregnancy	120-360	Preconception weekly
		Pregnancy twice weekly

*Source: data from van Spronsen, F.J., et al. (2017). Key European guidelines for the diagnosis and management of patients with phenylketonuria. *Lancet Diabetes Endocrinol.* doi: 10.1016/ S2213-8587(16)30320-5.

Low Phe diet—monitoring

A low Phe diet is monitored by regular measurement of plasma Phe concentrations. See Table 36.3 for frequency of monitoring and recommended plasma Phe concentrations at different ages. Patients or carers collect blood samples for Phe analysis (usually on a dried blood spot card and send by first class post to the biochemistry lab). Ideally, blood should be taken at the same time, in the morning before the amino acid supplement. Patients and carers need to be promptly advised of any necessary dietary changes depending on plasma Phe results.

Reasons for high plasma Phe concentrations:
• intercurrent illnesses;
• too much dietary protein or Phe;
• insufficient amino acid supplement;
• unintentional use of non-PKU amino acid supplement or gluten-free, rather than low protein manufactured foods.

Reasons for low plasma Phe concentrations:
• inadequate intake of protein or Phe;
• growth spurt;
• ↑ requirement post-illness.

Further reading

British Inherited Metabolic Group. Available at: ℘ www.bimdg.org.uk.

Dixon, M. (2014). Chapters 17-19. In: V Shaw (ed) *Clinical paediatric dietetics* 4th edn. Wiley-Blackwell, Oxford.

Saudubray, J.M., et al. (2016). *Inborn metabolic diseases: diagnosis and treatment* 6th edn. Springer-Verlag, Berlin.

Singleton, K. et al. (2019). Inherited metabolic disorders. In: J Gandy (ed) *Manual of dietetic practice* 6th edn. Wiley-Blackwell, Chichester.

Refsum's disease

Refsum's disease is a rare autosomal recessive disorder of lipid metabolism where the presence of a defective enzyme, phytanoyl-coenzyme A hydroxylase, results in accumulation of phytanic acid leading to neurological symptoms.

Treatment is based on restricting the dietary intake of phytanic acid from a typical intake of 50–100 mg/day to <10 mg/day, and minimizing release of endogenous phytanic acid.

- *Rich sources of phytanic acid:*[1] avoid in Refsum's disease, e.g. beef, lamb, meat from ruminant animals (e.g. venison), dairy products (including cow's and goat's), fish and fish oils, baked products with unknown sources of fat.
- *Foods containing little phytanic acid:* (or in bound form): acceptable in Refsum's disease, e.g. poultry, pork, fruit, vegetables, seafood with very low-fat content, e.g. crab and prawns, cereal products (unless prepared with dairy or fish oil), eggs, soya milk, vegetable oils, and margarine made exclusively from vegetable oils.
- *Nutritional adequacy of the diet:* must be checked to ensure sufficient energy and all other nutrients are provided.[2] A low energy diet will lead to weight loss and the accompanying lipolysis will mobilize endogenous phytanic acid. If necessary, supplements should be provided during periods of intercurrent illness to ensure an adequate intake is maintained.
- *Caffeine:* high intakes should be avoided as they are associated with hepatic lipolysis and phytanic acid release.

Adherence to the diet is associated with sustained reductions in serum phytanic acid and few acute complications that are associated with untreated Refsum's disease. It is recommended[3] that patients are reviewed 6-monthly and that dietary restrictions should be followed for life.

1 Roca-Saavedra, P., *et al.* (2017). Phytanic acid consumption and human health, risks, benefits and future trends: A review. *Food Chem.* **221**, 237-47.

2 Baldwin, E.J. *et al.* (2016). Safety of long-term restrictive diets for peroxisomal disorders: vitamin and trace element status of patients treated for adult Refsum disease. *Int. J. Clin. Pract.* **70**, 229-35.

3 Baldwin, E.J. *et al.* (2010). The effectiveness of long-term dietary therapy in the treatment of adult Refsum disease. *J. Neurol. Neurosurg. Psychiatry* **81**, 954-7.

Chapter 37

Food hypersensitivity

Food hypersensitivity 826
Management 828
Food labels 832

Food hypersensitivity

Classification

Food hypersensitivity (FHS) reactions can be categorized as immune-mediated (food allergies) and non-immune mediated (food intolerances).

IgE-mediated food hypersensitivity

- Includes classic primary and secondary sensitization to foods, causing a spectrum of symptoms from mild oropharyngeal symptoms through to anaphylaxis.
- Characterized by symptoms within 2 hours of eating.
- Prevalence of 4–8% in childhood and 1.3–4% in adults.

Non-IgE and non-immune mediated FHS

- Non-IgE mediated food allergy includes coeliac disease, food-induced proctitis and enterocolitis syndrome (FPIES), and eosinophilic oesophagitis.
- Non-immune mediated FHS includes enzymatic reactions such as lactose intolerance, pharmacological reactions such as hypersensitivity to vaso-active amines and salicylates, and reactions of unknown aetiology such as those to food additives.
- Onset of symptoms for non-IgE mediated or non-immune mediated FHS is usually delayed.
- Actual prevalence for many conditions is unknown, except for well-characterized disorders such as lactose intolerance and coeliac disease.
- 30% or more of the population perceive themselves or their child to have FHS, whereas the actual prevalence varies greatly according to the condition. Only 20% of children and adults presenting with food-related symptoms are diagnosed with an IgE mediated food allergy.

Diagnosis

- *Clinical history:* the cornerstone of diagnosis should include information on symptom type and speed of onset, suspect foods, current diet, and food exclusions, whether co-factors such as exercise, alcohol, or aspirin were involved in the reactions, the presence of eczema, asthma, or rhinitis, other relevant medical history, and family history of allergy.
- *Skin prick test (SPT):* good first-line test for all FHS. Is inexpensive, gives immediate results, with a 95% negative predictive value (NPV) and good sensitivity. However, SPT have poor specificity and positive predictive value (PPV) for plant foods; using fresh foods can improve this. A skin wheal over a certain size can have a high PPV for some foods, but this can vary between populations; PPVs have only been published for children and mainly for milk, egg, and peanut. This test will not provide reliable results if the patient has taken antihistamines and may not be a suitable first-line test for those who have experienced an anaphylactic reaction. Patients with extensive eczema may not have sufficient clear skin to allow testing.
- *Serum IgE:* good for validating SPT or if SPT is not advisable, although unlike SPT the result is not immediately available. Has good NPV and sensitivity but poor specificity and PPV. As with SPT, a high level of

specific IgE can be highly predictive of allergy for some foods, although the same caveats for PPV apply as for SPT. Not a useful test for some foods such as wheat (unless checking specifically for the wheat allergen omega-5 gliadin), soy, fruits, and vegetables.

- *Component-resolved diagnosis (CRD)*: similar to a specific IgE blood test, this method of diagnosis determines sensitization to individual allergens in a food. For example, sensitization to the casein allergen (Bos d 8) in milk, or the ovomucoid allergen (Gal d 1) in egg indicates continued milk or egg allergy. The test can also evaluate whether a positive food-specific IgE level or SPT is the result of a primary allergy to that food or is an indication of cross-reactivity from pollen or house dust mite sensitization. For example, the peanut allergen, Ara h 2, is a marker for primary peanut allergy, whereas Ara h 8 is the peanut allergen that cross-reacts to birch pollen.
- *Diagnostic diets*: 4-6 weeks avoidance of a food group, food additive, or naturally occurring substance in food followed by open or blinded challenge if symptoms improve. Useful if discordance between tests and clinical history and essential if no suitable tests available. Total exclusion, or 'few foods' diets are not advised for any type of diagnosis and unsupervised elimination diets may be unsafe. Targeted diagnostic elimination diets can be useful for non-IgE mediated and non-immune mediated FHS, but should be managed by a dietitian to ensure dietary adequacy.
- *Food challenge*: the gold standard of diagnosis. A food challenge is used to establish a diagnosis for IgE mediated FHS if discordance between history, test results, and diagnostic diet. Can also be used to check whether a childhood food allergy has resolved. May be the only diagnostic test for non-IgE mediated and non-immune mediated FHS. Speed of onset and symptom severity normally dictate whether a challenge should be carried out in the hospital setting and whether it should be open or blinded.

There are many non-validated tests available that claim to diagnose FHS. Patients should be discouraged from using the results of such tests as a basis for implementing dietary change.

Management

The main management for any FHS reaction is avoidance of the trigger food(s). For most foods, the avoidance advice will be similar but degree may vary depending on the severity of symptoms and type of reaction.

Cow's milk

- Milk is the most common cause of food allergy worldwide. The UK prevalence of IgE milk allergy is 2-3%. Milk can also be a trigger of non-IgE mediated food allergy such as FPIES and eosinophilic oesophagitis, and also non-immune mediated FHS such as lactose intolerance.
- Immune-mediated milk allergy resolves in 90% of cases, especially in those who can tolerate baked milk, and usually before adulthood. Lactose intolerance is often lifelong, although it can occur temporarily after severe illness.
- Lactose intolerant individuals may tolerate some forms of milk, such as hard cheese, yogurt (see ➔ Chapter 26, 'Lactose intolerance', p. 650).
- Those with immune mediated milk allergy need to exclude all mammalian milks (cow's, goat's, or sheep milk) and foods containing milk solids, lactose, casein, and whey, e.g. flavoured crisps, sausages, baked goods, baked beans, and breakfast cereals.
- Children with mild to moderate IgE or non-IgE mediated milk allergy require a milk substitute; usually an extensively hydrolysed formula (EHF) is appropriate.
- If EHF fails to improve symptoms, or if the infant has had anaphylaxis, faltering growth, and/or is exclusively breastfed, then an amino acid formula is indicated.
- The hypoallergenic formula should be continued until the child is 2 years old unless a full dietary review has indicated otherwise.
- Milk substitutes made from soya, rice, hemp, potato, nut, coconut, pea, or oat may be suitable for older children and adults, if the diet is nutritionally adequate.
- Rice milk is not recommended for children aged <4.5 years because of a high level of inorganic arsenic relative to the amount consumed.
- Soya yogurts, deserts, cream cheeses, hard cheeses, and cream are suitable for infants aged ≥6 months if tolerated.
- Calcium and vitamin D supplements may be required by both children and adults.
- Nutritional adequacy of milk-free diets that do not include a milk replacement may be compromised.

Eggs

- Affects 1.6–3.2% of children and most commonly presents in the first year of life.
- Two-thirds of children will become tolerant to egg by the age of 5 years and the majority of those with persisting allergy will be able to tolerate cooked egg. High level of cross-reactivity to other avian eggs such as duck and goose eggs; there is also cross-reactivity to allergens in chicken meat.

- Cooking reduces the allergenicity of eggs but raw or loosely cooked egg may still be present in foods, e.g. royal icing, marzipan, meringue (Pavlova), mayonnaise, Yorkshire pudding.

Fish and shellfish

- Fish allergy most commonly presents in children and shellfish allergy in adults. Seafood allergy is usually lifelong.
- Because of the presence of pan-allergens in fish and shellfish, allergy to more than one species is common. The main allergen in fish, β parvalbumin, is found in high levels in cod and herring, whereas swordfish and tuna have low levels. The main allergen in shellfish is tropomyosin, which is largely the cause of allergy to crustaceans (prawns, lobster, and crab). Although molluscs (mussels, squid, oysters, snails) contain tropomyosin, allergy to this group of shellfish is less common.
- Because the allergens in seafood allergy differ, there is no cross-reactivity between fish and shellfish, although co-sensitization and allergy can occur.
- Cross-contamination can be an issue, with avoidance of all seafood being prudent for people while eating away from home.
- Although some allergens in fish can be denatured during the canning process, standard cooking methods will not affect them. The allergens in shellfish are very robust and not affected by heat. Fish and shellfish allergens may also be present in cooking vapours.
- Certain species of fish such as tuna and mackerel, and fish/shellfish that is not completely fresh, may contain high levels of histamine that can precipitate a pseudo-allergy called scombroid poisoning, which may be mistaken for allergy.

Wheat and other grains

- Wheat allergy is more common in children than adults. Wheat is, however, implicated in a form of food allergy that does affect adults, known as food-dependent, exercise-induced anaphylaxis (FDEIA) where the reaction only occurs when the trigger food is eaten in conjunction with exercise; wheat is the most common precipitant.
- SPT and serum IgE are poor predictors of wheat allergy; a better choice is to test for the presence of IgE antibodies to the wheat allergen omega-5 gliadin which is highly predictive of wheat allergy in children and FDEIA triggered by wheat.
- There is a high degree of cross-reactivity between wheat and grass pollen, so that 80% of positive SPT to wheat have no clinical significance in people with a grass pollen allergy.
- Wheat is also involved in other FHS reactions such as coeliac disease (see ➲ Chapter 26, 'Coeliac disease', p. 656), and is often reported to precipitate symptoms in people with irritable bowel syndrome.
- Corn/maize, barley/malt, and rice have all been reported to cause food allergy, although less so than some other cereals.

Fruit and vegetables

- Can cause primary allergy with sensitization mediated though ingestion, but more commonly involved in cross-reactions between tree pollen and plant foods, known as Pollen Food Syndrome (PFS), part of a spectrum of conditions called Oral Allergy Syndrome.
- PFS affects 2% of the UK population, and two-thirds of those sensitized to birch pollen are likely to have PFS.
- Symptoms are most commonly triggered by apples, stone fruits, and tree nuts, with immediate oropharyngeal symptoms on consuming the fruit or vegetable in its raw state.
- Allergens from grass and weed pollens and latex can also cross-react to plant foods.
- There can also be cross-reactions between plant foods through lipid transfer proteins (LTP). This allergy is usually due to sensitization to peach LTP, and is associated with severe reactions. Co-factors such as exercise, alcohols and non-steroidal anti-inflammatory drugs often precipitate reactions to foods which can otherwise be consumed without any problems.

Peanuts, tree nuts, soya, and seeds

- In UK children, the cumulative prevalence of peanut allergy is 0.7-1.4%.
- Usually manifests in childhood, with the average age of onset 18 months. Resolution is less likely than it is for milk and egg; 20-39% of peanut allergy resolves, but <10% of tree nut allergy.
- Peanuts are the most common food to cause severe reactions including anaphylaxis.
- Better labelling with declaration of ingredients and nut trace warnings may help decrease accidental exposure.
- Peanut allergic individuals have a 25–40% risk of developing a co-allergy to tree nuts.
- IgE mediated tree nut allergy prevalence ranges from 0.05% to 4.9%. Tree nuts most usually involved are hazelnuts, Brazil nuts, almonds, and walnuts.
- Cashew nut allergy can cause severe reactions.
- Important to determine whether symptoms or positive allergy tests to peanuts or tree nuts are caused by a primary allergy or PFS, using CRD.
- Those with PFS to only one nut often tolerate other nuts and do not need to avoid those foods which state 'may contain nuts'.
- Those with a primary peanut and/or tree nut allergy need to avoid the trigger food and any foods that contain it. Peanut allergy sufferers have a greater risk of accidental exposure. Individual advice on the avoidance of tree nuts or peanuts other than the provoking food should be given depending on age, the presence of co-sensitizations, risk of cross-contamination, and implications of dietary restrictions.
- Individuals with a peanut allergy do not usually need to avoid other legumes unless symptoms have been reported.
- Foods most likely to contain nuts include pastries, biscuits, breakfast cereals, ice-cream, desserts, pesto (which may contain cashew

nuts), oriental and Asian cuisine, named nut oils such as hazelnut oil; refined oils containing peanut oil are usually allowed.

- Allergy to soya manifests in infancy and childhood, with a prevalence of 0.5%. It is a transitory allergy, usually resolving before adolescence. New-onset soya allergy in teenagers and adults manifests because of PFS; cross-reactions between soy and birch pollen can provoke severe oropharyngeal symptoms.
- Sesame seeds are the most common seed allergens. Sesame allergy usually manifests before the age of 2 years, with 80% continuing to be allergic into their adult life. Sesame seeds have similar allergens to tree nuts and peanuts and cross-reactions may occur.
- Reactions to mustard seeds, sunflower seeds, and pumpkin seeds are becoming more common.

Food additives

- Commonly perceived to cause FHS, but are likely to affect <0.1% of the population.
- People who have asthma and urticaria are more likely to report hypersensitivity to certain food additives.
- The following additives are the most likely to be implicated in FHS:
  - *Colourings:* both natural food colourings such as carmine (cochineal), annatto, turmeric, and saffron, and synthetic azo dyes such as tartrazine (E102) and sunset yellow (E110).
  - *Preservatives:* benzoates (E210–219) found in beer, jam, fruit products, pickled foods, yogurt, salad cream, berries, prunes, and spices such as cinnamon and cloves; sulphites (E220–E227) in wine, cider, lager, fruit juices and squashes, meat products, dried fruits, and vegetables.
  - *Flavour enhancers:* monosodium glutamate in soups, sauces, dried noodle snacks, gravy, ready-meals, and Chinese food.

Naturally occurring food hypersensitivity triggers

- *Salicylates:* occur naturally in plant foods, and have a similar chemical structure and properties to aspirin; foods containing the most salicylate include coffee, tea, wine, dried herbs and spices, black pepper, oil of wintergreen, spearmint, certain fruits, and vegetables.
- *Vaso-active amines:* can cause a type of FHS, which mimics IgE mediated FHS; histamine, the most common vaso-active amine, is found in red wine, strong and blue cheeses, oily fish especially tuna and mackerel, spinach, aubergines, and pork products.

Food labels

From December 2014, EU Regulation 1169/2011[1] has required that information is provided on the labels of all packaged food highlighting 14 allergens (Table 37.1) in the list of ingredients in a legible font size. Information on allergens must also be provided on non-pre-packaged foods including those sold in restaurants and cafés.

See → Chapter 8, 'Food labelling', p. 188.

Table 37.1 Allergens to be listed on packaging under EU Regulation 1169/2011

Celery	Molluscs (including mussels, scallops, squid and oysters)
Cereals containing gluten (including wheat, rye, barley, oats, spelt, and kamut)	Mustard
Crustaceans (including prawns, lobster, crab)	Peanuts
Eggs	Sesame seeds
Fish	Soya bean and products containing soy (but not refined soya bean oil)
Lupin flour	Sulphites and SO_2 >10 mg/kg
Milk and milk products including lactose	Tree nuts, i.e. almond, hazelnut, walnut, cashew, pecan, brazil, pistachio, macadamia, and Queensland nuts

Further information

Skypala, I., Venter, C. (2009). *Food hypersensitivity: diagnosing and managing food allergies.* Wiley-Blackwell, Oxford.

1 Food Standards Agency (2017). Allergen labelling for manufacturers. Available at: ℛ https:// www.food.gov.uk/business-guidance/allergen-labelling-for-food-manufacturers.

Chapter 38

Drug–nutrient interactions and prescription of nutritional products

Drug–nutrient interactions 834
Prescription of nutritional products 842

Drug–nutrient interactions

Practitioners should consider any possibility of interactions between food or enteric feed given to patients and prescribed or over-the-counter medication. Both micro- and macronutrients may interact with drug therapy and these interactions may be positive (enhancing the effects of the medication leading to medication toxicity) or detrimental (leading to a failure of therapy or drug ineffectiveness).

Herbal medicines, e.g. St. John's wort, ginkgo, dong quai, may also interact with prescribed medication or interfere with the patient's condition.

The risk of nutrient-drug interactions is greatest in those taking more than one medication, children, and elderly people. This raises particular concern about drugs with a narrow therapeutic index, i.e. those that require careful monitoring, for example:
• lithium;
• monoamine oxidase inhibitors (MAOI);
• phenytoin;
• theophylline;
• warfarin.

Food, enteral feeds, and herbal medicines can affect the main pharmaco-kinetic processes—absorption, distribution, metabolism, and excretion of drug therapy. Examples of each are given in Tables 38.1–3.

▶ Medication is best taken with a glass of water, as acidity of fruit juices, tea, and coffee can alter drug properties and its pH balance.

Interactions leading to alterations in drug therapy

The absorption of certain drugs may be delayed and reduced by the presence of food in the stomach or, in some cases, enhanced. Taking certain medication with food can reduce gastric irritation or damage. For example, it is advisable to take ibuprofen, naproxen, and diclofenac with or after food. It is for this reason that cautionary medication labels such as 'with or after food', 'an hour before food or an empty stomach', should be followed.

Warfarin and vitamin K containing foods

The anticoagulant, warfarin, is a vitamin K antagonist, and alterations in vitamin K intake may affect the levels of warfarin and its anticoagulant effect. For example, consumption of large amounts of beetroot, green leafy vegetables (spinach, brussels sprouts, lettuce), green tea, mango, large quantities of ice-cream and alcohol may ↓ anticoagulant effects of warfarin. Once patients are stabilized on warfarin they should avoid major variations in the consumption of these foods and diet overall.

Potentiation of drug action

Inhibition of drug metabolism by nutrients may enhance drug effects. For example:
• Cranberry juice has been implicated in death through enhancing the effects of warfarin leading to fatal bleeding.
• Grapefruit juice may enhance the actions of calcium-channel blockers (especially felodipine, nimodipine, nicardipine, and verapamil) used in hypertension, angina, and arrhythmias. It may also potentiate the effects

Table 38.1 Absorption drug-food/nutrient interactions*

Drug/class	Food and/or nutrient	Effect of interaction/advice
Bismuth Flucloxacillin Phenoxymethylpenicillin Rifampicin	Presence of food in the stomach	Absorption delayed and ↓ Advise to take on an empty stomach or 1 h before food
Ciprofloxacin Norfloxacin Tetracyclines	Milk and dairy products	Absorption ↓ Advise to leave 2-h gap between drug and dairy consumption
Theophylline	High protein diet High carbohydrate diet	Bioavailability ↓ by high protein diets Bioavailability ↑ by high carbohydrate diets
Ciprofloxacin Digoxin Phenytoin Rifampicin Tetracycline Theophylline	Enteral feeds	Absorption ↓ Leave time gap between giving medication and enteral feed

* These lists are not exhaustive—the reader should consult *Stockley's Drug Interactions* or *British National Formulary* for further details.

Table 38.2 Metabolism drug-food/nutrient interactions*

Drug/class	Food and/or nutrient	Effect of interaction/advice
Amiodarone Buspirone Calcium channel blockers Carbamazepine Ciclosporin Colchicine Corticosteroids Coumarins Digoxin Fexofenadine Simvastatin	Grapefruit juice	Metabolism of drug altered by liver enzyme, cytochrome P450, stimulation Advise to follow manufacturer's instructions
Warfarin	Large amounts of brussels sprouts, green vegetables, cabbage, lettuce, green tea, excess quantities of ice-cream, avocado, mango	Drug metabolism ↑ and anticoagulant effect of warfarin ↓

(Continued)

Table 38.2 (Contd.)

Drug/class	Food and/or nutrient	Effect of interaction/advice
Warfarin	Cranberry juice	Anticoagulant effect of warfarin ↑
		↑ fatal incident reported
Warfarin	High doses of vitamin E	Anticoagulant effect of warfarin ↑
Levodopa Phenobarbital, phenytoin	Vitamin B6 (pyridoxine)	Effects of levodopa ↓ by concurrent supplementation of pyridoxine
		Advise to avoid vitamin B$_6$

* These lists are not exhaustive—reader should consult *Stockley's Drug Interactions* or *British National Formulary* for further details.

Table 38.3 Excretion drug–food/nutrient interactions*

Drug/class	Food and/or nutrient	Effect of interaction/advice
Lithium	Salt (sodium containing)	Excretion of lithium affected by ↑ or ↓ sodium intake
		Advise that once stabilized on lithium, patients should keep sodium intake stable

* These lists are not exhaustive—reader should consult *Stockley's Drug Interactions* or *British National Formulary* for further details.

of simvastatin by reducing its metabolism. Amlodipine can occasionally interact with grapefruit juice.

- Grapefruit juice may enhance the actions of the antihistamine fexofenadine and the immunosuppressant ciclosporin. Increase in plasma drug concentrations of those drugs can lead to drug toxicity.
- Fish oils inhibit platelet aggregation and may ↑ bleeding when used together with antiplatelet drugs (aspirin) and anticoagulant, warfarin.
- High doses of vitamin E enhance the anticoagulant effects of warfarin.
- Dietary sodium influences the excretion of lithium (used in bipolar affective disorder) so that increasing salt intake may ↓ plasma lithium while salt-restricted diets may ↑ plasma lithium to toxic levels.

Interactions limiting therapy

- Diuretics such as bendroflumethiazide and furosemide used for hypertension and chronic heart failure cause salt and water excretion. Their therapeutic effects may be reduced by consuming a high salt intake.
- The antibiotics, tetracycline and quinolones (such as ciprofloxacin) should not be taken at the same time as antacids, milk, or substances containing zinc, iron, or calcium salts as these can lead to ↓ absorption and ↓ effectiveness of the antibiotic. Separate intake by 2 hours.

- The therapeutic actions of levodopa for the management of Parkinson's disease may be ↓ by supplements of vitamin B$_6$ (pyridoxine). This does not occur when the levodopa is combined with a dopa-decarboxylase inhibitor, e.g. carbidopa.

❶ Interactions with potentially serious events
- *Warfarin and vitamin K containing foods:* see Table 38.2.
- *Warfarin and cranberry juice:* see Table 38.2.
- *Grapefruit juice and fexofenadine or ciclosporin:* see Table 38.2.
- *Angiotensin converting enzyme (ACE) inhibitors/angiotensin II receptor antagonists or potassium supplements or salt substitutes:* ACE inhibitors (e.g. ramipril, enalapril) and angiotensin II receptor antagonists (e.g. losartan) may cause K$^+$ retention and this may be exacerbated by K$^+$ supplements or K$^+$-containing salt substitutes causing hyperkalaemia.
- *MAOI and tyramine:* patients taking MAOI (e.g. phenelzine, moclobemide) for depression (rarely used nowadays) should avoid tyramine-containing foods (e.g. mature cheese, yeast extracts, soya bean products, pickled herring, red wine) as this may lead to the 'cheese reaction' with a severe increase in blood pressure and palpitations.
- *Isotretinoin and vitamin A:* isotretinoin is a retinoid used in the treatment of acne and should not be used with vitamin A supplements because of the risk of a vitamin A overdose.

Drug therapies requiring nutritional supplements
Certain drug therapies may require nutritional supplements to limit adverse effects.
- *Corticosteroids:* long-term treatment with oral corticosteroids (e.g. prednisolone) or potentially high dose inhaled corticosteroids is a risk factor for the development of osteoporosis, and calcium supplements may be recommended.
- *Methotrexate:* this is a folate-antagonist used in rheumatoid arthritis, Crohn's disease, anticancer chemotherapy, and psoriasis. Folic acid 5 mg/day should be prescribed as appropriate prevention of megaloblastic anaemia.
- *Isoniazid:* this antibiotic used in treatment of tuberculosis may have anti-vitamin B$_6$ effects leading to peripheral neuropathy and so 10 mg/day pyridoxine is recommended.
- *Antiepileptic drugs in pregnancy:* many antiepileptic drugs are associated with birth defects and folic acid 5 mg/day is prescribed to ↓ risk of neural tube defects. Carbamazepine, phenytoin, and phenobarbital are associated with risk of neonatal bleeding (including intracranial bleeds) and vitamin K is given to the mother from the 36th week of pregnancy and to the baby at birth.
- *Proguanil:* if this antimalarial drug is prescribed in pregnancy, supplementation of folic acid 5 mg/day is required.

Drug therapy leading to nutritional deficiencies
Certain drug treatments may reduce the absorption of nutrients.
- *Colestyramine and orlistat:* colestyramine (for hyperlipidaemia or jaundice) and orlistat (for obesity) may both ↓ the absorption of

fat-soluble vitamins (A, D, E, and K). Supplements may be required and should be taken at a different time to the drug.
- *Antiepileptic drugs:* enzyme-inducing antiepileptic drugs (e.g. carbamazepine, phenytoin) may induce the metabolism of vitamin D and may be overcome by vitamin D supplementation.
- Diuretics such as bendroflumethiazide and furosemide, especially when used at higher doses for chronic heart failure, may cause hypokalaemia, and K^+ supplements or foods rich in K^+ such as bananas may be recommended.
- Metformin (for diabetes) may ↓ absorption of vitamin B_{12}.
- *Insulin and sulfonylureas:* e.g. gliclazide and glibenclamide, (for diabetes) may lead to hypoglycaemia if meals are skipped or insufficient (see ➔ Chapter 22, 'Hypoglycaemia', p. 512).
- *Methotrexate and folic acid:* see above.

Alcohol and drugs
- Alcohol may enhance the action of many drugs acting on the brain (e.g. antidepressants, benzodiazepines, and antiepileptic drugs) leading to impaired mental ability and increased sedation.
- It is a misconception that <u>all</u> antibiotics interact with alcohol. Of the commonly used agents, there is a significant interaction with metronidazole and tinidazole, which leads to a severe reaction including nausea, vomiting, and flushing.
- Even small amounts of alcohol consumed with disulfiram (used in treatment of alcohol dependence) will cause a reaction resulting in facial flushing, tachycardia, giddiness, hypotension, and potentially collapse. Some oral medicines and mouthwashes bought over the counter contain sufficient alcohol to precipitate this reaction.
- Major changes in alcohol intake will affect anticoagulant effect of warfarin.

Nutritional status and drug therapy
- Dehydration will enhance the actions of diuretics and other antihypertensives and may ↑ the risks of falls in the elderly.
- Low dietary protein intake as well as disease processes may cause hypoalbuminaemia. Many drugs are bound to plasma proteins; this does not necessarily lead to major changes in therapy although correction may be required in therapeutic drug monitoring.
- Enteral tube feeding provides the opportunity for drugs to interact with constituents of the feed. When changing from a tablet to a liquid preparation (e.g. digoxin), the bioavailability may be altered and the dose of drug may need to be changed. ❶ Clinically significant interaction exists between enteral feeds and the following drugs: phenytoin, theophylline, digoxin, ciprofloxacin, tetracyclines, and rifampicin. See ➔ Chapter 25, 'Enteral feeding and drugs', p. 590.

Metabolic effects of drugs

- Some drugs may alter plasma lipid or glucose levels.
- Drugs that may lead to dyslipidaemia: β-blockers, corticosteroids, thiazide diuretics, anabolic steroids, certain anti-HIV drugs, retinoids, and combined oral contraceptives.
- Drugs that may affect glucose tolerance: thiazide diuretics, corticosteroids.

Effects of drug treatment on appetite and feeding

Some drug treatments may affect appetite (Table 38.4) and thus influence intake.

Some drugs may adversely influence nutritional intake by causing:

- *Taste disturbances:* with ACE inhibitors, calcium-channel blockers, anticancer chemotherapy drugs.
- *Dry mouth:* antimuscarinic side effects (e.g. with tricyclic antidepressants).
- *Oral mucositis:* this is a common side effect of anticancer drugs (especially with alkylating agents, methotrexate, and fluorouracil) where interference with cell division leads to oral ulceration. This may be exacerbated by poor oral hygiene. Saline mouthwashes are often used for relief and, in the case of fluorouracil, sucking ice while it is infused is recommended.
- *Nausea and vomiting:* digoxin, anticancer chemotherapy, opioids (such as morphine), certain drugs for Parkinson's disease, selective serotonin re-uptake inhibitors (SSRIs), erythromycin, theophylline.
- *Gastric irritation:* use of non-steroidal anti-inflammatory drugs in particular is associated with gastric damage and ulceration.

Table 38.4 Examples of drugs causing changes in appetite

Drug	Appetite ↑/weight ↑	Appetite ↓/nausea + vomiting
Antidiabetic Sulfonylurea, insulin	✓	
Antiemetic Chlorpromazine	✓	
Antiepileptic Sodium valproate	✓	
Antimanic Lithium	✓	
Antipsychotic Olanzapine, mirtazapine	✓	
Digoxin		✓
Corticosteroids Prednisolone, dexamethasone	✓	
Antidepressants SSRIs		✓
Tricyclics	✓	

Common herb–drug interactions

There are an increasing number of herbal products available with the potential to interact with prescribed medication (see Table 38.5 for the most common). The use of herbal drug products is prevalent among cancer patients, elderly people, children, and adults who are trying to reduce their body weight but is often unreported to healthcare professionals.

For full details on herb-to-drug interaction, consult *Stockley's Herbal Medicines Interactions*.

As with conventional medicines, pharmacokinetic and pharmacodynamic type interactions can occur between herbal products and drugs leading to either enhancement or antagonism of drug effect.

St John's wort (*Hypericum perforatum*) used commonly as an antidepressant, is an important liver enzyme inducer and may reduce the effects of a number of drugs. Concomitant treatment should be avoided and the patient's GP or a pharmacist should be consulted.

Table 38.5 Most common herb-drug interactions*

Herb	Interacts with	Comment
St John's wort	Antidepressants	Plasma drug concentration ↓ ↑ ↓ therapeutic effect
	Antivirals: HIV protease inhibitors (atazanavir, indinavir, nelfinavir, ritonavir, saquinavir)	↓ Therapeutic effect
	HIV non-nucleoside reverse transcriptase inhibitors (efavirenz, nevirapine)	↓ Therapeutic effect
	Anticonvulsants (carbamazepine, phenobarbital, phenytoin)	↓ Control of seizures
	Ciclosporin, tacrolimus	↑ Risk of transplant rejection
	Digoxin	↓ Therapeutic effect
	Oral combined contraceptives, oestrogen-containing patches and vaginal rings	↓ Therapeutic effect
	Voriconazole	↓ Therapeutic effect
	Theophylline	↓ Asthma control
	Warfarin	↓ Anticoagulant effect
	SSRIs (fluoxetine, paroxetine, sertraline)	↑ Serotonergic effects
	Triptans (sumatriptan, naratriptan, rizatriptan, zolmitriptan)	↓ Therapeutic effect
Ginkgo biloba	Anticoagulant (warfarin) Antiplatelet (aspirin)	↑ Risk of bleeding
Ginseng	Anticoagulant (warfarin)	↑ Risk of bleeding
Dong quai	Anticoagulant (warfarin)	↑ Risk of bleeding
Echinacea	Immuno-suppressant	Possible immune-stimulation
Saw palmetto	Anticoagulant (warfarin)	Altered anticoagulation

*List is not exhaustive. The reader should consult Stockley's Herbal Medicines Interactions or British National Formulary for further details.

Prescription of nutritional products

All nutritional products within the UK can be bought without a prescription, i.e. none are classified as *prescription-only medication*, which can only be obtained if prescribed by a medical practitioner or other specified healthcare professional. However, some nutritional products may be prescribed for specific conditions and are then categorized as drugs, rather than food. This facility is important for patients with chronic conditions who may need expensive special products over a long period of time, e.g. phenylketonuria where low-protein products are required.

Prescribable nutrition products are listed in the *British National Formulary*, Appendix 2, borderline substances as foods that may be prescribed for clinical conditions, alphabetically by brand name of products in the following categories:

- A2.1 Enteral feeds (non-disease specific).
- A2.2 Nutritional supplements (non-disease specific).
- A2.3 Specialized formulas.
- A2.4 Feed supplements.
- A2.5 Feed additives.
- A2.6 Foods for special diets.
- A2.7 Nutritional supplements for metabolic diseases.

Doctors, and independent or supplementary non-medical prescribers who prescribe such products are advised to:

- Endorse the prescription with 'ACBS' i.e. prescribed in accordance with the guidelines from the Advisory Committee on Borderline Substances.
- Ensure that the patient will be adequately monitored in taking the products and that, where necessary, expert hospital supervision, usually by a dietitian, will be available. Good communication between healthcare professionals and patients is required to optimize the products provided and the cost to the prescribing budget.
- In the UK advanced dietetic practitioners with appropriate training can have supplementary prescribing rights.

Further information

British Dietetic Association (2016) *Dietitians prescribing*. Available at ℘ https://www.bda.uk.com/professional/practice/prescribing/home

The British National Formulary is published twice yearly in March and September. Available at ℘ http://bnf.org/. BMJ Group and Pharmaceutical Press, London.

Preston, C.L. (ed) (2019). Stockley's Drug Interactions (12th edition). Pharmaceutical Press, London.

Williamson, E., Driver, S., Baxter, K., (eds) (2013). *Stockley's Herbal Medicines Interactions*. Pharmaceutical Press, London.

Weights and measures

Volume *844*
Mass/weight *845*

Volume

1fl oz = 28.41 mL
1 pint = 568.3 mL
1 litre = 1.76 pint

Table A1.1 Approximate volume conversion

fl oz/pint	mL/L	mL/L	fl oz/pt
1 fl oz	28 mL	50 mL	1.75 fl oz
¼ pint (5 fl oz)	142 mL	100 mL	3.5 fl oz
½ pint	284 mL	200 mL	7 fl oz
1 pint	568 mL	500 mL	8.8 fl oz
2 pints	1.1 L	1 L	1.76 pints
3 pints	1.7 L		
4 pints	2.3 L		
5 pints	2.8 L		

Mass/weight

1 ounce = 28.35 g
1 pound (16 oz) = 454 g (0.45 kg)
1 stone (14 lb) = 6.35 kg
1 g = 0.0352 ounces
1 kg = 2.2 pounds

Table A1.2 Approximate weight conversion

g to oz		oz to g	
g	oz	oz	g
1	0.04	1	28
10	0.35	2	57
15	0.53	3	85
20	0.71	4	113
30	1.06	5	142
40	1.41	6	170
50	1.76	7	198
60	2.12	8	227
70	2.47	9	255
80	2.82	10	284
90	3.17	11	312
100	3.53	12	340
		13	368
		14	397
		15	425
		16	454

Anthropometrics

Length/height conversions *848*
Mass/weight conversions *850*
Body mass index *852*
Waist circumference cut-offs for risk of metabolic complications,
    and mindex and demiquet measures of adiposity *854*
Upper arm anthropometry *858*
Child growth foundation charts *860*

Length/height conversions

1 inch = 2.54 cm
1 foot (12 in) = 30.48 cm
1 yard (36 in) = 91.44 cm
1 cm = 0.394 inch
1 m = 39.37 inches

Table A2.1 Approximate length conversions

Inches to centimetres		Centimetres to inches	
in	cm	cm	in
1	2.54	1	0.39
2	5.08	2	0.79
3	7.62	3	1.18
4	10.16	4	1.57
5	12.70	5	1.97
6	15.25	6	2.36
7	17.78	7	2.76
8	2.32	8	3.15
9	22.86	9	3.54
10	25.40	10	3.94
20	50.80	20	7.87
30	76.20	30	11.81
40	101.60	40	15.75
50	127.00	50	19.69
60	152.40	60	23.62
70	177.80	70	27.56
80	203.20	80	31.50
90	228.60	90	35.43
100	254.0	100	39.37

Table A2.2 Approximate height conversions

m	ft and in	m	ft and in
1.22	4'0"	1.6	5'3"
1.23	4'½"	1.61	5'3½"
1.24	4'1"	1.63	5'4"
1.26	4'1 ½"	1.64	5'4½"
1.27	4'2"	1.65	5'5 "
1.28	4'2 ½"	1.66	5'5½"
1.29	4'3"	1.68	5'6"
1.31	4'3 ½."	1.69	5'6½"
1.32	4'4"	1.7	5'7"
1.33	4'4½"	1.71	5'7 ½"
1.35	4'5"	1.73	5'8"
1.36	4'5½"	1.74	5'8 ½"
1.37	4'6"	1.75	5'9"
1.38	4'6½"	1.76	5'9 ½"
1.4	4'7"	1.78	5'10"
1.41	4'7 ½"	1.79	5'10½"
1.42	4'8"	1.8	5'11 "
1.43	4'8 ½"	1.82	5'11½"
1.45	4'9"		
1.46	4'9 ½"	1.83	6'0"
1.47	4'10"	1.84	6'0 ½"
1.49	4'10½"	1.85	6'1"
1.5	4'11 "	1.87	6'1 ½"
1.51	4'11½"	1.88	6'2"
		1.89	6'2 ½"
1.52	5'0"	1.9	6'3"
1.54	5'0 ½"	1.92	6'3½"
1.55	5'1"	1.93	6'4 "
1.56	5'1 ½"	1.94	6'4½"
1.57	5'2"	1.96	6'5"
1.59	5'2 ½"	1.97	6'5½"
		1.98	6'6"

Mass/weight conversions

1 oz = 28.35 g
1 lb = 454 g or 0.45 kg
1 g = 0.0352 oz
1 kg = 2.2 lb

Table A2.3 Approximate weight conversions

kg	st	lb	kg	st	lb	kg	st	lb	kg	st	lb
0.5		1	44	6	13	83	13	1	122	19	3
1		2	45	7	1	84	13	3	123	19	
1.5		3	46	7	3	85	13	6	124	19	7
2		4	47	7	6	86	13	7	125	19	10
2.5		6	48	7	8	87	13	10	126	19	11
3		7	49	7	10	88	13	11	127	20	0
3.5		8	50	7	13	89	14	0	128	20	1
4		9	51	8	0	90	14	3	129	20	5
4.5		10	52	8	3	91	14	4	130	20	7
5		11	53	8	4	92	14	7	131	20	8
5.5		12	54	8	7	93	14	8	132	20	11
6		13	55	8	10	94	14	11	133	20	13
			56	8	11	95	14	13	134	21	1
10	1	8	57	9	0	96	15	1	135	21	3
15	2	6	58	9	1	97	15	4	136	21	6
20	3	1	59	9	4	98	15	6	137	21	8
21	3	4	60	9	6	99	15	8	138	21	10
22	3	7	61	9	8	100	15	10	139	21	13
23	3	8	62	9	11	101	15	13	140	22	0
24	3	11	63	9	13	102	16	1	141	22	3
25	3	13	64	10	1	103	16	3	142	22	5
26	4	1	65	10	3	104	16	6	143	22	7
27	4	3	66	10	6	105	16	7	144	22	10
28	4	6	67	10	7	106	16	10	145	22	11
29	4	8	68	10	10	107	16	11	146	23	0
30	4	10	69	10	13	108	17	0	147	23	1
31	4	13	70	11	0	109	17	3	148	23	5
32	5	0	71	11	3	110	17	5	149	23	6
33	5	3	72	11	4	111	17	7	150	23	8

Table A2.3 (*Contd.*)

kg	st	lb	kg	st	lb	kg	st	lb	kg	st	lb
34	5	6	73	11	7	112	17	8	151	23	11
35	5	7	74	11	8	113	17	11	152	23	13
36	5	10	75	11	11	114	17	13	153	24	1
37	5	11	76	12	0	115	18	1	154	24	3
38	6	0	77	12	1	116	18	5	155	24	6
39	6	1	78	12	5	117	18	6	156	24	7
40	6	3	79	12	6	118	18	8	17	24	10
41	6	7	80	12	8	119	18	10	158	24	13
42	6	8	81	12	10	120	18	13	159	25	0
43	6	11	82	12	13	121	19	0	160	25	3

Body mass index

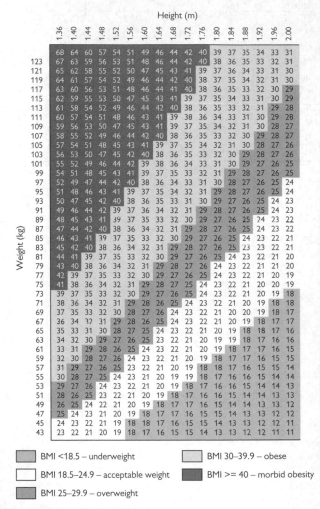

Fig. A2.1 Adult BMI ready reckoner.

Table A2.4 International BMI classification*

BMI		Weight status
< 18.5		Underweight
18.5–24.9		Normal
25.0–29.9		Pre-obesity
≥30.0		Obese
	30.0-34.9	Obese class I
	35.0-39.9	Obese class II
≥ 40		Obese class III

*Source: data from World Health Organization (2018). Body Mass Index-BMI. Available at http://www.euro.who.int/en/health-topics/disease-prevention/nutrition/a-healthy-lifestyle/body-mass-index-bmi.

Waist circumference cut-offs for risk of metabolic complications, and mindex and demiquet measures of adiposity

Table A2.5 International cut-off points for body mass index for overweight and obesity between 2 and 18 years*

Age, years	Body mass index 25 kg/m²		Body mass index 30 kg/m²	
	Males	Females	Males	Females
2	18.41	18.02	20.09	19.81
2.5	18.13	17.76	19.80	19.55
3	17.89	17.56	19.57	19.36
3.5	17.69	17.40	19.39	1923
4	17.55	17.28	19.29	19.15
4.5	17.47	17.19	19.26	19.12
5	17.42	17.15	19.30	19.17
5.5	17.45	17.20	19.47	19.34
6	17.55	17.34	19.78	19.65
6.5	17.71	17.53	20.23	20.0
7	17.92	17.75	20.63	20.51
7.5	18.16	18.03	21.09	21.01
8	18.44	18.35	21.6	21.57
8.5	18.76	18.69	22.17	22.18
9	19.10	19.07	22.77	22.81
9.5	19.46	19.45	23.39	23.46
10	19.84	19.86	24.00	24.11
10.5	20.20	20.29	24.57	24.77
11	20.55	20.74	25.10	5.42
11.5	20.89	21.20	25.58	26.05
12	21.22	21.68	26.02	26.67
12.5	21.56	22.1	26.43	27.24
13	21.91	22.58	26.84	27.76
13.5	22.27	22.98	27.25	28.20
14	22.62	23.34	27.63	28.57
14.5	22.96	23.66	27.98	28.87
15	23.29	23.94	28.30	29.11

(Continued)

Table A2.5 (*Contd.*)

Age, years	Body mass index 25 kg/m²		Body mass index 30 kg/m²	
	Males	Females	Males	Females
15.5	23.60	24.17	28.60	29.29
16	23.90	24.37	28.88	29.43
16.5	24.19	24.54	29.14	29.56
17	24.46	24.70	29.41	29.69
17.5	24.73	24.85	29.70	29.84
18	25	25	30	30

Table A2.6 Waist circumference cut-offs associated with disease risk*

Country or ethnic group	Gender	Waist circumference, cm
Europid	Men	>94
	Women	>80
South Asian	Men	>90
	Women	>80
Chinese	Men	>90
	Women	>80
Japanese	Men	>90
	Women	>80

*Source: data from WHO (2008). Waist circumference and waist hip ratio. WHO, Switzerland.

Mindex and demiquet

Measures of adiposity >64 years using demispan as proxy for height:

$$\text{Mindex (5)} = \text{wt (kg)}/\text{demispan (m)}$$

$$\text{Demiquet (4)} = \text{wt (kg)}/\text{demispan (m}^2)$$

Table A2.7 Deciles for mindex ($♀$)*

	10	20	30	40	50	60	70	80	90
64–74 years	68.3	73.3	77.8	82.2	84.8	88.4	92.3	99.9	110.6
75+ years	63.1	68.4	73.6	78.1	81.7	85.3	88.4	94.6	102.2

*Reproduced with permission from Lehmann, B., et al. (1991). Normal values for weight, skeletal size and body mass indices in 890 men and women aged over 65 years. *Clin. Nutr.* 1, 18–23. Copyright © 1991 Elsevier. All rights reserved.

Table A2.8 Deciles for demiquet ($♂$)*

	10	20	30	40	50	60	70	80	90
64–74 years	87.6	96.1	99.6	102.4	106.7	111.6	117.1	123.7	130.7
75+ years	84.5	92.8	98.9	103.1	106.3	109.1	113.4	119.3	125.3

*Reproduced with permission from Lehmann, B., et al. (1991). Normal values for weight, skeletal size and body mass indices in 890 men and women aged over 65 years. *Clin. Nutr.* 1, 18–23. Copyright © 1991 Elsevier. All rights reserved.

Table A2.9 Mid-arm circumference (MAC), cm*

Age group, years	Percentile						
	5th	10th	25th	50th	75th	90th	95th
♂							
18–74	26.4	27.6	29.6	31.7	33.9	36.0	37.3
18–24	25.7	27.1	28.7	30.7	32.9	35.5	37.4
25–34	27.0	28.2	30.0	32.0	34.4	36.5	37.6
35–44	27.8	28.7	30.7	32.7	34.8	36.3	37.1
45–54	26.7	27.8	30.0	32.0	34.2	36.2	37.6
55–64	25.6	27.3	29.6	31.7	33.4	35.2	36.6
65–74	25.3	26.5	28.5	30.7	32.4	34.4	35.5
♀							
18–74	23.2	24.3	26.2	28.7	31.9	35.2	37.8
18–24	22.1	23.0	24.5	26.4	28.8	31.7	34.3
25–34	23.3	24.2	25.7	27.8	30.4	34.1	37.2
35–44	24.1	25.2	26.8	29.2	32.2	36.2	38.5
45–54	24.3	25.7	27.5	30.3	32.9	36.8	39.3
55–64	23.9	25.1	27.7	30.2	33.3	36.3	38.2
65–74	23.8	25.2	27.4	29.9	32.5	35.3	37.2

*Source: data from Bishop, C.W., et al. (1981). Norms for nutritional assessment of American adults by upper arm anthropometry. *Am. J. Clin. Nutr.* **34**, 2530–9.

Upper arm anthropometry

Table A2.10 Mid-arm muscle circumference (MAMC), cm*

Age group, years	Percentile						
	5th	10th	25th	50th	75th	90th	95th
♂							
18–74	23.8	24.8	26.3	27.9	29.6	31.4	32.5
18–24	23.5	24.4	25.8	27.2	28.9	30.8	32.3
25–34	24.2	25.3	26.5	28.0	30.0	31.7	32.9
35–44	25.0	25.6	27.1	28.7	30.3	32.1	33.0
45–54	24.0	24.9	26.5	28.1	29.8	31.5	32.6
55–64	22.0	24.4	26.2	27.9	29.6	31.0	31.8
65–74	22.5	23.7	25.4	26.9	28.5	29.9	30.7
♀							
18–74	18.4	19.0	20.2	21.8	23.6	25.8	27.4
18–24	17.7	18.5	19.4	20.6	22.1	23.6	24.9
25–34	18.3	18.9	20.0	21.4	22.9	24.9	76.6
35–44	18.5	19.2	20.6	22.0	24.0	26.1	27.4
45–54	18.8	19.5	20.7	22.2	24.3	26.6	27.8
55–64	18.6	19.5	20.8	22.6	24.4	26.3	28.1
65–74	18.6	19.5	20.8	22.5	24.4	26.5	28.1

*Source: data from Bishop, C.W., et al. (1981). Norms for nutritional assessment of American adults by upper arm anthropometry. *Am. J. Clin. Nutr.* 34, 2530–9.

Table A2.11 Triceps skin-fold thickness, cm*

Age group, years	Percentile						
	5th	10th	25th	50th	75th	90th	95th
♂							
18–74	4.5	6.0	8.0	11.0	15.0	20.0	23.0
18–24	4.0	5.0	7.0	9.5	14.0	20.0	23.0
25–34	4.5	5.5	8.0	12.0	16.0	21.5	24.0
35–44	5.0	6.0	8.5	12.0	15.5	20.0	23.0
45–54	5.0	6.0	8.0	11.0	15.0	20.0	25.5
55–64	5.0	6.0	8.0	11.0	14.0	18.0	21.5
65–74	4.5	5.5	8.0	11.0	15.0	19.0	22.0
♀							
18–74	11.0	13.0	17.0	22.0	28.0	24.0	37.0
18–24	9.4	11.0	14.0	18.0	24.0	30.0	34.0
25–34	10.5	12.0	16.0	21.0	26.5	33.5	37.0
35–44	12.0	14.0	18.0	23.0	29.5	35.5	39.0
45–54	13.0	15.0	20.0	25.0	30.0	36.0	40.0
55–64	11.0	14.0	19.0	25.0	30.5	35.0	39.0
65–74	11.5	14.0	18.0	23.0	28.0	33.0	36.0

*Source: data from Bishop, C.W., et al. (1981). Norms for nutritional assessment of American adults by upper arm anthropometry. *Am. J. Clin. Nutr.* **34**, 2530–9.

Child growth foundation charts

Table A2.12 Normative values for handgrip strength in adults*

Age, years	Handgrip strength centiles, kg				
	10th	25th	50th	75th	90th
Men					
20	30	35	40	46	52
25	36	41	48	55	61
30	38	44	51	58	64
35	39	45	51	58	64
40	38	44	50	57	63
45	36	42	49	56	61
50	35	41	48	54	60
55	34	40	47	53	59
60	33	39	45	51	56
65	31	37	43	48	53
70	29	34	39	44	49
75	26	31	35	41	45
80	23	27	32	37	42
85	19	24	29	33	38
90	16	20	25	29	33
Women					
20	21	24	28	32	36
25	23	26	30	35	38
30	24	27	31	35	39
35	23	27	31	35	39
40	23	27	31	35	39
45	22	26	30	34	38
50	21	25	29	33	37
55	19	23	28	32	35
60	18	22	27	31	34
65	17	21	25	29	33
70	16	20	24	27	31
75	14	18	21	25	28
80	13	16	19	23	26
85	11	14	17	20	23
90	9	11	14	17	20

*Dodds, R.M., et al. (2014). Grip strength across the life course: Normative data from twelve British Studies. PLoS One. 9, e113637. doi: 10.1371.

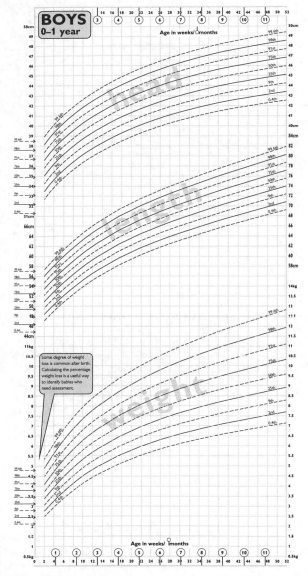

Fig. A2.2 UK-WHO growth chart for boys, 0–1 year. Reproduced with permission of Royal College of Paediatrics and Child Health. Copyright © 2009 Department of Health.

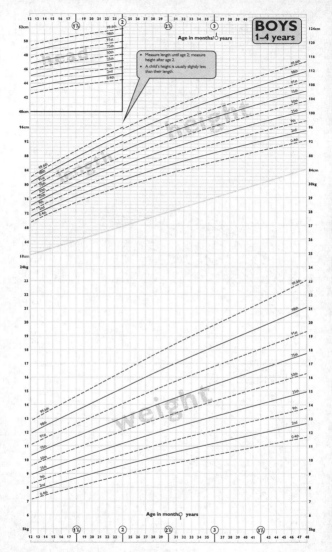

Fig. A2.3 UK-WHO growth chart for boys 1–4 years. Reproduced with permission of Royal College of Paediatrics and Child Health. Copyright © 2009 Department of Health.

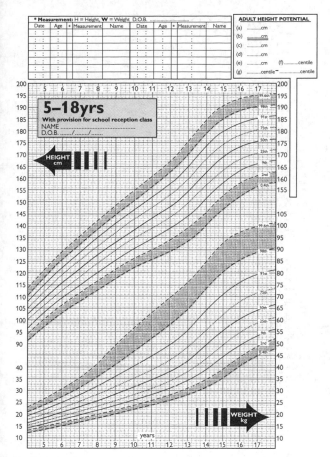

Fig. A2.4 Child Growth Foundation 9-centile growth chart for boys 5–18 years. Reproduced with the kind permission of the Child Growth Foundation.

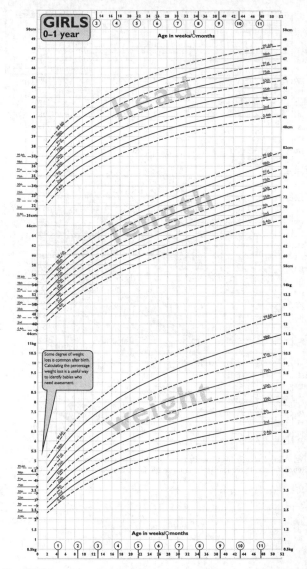

Fig. A2.5 UK-WHO growth chart for girls 0–1 year. Reproduced with permission of Royal College of Paediatrics and Child Health. Copyright © 2009 Department of Health.

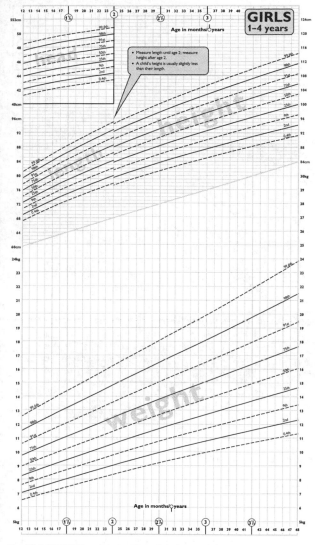

Fig. A2.6 UK-WHO growth chart for girls 1–4 years. Reproduced with permission of Royal College of Paediatrics and Child Health. Copyright © 2009 Department of Health.

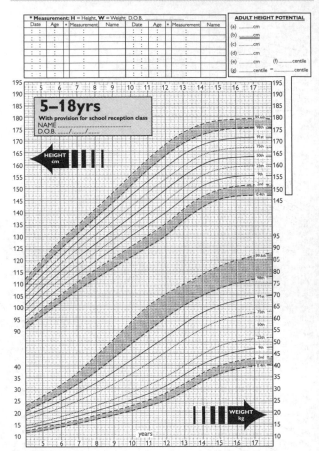

Fig. A2.7 Child Growth Foundation 9-centile growth chart for girls 5–18 years. Reproduced with the kind permission of the Child Growth Foundation.

Conversion factors

Dietary energy *868*
Protein/nitrogen *868*
Vitamin A *868*
Vitamin D *869*
Nicotinic acid/tryptophan *869*
Mineral content of compounds and solutions *869*

Dietary energy

Units used in energy balance
1000 J = 1 kJ
1000 kJ = 1 MJ
1 kcal = 4.184 kJ[1]
1 kJ = 0.239 kcal
1 W = 1 J/s
0.06 W = 1 kJ/min
86.4 W = 1 kJ.24 h

Table A3.1 Nutrient energy yields

Nutrient	Energy yield per gram	
	kcal	kJ
Protein	4	17
Carbohydrate	3.75	16
Fat	9	37
Alcohol	7	29
Medium chain triglyceride (MCT)	8.4	35

Protein/nitrogen

Dietary protein/dietary nitrogen
Dietary protein (g) = dietary nitrogen (g) × 6.25[2]
Dietary nitrogen (g) = dietary protein (g) ÷ 6.25[2]

Vitamin A

The active vitamin A content of a diet is usually expressed in retinol equivalents.
1 μg retinol equivalent = 1 μg retinol or 6 μg β carotene
1 IU vitamin A = 0.3 μg retinol or 0.6 μg β carotene

1 The Royal Society (London) recommended conversion factor.

2 This conversion factor is only appropriate for a mixture of foods. For milk or cereals alone, the factors 6.4 or 5.7 should be used.

Vitamin D

1 μg vitamin D = 40 IU
1 IU = 0.025 μg vitamin D

Nicotinic acid/tryptophan

1 mg nicotinic acid = 60 mg tryptophan
Nicotinic acid content mg equivalents = nicotinic acid (mg) + (tryptophan (mg)/60

Mineral content of compounds and solutions

Table A3.2 Mineral content of compounds and solutions

Solution/compound	Mineral content	
1 g sodium chloride	393 mg Na	17 mmol Na
1 g sodium bicarbonate	273 mg Na	12 mmol Na
1 g potassium bicarbonate	524 mg K	13.4 mmol K
1 g calcium chloride (hydrated)	273 mg C	7 mmol Ca
1 g calcium carbonate	400 mg Ca	10 mmol Ca
1 g calcium gluconate	93 mg Ca	2.3 mmol Ca
1 L normal saline	3450 mg Na	150 mmol Na

Energy expenditure prediction equations

The following equations are used as a basis for calculating energy expenditure (DRVs):[1] they have been derived from a large number of studies,[2] which measured energy expenditure in healthy subjects. In clinical practice, these are often referred to as the Henry equations.

Table A4.1 Formulae for the estimation of BMR

Age, years	BMR prediction equation, MJ/d†
<3	0.255 (W) − 0.141
3–10	0.0937 (W) + 2.15
10–18	0.0769 (W) + 2.43
18–30	0.0669 (W) + 2.28
30–60	0.0592 (W) + 2.48
>60	0.0563 (W) + 2.15
<3	0.246 (W) − 0.0965
3–10	0.0842 (W) + 2.12
10–18	0.0465 (W) + 3.18
18–30	0.0546 (W) + 2.33
30–60	0.0407 (W) + 2.90
>60	0.0424 (W) + 2.38

*W, Weight in kg.

Table A4.2 Calculated physical activity level (PAL) values for light, moderate, and heavy activity (occupational and non-occupational)*

Non occupational activity level	Occupational activity level					
	Light		Moderate		Heavy	
	♂	♀	♂	♀	♂	♀
Sedentary	1.4	1.4	1.6	1.5	1.7	1.5
Moderately active	1.5	1.5	1.7	1.6	1.8	1.6
Very active	1.6	1.6	1.8	1.7	1.9	1.7

*Source: data from Department of Health (1991). *Dietary reference values for food and nutrients for the United Kingdom.* HMSO, London.

1 SACN. (2011). Dietary reference values for energy. TSO, London.

2 Henry, C.J. (2005). Basal metabolic rate studies in humans: measurement and development of new equations. *Public Health Nutr.* **8**, 1133–52.

Energy expenditure prediction equation?

Appendix 5

Clinical chemistry reference ranges

Note. The values given are for guidance purposes only. Values will vary between laboratories. Check normal ranges in use at applicable setting before making clinical decisions.

Table A5.1 Adult normal values[*]

Substance	Value	Substance	Value
Albumin	32–50 g/L	Red cell count	
Bicarbonate	20–29 mmol/L	Males	$4.5–6.5\times10^{12}$/L
Bilirubin	<17 μmol/L	Females	$3.8–5.8\times10^{12}$/L
Calcium	2.15–2.55 mmol/L	Mean cell haemoglobin (MCH)	27–32 pg
Chloride	97–107 mmol/L	Mean cell volume (MCV)	77–95 fl
Non HDL-cholesterol	<2.5 mmol/L	Mean cell haemoglobin conc	32–36 g/dL
LDL-cholesterol	<1.8 mmol/L		
Creatinine	60–125 mmol/L	White blood count (WBC)	$4.0–11.0\times10^{9}$/L
Phosphate	0.14-0.46 mml/L	Neutrophils	$2.0–7.5\times10^{9}$/L
		Eosinophils	$0.04–0.4\times10^{9}$/L
Potassium	3.5–5.0 mmol/L	Monocytes	$0.2–0.8\times10^{9}$/L
Sodium	135–150 mmol/L	Basophils	$0.0–0.1\times10^{9}$/L
Triglycerides	0.55–1.90 mmol/L	Lymphocytes	$1.5–4.5\times10^{9}$/L
Urate	0.14–0.46 mmol/L	Platelets	$150–400\times10^{9}$/L
Urea	3.0–6.5 mmol/L	Erythrocyte sedimentation rate	2–12 mm/ 1st hour
Haemoglobin		Ferritin (varies with sex and age)	15–300 μg/L
Male	13.0–18.0 g/dL	Pre-menopausal women	14–200 μg/L
Female	11.5–16.5 g/dL	Serum B_{12}	150–700 ng/L
Haematocrit (PCV)		Serum folate	2.0–11.0 μg/L
Male	0.40–0.52	Red cell folate	150–700 μg/L
Female	0.36 0.47	Thrombin time (TT)	±3s of control

[*]Adapted from Provan, J. (2010). *Oxford handbook of clinical and laboratory investigation*, 3rd edn. By permission of Oxford University Press, Oxford.

Table A5.2 Values for the diagnosis of diabetes mellitus and other categories of hyperglycaemia[1,2]

	Fasting venous plasma glucose concentration		2-h venous plasma glucose concentration after 75 g glucose load		HbA1c	
	mmol/L	mg/dL	mmol/L	mg/dL	mmol/mol	%
Diabetes	≥7.0	≥126	≥11.1	≥200	≥48	≥6.5*
Impaired glucose tolerance**	<7.0	<126	≥7.8-<11.1	≥140-<200	-	-
Impaired fasting glucose	6.1-6.9	110-125	<7.8	<142	-	-

*In the absence of symptoms, diagnosis should not be made on the basis of a single HbA1c test. An additional test (HbA1c or plasma glucose) is required to confirm the diagnosis.

Impaired glucose tolerance is diagnosed in the presence of **both abnormal fasting glucose and 2-h glucose concentrations.

1 World Health Organization (2006). *Definition and diagnosis of diabetes mellitus and intermediate hyperglycaemia*. WHO, Geneva.

2 World Health Organization (2011). *Use of glycated haemoglobin (HbA1c) in the diagnosis of diabetes mellitus*. WHO, Geneva.

Dietary reference values (DRVs)

Estimated average requirements *876*
Reference nutrient intakes *878*

Estimated average requirements

Table A6.1 Estimated average requirements (EARs) (MJ/d) according to height and weight at BMI = 22.5 kg/m² and assuming a physical activity level (PAL) of 1.63†

	Height, cm	Weight (kg) BMI = 22.5 kg/m²	EAR, MJ/d
Males			
19–24	178	71.5	11.6
25–34	178	71.0	11.5
35–44	176	69.7	11.0
45–54	175	68.8	10.8
55–64	174	68.3	10.8
65–74	173	67.0	9.8
75+	170	65.1	9.6
Females			
19–24	163	29.9	9.1
25–34	163	59.7	9.1
35–44	163	59.9	8.8
45–54	162	59.0	8.8
55–64	161	58.0	8.7
65–74	159	57.2	8.0
75+	155	54.3	7.7

†Source: data from SACN. (2011). *Dietary reference values for energy.* TSO, London.

Table A6.2 Estimated average requirements (EARs) for energy of children 0–18 years*

Age	EAR MJ/d, kcal/d	
	Boys	Girls
0–3 months	2.6	2.4
4–6 months	2.7	2.5
7–9 months	2.9	2.7
10–12 months	3.2	3.0
1–3 years	4.1	3.8
4–6 years	6.2	5.8
7–10 years	7.6	7.1
11–14 years	9.9	9.1
15–18 years	12.6	10.2

*Source: data for EARs from SACN. (2011). *Dietary reference values for energy.* TSO, London.

Reference nutrient intakes

Table A6.3 Reference nutrient intakes for protein (RNI)*

Age	Weight, kg	RNI, g/day
0–3 months	5.9	12.5
4–6 months	7.7	12.7
7–9 months	8.8	13.7
10–12 months	9.7	14.9
1–3 years	12.5	14.5
4–6 years	17.8	19.7
7–10 years	28.3	28.3
Male		
11–14 years	43.0	42.1
15–18 years	64.5	55.2
19–50 years	74.0	55.5
50+ years	71.0	53.3
Female		
11–14 years	43.8	41.2
15–18 years	55.5	45.4
19–50 years	60.0	45.0
50+ years	62.0	46.5
Pregnancy		
Lactation		+6.0
0–4 months		+11.0
4+ months		+8.0

*Department of Health (1991). *Dietary reference values for food and nutrients for the United Kingdom*. HMSO, London.

Table A6.4 RNIs for vitamins*

Age	Thiamine, mg/d	Riboflavin, mg/d	Niacin, mg/d†	Vitamin B$_6$, mg/c‡	Vitamin B$_{12}$, µg/d	Folate, µg/d	Vitamin C, mg/d	Vitamin A, µg/d	Vitamin D**,
0–3 months	0.2	0.4	3	0.2	0.3	50	25	350	8.5–10.0††
4–6 months	0.2	0.4	3	0.2	0.3	50	25	350	8.5–10.0
7–9 months	0.2	0.4	4	0.3	0.4	50	25	350	8.5–10.0
10–12 months	0.3	0.4	5	0.4	0.4	50	25	350	8.5–10.0
1–3 years	0.5	0.6	8	0.7	0.5	70	30	400	8.5–10.0
4–6 years	0.7	0.8	11	0.9	0.8	100	30	400	8.5–10.0
7–10 years	0.7	1.0	12	1.0	1.0	150	30	500	8.5–10.0
Male									
11–14 years	0.9	1.2	15	1.2	1.2	200	35	600	10
15–18 years	1.1	1.3	18	1.5	1.5	200	40	700	10
19–50 years	1.0	1.3	17	1.4	1.5	200	40	700	10
50+ years	0.9	1.3	16	1.4	1.5	200	40	700	10

(Continued)

Table A6.4 (Contd.)

Age	Thiamine, mg/d	Riboflavin, mg/d	Niacin, mg/d†	Vitamin B₆, mg/d‡	Vitamin B₁₂, µg/d	Folate, µg/d	Vitamin C, mg/d	Vitamin A, µg/d	Vitamin D**,
Female									
11–14 years	0.7	1.1	12	1.0	1.2	200	35	600	10
15–18 years	0.8	1.1	14	1.2	1.5	200	40	600	10
19–50 years	0.8	1.1	13	1.2	1.5	200	40	600	10
50+ years	0.8	1.1	12	1.2	1.5	200	40	600	10
Pregnancy	+0.1§	+0.3	¶	¶	¶	200+100	+10	+100	10
Lactation									
0–4 months	+0.2	+0.5	+2	¶	+0.5	+60	~+30	+350	10
4+ months	+0.2	+0.5	+2	¶	+0.5	+60	+30	+350	10

* Data from Department of Health (1991). *Dietary reference values for food and nutrients from the United Kingdom.* HMSO, London. Table from appendix 6.2, pp.716–17 of Thomas, B. (2001). *Manual of dietetic practice.* 3rd edn. Blackwell science, Oxford.

† Nicotinic acid equivalent.

‡ Based on protein providing 14.7% of the EAR for energy.

§ Last semester only.

¶ No increment.

** People who stay indoors and are fully covered or live at high altitudes are at risk of deficiency because of a lack of ultraviolet radiation from sunlight. It is recommended that people consider taking a supplement of 10 µg in autumn and winter in the UK. Housebound/care home residents etc., those who cover their skin, and ethnic groups with dark skin should consider taking a supplement throughout the year.

††Safe level for 0–4 years.

Table A6.5 RNIs for minerals*

Age	Ca, mg/d	P, mg/d	Mg, mg/d	Na, mg/d	K, mg/d	Cl, mg/d	Fe, mg/d	Zn, mg/d	Cu, mg/d	Se, µg/d	I, µg/d
0–3 months	525	400	55	210	800	320	1.7	4.0	0.2	10	50
4–6 months	525	400	60	280	850	400	4.3	4.0	0.3	13	60
7–9 months	525	400	75	320	700	500	7.8	5.0	0.3	10	60
10–12 months	525	400	80	350	700	500	7.8	5.0	0.3	10	60
1–3 years	350	270	85	500	800	800	6.9	5.0	0.4	15	70
4–6 years	450	350	120	700	1100	1100	6.1	6.5	0.6	20	100
7–10 years	550	450	200	1200	2000	1800	8.7	7.0	0.7	30	110
Male											
11–14 years	1000	775	280	1600	3100	2500	11.3	9.0	0.8	45	130
15–18 years	1000	775	300	1600	3500	2500	11.3	9.5	1.0	70	140
19–50 years	700	550	300	1600	3500	2500	8.7	9.5	1.2	75	140
50+ years	700	550	300	1600	3500	2500	8.7	9.5	1.2	75	140

(Continued)

Table A6.5 (Contd.)

Age	Ca, mg/d	P, mg/d	Mg, mg/d	Na, mg/d	K, mg/d	Cl, mg/d	Fe, mg/d	Zn, mg/d	Cu, mg/d	Se, µg/d	I, µg/d
Female											
11–14 years	800	625	280	1600	3100	2500	14.8‡	9.0	0.8	45	130
15–18 years	800	625	300	1600	3500	2500	14.8‡	7.0	1.0	60	140
19–50 years	700	550	270	1600	3500	2500	14.8‡	7.0	1.2	60	140
50+ years	700	550	270	1600	3500	2500	8.7	7.0	1.2	60	140
Pregnancy	‡	‡	‡	‡	‡	‡	‡	‡	‡	‡	‡
Lactation											
0–4 months	+550	+440	+50	‡	‡	‡	‡	+6.0	+0.3	+15	‡
4+ months	+550	+440	+50								

‡ No increment.

‡ Supplements required if menstrual losses are high.

* Data from Department of Health (1991). Dietary reference values for food and nutrients from the United Kingdom. HMSO, London. Table from appendix. 6.2, pp. 716–17 of Thomas, B. (2001). Manual of dietetic practice, 3rd edn. Blackwell Science, Oxford.

Nutritional composition of common foods

Protein exchanges *884*
Carbohydrate exchanges *886*
Average portion sizes *888*

Protein exchanges

Table A7.1 Foods containing approximately 6 g protein

	Weight, g	Description
Meat—cooked, e.g. lean beef, lamb, pork	25	1 small slice
Sausage—cooked	40	1 large sausage
Poultry—cooked	25	1 small slice
Fish—cooked or tinned	40	1 tablespoon
Fish fingers—cooked	45	2 fingers
Egg	50	1 medium hen's egg
Cheese e.g. Cheddar	25	Matchbox-sized piece
Milk—full fat, semi-or skimmed	200	Average glass (1/3 pt)
Milk powder—skimmed	15	4 teaspoons
Yogurt	125	Small pot
Pulses—cooked e.g. lentils	100	3 tablespoons
Nuts, e.g. almonds, peanuts	25	15–25 nuts
Hummus	100	3 tablespoons

Table A7.2 Foods containing approximately 2 g protein

	Weight, g	Description
Bread—white/wholegrain	25	1 large thin slice
Potato—boiled	125	2 × size of hen's egg
Potato—mashed	110	2 scoops
Chips	50	8 large
Rice—boiled	75	1½ tablespoons
Pasta—boiled	50	1 tablespoon
Breakfast cereal—cornflake type	25	small average portion
Breakfast cereal—wheat biscuit type	20	1 biscuit
Biscuits, e.g. plain digestive	30	2 biscuits
Cream crackers	20	4 crackers
Cake—plain sponge	25	½ small average slice
Ice cream—plain	50	1 small scoop
Baked beans	40	1 tablespoon

Table A7.3 Foods containing little protein per typical portion

	Protein content*		
Butter	0.6	Apples, pineapple	0.4
Margarine	Trace	Pear	0.3
Cooking oil	Trace	Melon	0.6
Sugar	0.5	Apple juice	0.1
Golden syrup	0.3	Cranberry juice	Trace
Jam, honey	0.5	Boiled sweets	Trace
Marmalade	0.1	Peppermints	0.5
Carrots, boiled	0.6	Cola, lemonade	Trace
Celery, cucumber, lettuce	0.5–0.8	Tea, infusion	0.1
Swede, boiled	0.3	Coffee, infusion	0.2

*g/100 g food.

Carbohydrate exchanges

Table A7.4 Foods containing approximately 10 g carbohydrate

	Weight, g	Description
Wholemeal bread	25	1 thin slice/large loaf
White bread	20	1 thin slice/small loaf
Potatoes—boiled	60	1 size of hen's egg
Potatoes—mashed	60	1 scoop
Potatoes—roast	40	1 very small
Sweet potato—boiled	50	1 size of hen's egg
Rice—boiled, brown, white	30	¾ tablespoon
Pasta—boiled, e.g. spaghetti, macaroni	50	1 tablespoon
Pulses, e.g. lentils	60	2 tablespoons
Peas—frozen	100	3 tablespoons
Parsnip—boiled	80	1 medium
Sweetcorn—boiled	50	2 tablespoons
Thick soup, e.g. tinned vegetable	100	1 small tin
Thin soup, e.g. minestrone	250	1 standard mug
Sausages	100	2 large sausages
Beefburger, economy	100	1 economy burger
Beefburger, 100% meat = no CHO	—	—
Fish fingers	60	2 fish fingers
Breakfast cereals, e.g. branflakes	15	2 tablespoons
Breakfast cereals, e.g. wheat biscuit type	20	1 biscuit
Muesli, no added sugar	15	¾ tablespoon
Porridge—made with water	125	small average portion
Biscuits—plain digestive	15	1 digestive
Apple, pear	100	1 medium
Orange	120	1 small
Banana	45	½ small banana
Melon—galia, honeydew	200	1 medium slice
Pineapple, fresh	100	1 large slice
Grapes	70	15 large grapes
Orange juice—no added sugar	110	½ average glass

(Continued)

Table A7.4 (*Contd.*)

	Weight, g	Description
Apple juice—no added sugar	100	½ average glass
Cranberry juice	70	1/3 average glass
Milk—full fat, semi- or skimmed	200	1 average glass
Yogurt—low fat, fruit	70	½ small pot
Yogurt—low fat, plain	135	1 small pot
Ice cream—plain dairy, vanilla	50	1 small scoop
Lemonade	170	1 small glass
Lucozade®	60	1/3 average glass
Cola	90	½ average glass
Beer—best bitter	450	¾ pint glass
Lager—premium	400	¾ pint glass
Wine—medium white	330	2½ small wine glasses
Wine—red contains 0.2 g CHO/100 mL	—	—
Crisps	20	¾ small packet
Peanuts—dry roasted	100	1 large packet

Average portion sizes

Table A7.5 Examples of household measures of foods used commonly in the UK*

Food group	Household measure	Quantity	kcal/portion
Cereals and starchy foods	1 med. bowl breakfast cereal-sweet	40 g	149
	1 med. bowl breakfast cereal	40 g	132
	1 medium bowl porridge (whole)	200 g	232
	1 biscuit Weetabix	20 g	70
	1 medium slice of bread	35 g	76
	1 bread roll	50 g	134
	4 tablespoons of cooked pasta	60 g	52
	4 tablespoons of cooked white rice	60g	83
	2 egg-sized boiled potatoes	60 g	45
	1 medium plate of chips	100 g	239
	1 average jacket potato with skin	180 g	245
	1 croissant/brioche	50 g	180
	1 chapatti	55 g	100
	1 crumpet	40 g	79
	1 poppadum grilled	10 g	37
	1 naan bread	160 g	537
Fruit	1 medium apple (without core)	100 g	48
	1 medium banana (no skin)	100 g	95
	½ avocado (flesh only)	75 g	143
	1 cherry (no stone)	10 g	5
	1 medium clementine/mandarin	60 g	22
	1 apricot (without stone)	65 g	20
	1 slice melon (without skin)	180 g	34
	1 medium pear	170 g	68
	1 medium nectarine (no stone)	110 g	44
	1 medium kiwi (without skin)	60 g	29
	1 grape	5 g	3
	½ grapefruit (flesh only)	80 g	24
	1 medium plum (without stone)	55 g	20
	1 glass of fruit juice	200 mL	72

(Continued)

Table A7.5 (*Contd.*)

Food group	Household measure	Quantity	kcal/portion
Vegetables	1 average portion of vegetables, e.g. cauliflower, Brussels sprouts, carrots	90 g	38
	Medium boiled carrot	45 g	16
	1 slice cucumber	6 g	1
	1 spring onion	20 g	5
	1 average onion	90 g	32
	1 average portion of peas	65 g	45
	1 average tomato	85 g	15
	1 tablespoon sweetcorn	30 g	37
	1 broccoli spear	45 g	10
Dairy products	1 pint of whole milk	568 mL	375
	1 pint of semi-skimmed milk	568 mL	261
	1 pint of skimmed milk	568 mL	187
	1 pot of yogurt, low fat	125 g	113
	Hard cheese (small matchbox size)	30 g	122
	Cottage cheese—small pot	112 g	110
Protein sources	2–3 thin slices of beef-lean	90 g	193
	2–3 thin slices of pork-lean	90 g	371
	2–3 thin slices of lamb-lean	90 g	257
	1 medium burger	105 g	270
	1 rasher bacon-back	25 g	51
	1 medium chicken portion	150 g	223
	1 rump or fillet steak (5 oz.)	115 g	326
	1 medium slice of ham	50 g	60
	2 hot dog sausages	70 g	192
	1 medium piece of fish	120 g	115
	2 sardines (tinned in tom. sauce)	40 g	71
	2 fish fingers	60 g	128
	1 average serv. tuna in sandwich	45 g	45
	1 hen's egg	50 g	73
	1 omelette/1 serving scrambled egg	120 g	228
	Average portion of beans/lentils	120 g	105
	1 small tin of baked beans	170 g	143
	1 handful of nuts	40 g	243

(Continued)

Table A7.5 (Contd.)

Food group	Household measure	Quantity	kcal/portion
Fats and fat-rich	1 teaspoon of butter/margarine	5 g	37
	1 tablespoon of oil	11 mL	90
	1 packet of crisps	28 g	153
Sweet foods	1 sugar cube	5 g	20
	1 sachet of sugar	10 g	40
	2 squares of chocolate	5 g	26
	1 dessertspoon of jam	30 g	78
	1 sweet biscuit	20 g	91
	1 vanilla slice	110 g	305
	1 slice of chocolate/sponge cake	65 g	298
	1 slice of apple pie	115 g	214
	1 jam doughnut	75 g	252
	1 slice fruit cake	70 g	248
	1 jam tart	24 g	91
	1 fruit scone	48 g	156
Drinks	1 small glass	150 mL	
	1 medium glass	200 mL	
	1 mug	250 mL	
	1 can of fizzy sweet drink	330 mL	129
	1 average glass of wine	125 mL	88
	1 average bottle of wine	750 mL	525
	1 measure of spirits	23 mL	51
Composite meals	1 medium pizza	300 g	750
	1 slice of quiche/flan	120 g	377
	1 average portion of stew	330 g	396
	1 average portion of curry	330 g	677
	1 average portion of lasagne	450 g	460
	1 individual steak and kidney pie	200 g	646
	1 average portion of shepherd's pie	300 g	354
Spoon sizes	1 teaspoonful	~5 mL	
	1 dessertspoonful	~10 mL	
	1 tablespoonful	~15 mL	

*Source: data from Crawley, H. (1990). *Food portion sizes*, MAFF publication. HMSO, London; and Krebs, J. (2002). *McCance & Widdowson's the Composition of Foods*, 6th edn. FSA, London.

The National Statistics Socio-economic Classification (UK)

From 2001, the National Statistics Socio-economic Classification (NS-SEC) has been used for official statistics and surveys. It was rebased in 2010.[1] It replaces social class based on occupation and socio-economic groups. The information required to create the NS-SEC is occupation (coded to the Standard Occupational Classification 2000) and details of employment status (whether an employer, self-employed, or employee; whether a supervisor; number of employees at the workplace) (see Box A8.1). There are eight classes, the first of which can be subdivided.

A simpler, self-coded version of the NS-SEC has been developed with five classes for use in postal surveys or where detailed occupation information is not needed (Box A8.2).

Box A8.1 The National Statistics Socio-economic Classification Analytic Classes*

- 1 Higher managerial and professional occupations
  - 1.1 Large employers and higher managerial occupations
  - 1.2 Higher professional occupations
- 2 Lower managerial, administrative and professional occupations
- 3 Intermediate occupations
- 4 Small employers and own account workers
- 5 Lower supervisory and technical occupations
- 6 Semi-routine occupations
- 7 Routine occupations
- 8 Never worked and long-term unemployed

* For complete coverage, the three categories of students, occupations not stated or inadequately described, and not classifiable for other reasons are added as 'Not classified'.

---

1 ✍ Further information: https://www.ons.gov.uk/methodology/classificationsandstandards/otherclassifications/thenationalstatisticssocioeconomicclassificationnssecrebasedonsoc2010.

Box A8.2 Simpler National Statistics Socio-economic Classification Analytic Classes
- 1 Higher managerial and professional occupations
- 2 Intermediate occupations
- 3 Small employers and own account workers
- 4 Lower supervisory and technical occupations
- 5 Semi-routine and routine occupations

Index

Tables, figures and boxes are indicated by *t*, *f* and *b* following the page number

A

ABCDEF nutrition assessment 38
abetalipoproteinaemia 817*t*
absorption reduction, malnutrition 565
acarbose 511*t*
accelerometers 95, 96*b*
ACE (angiotensin converting enzyme) inhibitors 837
acetic acid 216*t*
achalasia 628
acidaemias 817*t*
aciduria, argininosuccinic aciduria 817*t*
acne 309
acute hepatitis 694
acute kidney injury (AKI) 704
  classification 705*t*
  contributing causes 705*b*
  nutritional support 730–1
acute pancreatitis 684*b*
AD (Alzheimer's disease) 790
additives see food additives
ADeH (alcohol dehydrogenase) 206
adequate intake (AI) 24*b*
ADHD (attention deficit hyperactivity disorder) 765–6
adolescents see children and adolescents
adults
  global nutrition problems 437
advertising regulation 410, 411*b*
AfN (The Association for Nutrition) 13–14
African-Caribbean, food restrictions 342*t*
agar 217*t*
age groups, global nutrition problems 436–7
ageing see older people
agriculture, WHO obesity prevention recommendations 400*b*
AI (adequate intake) 24*b*

air-displacement plethysmography 51
AKI see acute kidney injury (AKI)
albiglutide 511*t*
albumin
  kidney nutritional assessment 707*t*
  reference ranges 873*t*
alcohol 206–9
  acute effects of 208
  breastfeeding 272
  carbohydrates 82*t*
  cardioprotective diet 526*t*
  children and adolescents 309–10
  consumption of 208
  current dietary patterns 34–5
  diabetes 209
  drug–nutrient interactions 838
  energy values for oxidation 89*t*
  health effects 208, 209
  heart failure 530
  hypertension 538–9
  intake recommendations 207–8
  intoxication stages 207*t*
  metabolism of 206
  nutritional value 207
  preconceptual nutrition avoidance 238
  pregnancy 209, 242
  UK recommendations 28*t*
  various drinks 206*b*, 207*t*
alcohol dehydrogenase (ADeH) 206
alcoholic beverages
  alcohol by volume 206*b*
  folate (folic acid) 127*t*
  iodine 161*t*
  potassium 181*t*
  riboflavin (vitamin B_2) 117*t*
  vitamin B_6 132*t*
aldehyde dehydrogenase (ALDH) 206
alginic acid 217*t*
alkaline diets 232–6
allergenic ingredients, food labelling 190*b*
allergies

food see food hypersensitivity
  risk in weaning 282*b*
alogliptin 511*t*
alpha-glucosidase inhibitors 511*t*
alternative diets
  cancer 551
  HIV infection 751
  multiple sclerosis 783–4, 784*b*
aluminium 790
Alzheimer's disease (AD) 790
amaranth (red) colouring 215*t*
amino acids
  classification 66*t*
  disorders 817*t*
  essential (indispensible) 65, 66*t*
  intra-peritoneal amino acids 716–17
  metabolism 761–2
aminopterin, folate interactions 126
anaemia
  chronic kidney disease 719
  iron deficiency see iron-deficiency anaemia (IDA)
angiotensin converting enzyme (ACE) inhibitors 837
angiotensin II receptor antagonists 837
anorexia nervosa (AN) 769–71
Antabuse® (disulfiram) 206
anthropometry 54–8, 847–60
  adults 55–8
  biceps skin-fold measurements 55*t*
  body composition 41*t*, 53
  body mass index see body mass index (BMI)
  child growth foundation charts 860*t*, 861*f*, 862*f*, 863*f*, 864*f*, 865*f*, 866*f*

demi-span 56, 57t
height see height
knee height 56, 57t
length/height conversion 848, 849t
mass/weight conversions 850
mid-arm circumference (MAC) 857t
skin-fold measurements 55t
standard measurements 55t
triceps skin-fold measurements 55t, 58, 859t
UK 0–4 year charts 54
ulna length 56, 561f
upper arm anthropometry 858, 859t
waist circumference (WC) see waist circumference (WC)
weigh 476t
weight 55
WHO growth charts 54
Z-score 54
antibiotics
associated diarrhoea 199
nutrient interaction 836–7
anticarcinogenic phytochemicals 210
anticonvulsant drugs 757b
folate interactions 126
antidepressant drugs 757b
antiepileptic drugs 837–8
antioxidants 210
food additives 216, 217t
motor neuron disease 787
Parkinson's disease 789
antipsychotic drugs 757b
atypical 757b
appetite effects, drug–nutrient interactions 839t, 839
APs (assistant practitioners) 13
arachidic fatty acid 72t
arachidonic fatty acid 72t
arginine 620
argininosuccinic aciduria (ASA) 817t
Armed Forces 230
arm muscle measurements 55t, 58
artificial sweeteners 216–17
ASA (argininosuccinic aciduria) 817t
AS A24 (automated self-administered 24-hour recall) 47

ascorbic acid see vitamin C (ascorbic acid)
ASDs (autism spectrum disorders) 764–5
aspiration, enteral feeding 586
assistant practitioners (APs) 13
The Association for Nutrition (AfN) 13–14
asthma 736
food hypersensitivity 736
asylum seekers see refugees and asylum seekers
Atkins diet 232–6
atopic eczema 803
attention deficit hyperactivity disorder (ADHD) 765–6
atypical antipsychotics 757b
autism spectrum disorders (ASDs) 764–5
automated self-administered 24-hour recall (ASA24) 47
average portion sizes 888

B

Baby Friendly Initiative (BFI), breastfeeding 267b, 269
Bangladeshi, food restrictions 340t
BAPEN (British Association for Parenteral and Enteral Nutrition) 558–61
barbiturates 757b
bariatric surgery 486, 487t
basal metabolic rate (BMR) 86–7
estimation of 90–1, 871t
measurement 87
total energy expenditure 86–91
BDA see British Dietetic Association (BDA)
BED (binge eating disorder) 771
behavioural approaches, weight management 483
behaviour change wheel 382–4, 383f
behenic fatty acid 72t
benzoates 214–15
benzoic acid 214–15, 216t
Better Hospital Food (BHF) 222
Beverley Hills diet 232–6
BHA (butylated hydroxyanisole) 217t

BHF (Better Hospital Food) 222
BHT (butylated hydroxytoluene) 217t
BIA (bioelectrical impedance analysis) 41t, 52
bicarbonate 869t
kidney nutritional assessment 707t
reference ranges 873t
biceps skin-fold measurements 55t
biguanides 511t
bilirubin 873t
binge eating disorder (BED) 771
biochemical assessment
individual nutrition 48
bioelectrical impedance analysis (BIA) 41t, 52
biologically active dietary constituents 210–12
anticarcinogenic phytochemicals 210
antioxidants 210
caffeine 211–12
methylxanthines 211–12
polyphenols 210–11
vasoactive amines 212
biotin (vitamin B₇) 136b, 136t
bipolar affective disorder 761
birth weights, low 436
blanket supplementary feeding, LMICs 466–7
blended enteral feeding 591
Blood Group diet (Eat Right for Your Type) 232–6
blood sugars, burn injury 617
BMI see body mass index (BMI)
BMR see basal metabolic rate (BMR)
body composition 41t, 50–3
independent methods 50–2
theoretical models 50
body mass index (BMI) 57t, 852t
adult anthropometry 56
international classification 854t
obesity definition 470, 471t
undernutrition classification 562, 563t
bolus enteral feeding 580
bones
demineralization in HIV infection 749
loss in older people 330
bottle feeding

breastfeeding with 274
energy 275
establishment 274–6
formula choice 274–5
formula preparation 275
goat's milk infant
  formula 275
Healthy Start scheme 276
prolonged use of 283
soya-based infant
  formula 275
support literature 276
see also weaning
box schemes, food
  poverty 362–3
breakfast clubs 362–3
breakfast omission, children
  and adolescents 309
breast cancer 208
see also cancer
breastfeeding 262–4
Baby Friendly Initiative
  267b, 269
benefits of 262–3
bottle feeding with 274
dietary recommendations
  272, 273t
establishing of 269, 270b
help and support 271
hepatitis 694b
obstacles to 263–4
positions 269f
promoting 266–8
protective factors 262b
reasons for 268t
stopping reasons 268t
undernutrition 458
see also weaning
Bristol Approach to
  Healthy Eating 232–6
British Association
  for Parenteral and
  Enteral Nutrition
  (BAPEN) 558–61
British Dietetic Association
  (BDA) 12
  Parenteral and Enteral
    Nutrition Group
    see Parenteral and
    Enteral Nutrition
    Group (PENG)
buffering function,
  proteins 64
built environment, WHO
  obesity prevention
  recommendations 400b
bulimia nervosa 772
bulk hospital catering 223
buried bumper
  syndrome 577
burn injury 616–18
  feeding routes 617
  nutritional
    requirements 616–17

butylated hydroxyanisole
  (BHA) 217t
butylated hydroxytoluene
  (BHT) 217t
butyric fatty acid 72t

C

Cabbage Soup diet 232–6
caffeine 211–12
  breastfeeding 272
  Parkinson's disease 789
  pregnancy 242b
  Refsum's disease 824
  see also coffee
calciferols *see* vitamin D
  (calciferols)
calcimimetic agents 718
calcium 142–4, 143t, 144b
  breastfeeding RNI 273t
  child and adolescent
    RNIs 305t
  coeliac disease 658
  deficiency in children and
    adolescents 313
  infants and preschool
    children 259t
  kidney nutritional
    assessment 707t
  kidney stones
    management 732
  low fat diets in
    steatorrhoea 644
  milk 807t
  older people
    recommendations 321
  osteoporosis
    307–308t, 806–7
  reference ranges 873t
  requirement
    estimation 597t
  RNIs 881t
  vegetarian/vegan
    problems 350–1
calcium carbonate 869t
calcium chloride 869t
calcium gluconate 869t
calcium supplements
  gastrectomy/stomach
    surgery 638
  osteoporosis 808–9
caloric sweeteners 216–17
calorimetry
  direct calorimetry 87–8
  indirect *see* indirect
    calorimetry
canagliflozin 511t
cancer 541–54
  aetiology 542
  breast cancer 208
  childhood cancers 553t
  colorectal 673–4
  frequently asked
    questions 551

gallbladder 677
head and neck
  cancer 553t
late effects 553
living with 550
lung cancer 738
mouth cancer 622
neutropenia *see*
  neutropenia
nutritional status 547
oesophageal
  disorders 628–9
pancreas 685
pharyngeal cancer 622
stomach 633–4
upper gastrointestinal
  tract cancer 553t
see also World Cancer
  Research Fund
cancer cachexia 544–5
cancer treatment 546–7
  aims of 546
  diet/nutrition in 542,
    543f, 548, 548t
  nutritional
    requirements 547
  palliative care 554
capric fatty acid 72t
caprylic fatty acid 72t
capsaicin 635b
carbamazepine 757b
carbamoyl phosphate syn-
  thase deficiency (CPS 1
  deficiency) 817t
carbohydrate exchanges,
  food composition
  886, 886t
carbohydrates 78–84
  classification 78–81, 79t
  content calculation 9
  current dietary
    patterns 35t
  diabetes dietary
    management 503–4
  dietary treatment of
    disorders 817t
  energy conversion
    factors 9t
  fermentable, dental
    erosion 626b
  food-based dietary
    guidelines 27
  glycaemic index 81–3, 84t
  glycaemic load 84
  metabolism in cancer
    cachexia 544–5
  recommended intakes
    81, 82t
  requirements in critical
    care 607–8
  sources 82t
  structure 78–81
  sugars *see* sugars
  see also fibre; starch

cardioprotective diet 524–7
  advice about 525
  fats 524–5
  lifestyle interventions 527
  nutrient/food intake
    524–5, 526b
  peripheral arterial
    disease 540
cardiovascular disease
  (CVD) 519–40
  age-standardized death
    rates 522f
  cardioprotective diet see
    cardioprotective diet
  chronic kidney disease
    and 718–19
  classification 520
  deaths and
    morbidity 522t
  diabetes 496
  prevalence 520
  risk factors 521b
  see also cerebral infarc-
    tion; coronary heart
    disease (CHD)
cardiovascular system
  chronic kidney
    disease 718–19
  HIV infection 749
Care Act (2014) 779
Care and Quality
  Commission
  (CQC) 223
Care Co-Lactase® 293
α-carotene 207t
carotenoids 102–4, 210
carrageenan 217t
casein dominant formula,
  bottle feeding 274–5
CC see critical care (CC)
CCGs see Clinical
  Commissioning
  Groups (CCGs)
cellular injury,
  hyperkalaemia 714t
cereals
  carbohydrates 82t
  copper 158t
  fats 75t
  folate (folic acid) 127t
  iodine 161t
  iron 151t
  magnesium 165t
  manganese 167t
  niacin 120t
  nutrient profiles 5t
  phosphorus 147t
  potassium 181t
  proteins 73t
  riboflavin (vitamin
    B₂) 117t
  selenium 163t

staple foods as 6
  thiamine (vitamin B₁) 124t
  vitamin B₆ 132t
  vitamin D 109t
  vitamin E 110b
  zinc 155t
cerebral infarction 520
cerebrovascular system,
  alcohol effects 209t
CF see cystic fibrosis (CF)
Change4Life (PHE) 408
change panning, health behaviour models 386–7
Charlie Foundation
  (USA) 794
CHD see coronary heart
  disease (CHD)
cheese 807t
chemotherapy, cancer
  treatment 546–7
chief cells 16–17
child growth foundation
  charts 860t, 861f, 862f,
    863f, 864f, 865f, 866f
Child Growth Standards
  (2006, WHO) 462
childhood cancers 553t
childhood obesity 314–15
  classification 314
  health effects 314
  long-term effects 315
  prevalence 314–15
  prevention 316
  wellbeing effects 314
Child Obesity Plan 406–7
  advertising regulation 410
children
  adult height
    potential 259b
children and
  adolescents 304
  acne 309
  alcohol
    consumption 309–10
  breakfast omission 309
  dental health 316, 317b
  diabetes 517
  dietary
    recommendations 306
  food choice
    influences 318f
  food habits 308–10
  global nutrition
    problems 436
  healthy eating
    promotion 320
  HIV infection 750
  iodine deficiency 451b
  National measurement
    programme 315
  nutrient
    deficiencies 312–13

physical activity
  assessment 93
  pregnancy 254
  RNIs 305t
  sedentary behaviour 310
  snacks 307b, 309
  underweight
    individuals 315
  unnecessary dieting 315
  vegetarians 309, 352
Chinese communities, food
  restrictions 339t
chloride 182
  reference ranges 873t
chlorine 881t
chlorophyll 207t
choking risk, weaning 283
cholecystitis 677
cholecystosteatosis 677
cholesterol 74
  dietary sources 75t
  digestion 18
  disorders see familial
    hypercholesterol-
    aemia (FH)
  familial hypercholesterol-
    aemia 529t
  non HDL-cholesterol 873t
cholesterol gallstones 676b
colestyramine 837–8
Christians, food
  restrictions 342t
chromium 170
chronic diseases, older
  people 330
chronic hepatitis 694
chronic kidney disease
  (CKD) 704
  anaemia 716
  cardiovascular
    risk 718–19
  classification 704f
  contributing causes 705b
  diabetes 719
  exercise 720
  malnutrition in 716–17
  mineral and bone dis-
    order 718, 719t
  nutritional
    considerations 718–20
  nutrition in stages 1-3 710
  nutrition in stages
    4-5 712–13
  older people 713
  prevalence 704–5
  weight management 720
chronic obstructive
  pulmonary disease
  (COPD) 737
chronic pancreatitis
  682, 683b
chronic undernutrition 436

chylomicrons, lipid transport 75
circulatory system, alcohol effects 209t
circumferences, adult anthropometry 56
cirrhosis 695
citric acid 217t
citrullinaemia 817t
CKD see chronic kidney disease (CKD)
classical ketogenic diet 792
clean eating 232–6
climate change
  diet and 431–2
  obesity and 430–3, 431f, 432–3
  physical activity and 432
clinical assessment see ABCDEF nutrition assessment; medical assessment, weight management
clinical chemistry reference ranges 873
Clinical Commissioning Groups (CCGs) 392–3
  local nutrition policy 416, 417b
clinical history, food hypersensitivity 826–7
clinically functional nutrients 620
closed questions, open questions vs. 379t
close spacing, pregnancies 255
Clostridium difficile diarrhoea, probiotics 199
cloves 635b
CMAM (community-based management of acute malnutrition) 464–6
cobalamin see vitamin B₁₂ (cobalamin)
CoD (coeliac disease) 656–9
Codex Alimentarius Commission 214–17
cod liver oil, vitamin D 807t
coeliac disease (CoD) 656–9
cofactors 816
coffee 623t
  see also caffeine
cognitive behavioural therapy (CBT) 763
Colief® 293
colon disorders 672–4
  cancer 673–4
  constipation 672–3

diverticular disease 673
haemorrhoids 673
colostomy 664–5
colourings
  additives 207t, 214
  artificial and ADHD 766
  food hypersensitivity management 831
  synthetic 215t
COMA see Committee on Medical Aspects of Food and Nutrition (COMA)
combined monitors, physical activity assessment 57
Committee on Medical Aspects of Food and Nutrition (COMA) 393–4
  dietary reference values 22–5
communication
  nutrition education 378–80
  refugees and asylum seekers 358
community-based management of acute malnutrition (CMAM) 464–6
community-based projects
  community cafés 362–3
  community shops 362–3
  food poverty 363
  nutrition support in older people 332
community transport
  food poverty 362–3
  older people 332
comparative claims, food labelling 193t
component-resolved diagnosis (CRD) 826–7
The Composition of Food (McCance & Widdowson) 414–15
The Composition of Food Online Integrated Database (McCance & Widdowson) 414–15
computed tomography (CT), body composition 41t, 53
computer-based dietary assessment 47
conceptual models of public health 396
conjugated linoleic acid (CLA) 197t
constipation 672–3
  hyperkalaemia 714t
  infants and preschool children 292

Parkinson's disease 788
  pregnancy 251–2
  schizophrenia 761–2
  spinal cord injury 612–13
contamination, gluten-free products 657–8
contemporary diets, cancer 551
continuous infusion enteral feeding 580
continuous renal replacement therapy (CRRT) 730
continuous subcutaneous insulin infusion (CSSI) 506–9
conversion factors 867–9
  dietary energy 868
  mineral content 869
  nicotinic acid/tryptophan 869
  protein/nitrogen 868
  vitamin A 868
  vitamin D 869
cook–freeze, hospital catering 222–3
cooking clubs
  food poverty 362–3
  older people 332
COPD (chronic obstructive pulmonary disease) 737
copper 156–8, 157t, 158t
  breastfeeding RNI 273t
  burn injury 617
  child and adolescent RNIs 305t
  enzyme functions 157t
  infants and preschool childrens RNIs 259t
  RNIs 881t
coronary heart disease (CHD) 520
  alcohol 208
  deaths and morbidity 522t
corticosteroids
  nutrient interaction 837
  systemic lupus erythematosus 802
co-trimoxazole 126
counselling skills, nutrition education 378–80, 379t
country level dietary assessment 40–1, 41t
country of origin, food labelling 189
coupons, food poverty 362–3
cows' milk
  food hypersensitivity management 828
  protein allergy 293–4

CQC (Care and Quality Commission) 223
cranberry juice 834–6
CRD (component-resolved diagnosis) 826–7
C-reactive protein (CRP) 707t
creatine 789
creatinine
  kidney nutritional assessment 707t
  reference ranges 873t
cretinism 160
critical care (CC) 606–8
  feeding routes 606–7
  nutritional requirements 607–8
Crohn's disease (CD) see inflammatory bowel disease (IBD)
crossed grain symbol 657
CRRT (continuous renal re-placement therapy) 730
CSSI (continuous sub-cutaneous insulin infusion) 506–9
culture
  acceptability of food-based dietary guidelines 26
  refugees and asylum seekers 358
curcumin 635b
current dietary patterns 34–6, 35t
  adult energy intake 34
  alcohol 34–5
  fruit & vegetables 34
  vegetarianism/veganism 36
  vitamins & minerals 35
CVD see cardiovascular disease (CVD)
cycloserine 131
cystic fibrosis (CF) 740–3
  diabetes 743
  infants 742
  liver disease 743
  nutritional management 741
  undernutrition 740
  weight loss 740

D

dairy foods
  nutrient profiles 5t
  weaning 279t
  see also milk/milk products
dapagliflozin 511t
DASH (Dietary Approaches to Stop Hypertension) 539b

DDP-4 inhibitors 511t
Defence Catering Manual 230
DEFRA see Department for Environment, Food and Rural Affairs (DEFRA)
dehydration
  older people 330
  undernutrition treatment 456
dementia 774–6
  causes 774
  niacin deficiency 118
  nutrient uptake 775–6, 776t
  nutrition improvement 775
  older people 330
  prevalence 774
demiquet 856
demi-span, height surrogate measures 56, 57t
demi-vegetarian diets 347t
densitometry 41t
dental caries 624
  children and adolescents 316
dental erosion 624–5
dental health 624–5
  children and adolescents 316, 317b
  dental caries see dental caries
  dental erosion 624–5
Department for Education (DoE)
  nutrition policy 392
  School Food Plan 407
Department for Environment, Food and Rural Affairs (DEFRA)
  Green Food Project initiative 426
  nutrition policy 392
  organic food labelling 192
depression 760
derived prediction equations 53
dermatitis 118
dermatology 795–809
  atopic eczema 803
  epidermolysis bullosa 804b, 804–5
descending colon 16f
DESM (diabetes education and self-management) 514
DESMOND 514
detox diets 232–6
developmental mental disorders 764–6

DEXA (dual-energy X-ray absorptiometry) 41t, 52
DHA (docosahexaenoic acid) 72–3
diabetes 493–518
  alcohol 209
  biochemical values 874t
  cardiovascular disease in CKD 718–19
  children and adolescents 517
  chronic kidney disease 719
  classification 494
  clinical consequences 496
  co-morbidities 499
  contributing causes 496
  cystic fibrosis 743
  diagnosis 495–6
  dietary management 502–4, 503b
  eating disorders 773
  gestational diabetes 251, 494, 516
  glycaemic control 497b, 498–9
  hypoglycaemia 512, 513b
  management 500–1
  older people 518
  postnatal care 517
  preconception care 516
  pregnancies 255
  pregnancy 516
  pregnancy in see gesta-tional diabetes (GDM)
  prevalence 494
  risk factors 495
  structured education in 514
  weight management 515
diabetes education and self-management (DESM) 514
diabetes, gestational 251, 494, 516
diabetes type 1 494
  children and adolescents 517
  co-morbidities 499
  contributing causes 496
  glycaemic control 497b
  management 500, 506–9, 507t, 508b
  risk factors 495
diabetes type 2 494
  carbohydrate management 503–4
  children and adolescents 517
  co-morbidities 499
  contributing causes 496
  glycaemic control 497b

management 501, 510
risk factors 495
diabetes type 3c 494
diagnostic diets 826–7
dialysis
  hyperkalaemia 714t
  nutritional requirements
    705t, 724
diaries, physical activity
  assessment 94
diarrhoea
  antibiotic-associated 199
  enteral feeding 587, 588t
  niacin deficiency 118
  toddler diarrhoea 292–3
diet(s)
  alkaline diets 232–6
  alternative see
    alternative diets
  anorexia nervosa 770
  Atkins diet 232–6
  Beverley Hills diet 232–6
  biologically active con-
    stituents see biologic-
    ally active dietary
    constituents
  Blood Group diet
    (Eat Right for Your
    Type) 232–6
  Cabbage Soup diet 232–6
  cardioprotective see
    cardioprotective diet
  classical ketogenic
    diet 792
  climate change
    and 431–2
  components 4
  contemporary diets,
    cancer 551
  current patterns see cur-
    rent dietary patterns
  definition 4
  demi-vegetarian
    diets 347t
  detox diets 232–6
  diabetes management
    502–4, 503b
  Dukan diet 232–6
  environmental
    impacts of 425
  food combining
    diets 232–6
  fruitarian diets 347t
  Gerson diet 232–6
  gluten free see gluten free
    (GF) diet
  glycaemic index (GI)
    diet 232–6
  grapefruit diet 232–6
  Hay diet 232–6
  health and sustainable
    diets 423–34

jejunocolic anastomosis
  660–1, 661t
jejunostomy 660, 661t
ketogenic diet see
  ketogenic diet (KD)
kidney nutritional
  assessment 706
lacto-ovo-vegetarian
  diets 347t
lactose intolerance
  648–50, 649t
lacto-vegetarian
  diets 347t
long-term restrictions 667
low carbohydrate
  diet 478
low fat diets 644, 645t
low fat, plant-based
  diet 782–3
low FODMAP
  diet 669–70
low phenylalanine diet see
  low phenylalanine diet
low-sodium diet
  696–7, 697t
macrobiotic diets 347t
Mediterranean diet see
  Mediterranean diet
medium chain triglyceride
  ketogenic diet 792
modified Atkins diet 792
modified ketogenic
  diet 792
modified-texture
  diets 776
no-added salt diet 696–7
Parkinson's disease 788
pescatarian diets 347t
Pioppi diet 232–6
popular diets see
  popular diets
prisons 228
problems in
  pregnancy 250–2
Slimming World
  diet 232–6
South Beach diet 232–6
stroke prevention 552–3
Sugar Busters diet 232–6
vegan diets 347t
very low calorie diets
  (VLCD) 480
very low energy diets
  (VLED) 480
Weight Watchers
  diet 232–6
Zone diet 232–6
Dietary Approaches to
  Stop Hypertension
  (DASH) 539b
dietary assessment 40–2
  computer-based 47

  country level assessment
    40–1, 41t
  household-based
    surveys 42
  see also food intake
dietary change, counselling
  skills 380
dietary energy, conversion
  factors 868
dietary guidelines
  vegetarians 351
  WHO obesity preven-
    tion recommenda-
    tions 400b
dietary induced thermogenesis (DIT) 86–91
dietary reference values
  (DRVs) 22–5, 875–8
  affecting factors 22–4
  aged diet 322–3
  deficiency and 23f
  definition 23f
  derivation 23f
  estimated average re-
    quirements 876, 877t
  limitations 22
  pregnancy 242–3
  RNIs 878, 879t
  uses of 24–5
dietary value 4
diet history 47
diet-induced thermogenesis
  (DIT) 597b
dietitians 12
digestion 16–18
  fats 18, 19f
  large intestine 18
  mouth 16
  oesophagus 16
  small intestine 17–18
  stomach 16–17
dilution methods, body
  composition 41t
direct calorimetry 87–8
disaccharides 79t
disulfiram (Antabuse®) 206
DIT (dietary induced
  thermogenesis) 86–91
diuretics 836–7, 837–8
diversity sensitive diets 344
diverticulosis (diverticular
  disease) 673
docosahexaenoic acid
  (DHA) 72–3
DoE see Department for
  Education (DoE)
dong quai 841t
levodopa 131
doubly labelled
  water 89–90
  physical activity
    assessment 97b

Down syndrome 490
drinking yogurt 623t
drinks
  manganese 167t
  potassium 181t
  potassium limitation 714t
  sugar sweetened
    beverages 221–2
  see also alcoholic bever-
    ages; non-alcoholic
    beverages
drug–nutrient interactions
  335–336t, 834–40,
  835t
  alcohol 838
  appetite effects 839t, 839
  drug action
    potentiation 834–6
  drug therapy
    alterations 834
  herbs 840, 841t
  metabolic effects of
    drugs 839
  nutritional status 838
  nutritional
    supplements 837
  nutrition
    deficiencies 837–8
  serious interactions 837
  therapy limitation 836–7
  vitamin K 834
  warfarin 834
drugs
  hyperkalaemia 714t
  malabsorption 643b
DRVs see dietary reference
  values (DRVs)
dry beriberi 122
dry mouth
  (xerostomia) 622
  drug–nutrient
    interactions 839
  Parkinson's disease 788
dual-energy X-ray absorptiometry (DEXA) 41t, 52
Dukan diet 232–6
dulaglutide 511t
duplicate diets, nutrition
  assessment 41t, 44–5
dyslipidaemia 749
dysphagia 628
  cancer 548
  stroke 535

E

early satiety, cancer 548
EARs see esti-
  mated average
  requirements (EARs)
eating disorders 768–73
  anorexia nervosa 769–71

assessment 768–9
bulimia nervosa 772
diabetes 773
identification 768–9
pathogenesis 768
statistics 768
Eat Right for Your
  Type (Blood Group
  diet) 232–6
The Eatwell Guide 27–9,
  30f, 412
  breastfeeding 272
  children and
    adolescents 306
  HIV infection 749
  preconceptual
    nutrition 238
  sustainable nutrition
    and 426
EB (epidermolysis bullosa)
  804b, 804–5
Echinacea 841t
eczema, atopic 803
Education Act (2002) 224
education, nutrition see
  nutrition education
EE see energy
  expenditure (EE)
EFAD (European
  Federation of the
  Associations of
  Dieticians) 12
EFAs see essential fatty
  acids (EFAs)
eggs
  cardioprotective diet 525
  food hypersensitivity
    management 828–9
  nutrient profiles 5t
  vitamin D 807t
EHF (extensive hydrolysed
  formula) 828
eicosanoic fatty acid 72t
eicosapentaenoic acid
  (EPA) 72–3
elaidic fatty acid 72t
elderly see older people
electrolytes 176
  acute kidney injury 730–1
  burn injury 616–17
  critical care 607–8
  requirement estimation
    597t, 599–600
  see also chlorine;
    potassium
empagliflozin 511t
emulsifiers 216
endocrine system, alcohol
  effects 209t
energy
  acute kidney injury 730–1
  bottle feeding 275

breastfeeding RNI 273t
cardioprotective
  diet 526t
child and adolescent
  RNIs 305t
chronic kidney
  disease 712
consumption 91, 92f
conversion factors 9t
energy balance 91
food-based dietary guide-
  lines (FBDGs) 27
food labelling 193t
gastrectomy/stomach
  surgery 638
haemodialysis 705t, 725
infants and preschool
  childrens 259t
low fat diets in
  steatorrhoea 644
peritoneal dialysis
  705t, 724
requirement estimation
  600b, 596, 597b
value calculation 8–9, 9t
vegetarian/vegan
  problems 349
energy balance 86–97
energy consumption
  91, 92f
  energy intake 91
  energy requirements
    91, 93t
  units 86b
  units used 868
energy expenditure
  (EE) 86–91
  measurement 87–91
  prediction equations 871
energy requirements
  burn injury 616
  critical care 607–8
  energy balance 91, 93t
  estimation of 90–1, 91t
  head injury 614
engagement, motivational
  interviewing 384
enhanced recovery after
  surgery (ERAS) 610–11
enteral feeding 572
  blended enteral
    feeding 591
  complications 586–7,
    588t, 589t
  critical care 606–7
  cystic fibrosis 741
  drugs and 590
  gastrostomy feeding see
    gastrostomy feeding
  home enteral feeding 578
  intravenous feeding
    vs. 573b

jejunostomy feeding *see* jejunostomy feeding
monitoring 582–4, 583*t*
monitoring stable patients in community 584
nasogastric feeding 574–5
nasojejunal feeding 575
regimens 580
E numbers 214
environmental factors, kidney nutritional assessment 706
environmental impact of diet 425
enzymes
  inherited metabolic disorders 816
  insufficiency in malabsorption 643*b*
  proteins 64
EPA (eicosapentaenoic acid) 72–3
EPIC-SOFT, individual nutrition assessment 47
epidermolysis bullosa (EB) 804*b*, 804–5
epilepsy 792–4
epithelial tissue, vitamin A deficiency 102
ERAS (enhanced recovery after surgery) 610–11
erucic fatty acid 72*t*
erythrosine (red) 215*t*
ESPEN (European Society for Parenteral and Enteral Nutrition) 695*t*
essential fatty acids (EFAs) 65, 66*t*, 72–3, 74
  breastfeeding 262*b*
  low fat diets in steatorrhoea 644
estimated average requirements (EARs) 91, 92*t*, 93*t*, 876
  children 877*t*
  definition 24*b*
ethics
  palliative care 813–14
  undernutrition treatment 571*b*
ethnicity
  obesity and waist circumference 470, 471*t*
  see also minority ethnic communities
ethyl alcohols 9*t*
European Federation of the Associations of Dieticians (EFAD) 12
European Society for Parenteral and Enteral Nutrition (ESPEN) 695*t*

Europeans, waist circumferences 58*t*
European Union (EU), food labelling 188–92
Evidence into Action (PHE) 406
evoking, motivational interviewing 384–5
exenatide 511*t*
exercise *see* physical activity (PA)
extensive hydrolysed formula (EHF) 828
eyes, vitamin A deficiency 102

F

faeces 18
faltering growth 286–7
  causes of 287*b*
  management 286–7, 288*f*
  primary care assessment 286
familial hypercholesterolaemia (FH) 528–9
  cholesterol levels 529*t*
  dietary treatment 817*t*
FAO *see* Food and Agriculture Organization (FAO)
farmers' markets 362–3
fasting, intermittent 479
fat-free mass (FFM)
  body composition 50
  cardioprotective diet 526*t*
fat mass (FM)
  body composition 50
  energy values for oxidation 89*t*
fats 70–6
  adult average intake 73*t*
  cardioprotective diet 524–5
  children and adolescents 308–10
  content calculation 9
  current dietary patterns 35*t*
  digestion and absorption 18, 19*f*
  energy conversion factors 9*t*
  food-based dietary guidelines (FBDGs) 27
  food labelling 193*t*
  functions 70
  nutrient profiles 5*t*
  saturated *see* saturated fats
  sources of 75*t*
  sterols 74
  transport 74–6
  UK recommendations 28*t*

  see also fatty acids; lipid(s)
fat-soluble vitamins 741, 742*t*
fat spreads, vitamin E 110*b*
fatty acids 70–4
  essential fatty acids *see* essential fatty acids (EFAs)
  monounsaturated *see* monounsaturated (MUFAs)
  n-3 fatty acids 351
  nomenclature 72*t*
  omega (ω)-3 polyunsaturated fatty acid *see* omega (ω)-3 polyunsaturated fatty acid
  oxidation disorders 817*t*
  polyunsaturated *see* polyunsaturated fatty acids (PUFAs)
  saturated *see* saturated fatty acids (SFAs)
  stearic fatty acid 72*t*
  structure 71*f*
  trans fatty acids *see* trans fatty acids
  unsaturated fatty acids 790
FBDGs *see* food-based dietary guidelines (FBDGs)
feeding routes
  burn injury 617
  intestinal transplantation 666
fermentable carbohydrates, dental erosion 626*b*
ferritin 149*t*
5 A Day Programme 408
FFM *see* fat-free mass (FFM)
FFW (food for work) 466–7
FH *see* familial hypercholesterolaemia (FH)
fibre 80
  children and adolescents 305*t*, 308–10, 313
  current dietary patterns 35*t*
  dietary sources 81*t*
  food labelling 193*t*
  haemorrhoids 673
  peritoneal dialysis 724
  recommended intakes 81
  sources 83*t*
  UK recommendations 28*t*
finances, obesity 474
finger foods, dementia 776
FIRSSt (Food Intake Recording Software System) 47

fiscal measures, WHO obesity prevention recommendations 400b

fish
cardioprotective diet 526t
food hypersensitivity management 829
iodine 161t
milk 807t
niacin (nicotinamide, nicotinic acid, vitamin B₃) 120t
nutrient profiles 5t
preconceptual nutrition avoidance 239
pregnancy 242–3
proteins 73t
selenium 163t
vitamin B₁₂ (cobalamin) 135t
vitamin D 807t
vitamin D (calciferols) 109t
weaning 279t
see also seafood

fish oils 834–6
fistulae, small intestine disorders 662
fistuloclysis 662
fixation of the jaw 622–3
flavonoids 210–11
functional foods as 197t
flavour enhancers, food hypersensitivity 831
fluid balance 184–5
acute kidney injury 730–1
child and adolescent RNIs 305t
chronic kidney disease 712
fluid requirements 185, 186t
haemodialysis 705t, 725, 726t
hydrostatic pressure 184
kidney stones management 732
peritoneal dialysis 705t, 724, 726t
plasma osmolality 184
water balance 184–5, 185t
fluid intake
breastfeeding 272
infants and preschool childrens 259t
fluid requirements
burn injury 616–17
critical care 607–8
fluid balance 185, 186t
fluids
losses 184–5

requirement estimation 600b, 598
restriction in heart failure 530
fluoride 172t, 172, 173b
FM see fat mass (FM)
focus, motivational interviewing 384
folate (folic acid) 126, 127t, 128b
breastfeeding RNI 273t
child and adolescent RNIs 305t
food fortification 201
infants and preschool childrens 259t
older people recommendations 324
peripheral arterial disease 540
preconceptual nutrition 238, 239b
pregnancy 244, 245t
RNIs 879t
supplements in gas-trectomy/stomach surgery 638
folic acid see folate (folic acid)
follow-on milk 274–5
food(s)
access in undernutrition treatment 569
additives see food additives
aversions in pregnancy 250
avoidance see food avoidance
balance sheets 40b
choice influences in children and adolescents 318f
colourings see colourings
combining diets 232–6
composition see food composition
cravings in pregnancy 250
dairy foods see dairy foods
fortification 201
functional see functional foods
hypersensitivity see food hypersensitivity
intake see food intake
labelling see food labelling
policy in older people 332, 334, 335f
preparation in neutropenia 552
redistribution in food poverty 362–3

restrictions in minority ethnic communities 338, 339t, 340t, 342t, 347b
safety see food safety
safety in HIV infection 751
supplements see food supplements
supply quality, WHO 400b
food accounts 41t
household-based surveys 42
food additives 214–17
ADHD 766
antioxidants (E300-322) 216
colourings (E100-180) 207t, 214
emulsifiers, stabilizers, thickeners, and gelling agents (E400-495) 216, 217t
E numbers 214
food hypersensitivity management 831
food labelling 191
preservatives (E200-290) 214–15, 216t
sweeteners 216–17
synthetic colourings 215t
food aid 466–7
Food and Agriculture Organization (FAO)
dietary reference values 22–5
food intake, influences of 366–7
food security 429
food avoidance
neutropenia 552
weaning 281
food banks 354–5
food poverty 362–3
older people 332
food-based dietary guide-lines (FBDGs) 26–9, 28t, 40–1
development 26–7
food composition 883–8
carbohydrate exchanges 886, 886t
protein exchanges 884, 884t
food composition tables 8–10
carbohydrate content calculation 9
energy value calculation 8–9
fat content calculation 9

limitations of 10
micronutrients content
calculation 10
protein content
calculation 9
food co-operatives 362–3
food for work
(FFW) 466–7
food groups 4, 5t
food hypersensitivity 825–32
asthma 736
challenge in
diagnosis 826–7
classification 826
diagnosis 826–7
food labels 832
management 828–31
natural triggers 831
Food Information
for Consumers
Regulations 188–92
Food in Schools
Programme 2001
(FSP) 224
food intake
influences of 366f, 368f,
366
food intake 366–7, 368f
see also dietary assessment
Food Intake Recording
Software System
(FIRSSt) 47
food labelling 188–92, 411
food hypersensitivity 832
gluten-free products 657
legal requirements 188–91
nutrition and health claims
191–2, 192t, 193t
nutrition information
labelling 191
organic 192
signposting 192
food poisoning,
pregnancy 246b
food poverty 354–5, 357b
community
development 363
local projects 362–3
food safety
preconceptual
nutrition 239
pregnancy 246
food security 357b, 429
Food Standards
Agency (FSA)
food additives 214–17
food composition
tables 8–10
nutrition policy 392, 393
see also National Diet
and Nutrition
Survey (NDNS)

food supplements 202–3
health information 202
micronutrients 202
regulation 202–3
Food Supplements
Directive 202–3
food vouchers 362–3
FOS (fructo-
oligosaccharides) 201
free sugars 80–1
frozen meals, older
people 332
fructo-oligosaccharides
(FOS) 201
fructose 79
structure 78f
fruitarian diets 347t
fruit puree 623t
fruits
asthma 736
cardioprotective diet 526t
children and
adolescents 308–10
copper 158t
current dietary
patterns 34
food hypersensitivity
management 830
nutrient profiles 5t
potassium limitation 714b
UK
recommendations 28t
weaning 279t
FSA see Food Standards
Agency (FSA)
FSP (Food in Schools
Programme 2001) 224
functional foods 196–7
categories of 196t
examples 197b
ingredients 196
regulation of 197
fussy eaters, infants 300b

G

G A1 (glutaric aciduria type
I) 817t
galacto-oligosaccharides
(GOS) 201
galactosaemia 817t
galactose 79
gallates 217t
gallbladder
disorders 676–7
cancer 677
cholecystitis 677
cholecystosteatosis 677
gallstones see gallstones
gallstones 676
cholesterol
gallstones 676b

GAM see global acute
malnutrition (GAM)
garam masala 635b
gastrectomy 637f, 638
sleeve gastrectomy
486, 487t
total gastrectomy C26.
S26.6, 637f
gastric bands 486, 487t
gastric irritation 839
gastric residual volumes
(GRV) 606–7
gastritis 633
gastrointestinal
disease 621–77
colon see colon disorders
gallbladder disorders see
gallbladder disorders
gastrectomy 638
gastro-oesophageal reflux
disease see gastro-
oesophageal reflux
disease (GORD)
mouth disorders see
mouth disorders
oesophageal disorders see
oesophageal disorders
older people 330
small intestine see small
intestine disorders
stomach disorders see
stomach disorders
gastrointestinal stoma
664–5, 665b
gastrointestinal system
alcohol effects 207t
microbiota 198–9
gastrojejunostomy 578
gastro-oesophageal reflux
disease (GORD) 632–3
cause 294
diagnosis 294
feed adjustments 295
management 294–5
medication 296
gastrostomy feeding 576–8
complications 577
percutaneous endoscopic
gastrostomy 576
radiologically inserted
gastrostomy 576–7
surgical
gastrostomy 577–8
Gaviscon Infant™ 295
GDM (gestational diabetes)
251, 494, 516
gelling agents 216
general food distribution
(GFD) 466–7
genetically modified ingredients (GMOs) 191
Gerson diet 232–6

gestational diabetes (GDM) 251, 494, 516
GFD (general food distribution) 466–7
GF diet see gluten free (GF) diet
GHGE (greenhouse gas emissions) 424, 430b
GI see glycaemic index (GI)
ginger 635b
gingko biloba 841t
ginseng 841t
glibenclamide 511t
gliclazide 511t
glipizide 511t
global acute malnutrition (GAM) 458
anthropometric surveys 462
global nutrition problems 436
WHO classification of rates 463t
global nutrition 435–67
iodine deficiency 450, 451b
iron deficiency 448
malnutrition in emergencies 458
Millennium Development Goals (MDGs) 444b
nutrition emergencies 456
nutrition transition 454–5
problems in 436–7
undernutrition see undernutrition
vitamin A deficiency 452–3
World Health Assembly targets 445, 447b
glucose 79
energy values for oxidation 89t
impaired fasting glucose 874t
impaired glucose tolerance 874t
self-blood glucose monitoring 498
structure 78f
glucose tolerance factor (GTF) 170
glucosinolates 210–11
glutamine 620
burn injury 618
glutaric aciduria type I (G A1) 817t
gluten
avoidance of 659
sensitivity to 659
gluten free (GF) diet adherence to 658

coeliac disease 656–7
glycaemic control 497b
glycaemic index (GI) 81–3, 84t
diabetes dietary management 504
low treatment 792
glycaemic index (GI) diet 232–6
glycaemic index/glycaemic load (GI/GL) ratio 478–9
glycaemic load (GL) 84
glycerol 9t
glycogen storage diseases (GSDs) 817t
glycosylated haemoglobin 498
GMOs (genetically modified ingredients) 191
goal setting, health behaviour models 387
goat's milk infant formula 275
goblet cells 16–17
GORD see gastro-oesophageal reflux disease (GORD)
gout 800–1
grains 829
grapefruit diet 232–6
grapefruit juice 834–6
Green 5 215t
Green Food Project initiative (DEFRA) 426
greenhouse gas emissions (GHGE) 424, 430b
growth
disturbances in see faltering growth
stunting see stunted growth
growth reference charts 258–60
Grow Your Own
food poverty 362–3
older people 332
GRV (gastric residual volumes) 606–7
GSDs (glycogen storage diseases) 817t
GTF (glucose tolerance factor) 170
gums 217t
gynae-oncology 553t

H

haematocrit 873t
haematology
individual nutrition assessment 48

kidney nutritional assessment 707t
haemato-oncology 553t
haem enzymes, iron 149t
haemochromatosis, primary idiopathic 151
haemodialysis
nutritional requirements 705t, 725–6
haemoglobin
glycosylated haemoglobin 498
iron 149
kidney nutritional assessment 707t
reference ranges 873t
haemorrhoids 673
haemosiderin 149t
Hay diet 232–6
HCPC (Health & Care Profession Council) 12
HCU (homocystinuria) 817t
HDLs (high density lipoproteins) 76
HE (hepatic encephalopathy) 695t, 698
head and neck cancer 553t
head injury 614
energy requirements 614
nutritional support 614, 615b
protein requirements 614
health
childhood obesity effects 314
risks in vegetarians 346, 350b
sustainable diets and 423–34
Health and Social Care Act (2012) 392–3, 416–17
health behaviour models 382–7, 383f
behaviour change wheel 382–4, 383f
change panning 386–7
goal setting 387
motivational interviewing 384–6, 385t, 388b
Health Belief Model 382–7
Health & Care Profession Council (HCPC) 12
health claims/information
food labelling 191–2, 192t, 193t
food supplements 202
health departments, nutrition policy 392
Healthier Food Mark Scheme 426
Health Profession Council (HPC) 12

Health Survey for England (2014) 415
  mental health 754
Healthy Child Programme 266–8
Healthy Schools Programme 224
Healthy Start scheme 409
  bottle feeding 276
  low-income in pregnancy 255
heart, alcohol effects 220t
heartburn 632–3
  pregnancy 252
heart failure 530
heart monitors, physical activity assessment 95, 96b
height
  adult anthropometry 55–6
  length conversion 848, 849t
  length-for-age, malnutrition 438
  surrogate measures 56, 57t
Helicobacter pylori infection 633, 634b
HENRY project 290–1
hepatic encephalopathy (HE) 695t, 698
hepatic steatosis 743
hepatitis 694
  acute 694
  breastfeeding 694b
  chronic 694
hepatitis B 694b
hepatitis C 263–4, 694b
herbs 840, 841t
hiatus hernia 632–3
high density lipoproteins (HDLs) 76
Hindus, food restrictions 340t
hip circumference 55t
histamine 212
HIV infection see human immunodeficiency virus (HIV) infection
home delivery services, older people 332
homeless people 357b, 360, 361b
home parenteral nutrition (HPN) 593
  cancer 554
homocystinuria (HCU) 817t
hormones 64
  cancer treatment 546–7
hospital catering 220–3

initiatives 221–2
key characteristics 221
nutritional status 220b
regulation and monitoring 223
types of food production 222–3
types of service 223
household-based surveys
dietary assessment 42
food purchase surveys 414
household records 41t, 42
individual nutrition assessment 41t, 45
HPN see home parenteral nutrition (HPN)
human immunodeficiency virus (HIV) infection 745–51
  alternative therapies 751
  breastfeeding 263–4
  cardiovascular risk 749
  children 750
  food and drug interactions 750–1
  food and water safety 751
  lean tissue loss 748
  mother-to-child transmission prevention 750
  nutritional assessment 747
  nutritional goals 746
  weight loss 748
hydration assessment, stroke 534–5
hydro-densitometry 50
hydrostatic pressure, fluid balance 184
hypercalcaemia 143t
hypercholesterolaemia, familial see familial hypercholesterolaemia (FH)
hyperglycaemia 682
Hypericum perforatum (St John's Wort) 840, 841t
hyperkalaemia 714t
hyperlipidaemia
  cardiovascular disease in CKD 718–19
  nephrotic syndrome 722
  type I 817t
hypermetabolism 682
hypertension 538–9
  cardiovascular disease in CKD 718–19
  diet 538–9, 539b
hypoalbuminaemia 722
hypocalcaemia 143t
hypoglycaemia

diabetes 512, 513b
undernutrition treatment 456
hypoglycaemic agents 510, 511t
hypomagnesaemia 164
hypothermia 456

I

IBBD (irritable bowel disease) 199
IBS see irritable bowel syndrome (IBS)
ICCID (International Council for Control of Iodine Deficiency) 450
ICDA (International Confederation of Dietetic Associations) 12
ice cream 623t
IDA see iron-deficiency anaemia (IDA)
IDD (iodine deficiency disorder) 160
IDDSI (International Dysphagia Diet Standardization Initiative) 535–6, 536f
IDLs (intermediate density lipoproteins) 76
IDPN (intradialytic parenteral nutrition) 716–17
ileostomy 664
imaging, body composition 53
IMDs see inherited metabolic disorders (IMDs)
IMF (International Monetary Fund) 366–7
immune system
  protein function 64
  vitamin A deficiency 102
immunoglobulin E (IgE)
  mediated food hypersensitivity 826
serum measurements 826–7
immunological active components, breastfeeding 262b
immunosuppressive treatment 729b
impaired fasting glucose 874t
impaired glucose tolerance 874t
incretin mimetics 511t
Indians, food restrictions 340t
indigestion 632–3

indigo carmine (blue) 215t
indirect calorimetry 88, 89b
  equipment 88
indispensible (essential)
  amino acids 65, 66t
individual nutrition
  assessment
  biochemical and haemato-
    logical assessment 48
  choice of 46f
  dietary assessment 44–48
  new technology 47
  physical assessment 47–8
  prospective
    methods 44–5
  retrospective measure-
    ments 45t, 47
infant formula, soya-based
  see soya-based infant
  formula
infant growth and
  development 258–61
  adult height
    potential 259b
  delay in see
    faltering growth
  GOR 294–6
  growth reference charts
    258–60, 259b
  measurement 260–1
  nutritionally vulnerable
    babies 298
  obesity
    prevention 290–1
infants and preschool
  chuildren 257–300
  constipation 292
  cows' milk protein
    allergy 293–4
  cystic fibrosis 742
  dietary
    recommendations 258
  fussy eaters 300b
  global nutrition
    problems 436
  iron deficiency
    anaemia 284
  lactose intolerance 293
  milk hypersensitivity 293
  toddler diarrhoea 292–3
infections
  malabsorption 643b
  undernutrition
    treatment 456
inflammatory bowel disease
  (IBD) 652–5
infrared reactance, body
  composition 41t
ingredient list, food
  labelling 189
inherited metabolic dis-
  orders (IMDs) 815–24
  definitions 816

emergency regimens
  820, 821t
newborn screening 816
treatment 816, 817t
inositol 80
inpatient care, anorexia
  nervosa 770–1
INS (International
  Numbering System),
  food additives 214–17
instructions for use, food
  labelling 189
insulin
  diabetes type 1 man-
    agement 506–9,
    507t, 508b
  nutrient
    interaction 837–8
insulin resistance 494b
  HIV infection 749
intermediate density lipoproteins (IDLs) 76
intermittent fasting
  (intermittent energy
  restriction) 479
intermittent infusion, enteral feeding 580
International Council for
  Control of Iodine
  Deficiency (ICCID) 450
International Dysphagia
  Diet Standardization
  Initiative (IDDSI)
  535–6, 536f
International Monetary
  Fund (IMF) 366–7
International Numbering
  System (INS), food
  additives 214–17
intervention planning,
  behaviour change
  wheel 384
intestinal failure, small intestine disorders 660–1
intestinal
  transplantation 666–7
intradialytic parenteral nutrition (IDPN) 716–17
intra-peritoneal amino acids
  (IPAA) 716–17
intravenous feeding, enteral
  feeding vs. 573b
intrinsic sugars 80
inventories 41t
  household-based
  surveys 42
in vivo neuron activation
  analysis (IVNAA) 41t
iodine 160, 161b, 161t
  deficiency 450, 451b
  RNIs 881t
  vegetarian/vegan
  problems 351

iodine deficiency disorder
  (IDD) 160
IPAA (intra-peritoneal
  amino acids) 716–17
iron 148–51
  absorption 149t
  child and adolescent
    RNIs 305t
  compounds in the
    body 149t
  depletion 150
  dietary sources 151, 152b
  function 149
  gastrectomy/stomach
    surgery 638
  infants and preschool
    childrens 259t
  measurement 150
  metabolism 148f
  pregnancy 244, 245t
  requirements and intake
    150, 151t
  RNIs 881t
  supplements 638
  toxicity 151
  transport and
    absorption 148
  vegetarian/vegan
    problems 351
iron deficiency 150, 151
  children and
    adolescents 312b
  global nutrition 448
iron-deficiency anaemia
  (IDA) 150, 151
  infants and preschool
    children 284
  pregnancy 251
  prevention 448
irritable bowel syndrome
  (IBS) 199, 668–70
  diagnosis 668b
  probiotics 199
Islam, food restrictions
  340t, 342t
isoniazid
  nutrient interaction 837
  vitamin B$_6$ interactions 131
isotope dilution
  techniques 51
isotretinoin 837
isovaleric acidaemia
  (IVA) 817t
IVNAA (in vivo neuron ac-
  tivation analysis) 41t

J

jaw wiring 622–3
jejunocolic anastomosis
  660–1, 661t
jejunostomy 578
  diet 660, 661t

gastrointestinal stoma 664
jejunostomy feeding 578
gastrojejunostomy 578
jejunostomy 578
jejunum 16f
Jewish communities, food
restrictions 339t
Joined Up Clinical Pathways
for Obesity (NHS
England 2016) 417b
Joint Health and Wellbeing
Strategy (JHWS) 416

K

Kashin–Beck disease 162
Keshan disease 162
ketogenic diet (KD)
232–6, 792–4
availability and
support 794
classical ketogenic
diet 792
contraindications 793
implementation 793–4
indications 793
modified 792
traditional diets 792
kidney disease 703–34
chronic kidney disease
see chronic kidney
disease (CKD)
contributing causes 705
kidney stones see
kidney stones
nephrotic syndrome
722b, 723b
nutritional
assessment 706
transplantation see renal
transplantation
see also acute kidney
injury (AKI); chronic
kidney disease (CKD)
kidney stones 732
dietary treatment 732
formation 732
types of 733t
knee height, height surrogate measures 56, 57t
Korsakoff's psychosis 208
kwashiorkor 458,
459f, 460b

L

labelling
foods see food labelling
food supplements 203
WHO obesity preven-
tion recommenda-
tions 400b

lactase drops (Colief®/
Care Co-Lactase®) 293
lactic acid 216t
lacto-ovo-vegetarian
diets 347t
lactose 79
lactose intolerance 648–50
infants and preschool
children 293
lacto-vegetarian diets 347t
large intestine 18
lauric fatty acid 72t
LCHAD (long chain
3-hydroxyacyl-CoA
deficiency) 817t
LDL (low-density lipopro-
tein)-cholesterol 873t
LDLs (low density
lipoproteins) 76
lean body mass see fat-free
mass (FFM)
lean tissue loss, HIV
infection 748
learning outcomes 372, 373
learning theories 374
lecithins 217t
legumes 5t
length/height conversion
848, 849t
lentil soup 623t
lesson plans, nutrition education 374, 379t
levodopa 836–7
LGIT (low glycaemic index
treatment) 792
LIDNS (Low Income
Diet and Nutrition
Survey) 355–6
life expectancy, spinal cord
injury 612–13
lifestyle interventions
cardioprotective diet 527
cardiovascular disease in
CKD 718–19
LighterLife 232–6
linagliptin 511t
linoleic acid 72t
structure 71f
lipid(s)
kidney nutritional
assessment 707t
metabolism in cancer
cachexia 544–5
requirements in critical
care 607–8
see also fats
lipid disorders 817t
lipid-modifying drug
therapy 529
lipoatrophy, HIV
infection 749
lipoproteins 76t

liquid diets, jaw wiring
622–3, 623t
liraglutide 511t
listeriosis, pregnancy 246b
list-recall methods 41t
household-based
surveys 42
lithium salts 757b
nutrient interactions
836t
liver 16f
alcohol effects 209t
liver disease 689–701
ascites 696–7, 697t
cirrhosis 695
cystic fibrosis 743
hepatic encephalopathy
695t, 698
hepatic steatosis 743
hepatitis see hepatitis
non-alcoholic fatty liver
disease 692–3, 693b
non-alcoholic
steatohepatitis 692–3
nutritional assessment
690, 691b
nutritional screening 690
oedema 696–7, 697t
oesophageal varices 699
steatorrhoea 699
liver transplants 700–1
cystic fibrosis 743
LMICs see low- and middle-
income countries
(LMICs)
local authorities 416–17
local nutrition
policy 416–19
CCGs 416, 417b
evaluation of 420, 421b
food poverty 362–3
further
information 418–19
Health and Wellbeing
Boards (HWBs) 416
local authorities 416–17
national policy/guideline
input 417–19
obesity prevention 418
PHE centres 416
place-based local public
health 418
long chain 3-hydroxyacyl-
CoA deficiency
(LCHAD) 817t
long-term care,
stroke 536–7
long-term dietary
restrictions 667
long-term nutrition, liver
transplants 700–1
Look AHEAD trial 479–80

low- and middle-income
    countries (LMICs)
  breastfeeding 266–8
  undernutrition in 440,
    464–7, 465f, 466t
  see also low-income
    households
low birth weights 436
  global nutrition
    problems 436
low carbohydrate
    diet 478
low-density lipoprotein
    (LDL)-cholesterol 873t
low density lipoproteins
    (LDLs) 76
lower reference nutrient
    intake (LRNI) 24b
low fat diets 644, 645t
low fat, plant-based
    diet 782–3
low FODMAP
    diet 669–70
low glycaemic index/
    glycaemic load (GI/
    GL) 478–9
low glycaemic index treat-
    ment (LGIT) 792
Low Income Diet and
    Nutrition Survey
    (LIDNS) 355–6
low-income
    households 354–6
  children dietary
    deficiencies 313
  diet and nutritional
    consequences 355–6
  food poverty 354–5
  nutritionally vulnerable
    babies 298
  older people 356
  terminology 357b
  see also low- and middle-
    income countries
    (LMICs)
low-income,
    pregnancy 254–5
low phenylalanine
    diet 822
  monitoring 823
low-sodium diet
    696–7, 697t
LRNI (lower reference
    nutrient intake) 24b
luminal factors,
    malabsorption 643b
lunch clubs
  food poverty 362–3
  older people 332
lung cancer 738
lung transplantation 738
lycopene 197t

M

MAC (mid-arm
    circumference) 857t
MAC (biceps),
    anthropometry 55t
macrobiotic diets 347t
macronutrients, gas-
    trectomy/stomach
    surgery 638
MAD (modified Atkins
    diet) 792
magnesium 164b, 165t
  breastfeeding RNI 273t
  child and adolescent
    RNIs 305t
  deficiency 312, 313b
  infants and preschool
    childrens 259t
  requirement
    estimation 597t
  RNIs 881t
  supplements 602–3
magnetic resonance imaging
    (MRI) 41t, 53
malabsorption, chronic
    pancreatitis 682
malnutrition
  consequences of 565–6
  contributing causes 564–5
  emergency
    treatment 458
  prevalence 564
  self-screening tool 561
  types of 438
  see also global acute
    malnutrition (GAM);
    undernutrition
malnutrition universal
    screening tool
    (MUST) 558–61
  dementia 775
  management
    guidelines 560t
  steps of 559b
  use of 558b
MAMC (midarm muscle
    circumference) 58
manganese 166, 167b
mannitol 80
manufacturer details, food
    labelling 189
MAOIs see monoamine
    oxidase inhibitors
    (MAOIs)
maple syrup urine disease
    (MSUD) 817t
marasmus 458, 459f,
    460b
margarine, vitamin D 807t
MAS (milk alkali
    syndrome) 142–4

mass/weight 845
  conversions 850
  conversion tables 845t
  see also weight
maternal, infant and
    young child nutrition
    (MIYCN) 445
maternal weight gain 248–9
  multiple
    pregnancies 248–9
  overweight/obese
    women 248–9
Matthew's Friends
    (UK) 794
MCADD (medium
    chain acyl-CoA
    dehydrogenase
    deficiency) 817t
MCTs see medium chain
    triglycerides (MCTs)
MDGs (Millennium
    Development
    Goals) 444b
meal replacement
    232–6, 479–80
meals
  definition 6
  insulin in diabetes type 1
    management 508b
meals on wheels
  food poverty 362–3
  older people 332
meat
  copper 158t
  fats 75t
  iron 151t
  magnesium 165t
  niacin (nicotinamide,
    nicotinic acid, vitamin
    B₃) 120t
  nutrient profiles 5t
  phosphorus 147t
  potassium 181t
  proteins 73t
  riboflavin (vitamin
    B₆) 117t
  selenium 163t
  thiamine (vitamin B₁) 124t
  UK recommendations 28t
  vitamin A 103t
  vitamin B₆ 132t
  vitamin B₁₂
    (cobalamin) 135t
  vitamin D
    (calciferols) 109t
  vitamin E 110b
  weaning 279t
  zinc 155t
medical assessment, weight
    management 476t
  see also clinical
    assessment

medical history, kidney nutritional assessment 706
Medicines and Healthcare products Regulation Agency (MHRA) 658
Mediterranean diet 232–6
  cardioprotective diet 526b
  stroke prevention 533t
medium chain acyl-CoA dehydrogenase deficiency (MCADD) 817t
medium chain triglycerides (MCTs) 646b
  ketogenic diet 792
MEND project 290–1
Menkes disease 156
mental capacity 778–9
Mental Capacity Act (MC) 2005 778–9, 814
mental health 753–79, 754f
  developmental disorders 764–6
  nutritional care 755t, 758
  pharmacotherapy 756, 757b
MEOS (microsomal ethanol-oxidizing system) 206
metabolic disorders
  co-morbidities to obesity 474
  inherited see inherited metabolic disorders (IMDs)
metabolic response to injury 604, 605t
  starvation vs. 605t
metabolome/metabolomics 200b
metformin
  diabetes type 2 management 511t
  nutrient interaction 837–8
methotrexate
  folate interactions 126
  nutrient interaction 837
methylmalonic acidaemia (MMA) 817t
methylxanthines 211–12
MHRA (Medicines and Healthcare products Regulation Agency) 658
microbiological contamination, enteral feeding 587
micronutrients 100
  content calculation 10
  deficiency 436
  food-based dietary guidelines (FBDGs) 27
  food supplements 202

requirements in critical care 607–8
  see also minerals; vitamin(s)
microsomal ethanol-oxidizing system (MEOS) 206
mid-arm circumference (MAC) 857t
midarm muscle circumference (MAMC) 58
mid-upper arm circumference (MUAC) 562, 563t
migrants see refugees and asylum seekers
Military Dietary Reference Values (2008) 230
milk alkali syndrome (MAS) 142–4
milk/milk products
  drinking yogurt 623t
  fats 75t
  goat's milk infant formula 275
  ice cream 623t
  Infant hypersensitivity 293
  iodine 161t
  magnesium 165t
  niacin (nicotinamide, nicotinic acid, vitamin B$_3$) 120t
  phosphorus 147t
  potassium 181t
  proteins 73t
  riboflavin (vitamin B$_6$) 117t
  selenium 163t
  vitamin A 103t
  vitamin B$_{12}$ (cobalamin) 135t
  weaning 279t
  yogurt 807t
  zinc 155t
  see also cows' milk; dairy foods
Millennium Development Goals (MDGs) 444b
mindex 856
mineral and bone disorders, CKD 718, 719t
minerals 140
  acute kidney injury 730–1
  burn injury 617
  conversion factors 869
  current dietary patterns 35
  essentiality of 140
  food labelling 193t
  haemodialysis 726
  individual nutrition assessment 48
  RNIs 881t

UK recommendations 28t
mineral supplements
  breastfeeding 272
  cancer 551
  pregnancy 245t
minority ethnic communities 338–44
  food restrictions 338, 339t, 340t, 342t
  healthy diet promotion 344
  influences on diet 338, 348f
  nutrition interventions 347b
  traditional dietary habits 338
MIYCN (maternal, infant and young child nutrition) 445
MMA (methylmalonic acidaemia) 817t
MND (motor neuron disease) 786–7
modified Atkins diet (MAD) 792
modified ketogenic diet 792
modified-texture diets 776
molybdenum 168
monoamine oxidase inhibitors (MAOIs) 757b
  nutrient interaction 837
monosaccharides 79t
monounsaturated fatty acids (MUFAs) 71–2, 72t
  cardioprotective diet 524–5
mood stabilizers 757b
morning (pregnancy) sickness 250
mortality, undernutrition 440
mother-to-child HIV infection transmission 750
motivational interviewing 384–6, 385t, 388b
motor neuron disease (MND) 786–7
mouth disorders 622–3
  cancer of the mouth and pharynx 622
  jaw wiring 622–3
  salivary gland disorders 622
  see also dental health
MRI (magnetic resonance imaging) 41t, 53
MS see multiple sclerosis (MS)
MSUD (maple syrup urine disease) 817t

MUAC (mid-upper arm cir-
cumference) 562, 563t
mucosal insufficiency,
malabsorption 643b
MUFAs see monoun-
saturated fatty acids
(MUFAs)
multiple pregnancies 248–9
multiple sclerosis
(MS) 782–4
alternative diets
783–4, 784b
disease
progression 782–3
specific nutrition
concerns 783
MUST see malnutrition
universal screening
tool (MUST)
myoglobin 149t
MyPlate 29, 31f
myristic fatty acid 72t

N

n-3 fatty acids 351
N -acetyl glutamate
synthase deficiency
(NAGS) 817t
NAFLD (non-alcoholic
fatty liver disease)
692–3, 693b
NASH (non-alcoholic
steatohepatitis) 692–3
nasogastric feeding 574–5
burn injury 617
tube blockages 586
nasojejunal (NJ)
feeding 575
burn injury 617
tube blockages 586
nateglinide 511t
National Child
Measurement
Programme
(NCMP) 408
National Diet and
Nutrition Survey
(NDNS) 414–15
aged diet 322–3
children and
adolescents 308–10
current dietary patterns
34–6, 35t
household-based
surveys 42
low-income
households 355–6
older people obesity 331
see also Food Standards
Agency (FSA); Public
Health England (PHE)

National Health Service
(NHS) England
Five Year Forward
View 406
Joined Up Clinical
Pathways for Obesity
(NHS England
2016) 417b
nutrition policy 392, 393
National Heath and
Nutrition Examination
Surveys (NHANES) 42
National Institute for
Health and Care
Excellence (NICE)
breastfeeding 266–8
health behaviour
models 382–7
nutrition policy 392, 394
national measurement
programme 315
National Statistics Socio-
economic Classification
(UK) 891
analytic classes 891b
simple classes 892b
natural classification, food
labelling 193t
natural triggers, food
hypersensitivity 831
nausea and vomiting 632
drug–nutrient
interactions 839
nausea, cancer 548
NCMP (National Child
Measurement
Programme) 408
NDNS see National
Diet and Nutrition
Survey (NDNS)
nephrotic syndrome
722b, 723b
nervous system, alcohol
effects 209
neural tube defects
(NTDs) 238
neurological
conditions 781–94
Alzheimer's disease 790
motor neuron
disease 786–7
multiple sclerosis see multiple sclerosis (MS)
Parkinson's disease 788–9
neutropenia 552
food avoidance 552
food preparation 552
newborns, global nutrition
problems 436
NHANES (National
Heath and Nutrition
Examination Surveys) 42

NHS see National Health
Service (NHS) England
niacin (nicotinamide, nicotinic acid, vitamin B₃)
118–20, 119t, 120b
breastfeeding RNI 273t
child and adolescent
RNIs 305t
conversion factors 869
infants and preschool
childrens 259t
RNIs 879t
NICE see National Institute
for Health and Care
Excellence (NICE)
nicotinamide see niacin
(nicotinamide, nicotinic
acid, vitamin B₃)
nicotinic acid see niacin
(nicotinamide, nicotinic
acid, vitamin B₃)
nitrates 214–15, 216t
nitrites 214–15, 216t
nitrogen
requirements 607–8
NJ see nasojejunal (NJ)
feeding
no-added salt diet 696–7
non alcoholic beverages
folate (folic acid) 127t
riboflavin (vitamin
B₆) 117t
non-alcoholic fatty liver
disease (NAFLD)
692–3, 693b
non-alcoholic
steatohepatitis
(NASH) 692–3
non-caloric
sweeteners 216–17
non HDL-cholesterol 873t
non-immune me-
diated food
hypersensitivity 826
non-immunoglobulin
E-mediated food
hypersensitivity 826
non-milk extrinsic
sugars 308–10
non-starch polysaccharides
see fibre
non-statutorily
homeless 357b
NR-NCDs (nutrition-
related non-
communicable
diseases) 346
NTDs (neural tube
defects) 238
nucleotides 262b
nut allergy 282–3
nutmeg 635b

nutraceuticals 196–7
  categories of 196t
nutrient energy yields 868t
nutrients
  absorption in cystic
    fibrosis 740
  energy values for
    oxidation 89t
  supplements in gas-
    trectomy/stomach
    surgery 638
  see also macronutri-
    ents, gastrectomy/
    stomach surgery;
    micronutrients
nutrigenetics
  198–201, 199b
  nutrigenomics vs. 199f
nutrigenomics 198–201
  gastrointestinal
    microbiota 198–9
  nutrigenetics vs. 199f
  technologies 200b
nutritional assessment 38
  body composition see
    body composition
  HIV infection 747
  individuals see individual
    nutrition assessment
  individuals of see in-
    dividual nutrition
    assessment
  liver disease 690, 691b
  stroke 534–5
  weight management 476t
  see also ABCDEF nu-
    trition assessment;
    dietary assessment;
    nutritional status
nutritionally vulnerable
  babies 298
nutritional product
  prescription 842
nutritional requirements
  burn injury 616–17
  cancer treatment 547
  colorectal cancer 674
  critical care 607–8
  cystic fibrosis 740,
    741, 742t
  dialysis 705t, 724
  haemodialysis
    705t, 725–6
  peritoneal dialysis
    705t, 724
  renal transplantation 729b
nutritional screening
  556, 557b
  see also malnutrition
    universal screening
    tool (MUST)
nutritional status 220b

cancer treatment 547
drug–nutrient
  interactions 838
refugees and asylum
  seekers 358
see also nutritional
  assessment
nutritional supplements,
  undernutrition
  treatment 570–1
nutritional support
  555–620
  clinically functional
    nutrients 620
  head injury 614, 615b
  malnutrition in chronic
    kidney disease 716–17
  palliative care 813
  requirement estimation
    600b, 596–600
  surgery 610
Nutrition and Hydration
  Week 221
nutrition education 372–4
  communication
    skills 378–80
  counselling skills
    378–80, 379t
  learning outcomes
    372, 373
  learning theories 374
  lesson plans 374, 379t
  material design 376
  material readability 376
  message
    development 370
  patient material 376, 377b
  session planning 372–3
  teaching evaluation 374
nutrition information
  labelling 191
nutritionists 13
nutrition policy 391–421
  local policy see local
    nutrition policy
  national bodies 391
  national
    programmes 408–12
  surveys see nutrition
    surveys
nutrition-related non-
  communicable diseases
  (NR-NCDs) 346
nutrition-sensitive
  interactions,
  undernutrition 464
The Nutrition Society 13
nutrition surveys
  Health Survey for
    England 415
  household food purchase
    surveys 414

individual dietary
  surveys 414–15
Low Income Diet and
  Nutrition Survey
  (LIDNS) 355–6
National Diet and
  Nutrition Survey
  (NDNS) 414–15
nutrition transition, global
  nutrition 454–5

O

OA (osteoarthritis) 796–7
oats 658
obesity 469–91
  associated conditions 490
  asthma 736
  at-risk individuals 472
  causes 474
  children see childhood
    obesity
  chronic obstructive pul-
    monary disease 737
  climate change
    430–3, 431f
  climate change and 432–3
  co-morbidities 474
  definition 470, 471t
  Down syndrome and 490
  global nutrition
    problems 436
  gout 800
  maternal weight
    gain 248–9
  older people 331
  polycystic ovary syn-
    drome (POS) and 490
  Prader–Willi syndrome
    and 490
  preconceptual
    nutrition 240
  prevalence 472
  weight management see
    weight management
  see also overweight
obesity prevention 398–
  404, 399f, 488
  Joined Up Clinical
    Pathways for Obesity
    (NHS England
    2016) 417b
  local policies 418
  systems approach 398–404
  WHO recommenda-
    tions 400b
  see also weight
    management
obsessive compulsive dis-
  order (OCD) 762–3
OCD (obsessive compul-
  sive disorder) 762–3

oedema
liver disease 696–7, 697t
nephrotic syndrome 722
oesophageal
disorders 628–9
achalasia 628
cancer 628–9
dysphagia 628
oesophagitis 629
stents 629, 630b
strictures 629
varices 699
oesophago-gastrectomy
638, 637f
oesophagus 16f
digestion 16
oils, cardioprotective
diet 526t
oily fish
cardioprotective
diet 524–5
UK recommendations 28t
vitamin B₁₂
(cobalamin) 135t
older people 322–3
arthritis 330
bone loss 330
chronic diseases 330
chronic kidney
disease 713
community strategies for
healthy diet 332
dehydration 330
dementia 330
diabetes 518
diet 322–3
dietary
recommendations 324
food policy models
334, 335f
gastrointestinal
disease 330
low-income 356
obesity 331
older people
process 322
older people
malnutrition 326–7
consequences 327
risk factors 326–7
treatment 327, 328b
oleic fatty acid 72t
oligosaccharides 80
breastfeeding 262b
omega (ω)-3 polyunsatur-
ated fatty acid 73
attention deficit hyper-
activity disorder 766
autism spectrum dis-
orders (ASDs) 764–5
bipolar affective
disorder 761

cardioprotective
diet 524–5
depression 760
functional foods as 197t
schizophrenia 761–2
One You programme
(PHE) 408
open questions, closed
questions vs. 379t
operational ration packs
(ORPs) 230
oral feeding, burn
injury 617
oral mucositis 839
orange juice 623t
organic acidaemias 817t
organic labels 192
orlistat 484
nutrient interaction 837–8
ornithine carbamoyl
transferase deficiency
(OTC) 817t
ORPs (operational ration
packs) 230
OSFED 772
osteoarthritis (OA) 796–7
osteoporosis 806–9
dietary prevention
806–7, 808t
nutritional
management 808–9
nutritional risk
factors 806
OTC (ornithine
carbamoyl transferase
deficiency) 817t
overgranulation, gastros-
tomy feeding 577
overweight
global nutrition
problems 436
maternal weight
gain 248–9
see also obesity
oxalate-rich foods 733t
oxalates 732
oxandrolone 618

P

PA see physical activity (PA)
PA (propionic
acidaemia) 817t
packet front, food
labelling 188–90
PAD (peripheral arterial
disease) 520, 540
PAF (Population
Attributable
Fraction) 542
Pakistan, food
restrictions 340t

PAL see physical activity
level (PAL)
palliative care 812–14
artificial nutritional
support 813
cancer 554
ethics 813–14
nutritional
management 812–13
nutritional risk 812
oral nutrition support 813
palmitic fatty acid 72t
palmitoleic fatty acid 72t
pancreas 16f, 17–18
synthetic functions 680t
pancreatic disease 679–86
acute pancreatitis 684b
cancer 685
chronic pancreatitis
682, 683b
function disorders 680–5
pancreatic enzyme replacement therapy (PERT)
686, 687t
pancreatitis
acute 684b
chronic 682, 683b
pantothenic acid (vitamin
B₅) 138, 139b
Parenteral and Enteral
Nutrition Group
(PENG) 596–8
energy requirement
estimation 597b
protein requirement
estimation 599b
parenteral nutrition
(PN) 592–3
complications 593, 595t
critical care 607
HIV infection 748
home 593
indications 592
monitoring 593,
594t, 595t
regimens 592–3
routes 592
Parkinson's disease
(PD) 788–9
partial gastrectomy
638, 637f
patient-centred nutrition
education 378
Patient Generated
Subjective Global
Assessment
(PG-SGA) 544–5
patient material, nutrition
education 376, 377b
Pay as You Dine (PAYD) 230
PCR (protein catabolic
rate) 707t

PD (Parkinson's disease) 788–9
peanuts
  allergy in pregnancy 246b
  breastfeeding 272
  food hypersensitivity management 830–1
  preconceptual nutrition 240
pectin 217t
pedometers 94, 95b
PEG see percutaneous endoscopic gastrostomy (PEG)
PENG see Parenteral and Enteral Nutrition Group (PENG)
penicillamine 131
peptic ulcers 633
percutaneous endoscopic gastrostomy (PEG) 576
  HIV infection 748
  tube blockages 586
peri-conceptual nutrition 238–40
peripheral arterial disease (PAD) 520, 540
peristomal infections/ abscesses 577
peritoneal dialysis 705t, 724
PERT (pancreatic enzyme replacement therapy) 686, 687t
pescatarian diets 347t
PG-SGA (Patient Generated Subjective Global Assessment) 544–5
pharmacotherapy, weight management 484
pharyngeal cancer 622
PHE see Public Health England (PHE)
phenylalanine, low diet see low phenylalanine diet
phenylketonuria (PKU) 822–3, 823t
  breastfeeding 263–4
  dietary treatment 817t
phosphate
  haemodialysis 726
  kidney nutritional assessment 707t
  reference ranges 873t
  requirement estimation 597t
  supplements 602–3
phosphate binders 718
phosphorus 146b, 147t
  breastfeeding RNI 273t
  child and adolescent RNIs 305t

chronic kidney disease 712, 713t
CKD–mineral and bone disorder management 718
infants and preschool childrens 259t
peritoneal dialysis 705t, 724
RNIs 881t
physical activity (PA)
  chronic kidney disease 720
  climate change and 432
  insulin in diabetes type 1 management 508b
  kidney nutritional assessment 706
  total energy expenditure (TEE) 86–91
  weight management 482
  WHO obesity prevention recommendations 400b
physical activity assessment
  children 93
  definitions 94t
  objective instruments 94–7, 95b
  subjective instruments 94
  total energy expenditure (TEE) 92–3, 94t
physical activity level (PAL) 871t
  energy requirement estimation 597b
physical assessment, individuals 47–8
phytanic acid 824
phytoestrogens 210–11
  functional foods as 197t
phytosterols 210–11
pica 251
pioglitazone 511t
Pioppi diet 232–6
PKU see phenylketonuria (PKU)
place-based local public health 418
planning, motivational interviewing 385–6, 388b
plant programme 232–6
plant stanols/stenols
  cardioprotective diet 526t
  functional foods as 197t
plasma osmolality 184
plated meal service, hospital catering 223
plethysmography 51
PN see parenteral nutrition (PN)

PNI (protective nutrient intake) 24b
polycystic ovary syndrome (POS) 490
polyols 80
polyphenols 210–11
polysaccharides 79t
polyunsaturated fatty acids (PUFAs) 72–3
  cardioprotective diet 524–5
  multiple sclerosis 782–3
popular diets 232–6
  before starting 232b
Population Attributable Fraction (PAF) 542
porridge 623t
portion sizes, average 888
POS (polycystic ovary syndrome) 490
post-acute care, stroke 536–7
postnatal care, diabetes 517
post-operative nutrition, liver transplants 700
potassium 180, 181b, 181t
  chronic kidney disease 712
  depletion 180b
  haemodialysis 705t, 726
  intake limitation 714b
  kidney nutritional assessment 707t
  peritoneal dialysis 705t, 724
  reference ranges 873t
  requirement estimation 597t
  RNIs 881t
  supplements 602–3
  total body potassium 41t, 53
potassium bicarbonate 869t
potatoes
  copper 158t
  folate (folic acid) 127t
  magnesium 165t
  potassium 181t
  potassium limitation 714b
  thiamine (vitamin B₁) 124t
  vitamin B₆ 132t
poverty
  refugees and asylum seekers 358
  UK 354
Prader–Willi syndrome 490
prandial glucose regulators 511t
pre-albumin 707t
prebiotics 201
  functional foods as 197t

preconception nutrition, diabetes and 516
preconceptual nutrition 238–40
dietary advice 238
folic acid 239b
foods to avoid 238–9
healthy weight 240
importance of 238
peanuts 240
pregnancy
alcohol 209, 242
caffeine 212, 242b
diabetes 516
dietary problems 250–2
dietary reference values 242–3
fish consumption 242–3
food safety 246b
iodine deficiency 451b
maternal weight gain see maternal weight gain
mineral supplements 244, 245t
multiple pregnancies 248–9
RNI 243t
seafood 243
undernutrition 458
vegetarians 351–2
vitamin supplements 244, 245t
vulnerable groups 254–5
pregnancy (morning) sickness 250
pre-operative fasting 610–11
pre-operative nutrition 610
liver transplants 700
preschool children see infant growth and development
preservatives 214–15, 216t
food hypersensitivity management 831
preterm infants, weaning 283
primary idiopathic haemochromatosis 151
prisons 228, 229b
dietetic practice 228
probiotics 199
functional foods as 197t
product name, food labelling 188
proguanil 837
propionic acid 216t
propionic acidaemia (PA) 817t
propranolol 618
proprietary protein supplements 623t

protective nutrient intake (PNI) 24b
protein(s) 64–8
acute kidney injury 730–1
breastfeeding 262b, 273t
chronic kidney disease 712
content calculation 9
current dietary patterns 35t
deficiency 67–8
energy conversion factors 9t
energy values for oxidation 89t
food-based dietary guidelines 27
food labelling 193t
function 64
haemodialysis 705t, 725
individual nutrition assessment 48
kidney stones management 732
metabolic response to injury 605t
metabolism in cancer cachexia 544–5
nitrogen conversion factors 868
Parkinson's disease 789
peritoneal dialysis 705t, 724
sources 68, 73t
structure of 64, 65f, 66f
vegetarian/vegan problems 349
see also amino acids
protein catabolic rate (PCR) 707t
protein exchanges, food composition 884, 884t
protein requirements 600b, 65–7, 596–8
burn injury 616
child and adolescent RNIs 305t
critical care 607–8
head injury 614
infants and preschool childrens 259t
recommended daily intake 67t
RNIs 878t
proteinuria 722
proteomes/proteomics 200b
psychology
anorexia nervosa treatment 770
kidney nutritional assessment 706

refugees and asylum seekers 358
weight management 476t
psychosocial co-morbidities, obesity 474
public health
conceptual models 396
social inequalities 396
socio-economic models 396
systems approaches 396
weight management 488
Public Health England (PHE)
Change4Life 408
Evidence into Action 406
food composition tables 8–10
local nutrition policy 416
nutrition policy 392–3
One You programme 408
Sugar Reduction programme see Sugar Reduction programme (PHE)
see also National Diet and Nutrition Survey (NDNS)
public health nutrition 2
public information campaigns 400b
PUFAs see polyunsaturated fatty acids (PUFAs)
pulses 5t
potassium limitation 714b
purines 732, 733t
pyloric sphincter 17–18
pyridoxal see vitamin B$_6$
pyridoxamine see vitamin B$_6$
pyridoxine see vitamin B$_6$
pyrimethamine 126

Q

quantitative ingredient declaration, food labelling 189
questionnaires, physical activity assessment 94, 95b
quinolones 836–7

R

RA (rheumatoid arthritis) 798–9
radiologically inserted gas-trostomy (RIG) 576–7
radiotherapy 546–7
raffinose 80
rapidly digestible starch (RDS) 80

Rastafarian, food restrictions 342t
raw vegan diet 232–6
RDA (Recommended Daily Allowance) 24b
RDS (rapidly digestible starch) 80
ready to use therapeutic foods (RUTFs) 464
recall height 56
Recommended Daily Allowance (RDA) 24b
recommended intake 24b
rectum 16f
red tray/jug initiative, hospital catering 222b
REE (resting energy expenditure) 597b
refeeding syndrome (RfS) 602–3
    at-risk patients 603b
    clinical features 603b
reference intake (RI) 192, 195t
reference nutrient intakes (RNIs)
    adolescents in pregnancy 254
    aged diet 322–3
    breastfeeding 273t
    calcium 143t
    child growth and development 305t
    copper 157t
    definition 24b
    folate (folic acid) 127t
    infant growth reference charts 259t
    iodine 161t
    iron 150t
    magnesium 165t
    manganese 166t
    minerals 881t
    molybdenum 168
    niacin (nicotinamide, nicotinic acid, vitamin B₃) 119t
    phosphorus 147t
    potassium 181t
    pregnancy 243t
    protein 878t
    riboflavin (vitamin B₂) 117t
    selenium 163t
    sodium 179t
    thiamine (vitamin B₁) 123t
    vitamin A 103t
    vitamin B₆ 131t
    vitamin B₁₂ (cobalamin) 135t

vitamin D (calciferols) 109t
vitamins 879t
zinc 155t
Refsum's disease 824
refugees and asylum seekers 357b, 358
    migrant-specific diets 344
Registered Public Health Nutritionists (RPHNutr) 14
Regulation and Quality Improvement Authority (RQIA), hospital catering 223
renal disease see kidney disease
renal transplantation 728–9
    immediate post-transplant nutrition 728
    immunosuppressive treatment side effects 729b
    late nutrition 728
    long-term nutrition 729
    nutritional management 729b
repaglinide 511t
reproductive system, alcohol effects 209
resistance exercise, HIV infection 748
resistant starch (RS) 80
respiratory disease 735–43
    asthma see asthma
    chronic obstructive pulmonary disease 737
    ling cancer 738
    lung transplantation 738
    tuberculosis 738
respiratory system, alcohol effects 209
resting energy expenditure (REE) 597b
retinol see vitamin A (retinol)
RfS see refeeding syndrome (RfS)
rheumatoid arthritis (RA) 798–9
rheumatology 795–809
    osteoarthritis 796–7
    osteoporosis see osteoporosis
    rheumatoid arthritis 798–9
riboflavin (vitamin B₆) 116, 117b, 117t
    breastfeeding RNI 273t

child and adolescent RNIs 305t
food colourings (E100-180) 207t
infants and preschool childrens 259t
RNIs 879t
rickets 108
RIG (radiologically inserted gastrostomy) 576–7
RNIs see reference nutrient intakes (RNIs)
roots and tubers
    nutrient profiles 5t
    staple foods as 6
Roux-en-Y gastric bypass 486, 487t
Royal Free Hospital Global Assessment 690
Royal Free Hospital Nutrition Prioritization Tool 690
RPHNutr (Registered Public Health Nutritionists) 14
RQIA (Regulation and Quality Improvement Authority), hospital catering 223
RS (resistant starch) 80
RUTFs (ready to use therapeutic foods) 464

S

SACN see Scientific Advisory Committee on Nutrition (SACN)
salicylates 831
saline 869t
salivary gland disorders 622
salmonellosis, pregnancy 246b
salt (sodium chloride)
    asthma 736
    cardioprotective diet 526t
    chronic kidney disease 712
    food labelling 193t
    haemodialysis 726
    intake in hypertension 538–9
    kidney stones management 732
    mineral content 869t
    peritoneal dialysis 705t
    restriction in heart failure 530
    UK recommendations 28t
    weaning in 279t

saturated fats
  children and
      adolescents 308–10
  UK
      recommendations 28t
saturated fatty acids (SFAs)
    70–1, 71f, 72t
  current dietary
      patterns 35t
saw palmetto 841t
saxagliptin 511t
SBGM (self-blood glucose
    monitoring) 498
SCF (Scientific Committee
    for Food) 214–17
schizophrenia 761–2
School Food Plan (SFP)
    224, 225t, 407
School Food Trust
    (SFT) 224
The School Fruit and
    Vegetable Scheme 409
schools 224
  food poverty 362–3
  School Food Plan 224
  undernutrition in
      LMICs 466–7
SCI see spinal cord
    injury (SCI)
Scientific Advisory
    Committee on
    Nutrition (SACN)
    230, 393–4
  bottle feeding 276
  Carbohydrates and
      Health report 409
  dietary reference
      values 22–5
  nutrition policy 393–4
Scientific Committee for
    Food (SCF) 214–17
Scottish Commission
    for the Regulation of
    Care 223
scurvy 114
SDGs (Sustainable
    Development
    Goals) 447b
SDS (slowly digestible
    starch) 80
seafood
  preconceptual nutrition
      avoidance 239
  pregnancy 243
  shellfish 829
  see also fish
sedentary behav-
    iour, children and
    adolescents 310
seeds 830–1

selective serotonin re-
    uptake inhibitors
    (SSRIs) 757b
  obsessive compulsive
      disorder 763
selenium 162, 163b,
    163t
  breastfeeding RNI 273t
  burn injury 617
  child and adolescent
      RNIs 305t
  infants and preschool
      childrens 259t
  older people
      recommendations 324
  RNIs 881t
selenosis 162
self-blood glucose moni-
    toring (SBGM) 498
serotonin 212
serum immunoglobulin E
    (IgE) 826–7
session planning 372–3
Seventh Day Adventists,
    food restrictions 342t
SFAs see saturated fatty
    acids (SFAs)
SFP (School Food Plan)
    224, 225t, 407
SFT (School Food
    Trust) 224
SGA (subjective global
    assessment), kidney
    nutrition 706
SGLT-2 inhibitor 511t
shelf life, food labelling 188
shellfish 829
shopping trips, older
    people 332
shops, food poverty 362–3
short bowel 660–1, 661t
short stature,
    undernutrition 440
short-term dietary
    restrictions 667
short-term recovery, liver
    transplants 700
sibutramine 484
signposting, food
    labelling 192
Sikh, food restrictions 340t
sitagliptin 511t
skin-fold thickness meas-
    urements 55t, 58, 59f,
    see anthropometry
skin prick test (SPT) 826–7
SLE (systemic lupus
    erythematosus) 802
sleeve gastrectomy
    486, 487t

slowly digestible starch
    (SDS) 80
small intestine disorders 640
  coeliac disease 656–9
  fistulae 662
  gastrointestinal stoma
      664–5, 665b
  inflammatory bowel
      disease 652–5
  intestinal failure 660–1
  intestinal
      transplantation 666–7
  irritable bowel
      syndrome 668–70
  lactose
      intolerance 648–50
  malabsorption 642, 643b
  short bowel 660–1, 661t
  steatorrhoea 644
smoothies 623t
snacks
  children and
      adolescents 309
  definition 6
  insulin in diabetes type 1
      management 508b
  weaning 281b
social inequalities, public
    health 396
socio-economic
    models 396
sodium 178–9
  clinical restriction 179
  deficiency 178
  dietary sources 178
  drug interactions 834–6
  excess consumption 178
  food labelling 193t
  function 178
  kidney nutritional
      assessment 707t
  low-sodium diet
      696–7, 697t
  measurement 178
  reference ranges 873t
  requirement and
      intake 179t
  requirement
      estimation 597t
  RNIs 881t
  toxicity 178
sodium bicarbonate 869t
sodium chloride see salt
    (sodium chloride)
sodium valproate 757b
soft drinks industry
    levy 410
soft foods, dementia 776
The Soil Association 192

sorbic acid 216t
sorbitol 80
sore mouth, cancer 548
South Asian families
  nutritionally vulnerable
    babies 298
  waist circumferences
    55t
South Beach diet 232–6
soya-based infant formula
  bottle feeding 275
  food hypersensitivity
    management 830–1
soya isoflavones 210–11
special rules, food
  labelling 189–90
spicy food 635b
spinal cord injury
  (SCI) 612–13
  log-term issues 612–13
  short term nutritional
    issues 612
SPT (skin prick
  test) 826–7
SSBs (sugar sweetened
  beverages) 221–2
SSRIs see selective sero-
  tonin re-uptake inhibi-
  tors (SSRIs)
stabilizers 216
stachyose 80
standard deviation
  score (Z-score) 54,
  562–3, 563t
stanols see plant stanols/
  stenols
staple foods 6
starch 80
  classification 81t
  energy values for
    oxidation 89t
  recommended
    intakes 81
  weaning 279t
starchy foods,
  cardioprotective
  diet 526t
Start4Life campaign 291
starvation
  effects of 604, 605t
  metabolic response to
    injury vs. 605t
statutorily homeless 357b
Steamplicity® 222–3
stearic fatty acid 72t
steatorrhoea 644, 699
stenols see plant stanols/
  stenols
stents, oesophageal dis-
  orders 629, 630b
Still Hungry to be Heard
  campaign 222

St John's Wort (Hypericum
  perforatum) 840, 841t
stomach disorders 632–4
  cancer 633–4
  gastritis 633
  gastro-oesophageal reflux
    disease 632–3
  heartburn 632–3
  Helicobacter pylori infec-
    tion 633, 634b
  hiatus hernia 632–3
  indigestion 632–3
  nausea and
    vomiting 632
  peptic ulcers 633
  spicy food 635b
  surgery 638, 637f
storage instructions, food
  labelling 189
stress ulcers, burn
  injury 617
strictures, oesophageal
  disorders 629
stroke 532–7
  dysphagia 535
  food and fluid tex-
    ture modification
    535–6, 536f
  hydration
    assessment 534–5
  long-term care 536–7
  nutritional
    requirements 537
  nutrition
    assessment 534–5
  nutrition in
    prevention 532–3
  nutrition support
    following 533–7
  post-acute care 536–7
  secondary prevention by
    nutrition 533, 534b
  swallowing
    assessment 534
  tube feeding 535
structural proteins 64
structured fats,
  breastfeeding 262b
stunted growth
  adolescents 315
  global nutrition
    problems 436
subcapsular skin-fold
  measurements 55t
subjective global assess-
  ment (SGA), kidney
  nutrition 706
sucrose 79
  structure 78f
sugar alcohols, energy conversion factors 9t
Sugar Busters diet 232–6

Sugar Reduction pro-
  gramme (PHE) 409
advertising regulation 410
sugars
  cancer 551
  classification 79
  current dietary
    patterns 35t
  food labelling 193t
  free sugars 80–1
  intrinsic sugars 80
  nutrient profiles 5t
  oligosaccharides 80
  polyols 80
  recommended intakes 81
  sources 82t
  UK
    recommendations 28t
  see also disaccharides;
    monosaccharides
sugar sweetened beverages
  (SSBs) 221–2
sugary foods,
  weaning 279t
sulphides 210–11
sulfonylureas
  diabetes type 2
    management 511t
  nutrient
    interaction 837–8
sulphur dioxide
  214–15, 216t
sunset (yellow) 215t
supplements 203
  cystic fibrosis 741
  foods see food
    supplements
supra-iliac skin-fold
  measurements 55t
Sure Start 298
surgery
  cancer treatment 546–7
  gastrostomy 577–8
  nutritional support 610
sushi, pregnancy 243
Sustainable Development
  Goals (SDGs) 447b
sustainable nutrition
  policy 424
  development goals 428
  principles of 427b
  UK 426
swallowing
  disorders see dysphagia
  Parkinson's disease 788
  stroke assessment 534
systemic lupus erythema-
  tosus (SLE) 802
systems approaches
  obesity prevention
    398–404
  public health 396

T

Tacking Obesities: Future
   Choices 398–404
tannins 210–11
tartaric acid 217t
tartrazine 215t
taste changes
   cancer 548
   drug–nutrient
      interactions 839
TBK (total body potassium)
   41t, 53
teaching evaluation
   liquid diets 623t
   nutrition education 374
TEE see total energy
   expenditure (TEE)
tetracycline 836–7
texture modification, stroke
   535–6, 536f
Theory of Planned
   Behaviour 382–7
Theory of Reasoned
   Action 382–7
thiamine (vitamin B₁) 122,
   123t, 124b
   breastfeeding RNI 273t
   child and adolescent
      RNIs 305t
   infants and preschool
      childrens 259t
   refeeding syndrome
      management 602–3
   RNIs 879t
thiazolidinedione 511t
thickeners 216
thinness, adolescents 315
thioxanthenes 757b
thirst, water balance 184
thromboembolism, neph-
   rotic syndrome 722
TOBEC (total body elec-
   trical conductivity) 41t
tocopherol 217t
toddler diarrhoea 292–3
toddler milks 274–5
tolerable upper intake limit
   (UL) 24b
tomato juice 623t
tooth mottling, fluoride
   toxicity 172
total body electrical conductivity (TOBEC) 41t
total body potassium (TBK)
   41t, 53
total energy expenditure
   (TEE) 86–91
   energy requirement
      estimation 597t
   physical activity assess-
      ment 92–3, 94t

total gastrectomy
   638, 637f
toxin avoidance,
   pregnancy 246b
toxoplasmosis 246b
trace elements 140
   burn injury 617
   essentiality of 140
   haemodialysis 726
traditional dietary habits,
   minority ethnic
   communities 338
traffic light system, food
   labelling 192
transcriptomes 200b
trans fatty acids 74
   current dietary
      patterns 35t
transferrin, iron 149t
Transtheoretical Stages of
   Change Model 382–7
tree nuts 830–1
triacylglycerols 18
triceps skin-fold (TSF)
   measurements see
   anthropometry
tricyclic antidepressants 757b
triglycerides 873t
Trimtots study 290–1
tryptamine 212
tryptophan 869
tube blockages, enteral
   feeding 586
tube feeding
   dementia 776
   stroke 535
   see also nutritional support
tuberculosis 738
   breastfeeding 263–4
24-hour recall, individual
   nutrition assessment 47
tyramine 212
   nutrient interaction 837

U

ulcerative colitis (UC) see
   inflammatory bowel
   disease (IBD)
ulna length see
   anthropometry
   height surrogate meas-
      ures 56
   length measurement 561f
ultrasound, body
   composition 53
undernutrition 562–6
   chronic 436
   chronic obstructive pul-
      monary disease 737
   classification 562–3
   crisis as 456

cystic fibrosis 740
   global nutrition problems
      442, 443f
   inflammatory bowel
      disease 652–5
   kwashiorkor 458,
      459f, 466b
   low- and middle-income
      countries 440, 464–7,
      465f, 466b
   marasmus 458,
      459f, 460b
   motor neuron
      disease 786
   pregnancy and
      breastfeeding 458
   see also global acute
      malnutrition (GAM);
      malnutrition
undernutrition
   treatment 568–71
   assessment 568
   emergencies 456
   ethical issues 571b
   food access 569
   oral nutrition
      supplements 570–1
   supplementation with
      food 569
under-water weighing 50
underweight
   children and
      adolescents 315
   preconceptual
      nutrition 240
   see also weight loss
UNICEF (United Nations
   International Children's
   Emergency Fund) 366–7
United Kingdom (UK)
   Child Obesity Plan 406–7
   Evidence into
      Action 406
   national level nutrition
      policies 406–7
   NHS Five Year Forward
      View 406
   obesity prevalence 472
   poverty 354
   School Food Plan 407
   0–4 year anthropometry
      charts 54
United Nations
   International Children's
   Emergency Fund
   (UNICEF) 366–7
United Nations University
   (UNU) 22–5
unnecessary dieting, children
   and adolescents 315
unsaturated fatty acids,
   Alzheimer's disease 790

upper arm anthropometry
see anthropometry
upper gastrointestinal tract
cancer 553t
upper tolerable nutrient
intake level (upper limit
[UL]) 24b
urate 873t
urea
kidney nutritional
assessment 707t
reference ranges 873t
urea cycle disorders 817t
urinary metabolites 53

V

VAD (vitamin A
deficiency) 452–3
vagotomy 638
VAP (ventilator-associated
pneumonia) 606–7
vaso-active amines 212
food hypersensitivity 831
veganism 347t
current dietary
patterns 36
vitamin B$_{12}$ deficiency 134
vegetables
asthma 736
cardioprotective diet 526t
children and
adolescents 308–10
copper 158t
current dietary
patterns 34
fats 75t
folate (folic acid) 127t
food hypersensitivity
management 830
iron 151t
magnesium 165t
manganese 167t
nutrient profiles 5t
potassium 181t
potassium limitation 714b
riboflavin (vitamin
B$_6$) 117t
thiamine (vitamin B$_1$) 124t
UK recommendations 28t
vitamin A 103t
vitamin C (ascorbic
acid) 115t
vitamin E 110b
weaning 279t
vegetarianism 346–52
children and adolescents
309, 352
current dietary
patterns 36
dietary guidelines 351

dietary types 346, 347t
health risks 346, 350b
nutrients for special at-
tention 349–51, 350b
nutritionally vulnerable
babies 298
pregnancy 254, 351–2
trends in 346
vitamin B$_{12}$
deficiency 134
ventilator-associated pneumonia (VAP) 606–7
verbascose 80
very long chain acyl-CoA
dehydrogenase defi-
ciency (VLCAD) 817t
very low calorie diets
(VLCD) 480
very-low density lipopro-
teins (VLDLs) 75–6, 76t
very low energy diets
(VLEDs) 480
vildagliptin 511t
vitamin(s) 101
Alzheimer's disease 790
burn injury 617
current dietary patterns 35
fat-soluble vitamins
741, 742t
food labelling 193t
haemodialysis 726
individual nutrition
assessment 48
RNIs 879t
UK recommendations 28t
weaning 279t
vitamin A (retinol) 102–4
breastfeeding RNI 273t
child and adolescent
RNIs 305t
conversion factors 868
deficiency 102
function 102
infants and preschool
childrens 259t
low fat diets in
steatorrhoea 644
measurement 102
nutrient interaction 837
preconceptual nutrition
avoidance 239
pregnancy 244, 245t
requirements and intake
102, 103t, 104b
RNIs 879t
supplements 452, 453
toxicity 103–4
vitamin A deficiency
(VAD) 452–3
vitamin B$_1$ see thiamine
(vitamin B$_1$)

vitamin B$_3$ see niacin (nicotinamide, nicotinic acid,
vitamin B$_3$)
vitamin B$_6$ 130–1,
131t, 132b
older people
recommendations 324
RNIs 879t
vitamin B$_7$ (biotin)
136b, 136t
vitamin B$_{12}$ (cobalamin)
134, 135b, 135t
child and adolescent
RNIs 305t
gastrectomy/stomach
surgery 638
infants and preschool
childrens 259t
older people
recommendations 324
RNIs 879t
vegetarian/vegan
problems 349–50
vitamin C (ascorbic acid)
114, 115b, 217t
breastfeeding RNI 273t
child and adolescent
RNIs 305t
infants and preschool
childrens 259t
older people
recommendations 324
RNIs 879t
vitamin D
(calciferols) 108–10
child and adolescent
RNIs 305t
conversion factors 869
function 108
infants and preschool
childrens 259t
low fat diets in
steatorrhoea 644
measurement 108
older people
recommendations 324
osteoporosis 806–7
Parkinson's disease
789
peripheral arterial
disease 540
pregnancy 244, 245t
requirements and intake
108, 109t, 110b
RNIs 879t
sources of 807t
toxicity 110
UK
recommendations 28t
vegetarian/vegan
problems 350

vitamin D deficiency 108
  burn injury 617
  CKD–mineral and
    bone disorder
    management 718
vitamin D supplements
  gastrectomy/stomach
    surgery 638
  osteoporosis 808–9
vitamin E 107, 107t,
    109t, 110b
  Alzheimer's disease 790
  low fat diets in
    steatorrhoea 644
vitamin K 112–13
  low fat diets in
    steatorrhoea 644
  nutrient interactions 834
vitamin supplements
  breastfeeding 272
  cancer 551
  pregnancy 244, 245t
  refeeding syndrome
    management 602–3
VLCAD (very long chain
  acyl-CoA dehydro-
  genase deficiency) 817t
VLCD (very low calorie
  diets) 480
VLDLs (very-low density
  lipoproteins) 75–6, 76t
VLEDs (very low energy
  diets) 480
volumes 844
  conversion table 844t
  food labelling 188
vulnerable groups,
  pregnancy 254–5

W

waist circumference (WC)
    55t, 854–6, 855t
  adult anthropometry
    51t, 56
  cut-offs and associated
    disease 856t
  obesity definition
    470, 471t
  waist–hip ratio 56
warfarin 834
warnings, food
  labelling 188–9
water balance
    184–5, 185t
water safety in HIV
  infection 751

WC see waist
  circumference (WC)
weaning 278–83
  allergy risk 282b
  choking risk 283
  common problems 283
  delay in 283
  food avoidance 281
  healthy snacks 281b
  nut allergy 282–3
  preterm infants 283
  solids introduction 278
  suggested foods 278–81,
    279t, 281b
  support literature 283
  see also bottle feeding;
    breastfeeding
weight
  adult anthropometry 55
  food labelling 188
  preconceptual
    nutrition 240
  under-water 50
  see also mass/weight
weighted inventory, indi-
  vidual nutrition assessment 41t, 45
weight-for-age,
  malnutrition 438
weight-for-height/length,
  malnutrition 438
weight gain
  maternal see maternal
    weight gain
  schizophrenia 761–2
  spinal cord injury 612–13
weight loss
  attention deficit hyper-
    activity disorder 766
  cystic fibrosis 740
  HIV infection 748
  Parkinson's disease 788
  see also underweight
weight management 477
  assessment 476
  bariatric surgery
    486, 487t
  behavioural
    approaches 483
  cancer 551
  cardiovascular disease in
    CKD 718–19
  chronic kidney
    disease 720
  diabetes 515
  diet 478–80
  maintenance of loss 488

pharmacotherapy 484
  physical activity 482
  public health 488
  treatment structure 488
Weight Watchers
  diet 232–6
wellbeing effects, childhood
  obesity 314
Wernicke–Korsakoff
  syndrome 122
Wernicke's
  encephalopathy 208
wet beriberi 122
wheat 829
whey dominant
  formula 274–5
Wilson's disease 158
Working Group on Science
  and Evidence for Ending
  Childhood Obesity
  (WHO) 398–404
World Cancer
  Research Fund
  cancer
    recommendations 542
  living with cancer 550
World Health Assembly
  targets 445, 447b
World Health
  Organization (WHO)
  Ad hoc Working Group
    on Science and
    Evidence for Ending
    Childhood Obesity
    398–404
  Child Growth Standards
    (2006) 462
  dietary reference
    values 22–5
  food intake, influences
    of 366–7
  global acute malnutrition
    rates 463t
  growth charts 54
  infant growth reference
    charts 258–60
  obesity prevention re-
    commendations
    400b
  Working Group
    on Science and
    Evidence for Ending
    Childhood Obesity
    398–404
World Public
  Health Nutrition
  Association 453

World Trade
    Organization
    (WTO) 366–7
WRAP 426

X

xerostomia see dry mouth
    (xerostomia)
X-PERT 514

Y

yogurt 807*t*

Z

zinc 154, 155*t*, 155*t*
    breastfeeding
        RNI 273*t*
    burn injury 617

child and adolescent
    RNIs 305*t*
infants and preschool
    childrens 259*t*
    RNIs 881*t*
vegetarian/vegan
    problems 351
Zone diet 232–6
Z-score (standard deviation
    score) 54, 562–3, 563*t*